ESSENTIALS OF
NURSING CHILDREN AND YOUNG PEOPLE

Sara Miller McCune founded SAGE Publishing in 1965 to support the dissemination of usable knowledge and educate a global community. SAGE publishes more than 1000 journals and over 800 new books each year, spanning a wide range of subject areas. Our growing selection of library products includes archives, data, case studies and video. SAGE remains majority owned by our founder and after her lifetime will become owned by a charitable trust that secures the company's continued independence.

Los Angeles | London | New Delhi | Singapore | Washington DC | Melbourne

ESSENTIALS OF NURSING CHILDREN AND YOUNG PEOPLE

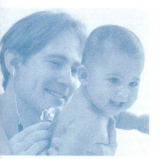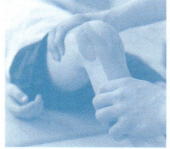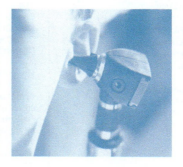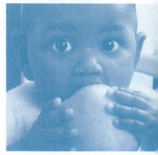

EDITED BY
JAYNE PRICE AND ORLA McALINDEN

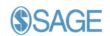
SAGE

Los Angeles | London | New Delhi
Singapore | Washington DC | Melbourne

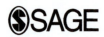

Los Angeles | London | New Delhi
Singapore | Washington DC | Melbourne

SAGE Publications Ltd
1 Oliver's Yard
55 City Road
London EC1Y 1SP

SAGE Publications Inc.
2455 Teller Road
Thousand Oaks, California 91320

SAGE Publications India Pvt Ltd
B 1/I 1 Mohan Cooperative Industrial Area
Mathura Road
New Delhi 110 044

SAGE Publications Asia-Pacific Pte Ltd
3 Church Street
#10-04 Samsung Hub
Singapore 049483

Editor: Becky Taylor
Assistant editor: Charlène Burin
Editorial assistant: Jade Grogan
Assistant editor, digital: Chloe Statham
Production editor: Katie Forsythe
Copyeditor: William Baginsky
Proofreader: Clare Weaver
Indexer: Gary Kirby
Marketing manager: Tamara Navaratnam
Cover design: Wendy Scott
Typeset by: C&M Digitals (P) Ltd, Chennai, India
Printed in the UK

Library of Congress Control Number: 2017939757

British Library Cataloguing in Publication data

A catalogue record for this book is available from the British Library

ISBN 978-1-4739-6484-6
ISBN 978-1-4739-6485-3 (pbk)

Orla: For Alex, Sharon, James and Oisin. Thank you for all you do

Jayne: For Zarah and the Brightness student fundraisers – all inspirational

CONTENTS

About the Editors and Contributors   x

Publisher's acknowledgements   xiv

Foreword   xviii
    Kath Evans

Guide to your Book   xx

Introduction   xxiv
    Jayne Price and Orla McAlinden

PART 1   PRINCIPLES OF NURSING CHILDREN AND YOUNG PEOPLE   **1**

1   Involving children, young people and families in care and care decisions   3
    Jackie Vasey, Joanna Smith, Nicola Mitchell

2   Effective communication with children and young people   20
    Jean Shapcott

3   Assessment and management of pain in children and young people   36
    Alison Twycross and Becky Saul

4   Medication: management, administration and compliance   55
    Mary Brady and Linda Moore

5   Interprofessional working with children and young people   66
    Debbie McGirr and Scott Richardson-Read

6   Organisation and settings for care of children and young people   81
    Jane Hughes, Amanda Kelly and Tracey Jones

7   Community care and care in non-hospital settings for children and young people   101
    Sarah Price

8   Law and policy for children and young people's nursing   119
    Marc Cornock and Orla McAlinden

9   Safeguarding children and young people   133
    Zoe Clark and Cameron Cox

PART 2   CHILD AND INFANT WELLBEING AND DEVELOPMENT   **149**

10   Genetics and epigenetics: effects on children and young people   151
    Gill Langmack and Elisabeth O'Brien

11 Infant mental wellbeing and health or 'how to grow a healthy adult' 164
   Orla McAlinden

12 Complexities of the developing and differing needs of children and young people 182
   Tim McDougall

13 Factors influencing wellbeing and development in children and young people 194
   Melanie Robbins and Cilla Sanders

14 Universal screening and the role of the health visitor 210
   Mandy Brimble and Sarah Reddington-Bowes

PART 3   CARING FOR CHILDREN AND YOUNG PEOPLE WITH ACUTE HEALTHCARE NEEDS AND INJURY 223

15 Assessment and care of children and young people with acute needs 225
   Rachael Bolland

16 Preparing children and young people for hospitalisation 247
   Lorna Ashbrooke and Jim Richardson

17 Care of children and young people in the peri- and postoperative recovery period 257
   Dawn James

18 Care of children and young people with respiratory problems 270
   Zoe Veal, Orla McAclinden and Doreen Crawford

19 Care of children and young people with cardiovascular problems 285
   Zoe Veal and Jo Bailey

20 Care of children and young people with neurological problems 301
   Stuart Hibbins

21 Care of children and young people with urinary and renal problems 318
   Mary Brady and Linda Moore

22 Care of children and young people with endocrine problems 330
   Kate Davies

23 Care of children and young people with immunological problems 350
   Katie Warburton

24 Care of children and young people with musculoskeletal problems 361
   Julia Judd

25 Care of children and young people with haematological problems 386
   Louise Holliday and Carla Kierulff

26 Care of children and young people with dermatological problems 397
   Joan Myers and Dolores D'Souza

27 Care of children and young people with a thermal injury 409
   Shirin Pomeroy

28 Care of children and young people with fluid and electrolyte imbalance 426
   Zoe Veal and Colin Veal

29 Care of children and young people with gastrointestinal problems 438
Zoe Veal, Orla McAlinden and Doreen Crawford

30 Discharge planning and transfer for children and young people 456
Elizabeth Gillespie and Sue Dunlop

PART 4 CARING FOR CHILDREN AND YOUNG PEOPLE WITH COMPLEX AND HIGH DEPENDENCY NEEDS 473

31 Care of highly dependent and critically ill children and young people 475
Usha Chandran and Fiona Lynch

32 Care of the neonate 493
Elisabeth Podsiadly and Mary Goggin

33 Care of children and young people with a malignant condition 512
Jayne Price and Suzanne Coulson

34 Care of children and young people with life-limiting illness 529
Antoinette Menezes and Tracie Lewin-Taylor

35 Care of children and young people at the end of life 539
Jayne Price and Melissa Heywood

36 Care of children and young people with learning disabilities 556
Trish Griffin and Jane Lopez

37 Care of children and young people with mental health issues 576
Orla McAlinden and Julia Pelle

PART 5 ON BEING A PROFESSIONAL CHILDREN'S NURSE 589

38 Leadership and management in children and young people's nursing 591
Jackie Phipps

39 Lifelong learning and continuing professional development for the children and young people's nurse 602
Claire Anderson

40 Decision-making and accountability in children and young people's nursing 616
Lorraine Highe

41 Being politically aware and professionally proactive in children and young people's nursing 626
Jim Richardson

Index 636

ABOUT THE EDITORS AND CONTRIBUTORS

ABOUT THE EDITORS

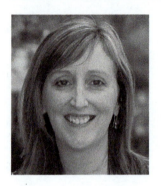

Jayne Price is Professor of Children's Nursing at Kingston University/ St George's University London and is the professional lead for children's nursing. She qualified as a general nurse in 1991 (Belfast) and as a children's nurse (Leeds) in 1995. Her clinical background within children's nursing includes a strong focus on oncology and palliative care. Having taught as a Senior Lecturer (Education) at Queen's University Belfast since 2001, Jayne moved to Kingston/St George's in 2014. In her current sole, Jayne teaches and facilitates student learning from foundation degree through to PhD level and has received a number of awards for teaching/educational developments. Throughout her career to date Jayne has made stringent efforts to enhance care for children requiring a palliative approach and their families, through practice, education and research. She is a Trustee of Shooting Star Chase and has published and presented widely nationally and internationally.

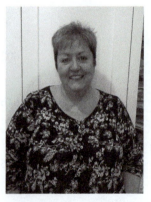

Orla McAlinden has been an adult nurse since 1979 (Royal Victoria Hospital Belfast, Northern Ireland, working through the period of civil and political turbulence known as 'the Troubles') and a children's nurse since 1986 (Queen Mary's Hospital Carshalton) and a Lecturer in Children's Nursing at Queen's University Belfast in Northern Ireland since 1992. Her clinical background with children includes medical/surgical nursing, education and clinical experience in PICU and NICU (Lewisham & Evelina Children's Unit at Guy's Hospital London). Orla's clinical and professional interests lie in ethical, legal and professional aspects of children's nursing, with a particular interest in infant mental health, emotional/mental health and wellbeing, complex needs and CAMHs-related issues.

Currently, Orla works in the Criminal Justice System in Northern Ireland in a Category A Prison, and as a Teaching Assistant at Queens University Belfast, Northern Ireland. She is a member of the Editorial Advisory Panel for the *Nursing Children and Young People's Journal*, a Specialist Advisor with the Care Quality Commission (CQC), a Steering Group member for RCN Community & Continuing Care Forum, and a Social Media Moderator for that Forum's Facebook/Twitter pages. She is a keen participant with the @WeCYPNurses community on Twitter and an advocate for professional social media use.

ABOUT THE CONTRIBUTORS

Dr Claire Anderson EdD; MSc; PGCHE; BSc; Senior Fellow HEA, Head of Work Force Development, University of West London.

Lorna Ashbrooke RSCN, RCNT, Bed (Hons), RNT.

Jo Bailey RN (Children) BSc(Hons), Assistant Cardiac Nurse Specialist, Bristol Royal Hospital for Children.

Rachael E. Bolland RGN, RSCN, MA, MSc, PG Cert Ed, Fellow of HEA.

Mary P. Brady RGN, RSCN, BSc (Hons.), CHSM, PGCLT HE, MSc, Senior Fellow HEA.

Mandy Brimble Senior Lecturer in Children's Nursing and Health Visiting at the School of Healthcare Sciences, Cardiff University.

Usha Chandran PICU Lecturer/Practitioner, Kingston University and St Georges, University of London and Paediatric Intensive Care Unit, St Georges University Hospitals NHS Foundation Trust.

Zoe Clark RN Adult, SCPHN (HV), BSc (Hans), PgDip, Msc, Fellow of HEA.

Marc Cornock academic lawyer and Senior Lecturer in the Faculty of Wellbeing, Education and Language Studies at The Open University.

Suzanne Coulson RSCN, BHSc (Hons), Clinical Educator, Children & Young People's Haematology & Oncology, Leeds Children's Hospital, Leeds Teaching Hospitals NHS Trust.

Cameron Cox RN Child, SCPHN (SN), BA (Hans), PgDip, MSc, Fellow of HEA.

Doreen Crawford MA, PGCE, BSc (Hons) SRN, RSCN, Fellow Royal Society Medicine, Fellow Academy Higher Education, Consultant Nurse Editor *Nursing Children and Young People*, Nurse Advisor Crawford-McKenzie Health Care Consultancy.

Kate Davies RN (Child), DipHE, BSc (Hons), MSc, NMP, PGCert Ed, Fellow of HEA, Senior Lecturer in Children's Nursing.

Dolores D'Souza Paediatric Advanced Nurse Practitioner, Community Children's Nursing.

Sue Dunlop Senior Lecturer child health and community nursing. University of South Wales. RGN, RSCN. Diploma Community Health Studies. BSc Professional Practice. PGCed. MSc Paediatrics and child health.

Elizabeth Gillespie RGN, RSCN, Specialist Practitioner Community Children's Nursing , MSc, PG Cert Ed, Fellow of HEA.

Mary Goggin Practice Educator at the Neonatal Unit at St. George's University Hospitals NHS Foundation Trust, London, UK.

Trish Griffin RNLD, RMN, DipCPN, RNT, MA, Fellow HEA,

Stuart Hibbins RGN, RSCN, MSc, PGCAP, Senior Lecturer, London South Bank University.

Lorraine Highe MA, PG Cert Ed, BSc(Hons), RN (Adult), RN(Child). Lecturer Practitioner, Great Ormond Street NHS Foundation Trust and Senior Lecturer, London South Bank University.

Louise Holliday, MSc Advanced Practice (Practice Education), RSCN/RGN. Lecturer in the School of Nursing and Midwifery, Robert Gordon University, Aberdeen (2013–2016).

Jane Hughes RN (Adult and Child) MA (Econ), Bsc Hon, Dip N, PG Dip, Fellow HEA, Senior Lecturer in Children and Young People's Nursing, The University of Manchester.

Dawn James Registerd Child Nurse, Lecturer in Children and Young People's Nursing, Cardiff University.

Tracey Jones RN Child, BSc, MSc, PGDip in HE, Senior Fellow of the HEA, Lecturer in Nursing, University of Manchester.

Julia Judd RSCN, RGN, MSc. Advanced Nurse Practitioner, Children's Orthopaedics.

Amanda Kelly RN Child, MSc. Senior Specialist Nurse for Looked After Children, Manchester University Foundation Trust, Manchester.

Carla Kierulff BSc (Hons), PG Cert Public Health and Health Promotion, DipHE Nursing (Child), ENB240 (Paediatric Oncological Nursing) Paediatric Oncology Research Nurse, Royal Aberdeen Children's Hospital.

Gill Langmack RGN, RSCN, MSc, BSc, PG Cert Higher Ed, Fellow of HEA.

Tracie Lewin-Taylor team leader of Shooting Star Chase's Symptom Care Team

Jane Lopez MA, B.Ed(Hons), RNT, RNLD, Dip. N.

Fiona Lynch RGN, RSCN, BSc (Hons), MSc (Adv Pract) MSc (Health Res) PICU Consultant Nurse, Evelina London.

Tim McDougall Associate Director of Nursing and Governance at Greater Manchester Mental Health NHS Foundation Trust.

Deborah J McGirr RGN, RSCN, BA Community Health, DN, MSc Advanced Nursing and Higher Education, Fellow of the HEA.

Antoinette Menezes PhD. MSc. PG Cert HE. RGN.

Nicola Mitchell RNC, Adv DPSN, MSc, Lecturer in children's nursing at University of Huddersfield. Nicola was a lecturer practitioner at the University of Huddersfield at the time of writing her chapter.

Linda Moore, RGN, RSCN, PGDipEd, FHEA.

Joan Myers OBE QN, Associate Director for Health Services and Chief Nurse at Moor Lane Centre, Chessington.

Elisabeth O'Brien B.Sc (Hons) M.Ed., RGN, RHV, PGCHE, FHEA, Lecturer, Child Health and Deputy Lead for Safeguarding, University of Nottingham.

Julia E Pelle RGN, RMN, PhD, MSc Health Psychology, BSc (hons) Nursing Studies, PG Cert Academic Practice, Fellow of HEA.

Jacqueline Phipps RGN, RSCN, BA (Hons) MA.

Shirin Pomeroy, RN (Child), BA (Hons), MSc, PG Cert Burn Care.

Elisabeth Podsiadly Senior Lecturer in Neonatal Nursing at the Faculty of Health, Social Care and Education at Kingston University and St. George's University of London.

Sarah Price RSCN, SCPHN, M.Ed, Senior Lecturer for Children and Young People's Health at Birmingham City University.

Sarah Reddington-Bowes Vice Chair CPHVA Executive and PT Health Visitor.

Jim Richardson, BA, RN (Child), RN (Adult), PGCE, PhD, FHEA, Senior Lecturer (Children's Nursing), Kingston University and St George's, University of London.

Scott Richardson-Read ASW. MSw/MSc.

Melanie Robbins RGN, RSCN, RHV, DNcert, RNT, BSc, MSc, Fellow of HEA, Professional Lead for Nursing (Child).

Katie Warburton (Rowson) Senior Lecturer at the University of Central Lancashire and Health Lead for Children's HIV Association in the UK.

Cilla Sanders RGN, RN (Child), BSc(Hons) Nursing, BSc (Hons) Specialist Practitioner Children's Community Nursing, PG Cert Clinical Education, MEd. Programme Lead for Child Nursing at the University of Leeds.

Rebecca Saul RGN, RSCN, MSc (Children's Advanced Nurse Practitioner), PgCert (Inter-professional Practice Education), PgCert (Non-Medical Prescribing), Clinical Nurse Specialist, Pain Control Service, Great Ormond Street Hospital for Children NHS Foundation Trust, London, UK.

Jean Shapcott SRN, RSCN, PGCEA, MSc formerly Senior Lecturer in Children's Nursing, Kingston University.

Dr Joanna Smith (PhD, MSc (Hons), BSc (Hons), RSCN, RGN) Lecturer in children's nursing at the University of Leeds.

Alison Twycross RGN RMN RSCN MSc DMS CertEd(HE) PhD, Deputy Dean and Lead Nurse and Professor of Children's Nursing at London South Bank University.

Dr Jackie Vasey RGN, RSCN, BSc (Hons), PG Dip HPE, Doctor of Nursing, Principal Lecturer (child nursing) and Head of Pre-Registration Nursing, University of Huddersfield.

Colin Veal RN (Child), BSc, Advanced Transport Nurse Practitioner, Wales and West Acute Transport for Children and PICU Bristol Royal Hospital for Children.

Zoë Veal RN (Child), RNT, MSc, BSc(Hons) BA (Hons), Senior Fellow of HEA.

PUBLISHER'S ACKNOWLEDGEMENTS

The editors and SAGE would like to thank all the students, patients/service users and nurses who contributed their stories to the book and online resources. The book is much richer for your contribution. We would also like to thank all the students, lecturers and practitioners who helped to review this book's content, design, and online resources to ensure it is as useful as possible.

VOICES

We would like to give special thanks to all the families who contributed their voices to this book, the book is richer for your contributions. We would also like to thank the students and nurses who also contributed their voices. All voices have been anonymised to protect privacy unless otherwise requested.

REVIEWERS

Bernie Carter

Joan Simons

Irene Kennedy

Lisa Abbott

Honor Nicholl

Prof Jocelyne Tourigny

Mark Broom

Manon Gravell

Elin Evans

Dean Snipe

Brian McGowan

Mark Broom

Anne Finnegan

Irene McTaggart

Carol Hall

Margaret Crowley

Robert Muirhead

Karen Blair

Joy Grech

Karen Tosh

Peter McNee

Jane Roberts

Ann L Bevan

Alison Warren

Marie Bodycombe-James

Emma Williams

Jane Leaver

Anne-Marie England

Sharon Pagett

STUDENT PANEL

We would like to give special thanks to our student review panel: Amy, Fatou, Justine and Monique, all children's nursing students at Kingston University.

PUBLISHER'S ACKNOWLEDGEMENTS

The authors and publisher are grateful to the following parties for permission to reproduce their material:

Figure 1.1 National Service Framework for Children Standards (DfES and DH, 2004) © Crown copyright.

Figure 3.2 Revised FLACC Scale, reproduced with kind permission, © The Regents of the University of Michigan.

Figure 3.3 Faces Pain Scale, reproduced with kind permission, © 2001, International Association for the Study of Pain.

Figure 9.1 MASH, Multi Agency Working and Information Sharing Project: Final Report. London: Home Office © Crown copyright.

Table 9.1 A MASH team comprises five core elements, London Safeguarding Children Board London MASH Project: The Five Core Elements © Crown copyright.

Table 9.2 Different types of FGM, reproduced with permission of the World Health Organization (WHO).

Table 9.3 Overall effects of FGM, NHS Choices (2014) *Female Genital Mutilation*. Used with permission under the terms of the Open Government Licence www.nationalarchives.gov.uk/doc/opengovernment-licence.

Table 11.1 Baby bonds, adapted from Moulin, S., Waldfogel, J. and Washbrook, E. (2014) *Baby Bonds: Parenting, Attachment and a Secure Base for Children*. London: The Sutton Trust. Reproduced with kind permission of The Sutton Trust.

Figure 13.1 The Assessment Framework (HM Government, 2015, p.22) © Crown copyright.

Table 13.1 Percentage of children classified as obese in the UK, adapted from House of Common Library briefing paper Number 3336 © Crown copyright.

Table 14.1 4, 5, 6 health visiting model (DH, 2015), used with permission under the terms of the Open Government Licence www.nationalarchives.gov.uk/doc/opengovernment-licence.

Table 15.1 Summary of symptoms and signs suggestive of specific diseases (NICE, 2013), reproduced with permission of the National Institute for Health and Care Excellence.

Table 15.2 Sites and devices to be used when measuring body temperature in infants and children, (NICE, 2013) reproduced with permission of the National Institute for Health and Care Excellence.

Table 15.3 Management according to risk of serious illness (NICE, 2013), reproduced with permission of the National Institute for Health and Care Excellence.

Table 15.4 Assessing dehydration in children under 5 years (NICE, 2009), reproduced with permission of the National Institute for Health and Care Excellence.

Table 15.6 Risk stratification tool for a 7-year-old with suspected sepsis (Adapted from NICE, 2016a). Reproduced with kind permission of the UK Sepsis Trust.

Table 15.7 Emergency department Red Flag Sepsis criteria for children aged 5–11 years. Reproduced with kind permission of the UK Sepsis Trust.

Table 15.8 Example of Paediatric Sepsis 6 chart: Complete all elements within one hour. Reproduced with kind permission of the UK Sepsis Trust.

Figure 15.1 Poster from the UK Sepsis Trust who provide support and advice to healthcare professionals and families. Reproduced with kind permission of the UK Sepsis Trust.

Table 22.1 Conditions seen in paediatric endocrinology, Raine, J.E., Donaldson, M.D.C., Gregory, J.W. & van Vliet, G. (2011) *Practical Endocrinology and Diabetes in Children*, 3rd edn. Chichester Wiley-Blackwell. Reproduced with kind permission of John Wiley and Sons Inc.

Page 337 Hypoglycaemia or 'hypos', bullet point list, adapted from Hanas, R. (2015) *Type 1 Diabetes in Children, Adolescents and Young Adults*, 6th edn. Somerset, Class Health. Reproduced with kind permission of Class Publishing.

Table 22.3 How diabetes interferes with normal adolescence, Dmitri, P. (2012) 'Endocrine and Metabolic Disorders'. In *Illustrated Textbook of Paediatrics*, 4th edn (Lissauer T & Clayden G eds.). Mosby/Elsevier, Edinburgh. Reproduced with permission of Elsevier under STM Guidelines: http://www.stm-assoc.org/copyright-legal-affairs/permissions/permissions-guidelines/.

Figure 22.2 Correct measurement of head circumference, photo reproduced with kind permission of Lee Martin.

Figure 22.3 Measuring a child, photo reproduced with kind permission of Lee Martin.

Table 22.5 Causes of short stature, Laing, P. (2014): 'Growth failure and hormone therapy'. *British Journal of Nursing* 23, S3-9. Reproduced with kind permission, © 2015 MA Healthcare Ltd.

Figure 24.3 Pavlik Harness, reproduced with permission from Clarke and Santy-Tomlinson, *Orthopaedic and Trauma Nursing: An Evidence-based Approach to Musculoskeletal Care*, 2014, Wiley.

Figure 24.5 Left club foot, reproduced with permission from Clarke and Santy-Tomlinson, *Orthopaedic and Trauma Nursing: An Evidence-based Approach to Musculoskeletal Care*, 2014, Wiley.

Figure 25.1 X-linked inheritance, reproduced with kind permission of the Genetic Support Foundation.

Figure 27.1 Image created from: St Helens and Knowsley Teaching Hospitals NHS Trust (2010–13) *Mersey Burns*. Reproduced with kind permission of *Mersey Burns*.

Figure 27.2 Lund and Browder chart, Harwood-Nuss A., Wolfson, A. and Linden, C. *The Clinical Practice of Emergency Medicine*. Philadelphia: Wolters Kluwer; 2015. Reproduced with permission.

Table 28.3 Assessing dehydration in children under 5 years, National Institute for Health and Clinical Excellence (2009) *CG84 Diarrhoea and Vomiting Caused by Gastroenteritis in Under 5s: diagnosis and management*. London: NICE. Reproduced with permission.

Table 28.4 Treatment of clinical dehydration and clinical shock based on NICE guidelines, National Institute for Health and Clinical Excellence (2009) *CG84 Diarrhoea and Vomiting Caused by Gastroenteritis in Under 5s: diagnosis and management.* London: NICE. Reproduced with permission.

Figure 30.1 Description of closed-loop communication (CLC), *Emergency Medicine*, Härgestam, M. et al. volume 3, Issue 10, page 2, 2013, reproduced with kind permission of BMJ Publishing Group Ltd.

Figure 33.1 Incidence of types of cancer in children. Reproduced with kind permission of Children with Cancer UK.

Figure 33.2 Symptoms of childhood cancer, Ped-Onc Resource Center (2015) *Signs of Childhood Cancer.* Reproduced with permission.

Figure 35.1 End-of-life care pathway, Widdas, D., McNamara, K. and Edwards, F. (2013) *A Core Care Pathway for Children with Life-limiting and Life-threatening Conditions* (3rd edn). Bristol: Together for Short Lives. Reproduced with permission.

Figure 35.2 Paediatric Pain Profile, Hunt, A., Goldman, A., Seers, K., Crichton, N., Mastroyannopolou, K., Moffat, V. et al. (2003) 'Clinical validation of the paediatric pain profile', *Developmental Medicine & Child Neurology*, 46(1): 9–18. Reproduced with permission of UCLB.

Figure 38.1 The nine dimensions of the NHS Healthcare Leadership Model, reproduced with kind permission © NHS Leadership Academy.

Figure 39.2 Driscoll's model of reflection, Driscoll, J. (2007) *Practising Clinical Supervision: A Reflective Approach for Healthcare Professionals*, 2nd edn. Edinburgh: Bailliere Tindall Elsevier. Reproduced with permission of Elsevier under STM Guidelines: http://www.stm-assoc.org/copyright-legal-affairs/permissions/permissions-guidelines/.

FOREWORD

KATH EVANS

> **“** There can be no keener revelation of a society's soul than the way in which it treats its children
>
> **Nelson Mandela** **”**

Caring for children, young people and their families is perhaps one of the most privileged roles in society. The care we deliver matters, not only for today but for the future too. We influence experiences and health outcomes with our knowledge, actions, behaviours and attitudes. All nurses need to know the essential principles and differences of caring for children and their families and understand the rich contribution we make to overall health and wellbeing.

Do you remember the story of *The Wizard of Oz*? Dorothy and her dog are picked up by a tornado and are deposited in the Land of Oz, things are very strange and Dorothy just wants to get home. Landing in the world of health can be very strange too, not only for the child or young person but also for their family. On Dorothy's journey to get home she meets some friends, a scarecrow who is seeking a brain, a tin man seeking a heart and a cowardly lion seeking courage. It's a reminder that children and families in our care require knowledgeable, compassionate and courageous practitioners to assist them on their journey; these are elements that mature as we progress on our lifelong learning careers as nurses.

This contemporary text and online resources will certainly assist all nurses in developing the critical requirements to support the children and families that we care for. The range of knowledge offered in this text spans the life of infants, children and young people, addressing acute short-term episodes of ill health as well as considering those with more complex and long-term health needs. Knowing what we're doing and the evidence base on which our practice is formed are the foundation for the care we deliver. The environments in which care is provided are diverse – homes, schools, primary care services, Accident and Emergency Departments, outpatient departments, child development settings as well as the more traditional environments of general and specialist inpatient units. All are duly considered, recognising the agile nature of contemporary children's nursing.

A strong focus on the experience of care within the text complements the need for knowledge and competence. The famous quote of Maya Angelou (an American poet and civil rights activist), 'I've learned that people will forget what you said, people will forget what you did, but people will never forget how you made them feel' reminds us of how we need to seek out and actively listen to children and families to ensure that they have choice and control over their care. Thines, a young man with osteogenesis imperfecta or brittle bones, shared recently that 'in my 19 years of using NHS services no one has ever once asked "What matters to you Thines?" and I've used all manner of health services in my life'. And Daniel, who is 14 years old, shared that 'in my hospital stay for pneumonia, the staff did the clinical things, they gave me my intravenous antibiotics, did my observations, but no one seemed to get how worried and scared I was, no one sat and spent time will with me'. Emily, a 10-year-old, asked me, 'Is it too much to ask that staff speak to me directly and call me by my name?'

Parents too need to be cared for with compassion and empathy. Mark, father to a child who has complex needs shares that 'Challenge (to healthcare professionals) in reality is seen as an attack and defensive positions are often taken'. We need to shift from only asking, 'What's the matter with you?' to 'What matters to you?' so that we can understand the complexity of physical and emotional needs.

As more children and families are more deeply involved, not only in their care but in interviewing new staff, are encouraged to offer insight on their experiences and are actively participating in children and parent carer forums, our responsibility is to use their insight to drive improvement. This requires professional courage. This text highlights the challenges of leadership, lifelong learning, decision-making, accountability and the need for political astuteness which ensures that we reflect on how we use our advocacy roles to best effect. Nurses are well placed to speak up and deliver excellent child and family-centred care. To do this we must foster our critical thinking, work across boundaries to promote integration of services and foster collaborative working with a wide range of colleagues.

Dorothy needed the good fairy to help her get home; this resource gathers knowledge, evidence, wisdom and insight from a range of highly regarded Children's Nursing professionals to support practitioners who care for and with children and families whilst they are on their healthcare journeys.

Adam Bojelian (2000–2015) blogged on things that mattered to him. Here he reflects on what good care looks like:

In the good hospitals:

1. Staff talk to me and involve me in decisions about my care. They ask me about what I want and don't want;
2. Staff talk to mum and dad and ask them about me;
3. Staff talk to each other and pass on important information about me;
4. If staff don't know something they are not afraid to say and ask someone who does know, sometimes that might even be me or mum and dad;
5. Staff treat me as an individual and recognise the things I can do, they don't jump to negative stereotypes and prejudices about me, because I am physically impaired;
6. Staff have time for me, they are friendly and chatty and make me feel as if I matter;
7. Staff are friendly and chatty to mum and dad, they work with them, they treat us all as if we matter;
8. I'm never left alone when I'm seriously ill and never in a room with the door closed so staff can't see me;
9. When I'm really ill doctors come quick and do everything necessary to make me better, I'm not left critically ill for hours without care;
10. I always feel that I am getting the best care possible, I'm never made to feel like a second class citizen for whom it doesn't matter if I live or die.

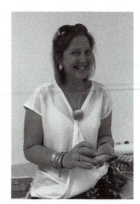

(http://intheblinkofaneyepoemsbyadambojelian.blogspot.co.uk/2013/04/what-does-good-care-look-like_2880.html)

(Shared with the kind permission of Adam's mum, Zoe, and his dad, Paul)

Kath Evans, Experience of Care Lead and Patient Experience Team Coordinator – Maternity, Infants, Children and Young People, NHS England

GUIDE TO YOUR BOOK

> We are the student panel for this book and we are all currently children's nursing students. We've road tested the features in this book and the online resources at **https://study.sagepub.com/essentialchildnursing** to make sure they work for you – wherever you are in your journey to becoming a children and young people's nurse. We hope you enjoy the book and the online resources, and that it helps you succeed in your degree and your future career. Good luck!

AMY, FATOU, JUSTINE AND MONIQUE

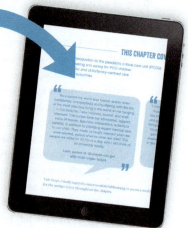

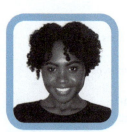

'The "voices" give valuable insight into true experiences from children and their families, as well as students and practitioners. I found these particularly useful in helping me empathise with children and their families and ensuring that I enhance their overall experience.'
- **Fatou**

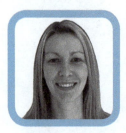

'Knowledge links in each chapter show where topics are related in other chapters. This helped me to reinforce my knowledge on how many things can relate to each other when providing holistic care.'
- **Justine**

ALSO IN
CHAPTER 15

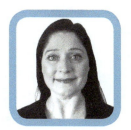

'You will learn a lot in the three years at university. The activities, and the online answers, helped me to assess my own knowledge and expand on it, before I needed to implement it in practice. There are also multiple choice questions for each chapter online to further test your knowledge.' - **Monique**

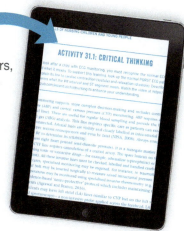

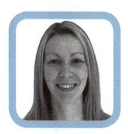

"The scenarios are very beneficial as they will help you reflect on what you would do if you were in this situation during placement. I found they helped me prepare for possible challenges. There are extra scenarios online for even more practice.' - **Justine**

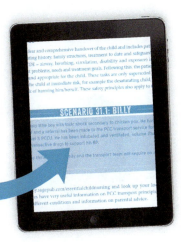

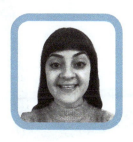

'Stopping to think about safeguarding, as this feature reminds you to do, is really important and is, I think, key when preparing for placement.'- **Amy**

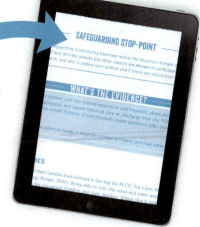

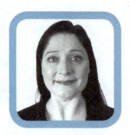

'Our entire practice throughout our career is based on evidence. "What's the Evidence" boxes in this book make learning about the evidence and contentious grey areas easy, and enabled me to be more confident in my knowledge and practice.' - **Monique**

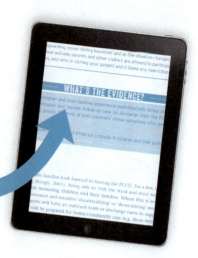

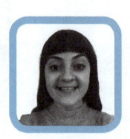

'If you find a certain topics of the book confusing or difficult, reading the chapter summary first will help. It is also useful when revising for an exam, writing an essay or in structuring your notes.' - **Amy**

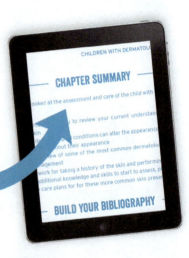

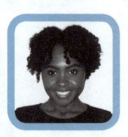

'I love the further reading and links to websites and videos. They save me from searching around for what I need - plus the video links are great to get a break from reading. ' - **Fatou**

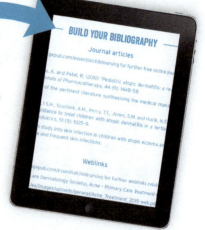

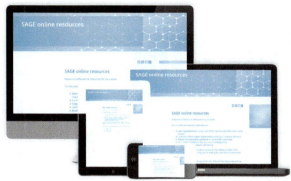

'**Don't forget** – you can find great online resources at **https://study.sagepub.com/essentialchildnursing** for more help with your learning, whether you are revising, doing assignments or preparing for placement. We've found these really helpful when you want a break from reading and to reinforce your learning in a different way –from watching a video to taking a quiz. The icons throughout the book will remind you where there is a resource available on the website.'

Answer available: When you see this icon, you'll be able to find an answer or guidance to an activity online so you can be sure you are on the right track.

A&P link: A&P revision relevant to the chapter will be available on where you see this.

Further reading and useful websites, including selected free journal articles, can be found online whenever you see this icon. This will help you when writing assignments or if you are interested in exploring a topic further.

Links to useful videos: the book has links throughout to useful and trustworthy videos – wherever you see this you can take a break from reading and watch a video instead by going online.

Preparing for placement is often quite nerve racking for students. When you see this icon **go** online to find extra placement support.

Revise - MCQs and extra scenarios: each chapter has a set of MCQs and an additional scenario to test your knowledge online

Health promotion is a fundamental part of the nursing role. Where you see this icon, you'll find extra health promotion tips and guidance online

INTRODUCTION

JAYNE PRICE AND ORLA McALINDEN

This book and the online resources (http://study.sagepub.com/essentialchildnursing) have been written for nurses everywhere who look after children and young people with a healthcare need.

Whilst the book is primarily aimed at children's nursing students in years 2 and 3 of their degree programme, it also presents a solid foundation of relevant material for any nurse and in particular those registered nurses (RNs) who may be working in a children's area which is not familiar to them. It should serve as an excellent source of reference material throughout your degree and beyond.

This book was developed by a dedicated team of lecturers, practitioners, students and of course by children and their families/carers to support your study, practice and future continuing lifelong learning. All contributors have been keen to be involved because they know how important good nursing care is and are aware of the challenges you will face in providing quality care. Everyone involved in this book is passionate about providing you with the knowledge, skills and confidence to be the type of children's nurse who inspires and provides best evidence-based care to children and their families. In addition we aim to enable you to create an environment for practice that prevents the negative situations you may see in the media from time to time.

The care of the child is first and foremost in all considerations; you will notice that the design and content of the book promote listening to what children tell us as well as signposting further information for you to read widely and deeply around topics. We recognise that no one text or resource can meet all your learning needs and for that reason this textbook and the accompanying online resources (http://study.sagepub.com/essentialchildnursing) use a variety of features to lead you towards other evidence and learning opportunities, not least of which is respecting the needs, views and wishes of children, young people and their families at all times.

Eight key themes underpin the entire text:

1. Child and family-centred care
2. Critical thinking and depth of theoretical thinking
3. Integration of acute and community care
4. Interprofessional working and collaboration
5. Evidence-based nursing
6. Preparation for practice placements
7. Health promotion
8. Safeguarding

These themes have been selected in consultation with a large number of course leaders in children's nursing degree programmes, and represent what they feel are essential areas of focus to be a successful children's nursing student. Keep these in mind and reflect on how you might develop your skills in these areas as you read through the text, and throughout your degree programme and practice placements.

Becoming a competent children's nurse is a long journey, and as students you are at the start. The contributors are all companions, and are at different stages of that journey. Their insight, experience and skills are freely shared with you to make you the best you can be as a children's nurse. The voices of children, young people and their families will serve as a reminder to keep them always at the heart of decisions and interventions. To care for children and young people is both a privilege and a big responsibility which will require you to be honest, transparent, inclusive and willing to be open to challenge and change. Advocacy and accountability are needed alongside excellent interpersonal and clinical skills.

A note on terminology: throughout the text we have usually referred to 'children' in place of the longer 'children and young people', and, in some cases, infants too. This is for reason of brevity and to prevent repitition; however, in most cases (unless specified), the shorter term should be understood to refer to both children *and* young people. In the same way, the term 'family' should be understood to refer to family and/or carers.

We hope that this book and its online resources (http://study.sagepub.com/essentialchildnursing) will give you a great start in the practice of children's nursing. We wish you much joy and success in this wonderful field of nursing.

Professor Jayne Price
Orla McAlinden, RN Adult and Child

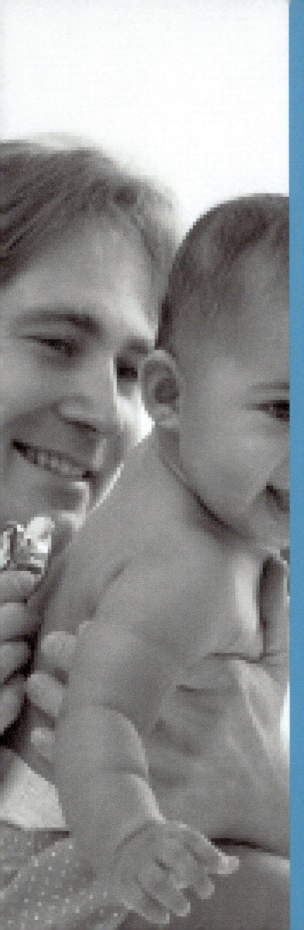

PART 1 PRINCIPLES OF NURSING CHILDREN AND YOUNG PEOPLE

1   Involving children, young people
    and families in care and care decisions   3

2   Effective communication with children
    and young people   20

3   Assessment and management of pain in
    children and young people   36

4   Medication: management, administration
    and compliance   55

5   Interprofessional working with children
    and young people   66

6   Organisation and settings for care of
    children and young people   81

7   Community care and care in non-hospital
    settings for children and young people   101

8   Law and policy for children
    and young people's nursing   119

9   Safeguarding children and
    young people   133

INVOLVING CHILDREN, YOUNG PEOPLE AND FAMILIES IN CARE AND CARE DECISIONS

1

JACKIE VASEY, JOANNA SMITH, NICOLA MITCHELL

THIS CHAPTER COVERS

- Social and political contexts underpinning the nursing care of children, young people and families
- Involving children and young people in care and care decisions
- Family involvement in care and care decisions
- Key skills required when involving children, young people and families in care and care decisions
- Involving children, young people and their families in care and care decisions – where next?

> Historically, involving children and young people, as appropriate, and parents in care has not been embedded into every day practice. In the 1990s parental participation in care was described as 'one of paediatric nursing's most amorphous and ill described concepts'.
>
> **Darbyshire, 1993, p.1672**

> Challenges to the implementation of family-centred care approaches persist.
>
> **Coyne, 2015**

Visit https://study.sagepub.com/essentialchildnursing to access a wealth of online resources for this chapter – watch out for the margin icons throughout the chapter.

FIND OUT MORE!

WEBLINK: RCPCH

INTRODUCTION

A key role of the children's nurse includes supporting children, young people and their families to be involved in care and care decisions; yet the opening quote to this chapter is part of the two decades of evidence that suggests working in partnership with the child and family remains challenging (Darbyshire, 1993; Coyne, 2015). While involving the whole family in the child's care has been widely advocated, historically children have not always been encouraged to contribute to decisions about their care (Royal College of Paediatrics and Child Health (RCPCH), 2011). Children's nurses are in an ideal position to advocate on behalf of the child and enable children's views to be heard. Models of care have evolved to support children's nurses to foster a collaborative approach to working with children, young people and families. Evidence suggests that involving children, young people and parents in care has the potential to improve satisfaction with care and may have a positive impact on health outcomes for children and young people (Shields et al., 2012). This chapter will help you develop a critical approach when considering how to involve children, young people and families effectively in care and care decisions, and build on your clinical experiences of working with families.

ACTIVITY 1.1: CRITICAL THINKING

Research that explored parent-professional interactions has found that the way information is communicated is not always conducive to involving families in care and care decisions (Smith et al., 2015a), highlighted in the followed extracts:

> I needed to know what was happening so I could let family know back at home. I was just having to guess because nobody told me anything. (*Admission 7, dad*)

> There is so much conflicting information really. They (doctors and nurses) don't seem to take on board what you're saying, that's my feeling. No they really have their own agenda and that's what we are on now – their agenda. (*Admission 2, mum*, Smith et al., 2015a, p.1308)

- What can nurses do to ensure parents are fully informed about all aspects of their child's condition and care?
- What can nurses do to involve parents in care and care decisions?

ACTIVITY ANSWER 1.1

Involvement in care and care decisions enables parents, and children as appropriate, to contribute to choosing care interventions that meet their needs, and ultimately empowers them to contribute to the child's care (Shields et al., 2012). Giving children a voice in decisions about them enables them to develop a sense of self, and improves their confidence and communication skills. In contrast, lack of involvement can lead to children and young people being fearful and anxious, and unprepared for procedures, and reduces their self-esteem (Coyne and Cowley, 2007). Furthermore, parents bring with them knowledge, experience and expertise about their child that is unique to them, thus contributing to improved care experiences for the child and family (Smith et al., 2015a).

SOCIAL AND POLITICAL CONTEXTS UNDERPINNING THE NURSING CARE OF CHILDREN, YOUNG PEOPLE AND FAMILIES

Understanding the historical and political contexts that have shaped and continue to shape children's nursing and service and care delivery will help you to contextualise the changing role of the children's nurse in optimising the health and wellbeing of children. Care delivery is influenced by a range of factors including: societal norms and values; national and international health policy and the alloca-tion of health resources; changing disease profiles; technological advancements; and the impact of lifestyle choices on health. Children's health and wellbeing are often viewed as an important marker of a nation's wellbeing and prospects. In England around 3.5 million children per year attend Emergency Departments, representing around 28 per cent of the child population, 1 in 11 children are referred to a hospital outpatient clinic and 1 in 10 children will be admitted to hospital (NHS England, 2016). Proportionally, children are high users of health services, yet the development of health services for children has historically been inconsistent.

In England, from the 17th to the late 19th centuries most workhouses and housing offering employ-ment to people who required support had infirmaries that cared for the sick and were the precursor of the modern hospital. Patients, including children, often shared spaces, including beds, with care delivered by female patients/residents. In the mid-19th century both large public and private modern hospitals proliferated. Some early hospitals did not treat children, partly because of poor response to treatments and high mortality rates; others treated children alongside adults. One of the first hospi-tals specifically for children opened in Paris in 1802, with London's Great Ormond Street Hospital opening in the 1850s. However, the movement to care for children separately from adults began with dispensaries offering advice to mothers and providing medicines for children, based on the belief that treatments for children would be best achieved by mothers caring for ill children at home. Despite promising developments during the early and mid-20th century, many children were admitted to hos-pital for extensive periods of time, often to recuperate from infectious diseases or minor surgery. Many wards admitted both adult patients and children, with restricted visiting for parents, and few nurses were trained in the specific needs of children.

Greater understanding about the impact of separating children from their families and reduced in-patient and institutional care influenced the approach to caring for children (Alsop-Shields and Mohay, 2001). The seminal work of Bowlby (1953) and Robertson (1958), a psychiatrist and psy-choanalyst respectively, highlighted the emotional plight of children when separated from their mothers. Although Bowlby's and Robertson's classical theories on young children's responses when separated from their mother have been criticised, they were a catalyst for change (Alsop-Shields and Mohay, 2001). The plight of children in hospital was highlighted in *The Welfare of Children in Hospital* report (Ministry of Health, 1959), commonly known as the 'Platt Report', which was her-alded as one of the most influential documents of its time. Among the key messages were that staff caring for children should have a detailed understanding of child development, recognise the fam-ily's role when a child is in hospital and provide unrestricted visiting for parents (Smith and Long, 2002). Increased parental presence in hospital contributed to the impetus for parents to become more involved in their child's care.

The slow adoption of the Platt Report recommendations resulted in a group of parents forming the National Association for the Welfare of Children in Hospital in 1961, which campaigned for the spe-cific needs of the hospitalised child to be recognised. Rebranding as Action for Sick Children (ASC) in 1991 coincided with the launch of the *Welfare of Children and Young People in Hospital* report (DH, 1991), which outlined the principles underpinning services for children, emphasising meeting both the physical and emotional needs of children. To celebrate the re-launch, ASC unveiled its *Charter for Children in Hospital* (ASC, 1991), updated at the beginning of the 21st century as the *Millennium Charter for Children's Health Services*, (ASC, 1999). Many of the principles in *Welfare of Children in Hospital* and the *Millennium Charter for Children's Health Services* remain relevant, and were reflected in the *National Service Framework for Children, Young People and Maternity Services* (DfES and DH, 2004; see Figure 1.1).

The profile of childhood diseases, particularly in developed countries, significantly changed during the latter part of the 20th century, with a decline in the incidence and outcome of previously fatal communicable infectious diseases and an increase in long-term conditions. Children with life-limiting

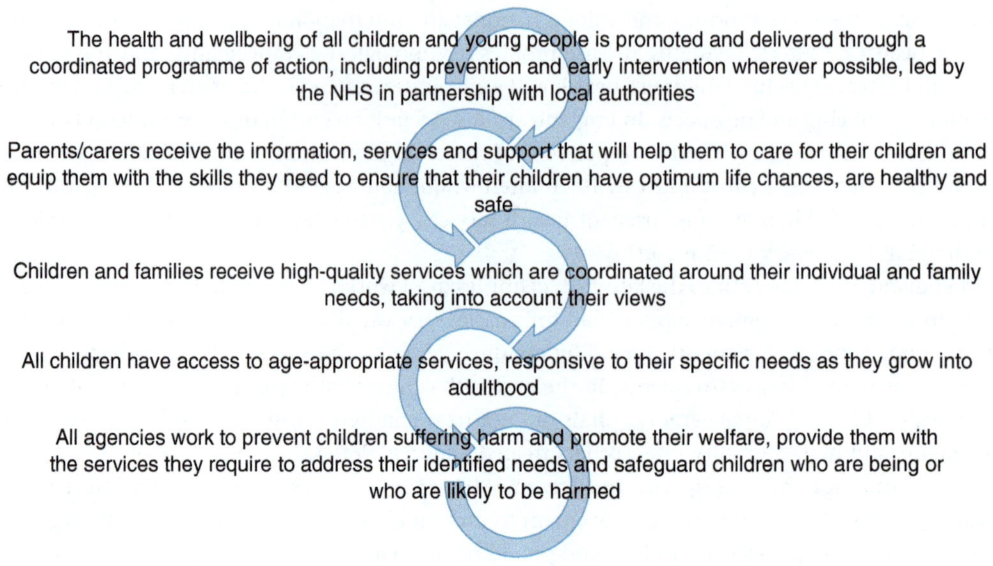

The health and wellbeing of all children and young people is promoted and delivered through a coordinated programme of action, including prevention and early intervention wherever possible, led by the NHS in partnership with local authorities

Parents/carers receive the information, services and support that will help them to care for their children and equip them with the skills they need to ensure that their children have optimum life chances, are healthy and safe

Children and families receive high-quality services which are coordinated around their individual and family needs, taking into account their views

All children have access to age-appropriate services, responsive to their specific needs as they grow into adulthood

All agencies work to prevent children suffering harm and promote their welfare, provide them with the services they require to address their identified needs and safeguard children who are being or who are likely to be harmed

Figure 1.1   National Service Framework for Children Standards (DfES and DH, 2004)

conditions and complex health needs are now surviving into adulthood. The management of children with long-term conditions, complex needs and those dependent on advanced technologies primarily takes place in the home environment, with the responsibility for monitoring symptoms and responding to changes in the child's condition becoming primarily the role of parents (Wang and Barnard, 2004). Changes in services and care delivery require health professionals to move from a position of care giver to one of collaborator, involving children and young people as appropriate and families in care and care decisions. Case Study 1.1 outlines care of a child called Molly who has a long-term condition and is being cared for by Nicola, a senior children's nurse in the acute care setting.

CASE STUDY 1.1: MOLLY

While working on a busy children's ward I cared for a 9-year-old girl I will call Molly with acute abdominal pain. Molly was known to the ward and had type 1 diabetes mellitus requiring frequent hospital admissions. Molly and her family were competent in managing her diabetes and delivering treatments. However, during acute illness parents can experience exclusion from the care they normally deliver, with nurses taking over care responsibilities. Nurses can find parents' expert knowledge threatening, particularly if they are recently qualified. This was frustrating for Molly's family. Although she presented to the hospital with abdominal pain, they were unable to provide the care they usually delivered in relation to her diabetes.

Although Molly and her family did not have skills to manage the intravenous insulin, I realised that they could retain responsibility for her blood glucose monitoring and interpret and report the result to the nurses, who could then adjust the infusion rates. With closer partnership working between the nurses, Molly and her family, I was able to support them to be involved in the delivery of the insulin, which allowed them to continue managing Molly's diabetes.

Molly and her mum reported that this involvement alleviated their distress during Molly's illness. Retaining usual care responsibilities made them feel safe, valued and gave them confidence in the nurses who provided the care they could not deliver.

- Reflect on the challenges in the case study that arose when collaborating with families of children with long-term conditions in acute care settings
- Consider any similar experiences you have had when in practice

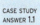

CHECK YOUR
ANSWERS
ONLINE!

CASE STUDY
ANSWER 1.1

INVOLVING CHILDREN AND YOUNG PEOPLE IN CARE AND CARE DECISIONS

The social constructs of childhood influence how children are viewed and beliefs about the skills, competencies and abilities of children to participate in care decisions. Traditionally, society has been divided into two broad groups, namely childhood and adulthood, with the passage into adulthood synonymous with rights, privileges and obligations (Franklin, 1995). The concept of 'agency' is particularly relevant to the children's nurse, and can be thought of in terms of the child's ability to reflect and act on information and an understanding that any decisions made have consequences (Mayall, 2002). The concept of child agency is complicated because children are often perceived as lacking adult reasoning and the cognitive capacity to participate in complex decisions.

The philosophical perspectives of paternalism, interventionalism and libertarianism can offer explanations about how individuals view the child's ability to participate in decisions and the rights bestowed on them (Franklin, 1995). Paternalists make choices on behalf of the child because they perceive that children are vulnerable and not capable of making autonomous rational decisions. Interventionists, such as the health professional, assume it is the responsibility of the decision-maker to act in a child's best interests and is similar to paternalism but the power balance has shifted to the health professional. Evidence suggests that children want to be heard but view health professionals as interventionists who do not support their involvement in care decisions (O'Quigley, 2000).

Unlike paternalists, libertarians advocate that children are capable of making informed choices and through experience would learn to contribute to decision-making processes (Franklin, 1995). Intuitively a libertarian approach for a very young child, who is unlikely to have the cognitive capacity to make complex healthcare decisions, seems inappropriate. However, young children can be involved in some choices about their care, which may depend on the relative importance of the decision. A more pragmatic approach to involving children and young people in care and care decisions that considers the differences in the way children think and process information is required. Children and young people should be supported to make decisions as appropriate and their participation in care valued, whilst recognising that the level of agency will evolve as the child matures (Mayall, 2002). Ravi Mistry, the Youth Advisory Panel Member at the Royal College of Paediatrics and Child Health (RCPCH), who actively promotes the inclusion of young people in healthcare, stated:

Participation encourages integration and inclusion, lets youth feel valued and ultimately leads to progress. It is a right and should not be tokenistic, where services merely ask youth for their views just so they fit in with a trend. I would urge all to include the views of children and young people wherever possible, the benefits are clear. (Ravi Mistry, Youth Advisory Panel Member, RCPCH, 2011, p.3)

WEBLINK:
OCC

VIDEO
LINK 1.1:
CHILDREN'S
EXPERIENCE
OF CARE

SEE ALSO
CHAPTER 8

Valuing children and young people's contribution to care is important because they have a right to have their views heard in all matters affecting them and their views taken seriously (Office of the Children's Commissioner, 2013). Children enjoy being involved in care decisions (Garnett et al., 2016). Engaging children and young people improves the relationship between children/young people and health professionals, which can enhance the quality of care and service delivery because issues important to children are more likely to be addressed (RCPCH, 2011). Young people should be involved in decisions about their care and be provided with age-appropriate information, including health advice following an acute illness episode (Care Quality Commission, 2015). Involvement in care and care decisions is particularly important in the context of childhood long-term conditions, where the young person will be preparing to make the transition to adult services. Case Study 1.2 highlights how Marta perceived her son was involved in care on a Teenage Cancer Unit. Sadly, Alex died at 16 years old as a result of his cancer returning.

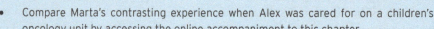

CASE STUDY 1.2: ALEX

We were asked at the time of Alex's diagnosis, 'What do you want to tell Alex?' Al was 14-and-a-half years old, sensible, able to verbalise emotions and debate the rationale for decisions made. So we took the view he should be included in everything – nothing to be hidden from him. We did not want to have discussions in secret or whisper behind closed doors. Al could consent to everything himself, although we were all involved in the discussions about whether he would go on a drug trial treatment protocol or offered alternative options, and what the pros and cons for all care and treatments were so he (and we) could make informed decisions. Al was the one who knew how he was feeling and Al was the one to live with the consequences of decisions made so it seemed right he should be involved.

PRACTICE
SCENARIO 1:
ALEX

SEE ALSO
CHAPTER 2

- Compare Marta's contrasting experience when Alex was cared for on a children's oncology unit by accessing the online accompaniment to this chapter
- How can nurses communicate effectively with children, young people and their families?

CASE STUDY
ANSWER 1.2

A shift from a paternalistic model of involving children and young people in care was reflected in the 1989 United Nations Convention on the Rights of the Child. Articles 12 and 13 are particularly relevant to children's nurses as they focus on children's right to participation, right to articulate an opinion and right to freedom of expression. For example, Article 12 states that 'the child who is capable of forming his or her own views has the right to express those views freely in all matters affecting the child: the views of the child being given due weight in accordance with age and maturity of the child' (United Nations, 1989). In relation to involving children and young people in care and care decisions, children's nurses are often faced with a range of dilemmas including the differences in opinions about care between the child/young person and parent, where choices exist. There are additional activities related to dilemmas when involving children and young people in care and care decisions in the online accompaniment to this chapter.

SEE ALSO
CHAPTER 8

The principle of involving children and young people in care and care decisions has been embedded within UK health policy over the past two decades including *Working Together to Safeguard Children*

(DH et al., 1999) and the *National Service Framework for Children, Young People and Maternity Services* (DfES and DH, 2004). The extent to which children can be fully involved in care depends on their age and developmental stage: children's nurses must be an advocate for the child and young person, ensuring that they and their families are at the centre of decisions about care. Involving children and young people to participate in care and care decisions requires health professionals to hear, value and appreciate their views, which can be achieved by:

- Providing age-appropriate information in order for the child to express their views
- Allowing children to tell the 'whole story' without interrupting
- Remaining open-minded and non-judgmental
- Viewing children's abilities and competencies as being different rather than of less importance to those of adults
- Being alert to signs of distress in the child
- Being aware of the impact of developmental and cultural factors, and that some children will not want to be involved in care and care decisions
- Assuring or clearly identifying limits of confidentiality (O'Quigley, 2000)

A UK national survey of almost 19,000 children's experiences of being in hospital (CQC, 2015) identified that:

- 43 per cent of 12-year-olds felt they were not fully involved in decisions about their care
- Only 35 per cent of parents reported being involved in decisions about their child's care
- Children with physical, learning or mental health needs reported poorer experiences of care

SAFEGUARDING STOP POINT

The views of children or young people with a learning disability have not always been actively sought or valued (Children and Young People's Health Outcomes Strategy, 2012). Yet these children are particularly vulnerable members of society.

SEE ALSO
CHAPTER 36

FAMILY INVOLVEMENT IN CARE AND CARE DECISIONS

Evidence suggests that parents want and expect to be involved in their child's care, share care decisions and work in collaboration with health professions but want choices about their level of involvement (Power and Franck, 2008; Smith et al, 2015a). Parents who make autonomous decisions and manage their child's care at home perceive that their expertise is not valued when their child is admitted to hospital (Smith et al., 2015b). Involving parents in care can reduce their anxiety and feelings of helplessness when their child is acutely ill (Twycross and Stinson, 2014), and is essential when the child has a long-term condition and parents have responsibility for delivering treatments and care at home (Smith et al., 2015b). Parental involvement in care is particularly salient for the pre-verbal child and children who have difficulties with communicating where parents' unique understanding of their child must be incorporated into care.

SEE ALSO
CHAPTER 2

WHAT'S THE EVIDENCE?

Research continues to identify that involving parents in their child's care is challenging, as highlighted in the evidence presented in Table 1.1; you may wish to discuss with peers and mentors the reasons why implementing research about involving families in care in practice is challenging.

FURTHER
READING:
COYNE ET AL.

Table 1.1   Findings from studies about involving parents in their child's care

Author	Study aim	Key findings
Coyne (2015), Ireland	Qualitative study exploring children, their parents and health professionals' perspectives and expectations of family-centred care	• Family-centred care was essential to reduce children's distress when in hospital and improve the quality of care • Nurses perceived that family-centred care was central to care delivery but the roles and boundaries between parent and nurse were unclear • Family-centred care operated in the context of minimal collaboration or negotiation with parents
Coyne et al., (2013), Ireland	Survey of nurses' perceptions and practices of family-centred care	• Family-centred care was identified as being central to valuing family individuality • Family is a resource in providing information about the unique needs of the child • Although nurses supported the philosophy of family-centred care they struggled to apply the principles to practice
Macdonald et al., (2012), Canada	Observational study that explored the family's experience of family-centred care	• Embedding family-centred care into practice is challenging; differences exist in the way family-centred care operated between families and professionals • Care practices should not solely rely on better information exchange but require health professionals to consider reducing the barriers to involving the family in care
Sousa et al., (2013), Portugal	Survey of parents' perspectives about being involved in their child's care	• Gaining information about their child's condition was an overwhelming priority for parents • Parents wanted to participate in their child's care but did not want to disrupt nursing routines • Being present during their child's hospital stay was thought to be essential to their child's safety and wellbeing
Uhl et al., (2013), USA	Mixed methods study exploring parents' experiences of family-centred care following their child's admission to hospital	• A child's admission to hospital is a stressful event, associated with uncertainty, fear and lack of control in relation to meeting their child's needs; involving parents in care can ameliorate their emotions, anxiety and stress • Characteristics valued in health professionals included treating parents with dignity, being courteous and actively listening to parents' concerns • Information sharing was identified as central to involving parents in care

Despite the development of a range of models and frameworks that aim to foster the family's involvement in care over the past two decades, concepts such as 'parental participation', 'partnership with parents' and 'family-centred care' remain poorly defined and are often used interchangeably (Hutchfield, 1999; Franck and Callery, 2004; Coyne et al., 2013; Smith et al., 2015a). While lack of clarity and understanding of terminology have contributed to the problematic implementation of parent–nurse partnership working, establishing the level of involvement in care and care decisions

Table 1.2 Levels of parental involvement care

Hierarchy of care (Hutchfield, 1999)	Level of involvement (Smith et al., 2010)
Family-centred care • Parents lead care and are fully involved in all decision-making as equal partners • Parents are expert and knowledgeable in all aspects of care for their child, which is respected • The nurse's role is one of consultant and counsellor • The child and other family members are involved in care	**Parent, and child as appropriate, lead care** Family leads care with support from health professionals
Partnership with parents • Parents have equal status as care givers, are knowledgeable and have skills required to deliver care • Parents are empowered to give care; parents and nurses negotiate roles parents undertake • Parents are primary, but not total, care givers • Nurses support, advise and facilitate parents to care for their child	**Parents and nurses work in partnership** Parents and nurses have equal status for care and in decisions about care delivery
Parental participation • Parents participate in usual child care and through negotiation undertake some aspects of nursing care • Nurses remain responsible for ensuring all care is given, and often act as gatekeepers for the care parents undertake • Nurses act as primary care givers, but support and teach parents how to provide care as appropriate	**Involvement of parents in care** The nurse involves parents in care but retains responsibility for care and leads care delivery
Parental involvement • Nurses respect parents as a constant in the child's life and their unique knowledge of their child • Nurses provide care and support parents to undertake usual child care and emotional support to their child • Nurses ensure parents have appropriate information and are advocates for the child and family	**No/minimal involvement of parents in care** The nurse leads and delivers care

that children, young people and parents are willing and/or able to undertake is fundamental to working in partnership with the family. At times parents may have minimal involvement in their child's care – for example, on first contact with services or during emergency care, while at the opposite end of the spectrum parents may lead care – for example, in the context of childhood long-term conditions (Smith et al., 2010). However, being valued, effective information exchange and, if desired, supported to undertake usual childcare activities, should be the minimal involvement parents can expect (Hutchfield, 1999). Individual family needs and preferences are unique and may change over time, reflecting changing levels of involvement in care. Table 1.2 highlights the relationship between the terminology associated with involving parents in care and levels of involvement.

VIDEO LINK
1.2: PARENT
INVOLVEMENT
IN CARE

Partnership in care

The provision of hospital 'rooming-in' facilities for mothers, who were encouraged to provide emotional support for their sick child, occurred in the wake of the Platt Report (Ministry of Health, 1959). The emergence of 'care by parents units' in the early 1980s, although perceived as radical, was criticised because the underpinning philosophy of many units centred around the belief that it was a privilege for mothers to be allowed to undertake care tasks delegated by nurses and be offered facilities to stay with their child in hospital (Webb, 1993). Consequently, questions about 'care by parents units' as the ideal model to involve parents resulted in the term 'partnership in care' appearing within children's nursing literature, with 'mother' being replaced by 'the family', 'parents' or 'carers'.

You may be familiar with the 'partnership in care model of paediatric nursing', widely adopted within the UK, as the underpinning philosophy for the care of children (Casey, 1995). Central to the model was the interconnected relationship between the four dimensions associated with nursing: person (or in this case child and family), health, environment and nursing. The model emphasised that care is best undertaken by the family with support from skilled health professionals by empowering parents, and children and young people as appropriate, to contribute to care (Casey, 1995). However, there were concerns that a shift from parent involvement in care to one of partnership occurred in the absence of the essential component of negotiation, and that parents may not have been empowered to become responsible for delivering treatments and care, but expected to undertake new roles delegated to them by the nurse (Coyne, 1996).

Parent participation in care has been widely researched in hospital settings with key findings suggesting: a coercive system of involving parents exists that hinders the development of effective parent–professional partnerships (Corlett and Twycross, 2006); parents are disempowered with care delegated to them by health professionals, resulting in anxiety when undertaking complex care tasks (Coyne and Cowley, 2007); and different perspectives about what constitutes collaboration and participation between parents and health professionals (Power and Franck, 2008). For participation in care to be meaningful, health professionals need to understand parents' perspectives (Power and Franck, 2008), which can be challenging because healthcare is increasingly varied with patients' expectations, experiences, knowledge of health and heath-related issues, and the degree they wish to participate in care being highly diverse. Although partnership in care has been positioned as a philosophy underpinning the care of children and young people (Casey, 1995), there is increasing consensus that partnership in care is a central component of family-centred care (Shields et al., 2012; Smith et al., 2015a).

Family-centred care

SEE ALSO
CHAPTER 6

The Institute for Patient- and Family-Centered Care (2017, p.2) define family-centred care as 'an approach to the planning, delivery, and evaluation of healthcare that is grounded in mutually beneficial partnerships among healthcare providers, patients, and families'. Family-centred care both guides care delivery based on recognising the importance of the family in optimising the child's health and wellbeing, and is a philosophy that shapes policy and health services (Shields et al., 2012). The eight core elements central to family-centred care developed by the American Association for the Care of Children's Health (Harrison, 2010, p.336) are:

1. Recognition that the family is the constant in a child's life is incorporated into child health policy
2. Facilitating family/professional collaboration at all levels of hospital, home and community care
3. Exchanging complete and unbiased information between families and professionals
4. Honouring cultural diversity, strengths, and individuality within and across all families, including ethnic, racial, spiritual, social, economic, educational, and geographic diversity
5. Recognising and respecting different ways of coping and provide developmental, educational, emotional, environmental, and financial supports to meet diverse needs

6. Encouraging and facilitating family-to-family support and networking
7. Ensuring that hospital, home, and community service and support systems for children needing specialised health and developmental care and their families are flexible, accessible, and comprehensive in responding to diverse family-identified needs
8. Recognising families have strengths, concerns, emotions, and aspirations beyond their need for specialised health and developmental services and support

Embracing family-centred care requires that nurses caring for children view the family as an integral part of the child's life (Smith et al., 2010), which is reflected in the way care is organised, planned, delivered and evaluated around the whole family (Shields et al., 2012; Coyne et al., 2013). While many children's nurses endorse family-centred care and are passionate about involving families in care, evidence suggests that family-centred care is not consistently and effectively embedded into practice (Shields et al., 2012; Coyne et al., 2013). Furthermore, there is a lack of robust evidence to support the impact of family-centred care on the health of children and the impact on the child and family experiences (Shields et al., 2012). Consequently, family-centred care has been criticised for being espoused rather than embedded into care delivery (Coyne et al., 2013). Lack of understanding of how to implement and embed family-centred care into practice hinders parental involvement in care. Nurses need to adopt the principles of empowerment, negotiation and participation, integral to family-centred care, to actively involve parents in their child's care (Smith et al., 2010).

Activity 1.2 helps you to consider ways to work in partnership with children, young peopleand families.

WEBLINK: IPFCC

WEBLINK: IFNA

ACTIVITY 1.2: CRITICAL THINKING

What is meant by the term 'family'?

- What is patient and family-centred healthcare?
- What is family nursing and how does this differ from family-centred care?
- How does family-centred care relate to nursing and nursing practice?

Think about the questions above and discuss with peers. Then go to https://study.sage pub.com/essentialchildnursing to access weblinks to the Institute for Patient- and Family-Centered Care and International Family Nursing Association websites to enable you to explore your answers further.

ACTIVITY ANSWER 1.2

KEY SKILLS REQUIRED WHEN INVOLVING CHILDREN, YOUNG PEOPLE AND FAMILIES IN CARE AND CARE DECISIONS

Valuing children's, young people's and parents' contribution is central to their involvement in care and care decisions. The relationship between the family and health professional must be based on developing mutual trust and respecting each other's skills, experiences and perspectives, and reducing the power imbalance by facilitating partnership working rather than adopting a paternalistic approach to care delivery. Involving parents as partners in care requires health professionals to recognise and embrace parents' unique knowledge of their child and incorporate that knowledge into clinical decisions (Smith et al., 2015a). The principles of involving children, young people and families in care and care decisions include:

- Developing a trusting relationship with the child and family by getting to know the family, and valuing their knowledge and experiences
- Respecting and being sensitive to the individual family context
- Focusing on problem-based communications by listening and responding to the child and family's concerns and drawing on their expertise
- Providing regular opportunities for a mutual exchange of information that is meaningful and delivered in a way that meets the child and family's needs
- Facilitating children and parents to be involved in the child's care; clarifying and negotiating roles to reach a mutual agreement about care responsibilities
- Including children and parents as members of the interdisciplinary care team and valuing their contribution
- Collaborating and sharing decisions about care; maintaining contact and offering ongoing support (Smith et al., 2015a, 2015b)

SEE ALSO
CHAPTER 2

Effective communication with children and families enables them to make informed choices about their involvement in care and the delivery of treatments (Smith et al., 2010). Effective communication skills are at the core of all nursing activities and can be explored further by accessing the online accompaniment to this chapter. Case study 1.3, based on a student's perspective of family-centred care, and undertaking the activities in the online accompaniment to this chapter will help develop your understanding of involving parents in care.

CASE STUDY 1.3: EMMA

Family-centred care is a topic that has been extensively taught during our nursing course, beginning in year 1 and its importance reinforced each year, including reflecting on how we practise family-centred care during placements. As a third-year student and currently undertaking my fifth placement, I have come to realise the importance of family-centred care. One occasion where I observed family-centred care in practice was when a family were given the devastating news that their daughter, 10 years of age, had been diagnosed with type 1 diabetes mellitus. The condition affects the whole family, as the child will need support with dietary restrictions, lifestyle, monitoring blood glucose levels, calculating doses and administering insulin. It was vital to support the whole family suddenly facing their child's life-changing illness. Even though as students we had been taught about family-centred care in lectures, it is very different to put into practice when you have a very sick child needing immediate care, and distraught family members requiring answers as to why their daughter had developed diabetes, and wanting information about diabetes and its treatment.

- Based on the scenario outlined, discuss with your peers and mentors the key skills required to involve the child and family in care decisions, and how care can be negotiated and an agreement reached about roles and responsibilities

CASE STUDY
ANSWER 1.3

INVOLVING CHILDREN, YOUNG PEOPLE AND FAMILIES IN CARE AND CARE DECISIONS - WHERE NEXT?

International health policy advocates that health services and care delivery are patient centred and that patient–professional interactions are participatory and collaborative in nature (International Alliance of Patients' Organizations, 2007). A concept synthesis of partnership in care and family-centred care highlighted that the foundations underpinning these concepts lack clarity and a framework of involvement that focused on valuing parents' expertise, effective relationship building and involving parents in care and care decisions might be more meaningful to nurses (Smith et al., 2015a). You can access the online accompaniment to this chapter for further information about the 'Framework for involvement' and its limitations.

Central to the patient-centred care agenda is supporting individuals to contribute to the management of their own condition through a process of shared decision-making. Shared decision-making is gaining prominence in clinical practice, and is based on the premise that the patient has unique experiences and insights, while health professionals have experiences and knowledge of care in similar situations, with the aim that treatment and care decisions are mutually agreed (Entwistle, 2009). Empowering patients to self-manage their care has the potential to improve health outcomes. For example, patients are more likely to respond and act on illness symptoms, use medicines and treatments more effectively, have greater understanding of the implications of professional advice and are better able to cope with their condition (Coulter et al., 2008). Shared decision-making is based on a collaborative approach to care delivery and can address the power imbalance between patients and professionals (Entwistle, 2009).

When the patient is a child, communication dyads are different when compared to the adult patient. Shared decision-making involves health professionals engaging with parents who are making decisions on behalf of their child. Older children may be involved in decision-making processes, with or without their parents. Although the literature on shared decision-making is primarily focused on adult patients, parents and children want to be involved in care and care decisions. Parents want their expertise and knowledge of their child, and child's condition, to be valued and inform health decisions (Smith et al., 2015a).

Parents perceive decision-making processes as based primarily on the provision of information and ensuring consent for treatment rather than encouraging active participation in decisions about their child's care (Alderson et al., 2006). Mutual information exchange is central to involving parents in care and care decisions. Parents want timely, consistent, up-to date, tailored information coupled with the need to talk to others in similar situations providing opportunities to share experiences (Jackson et al., 2008). The use of professionally endorsed, accessible and reliable online resources that meet parents' learning needs and preferences can help parents provide clinical care at home for children. Parents are increasingly becoming involved in research that develops and evaluates these resources as co-researchers, co-authors and co-presenters because the parent voice should be central to the creation of parent information (Nightingale et al., 2015).

Young people need support to develop the communications skills to participate in decisions about their health in consultation with health professionals. Interventions to promote participation in consultations and support young people to develop communication skills when interacting with health professionals are emerging with positive outcomes (Milnes et al., 2014). Younger children have the capacity to make complex decisions about the management of their condition but many children want to share decisions with parents (Garnett et al., 2016).

─────────────── **CHAPTER SUMMARY** ───────────────

- Involving and supporting children and young people, as appropriate, and their families in care and care decisions should be embedded within children's nursing
- The models and frameworks to support children's nurses to work effectively with children, young people and families appear difficult to embed into everyday practice
- However, the underpinning principles of involvement are essential to effective care delivery and include: valuing parents' expertise and knowledge about their child; forming effective partnerships with the child and family; facilitating the child and family to participate in care delivery
- Successful involvement as highlighted in this chapter can be achieved through the process of negotiation, empowerment and shared goal setting, and ensuring effective information provision to enable the child and family to collaborate in care decisions

─────────────── **BUILD YOUR BIBLIOGRAPHY** ───────────────

Books

- Smith, L. and Coleman, V. (eds) (2010) *Child and Family-centred Healthcare: Concept, Theory and Practice.* 2nd edn. Basingstoke: Palgrave Macmillan.

  This book provides a useful introduction to the concept of child and family-centred care from a range of perspectives against the backdrop of current child healthcare in the UK.

- Darbyshire, P. (1994) *Living with a Sick Child in Hospital: The Experiences of Parents and Nurses.* London: Chapman Hall. Chapter 2: Becoming a live-in parent 'parenting in public'.

  Although dated, this book presents an insight into a parent's experiences of their sick child in hospital.

- Lambert, V., Long, T. and Kelleher, D. (eds) (2012) *Communication Skills for Child Health Nurses.* Maidenhead: Open University Press.

  This book provides a comprehensive overview of essential communication skills for children's nurses.

Journal articles

FURTHER
READING:
ONLINE
JOURNAL
ARTICLES

Go to https://study.sagepub.com/essentialchildnursing for further free online journal articles related to this chapter.

These articles will help you to explore some key concepts of child and family involvement in care and decision making.

- Kelly, M., Jones, S., Wilson, V. and Lewis, P. (2012) 'How children's rights are constructed in family-centred care: a review of the literature'. *Journal of Child Health Care*, 16 (2): 190–205. http://chc.sagepub.com/content/16/2/190.full.pdf+html
- Lipstein, E.A., Brinkman, W.B. and Britto, M.T. (2012) 'What is known about parents' treatment decisions? A narrative review of pediatric decision making'. *Medical Decision Making*, 32 (2): 246–58. http://mdm.sagepub.com/content/32/2/246.full.pdf+html
- Hagvall, M., Ehnfors, M. and Anderzén-Carlsson, A. (2016) 'Experiences of parenting a child with medical complexity in need of acute hospital care'. *Journal of Child Health Care*, 20(1): 68–76. http://chc.sagepub.com/content/20/1/68.full.pdf+html

Weblinks

Go to https://study.sagepub.com/essentialchildnursing for further weblinks related to this chapter.

FURTHER
READING:
WEBLINKS

- Office of the Children's Commissioner, *We Would Like to Make a Change: Children and Young People's Participation in Strategic Health Decision-making*

  www.childrenscommissioner.gov.uk/publication-We-would-like-to-make-a-change

  About how children and young people were involved in strategic healthcare decision making.

- The Royal College of Paediatrics and Child Health, *Improving Child Health*

  www.rcpch.ac.uk/

  Website designed for health professionals, children and families as a resource to highlight the importance of child and family participation in healthcare decisions and delivery.

- Institute for Patient- and Family-Centered Care

  www.ipfcc.org

  The Institute for Patient- and Family-Centered Care (IPFCC) is an American-based non-profit organisation founded in 1992 and aims to enhance understanding and practice of patient- and family-centered care. IPFCC serves as a central resource for policy makers and patient and family leaders.

ACE YOUR ASSESSMENT

ONLINE
QUIZZES &
ACTIVITY
ANSWERS

Revise what you have learned by visiting https://study.sagepub.com/essentialchildnursing

- Test yourself with multiple-choice and short-answer questions
- Do the chapter activities in the book and check your answers online

REFERENCES

Action for Sick Children (ASC) (1991) *Working Together for Change. Cascade1*. London: ASC.

Alderson, P., Hawthorne, J. and Killen, M. (2006) 'Parents' experiences of sharing neonatal information decisions: consent, cost and risk'. *Social Science and Medicine*, 62: 1319–29.

Alsop-Shields, L. and Mohay, H. (2001) 'John Bowlby and James Robertson: theorists, scientists and crusaders for improvements in the care of children in hospital'. *Journal of Advanced Nursing*, 35 (1): 50–58.

Bowlby, J. (1953) *Child Care and the Growth of Love*. Harmondsworth: Penguin.

Care Quality Commission (2015) Children and Young People's Inpatient and Day Case Survey 2014 – Key Findings. London: Care Quality Commission.

Casey, A. (1995) 'Partnership nursing: influences on involvement of informal carers'. *Journal of Advanced Nursing*, 22: 1058–62.

Children and Young People's Health Outcomes Strategy (2012) *Report of the Children and Young People's Health Outcomes Forum*. London: Children and Young People's Health Outcomes Strategy Group.

Corlett, J. and Twycross, A. (2006) 'Negotiation of parental roles within family-centred care: a review of the literature'. *Journal of Clinical Nursing*, 15: 1308–14.

Coulter. A, Parsons, S. and Askham, J. (2008) *Where are the Patients in Decision-making about Their Own Care?* Copenhagen: WHO.

Coyne, I. (1996) 'Parent participation: a concept analysis'. *Journal of Advanced Nursing*, 23: 733–40.

Coyne, I. (2015) 'Families and health-care professionals' perspectives and expectations of family-centred care: hidden expectations and unclear roles'. *Health Expectations*, 18 (5): 796–808.

Coyne, I. and Cowley, S. (2007) 'Challenging the philosophy of partnership with parents: a grounded theory study'. *International Journal of Nursing Studies*, 44: 893–904.

Coyne, I., Murphy, M., Costello, T., O'Neill, C. and Donnellan, C. (2013) 'A survey of nurses' practices and perceptions of family-centered care in Ireland'. *Journal of Family Nursing*, 19: 469–88.

Darbyshire, P. (1993) 'Parents, nurses and paediatric nursing: a critical review'. *Journal of Advanced Nursing*, 18: 1670–80.

Department for Education and Skills (DfES)/Department of Health (DH) (2004) *National Service Framework for Children, Young People and Maternity Services*. London: Department of Health.

Department of Health (DH) (1991) *Welfare of Children and Young People in Hospital*. London: HMSO.

Department of Health (DH), Home Office and Department for Education and Employment (1999) *Working Together to Safeguard Children*. London: TSO.

Entwistle, V. (2009) 'Patient involvement in decision-making: the importance of a broad conceptualization', in A. Edwards and G. Elwyn (eds), *Shared Decision-making in Health Care: Achieving Evidence-based Patient Choice*. Oxford: Oxford University Press. pp. 17–22.

Franck, L.S. and Callery, P. (2004) 'Re-thinking family-centred care across the continuum of children's healthcare'. *Child: Care, Health and Development*, 30 (3): 265–77.

Franklin, B. (1995) *The Handbook of Children's Rights: Comparative Policy and Practice*. London: Routledge.

Garnett, V., Smith, J. and Ormnady, P. (2016) 'Child–parent shifting and shared decision-making for asthma management – a qualitative interview based study'. *Nursing Children and Young People*, 28 (4): 16–22.

Harrison, T.M. (2010) 'Family-centered pediatric nursing care: state of the science'. *Journal of Pediatric Nursing*, 25: 335–43.

Hutchfield, K. (1999) 'Family-centred care: a concept analysis'. *Journal of Advanced Nursing*, 29: 1178–87.

Institute for Patient- and Family-Centered Care (IPFCC) (2017) *Advancing the Practice of Patient and Family-Centered Care in Hospital Settings*. Bethesda, MD: Institute for Patient- and Family-Centered Care. Available at: www.ipfcc.org/resources/getting_started.pdf (accessed 19 June 2017).

International Alliance of Patients' Organizations (2007) *Patient-centre Healthcare Review*, 2nd edn. International Alliance of Patients' Organizations.

Jackson. C., Cheater, F.M. and Reid, I. (2008) 'A systematic review of decision support needs of parents making child health decisions'. *Health Expectations*, 11: 232–51.

Macdonald, M.E., Liben, S., Carnevale, F.A. and Cohen, S.R. (2012) 'An office or a bedroom? Challenges for family-centered care in the pediatric intensive care unit'. *Journal of Child Health Care*, 16: 237–49.

Mayall, B. (2002) *Towards a Sociology of Childhood: Thinking from Children's Lives*. Buckingham: Open University Press.

Milnes, L.J., Mcgowan, L., Campbell, M. and Callery, P. (2014) 'A qualitative evaluation of a pre-consultation guide intended to promote the participation of young people in asthma review consultations'. *Patient Education and Counseling*, 91: 91–6.

Ministry of Health and Central Health Services Council (1959) *The Welfare of Children in Hospital*. *Platt Report*. London: HMSO.

NHS England (2016) *The NHS in England*. Available at: www.nhs.uk/NHSENGLAND/Pages/NHSEngland.aspx (last accessed 3 May 2017).

Nightingale, R., Friedl, S. and Swallow, V. (2015) 'Parents' learning needs and preferences when sharing management of their child's long-term/chronic condition: a systematic review'. *Patient Education and Counseling*, 98 (11): 1329–38.

O'Quigley, A. (2000) *Listening to Children's Views*. York: Joseph Rowntree Foundation.

Office of the Children's Commissioner: Children's Commissioner (2013) *We Would Like to Make a Change. Children and Young People's Participation in Strategic Health Decision-making*. London: Office of the Children's Commissioner.

Power, N. and Franck, L. (2008) 'Parent participation in the care of hospitalised children: a systematic review'. *Journal of Advanced Nursing*, 62 (6): 622–41.

Robertson, J. (1958) *Young Children in Hospital*. London: Tavistock Publications.

Royal College of Paediatrics and Child Health (2011) *Involving Children and Young People in Health Services*. London: Royal College of Paediatrics and Child Health.

Shields, L., Zhou, H., Pratt, J., Taylor, M., Hunter, J. and Pascoe, E. (2012) 'Family-centred care for hospitalised children aged 0–12 years'. *Cochrane Database of Systematic Reviews* DOI:10.1002/14651858.CD004811.pub3

Smith, J. and Long, T. (2002) 'Confusing rhetoric with reality: achieving a balanced skill mix of nurses working with children'. *Journal of Advanced Nursing*, 40 (3): 258–66.

Smith, J., Cheater, F., Bekker, H. and Chatwin, J. (2015a) 'Are parents and professionals making shared decisions about a child's care on presentation of a suspected shunt malfunction: a mixed method study?' *Health Expectations*, 18 (5): 1299–315.

Smith, J., Swallow, V. and Coyne, I. (2015b) 'Involving parents in managing their child's long-term condition – a concept synthesis of family-centered care and partnership-in-care'. *Journal of Pediatric Nursing*, 30 (1): 143–59.

Smith, L., Coleman, V. and Bradshaw, M. (2010) 'Family-centred care: A practice continuum', in L. Smith and V. Coleman (eds), *Child and Family-centred Healthcare: Concept, Theory and Practice*, 2nd edn. Hampshire: Palgrave.

Sousa, P., Antunes, A., Carvalho, J. and Casey, A. (2013) 'Parental perspectives on negotiation of their child's care in hospital'. *Nursing Children and Young People*, 25: 24–8.

Twycross, A. and Stinson, J. (2014) 'Physical and psychological methods of pain relief in children', in A. Twycross, S. Dowden and J. Stinson (eds), *Managing Pain in Children: A Clinical Guide for Nurses and Healthcare Professionals*, 2nd edn. Chichester: Wiley Blackwell.

Uhl, T., Fisher, K., Docherty, S.L. and Brandon, D.H. (2013) 'Insights into patient and family-centered care through the hospital experiences of parents'. *Journal of Obstetric, Gynecological and Neonatal Nursing*, 42: 121–31.

United Nations (1989) United Nations Convention on the Rights of the Child. Geneva: United Nations.

Wang, K. and Barnard, A. (2004) 'Technology dependent children and their families: a review'. *Journal of Advanced Nursing*, 54 (1): 36–46.

Webb, B. (1993) 'Trauma and tedium: an account of living on a children's ward', in J. Walmsley, J. Reynolds, P. Shakespeare and R. Wolf (eds) (1993) *Health, Welfare and Practice: Reflecting on Roles and Relationships*. London: Sage.

EFFECTIVE COMMUNICATION WITH CHILDREN AND YOUNG PEOPLE

JEAN SHAPCOTT

THIS CHAPTER COVERS

- Developmental aspects of communication
- Communication in the context of family-centred care – the triad of communication
- Play as a means of communication
- Communicating with children in difficult circumstances
- Communicating using technology and social media

> When I told my parents that I was going to try to get into children's nursing (I was already a qualified adult nurse), my mother's response was classic – 'You're only doing that so that you can play all day and get paid for it'! In many ways she wasn't far wrong – OK, not every minute of every day is spent playing, but there is an element of play in almost every interaction that a nurse has with a child or young person and that is what makes every situation encountered by a children's nurse different.
>
> **Sadia, children's nurse**

Visit https://study.sagepub.com/essentialchildnursing to access a wealth of online resources for this chapter – watch out for the margin icons throughout the chapter.

INTRODUCTION

Children have a right to be involved in all decisions that involve them and their healthcare (UN, 1989). Children must therefore receive adequate and appropriate information in order to enable them to make sense of their situation. Inability to fully understand does not justify lack of discussion with a child who wishes to be involved in their care. Opportunities for interactions provided by undertaking assessments, providing advice and information, and facilitating the expression of feelings can only be successful if children's nurses fully understand how communicative abilities develop in children and use developmentally appropriate language (Hayes and Keogh, 2012). In addition, for successful and effective communication with children it is necessary to establish a good relationship with them, even when the healthcare encounter is short, since the development of therapeutic relationships between nurses, children and their families is a fundamental principle of children's nursing (Roberts et al., 2015).

Working with children requires active engagement with families in order to help them cope with the reality of illness and its consequences. Communication occurs both formally and informally in healthcare settings. While adults frequently communicate in a neutral and objective manner while gathering or imparting facts as they seek to find solutions, children are more likely to communicate when they are engaged and busy with another activity. Children respond better to nurses who display warm, caring, engaging and trusting behaviours as well as clear and developmentally appropriate verbal language. Children themselves have individual characteristics that are expressed both verbally and non-verbally in the way they speak, use gestures and apply and respond to touch. This can be observed in their play as well as other formal and informal interactions.

This chapter will enable you to explore a range of aspects of communicating with children and their families. Developmentally appropriate communication is essential if interactions with children and young people are to be effective, but it is also important to consider the role of the child when those interactions are triadic (three-way) and involve a parent too. The quote from a practitioner at the start of the chapter shows how some lay people might see play, simply as a means of occupying a child, but it is in, in fact, a really important communication tool for the children's nurse. Not all communication with children and families is easy – it is often complex and sometimes difficult – but one aspect often seen as particularly challenging, breaking bad news, will be explored in the chapter. Finally, it is impossible to consider communication in 21st-century children's nursing without addressing technology and social media, which can be very useful but may also create problems as noted in the safeguarding concern identified within the chapter.

DEVELOPMENTAL ASPECTS OF COMMUNICATION

In order to maximise opportunities presented by interactions with children and young people it is essential that nurses understand child development, as communication techniques vary according to the age and developmental stage a child has reached (Hayes and Keogh, 2012). The psychosocial conflicts (Erikson, 1959, cited in Mooney, 2013) and type of thinking (Piaget, 1936, cited in Mooney, 2013) which are present in every stage of development influence the way in which children perceive healthcare encounters, which can lead to age-specific fears, misconceptions and other psychosocial issues, all of which can have an impact on communication (Desai and Pandya, 2013) (see Chapter 12).

Development of language and communicative ability

Optimal development of communication skills in infancy depends on a range of intrinsic and extrinsic factors in the life of a child. Intrinsic factors are those 'pre-programmed', often biological, influences that arise from within the children themselves and about which very little can be done. Extrinsic factors include issues such as mother to child attachment and the social environment in which the child grows up (Prior et al, 2008).

WATCH A VIDEO ONLINE!

VIDEO LINK 2.1: LANGUAGE DEVELOPMENT

WEBLINK: CDI

The very first form of social interaction involves crying, through which the infant seeks to get the attention of others or have their needs met. In their first months, infants rapidly learn that the gaze and looking behaviour of others contains vital information from which relationships with others can begin to form. In addition they can also recognise the emotions of those close to them through facial expression. Around the age of six or seven months, infants begin babbling and using vocal utterances, in addition to crying, to gain the attention of others.

Typically children pass through three phases of communication development (Brown and Elder, 2014). The first of these is known as intentional communication and involves the use of vocalisation. The very early stage of this is seen in the final months of infancy when babies begin to gesture to express their needs or wants.

The second stage is symbolic communication where toddlers and young children begin to use early language to interact with others, gain attention and meet needs. Children at this age engage in three types of behaviours that assist in the development of communication: social and language skills, namely participation in motor imitation; joint attention; and symbolic play. Joint attention is the capacity to engage in coordinated social interaction (Beuker et al., 2013). This includes sharing attention, for example through the use of alternating gaze, following the attention of others by, for example, following where another person is pointing and directing the attention of another.

The final and most sophisticated phase of communication development is linguistic communication, in which children and young people are able to engage in full discourse with another person using many

Table 2.1 Communication and development

Early communication skill	Description	Development
Sharing attention	A triadic interaction involving the infant alternating their gaze between the adult and an object with the intention of integrating attention to the person and the object into one interaction	Sharing attention emerges around 9 months of age
Following attention	Following the direction of the gaze or manual pointing gesture of an adult to an external object	6 months: following the head movement of an adult with their eyes or turning their head in the appropriate direction
		Until 12 months: fixating on the first object along the path being followed by the infant's gaze, even if it is not the target object
		12-18 months: more and longer joint attention and is now able to follow attention to objects outside their visual feed
		Following a manual pointing gesture tends to emerge before following a gaze
Directing attention	By showing, giving, reaching and/or pointing with a clear imperative or declarative intention, the infant directs the attention of others towards objects or situations	The first declarative and imperative gestures with or without gaze alternation emerge around 9 months and become more frequent between 12 and 15 months
Language	Making sounds, speaking and understanding words to become a system of communication	First year of life: babbling and cooing
		12 months: first simple words
		18 months: productive vocabulary of 10-20 words
		2 years: words represent or symbolise actions, objects and thoughts; productive vocabulary grows to around 100 words

forms of communication, which is seen in late childhood and adolescence. Whatever a child or young person's stage of communication development, children's nurses need to be able to communicate effectively with those in their care. This final phase may be seen by many as the point where communication becomes easier, but other phases of development must also be addressed, as you can see in Table 2.1 above.

Developmentally appropriate communication

Children's nurses need to be able to adapt their communication to the developmental needs of the children in their care. Crying is a powerful pre-verbal signal that infants use to communicate and gain an immediate response. Even at this very early age, it is important to be aware of cultural and family norms for responding to crying, noting how parents respond to their baby's crying behaviour, but generally nurses should respond to crying in a timely manner. A soothing and calming tone when talking to a baby helps to allay their anxiety (and that of their parents) and can be effective in stopping them crying.

VIDEO LINK 2.2:
A CHILD'S
PERSPECTIVE

Toddlers (1–3 years) should be approached carefully as they are often fearful of strangers. Time spent observing a toddler with their parent is time well spent as they become used to the nurse's presence and gradually accept them into their communicative world. Children of this age often have their own particular words for objects and actions and it is important for the nurse to familiarise him/herself with these so that the toddler feels heard and understood.

Children between the ages of 3 and 5 years like to establish good relationships with adults and peers. They are curious and love to explore and create, so play (which will be addressed later in this chapter) is an important means of communication with this age group. It is important to be honest with children of this age and use simple connected terms when talking to them since, despite their growing vocabulary, the ability to understand complex sentences should not be assumed.

School-age children can utilise material presented in the form of age-appropriate diagrams, illustrations and books. Third-party stories can be used effectively to gather information such as asking, 'How might you...?' or 'Do you think that...?' particularly when direct questioning, careful observation or informal chatting are not working. This less direct approach can enable children to voice concerns or ask questions they may not otherwise have felt able to do.

SCENARIO 2.1: TONI

Toni is 6 years old. She has a chronic renal condition whereby she has only recently started gaining bladder control and, even now, when she needs to pass urine, she has to go straight away. As a result of this, Toni has had many hospital admissions with urinary tract infections (UTIs). Her perineal area is also prone to becoming very sore when she has little 'accidents' and has to wear slightly wet underwear.

Toni's school was reluctant to take her at the outset, believing that she could and should be dry at the age she started with them. Her parents were forced to get medical evidence before the school would take her in and, even now, some staff refuse to allow her to leave the classroom to go to the toilet, resulting in soreness and embarrassment as well as frequent UTIs.

In hospital, Toni is very clingy to whichever parent is present. Although she is generally a very bubbly and confident little girl, when she enters any healthcare environment she changes and becomes very quiet. When asked what makes a good nurse Toni gave two answers – 'the one who hasn't got a needle in her hand' and 'the one who plays with me and doesn't just talk to mummy or daddy'.

- Why do you think Toni changes so much when she enters hospital?
- How could nurses improve Toni's experience of healthcare through effective communication?

SCENARIO
ANSWER 2.1

When nurses communicate with young people it is important that they recognise that the stereo-typical views of adolescents held by society in general are just that, stereotypes, and therefore not applicable to every individual. Such views can foster a negative attitude and create a barrier to effective communication. Young people expect nurses to be available, accepting, informed and informative and empathic. Children's nurses therefore need to make opportunities and invest time in building a rapport with a young person (Fallon, 2012).

ACTIVITY 2.1: CRITICAL THINKING

The development of communication in children with autistic spectrum disorder (ASD) follows a very different pattern to that of normally developing children (Brown and Elder, 2014). A minority will not develop any form of functional communication, while those who do often display atypical communi-cation styles. It is likely that these develop because the children have limited understanding of the meanings and interactions of symbolic forms of language. These children may have the vocabulary and may even have learned sufficient syntax to pass standardised language screening, but they struggle in real world communication settings because they lack true understanding of meaning.

- How might children's nurses communicate effectively with children with ASD?

When answering this question, think creatively and reflect on ways that you have seen other health-care professionals communicate in difficult circumstances.

COMMUNICATION IN THE CONTEXT OF FAMILY-CENTRED CARE - THE TRIAD OF COMMUNICATION

Many interactions in the care of children are 'triadic', that is they involve three parties – the child, the parent/carer and the nurse. Interactions primarily occur between two parties at any one time, with the other person as an observer, therefore nurse–parent interaction is just one of the dyads that can occur. These dyads interact to form the triadic relationship which itself has features of a therapeutic alliance, whilst also possessing the potential for both cooperation and conflict in each of these alliances.

VIDEO LINK 2.3:
COMMUNICATING
WITH CHILDREN

WEBLINK:
UNICEF

ACTIVITY 2.2: REFLECTIVE PRACTICE

On your placement take the time to observe the interactions between nurses, children and families in the clinical areas.

- What do you notice about the focus of these interactions?
- Who are most involved in the interactions?
- How satisfying do you think the interactions were for a) the nurse, b) the parent and c) the child? And why?

It is important to develop a positive parent–nurse relationship since this is the key to the successful development of alliances within the triad which will ultimately improve the quality of care provided to the child. Nurse–parent interactions take place in the context of the parent's expectations, motivation and health beliefs (Callery and Milnes, 2012). Taking the time to listen to a parent, being attentive, validating their perspective and providing comfort ensures that parents feel supportive. Children's nurses need to be aware of the importance of attitude and approach as facilitators of communication (Fisher and Broome, 2011). Ammentorp et al. (2005) note that the two factors identified by parents as having the highest priority are the need to get answers to their questions and the behaviours of nurses caring for their child including expressing warmth, being kind, caring and taking parents' experiences seriously.

SCENARIO 2.2: JOSH

Josh is a 2-year-old boy. He lives with his mother Kelly, older sister Jemma and baby sister Jasmine. Josh has recently started attending a local nursery. Four weeks ago Kelly noticed that Josh's left leg seemed very swollen and he was not putting any weight on it. The local hospital said that there was no fracture, but the leg remains swollen and painful, so Kelly took him back to the Children's Emergency Department (CED). The first nurse they encountered was very abrupt, but reluctantly agreed to book them into the department. Another nurse came into the cubicle and told Kelly that she had to take the bandage off. Josh immediately started to cry and became more and more distressed as the nurse cut away the bandage and pulled it off his leg. She told him to be quiet and made Kelly hold onto his toy rabbit as it was getting in her way.

Kelly and Josh were then left alone in the cubicle until another nurse, Melanie, arrived to take them off to x-ray. Seeing Josh on the trolley, she very gently picked him up and put him in his mother's arms. Seeing how upset both Kelly and Josh were, she stayed with them throughout the x-ray, gently stroking Josh's hair and putting a comforting arm around Kelly's shoulders. When the x-ray was completed, Melanie stayed with Kelly and Josh while the doctor gave them the news that Josh's leg was, in fact, fractured and that the initial diagnosis had been wrong.

- Which nurse demonstrated more effective communication skills?

SCENARIO
ANSWER 2.2

Children's nurses generally seek to involve children in the interactions, but it is important to recognise that a child's willingness to participate cannot be assumed. Some children simply do not wish to be involved and would prefer to be 'passive bystanders' in any interactions (Lambert et al., 2010). Others may wish to be active participants at all times but, most commonly, a child's desire to be involved in any given interaction is dependent on its nature and the context within which it is taking place.

Children's nurses want to hear from the children themselves, not just parents speaking on their behalf and most parents value nurses' communication with their children. As well as putting the child at ease, parents see that communication between nurses and children could uncover information that might not otherwise have been available (Callery and Milnes, 2012). Children's nurses can employ a number of strategies to structure interactions with children, including direct questions to the child, making it clear that they are the person expected to speak next, and tacitly selecting the child by limiting eligible respondents through using phrases such as 'your diabetes', 'your medication'.

There are some situations in which the nurse–child dyad may not be effective, when, for example, younger children do not possess sufficient vocabulary to participate and situations in which children may defer to their parents or parents may respond on the child's behalf. While the majority of parental interventions during nurse–child interactions aim to supplement or clarify information provided by the child, parents might sometimes contradict their child or answer a question directed at the child, reflecting their own concerns about balancing protection (from hearing things that are too frightening or that the child may not understand) and encouraging independence.

Young people's contribution to triadic consultations is often limited despite them frequently having both the desire to participate and feelings of competence to be regarded as partners in their own care (van Staa, 2011). The most common reasons for this are considered to be the way in which the nurse controls turn-taking in the interaction and the way in which parents tend to 'jump in' to fill the gaps in information given by the young person. As a consequence, the young person is more likely to act as a 'passive bystander' because their participation has been neither requested nor encouraged.

This children's nurse recalls the experience she had with a 14-year-old boy named Rashid:

His father was killed in a road accident when he was 5 years old and he now lives with his mother and younger sisters. Despite having quite severe asthma, as the oldest child and the only boy, Rashid has taken on many of the male roles in the family. He went to see the practice nurse with his mother for his routine review and throughout the consultation, the nurse focused on his mother. Never once did she look at Rashid or direct a question to him. When he tried to speak up, the nurse cut him short and once again focused on his mother. As he left the consultation Rashid was heard to say, 'Next time, come without me. It is pointless me being here because you and the nurse seem to believe you know about my asthma better than me, so you don't need me.'

WHAT'S THE EVIDENCE?

Lambert et al. (2008) coined the term 'visible-ness' to reflect a continuum on which children's communication with nurses lies between 'being overshadowed' and 'being at the forefront'. Those children considered to be 'overshadowed' are marginal to the communication process as interactions were primarily between their parents and the healthcare professional. However, those 'at the forefront' of communication were the focal point of communication, holding a leading position in interactions as healthcare professionals communicated directly with them as well as their parents. Children's 'visible-ness' in communication is contingent on three factors:

- The child themselves in terms of their ability to articulate their thoughts and ideas or desire to participate in interactions
- Healthcare professionals' and parents' recognition of the child as part of the communication process, as well as their perception of the child's need to be involved
- The nature of the healthcare environment

In a second paper Lambert et al. (2010) used their earlier findings to develop the Child Transitional Communication Model which explains children's roles in healthcare interactions. Within their model the authors recognised a number of conflicting perspectives:

- Child as family member versus child as independent entity
- Child as powerless versus empowered child

- Child as immature, incompetent and dependent versus child as mature, competent and independent
- Child as having the right to protection versus child as having the right to liberation
- Child as becoming versus child as being

How might a better understanding of the communicative position of a child (as opposed to that of their parent/carer) improve the quality of the care they receive?

WHAT'S THE EVIDENCE? ANSWER 2.1

PLAY AS A MEANS OF COMMUNICATION

Play is a central activity in the lives of most children (Hayes and Keogh, 2012), providing a context for communication, understanding and catharsis. Symbolic or object play in childhood helps to develop symbol representation and is critical to the development of language skills. Pretend play with objects develops naturally in most children, becoming more complex over time with the understanding of symbols during play contributing to the comprehension of language (Brown and Elder, 2014).

ACTIVITY 2.3: REFLECTIVE PRACTICE

On every placement, observe children at play and ask yourself the following questions:

- Are they playing alone, with an adult or another child or children?
- What communication skills are they employing within their play?
- Does their play tell you anything about them or how they are feeling?

Ask to spend a day or two with the play specialists and observe their work with the children. Discuss with them how they utilise play to assist children in that particular care setting?

Developmental aspects of play

At first sight, play may appear to be simple and enjoyed only for its entertainment value. However, beneath its apparent simplicity lies a complexity in which ideas, understanding, exploration and communication are pursued with enthusiasm and developing skill (Binns and Hicks, 2012). Through play children can experience, connect and interact with the world in order to make sense of their experiences, practise for their future life and communicate feelings they may not be able to verbalise. Have a look at the different type of play identified and described in Table 2.2.

The importance of play in children's nursing

Observing children at play can give children's nurses insight into how the child is thinking and dealing with experiences and new situations. When a child is unwell or in a healthcare setting for the first

Table 2.2   Six different types of play

Type of play	Description
Unoccupied	The child is not playing, just observing. A child may be standing in one spot or performing random movements
Solitary (independent) play	The child is alone and maintains focus on its activity. Such a child is uninterested in or is unaware of what others are doing – most common in younger children (age 2-3)
Onlooker play (behaviour)	The child watches others at play but does not engage in it themselves – also more common in younger children
Parallel play (adjacent play)	The child plays separately from others but close to them, mimicking their actions. This type of play is seen as a transitory stage as a child moves to a more socially mature associative and cooperative type of play
Associative play	The child is interested in the people playing but not in coordinating their activities with those people, or when there is no organised activity at all
Cooperative play	The child is interested both in the people playing and in the activity they are doing. The activity is organised, and participants have assigned roles. There is also increased self-identification with a group, and a group identity may emerge

time, play has a particular role in helping them to understand and cope with what is happening to them. An example of this is the way in which play can help to address the negative consequences of being in hospital, which include:

- Decreasing stress
- Providing an outlet for anxiety
- Offering a diversion from unpleasant procedures and treatments
- Bringing meaning to the chaos of the experience
- Keeping memories of home and everything that is important to the child alive

Playing with dolls, books and equipment prior to a procedure can help to ease fear of the unknown and help children to become familiar with medical routines. Such carefully planned play opportunities allow children to express their feelings and promote positive coping strategies. Most play can be adapted to meet the needs of different children, but it takes time and planning as well as a real regard for play. Play specialists can provide advice on how best to create interesting play opportunities for children and develop exciting play and learning environments (Hayes and Keogh, 2012) and children's nurses should work closely with play specialists to ensure that opportunities provided by play can be used to maximise the effectiveness of both communication and treatment. One example of how this can be achieved is through the use of distraction therapy which aims to take the child's mind off a procedure by concentrating on something else that is happening. Distraction can be as simple as the children's nurse who has a pen shaped in the form of an animal which can be used as a puppet to distract the child or as sophisticated as projections of space scenes or a princess castle on the walls and ceiling of a treatment room.

Therapeutic play utilises play as a means of communication as well as a mode of therapy (Binns and Hicks, 2012). At times play may simply be a means for a child to express their needs and desires, but at others it may be used to affect a positive therapeutic outcome, with these often being closely linked since developing a means of communication can be therapeutic in itself. Therapeutic play can be categorised as non-directive and directive, both of which can be facilitated effectively by children's nurses. Non-directive play occurs when the practitioner assumes the role of an observer whilst the child plays freely, and directive play involves the nurse becoming actively engaged and directing the child's play in order to achieve a specific aim.

Play is a very important means of communication for children and cannot be ignored by children's nurses. While it is often seen as one of the more enjoyable aspects of nursing children, it is important to recognise its value as a therapeutic tool, not simply as a means of keeping children occupied.

COMMUNICATING WITH CHILDREN IN DIFFICULT CIRCUMSTANCES

Inevitably these aspects of care evoke many emotional issues and reactions, but they are also care situations where effective communication is even more important than normal. All the communications skills that a children's nurse possesses are required including supporting, observing, interviewing and listening. In addition it is essential that the nurse has self-awareness, emotional maturity, empathy and sensitivity. Children and families often note a link between inadequate or ineffective communication and an increase in their confusion and distress.

Breaking bad news

Barriers to communication in these situations include those related to the care environment, for example the multiple distractions inherent in a busy children's ward, physical factors and emotional issues inherent in the situation. Knowing that a child is very unwell or approaching the end of their life is inevitably stressful for their family. They may be afraid of what the future holds or even angry and frustrated with healthcare staff who they feel have 'given up' on their child. Family members often experience these situations in different ways leading to tensions within the family, while different healthcare professionals approach breaking bad news and the end of a child's life in their own individual ways.

ACTIVITY 2.4: CRITICAL THINKING

If you have been present when a child and family have received bad news, or even if you have not, consider how best the children's nurse might support them after their meeting with the doctor. What aspects of communication are going to be the most useful at this crucial time? What do children and parents need in order to absorb and assimilate the information they have just received?

- Read on to find out more about this
- Watch the video of profession sharing strategies for telling parents their child has a life-limiting illness at https://study.sagepub.com/essentialchildnursing

PRACTICE SCENARIO 2: SOLOMON

VIDEO LINK 2.4 BREAKING BAD NEWS

Breaking bad news is often considered one of the most complex and challenging aspects of communication in children's nursing. While any discussion of this aspect of communication emphasises the need for appropriate, honest communication with both the child and the family, it has already been noted that the child is often peripheral to such interactions. One of the reasons often quoted for this is lack of certainty regarding what children will understand in relation to the words 'death' and 'dying'. A number of approaches to breaking bad news to children have been noted (Kopchack Sheehan et al., 2014). Many choose to tell the truth to children while adjusting the content and timing of the message to their age and physical condition. Others 'skirt around' the facts, telling the truth but in an indirect or ambiguous way or in a way that is devoid of emotion, focusing instead on practical issues. A minority choose not to tell the child the full truth at any time during their illness.

While there is no right or wrong way to break bad news to children and families, the level of satisfaction reported by children decreases with their perception of the honesty of those involved. However, each situation is unique, with every child and family experiencing it through the lens of their own beliefs, values and knowledge. Breaking bad news must occur within a partnership approach to care. While the children's nurse is often the healthcare professional who has developed a therapeutic relationship with the child and family, often over a number of years, breaking bad news is traditionally seen as the remit of the doctor. The role of the children's nurse in this situation includes facilitation, support, counselling, educating and advocating for the child and their family (Price et al., 2006).

> I was on a long placement on a children's ward. I got to know a young man with a rare progressive genetic condition very well and his family always said that the best days on the ward were when I was looking after him. On this admission he had come in with a chest infection, but, despite several changes of antibiotics, he wasn't getting any better. The doctors told us (the nurses) that it was likely that he was going to die and asked who would accompany them when they told his parents. My mentor immediately said that I should be there, as I had a good relationship with them, and she would go with me. I wasn't so sure as I was only in my second year, but she persuaded me. It was really, really hard and I couldn't hold back the tears at one point, but I was glad I was there. His mother kept looking at me and, in the end, I just took hold of her hand, just to reassure like… Once the meeting was over, I wanted to run away, but my mentor said to me, 'Stay with them for a while. Don't worry if you don't talk, just be there for them', so I sat with them for about 15 minutes until they decided they could face going back into the ward. I didn't want to be in that meeting, but I am so glad my mentor changed my mind.
>
> **Tammy, children's nursing student**

> Our son Mikey has a very rare condition and the children's ward is his second home. We got to know a nursing student (Asha) very well over his last three admissions. She kept telling us that she was only in her second year, but you would not have thought it. She just seemed to know what Mikey needed and how to make me feel better too. I remember the day we were told that he was going to die. Although we always knew it would happen, we were not ready for it yet. It was a great relief to have Asha there when the doctor told us. I don't remember much of what was said, but I did feel that the doctors and nurses there really cared, not just about Mikey, but about us too. When Asha cried I just knew how much she cared about my son and then she just reached across and took my hand – I'm not usually a great one for touch, but that just felt right. I expected the nurses to leave when the doctor had finished talking to us, but Asha stayed, in silence, and somehow her presence gave me the courage to go back to see Mikey. Thank you Asha!
>
> **David parent**

CHECK YOUR
ANSWERS
ONLINE!

ACTIVITY 2.5: CRITICAL THINKING

Read carefully both voices above. Why do you think Mikey's parents valued Asha and the care she provided so highly?

ACTIVITY
ANSWER 2.5

Non-verbal communication is very important in breaking bad news. Every nuance of a nurse's posture, facial expression, etc. is a key communication message that will be noted and remembered by the child and family. The ability to listen actively to any information given by the doctor to the child/parents, but also to child/parental responses and questions, is also required alongside the use of observational skills to note and interpret their reactions in order to be able to support the child and family after their meeting with the doctor.

COMMUNICATING USING TECHNOLOGY AND SOCIAL MEDIA

In today's society one of the most influential factors on children of all ages is technology. With this increase in technology comes an increase in skills as well as social benefits, but also the potential for harm from 'sexting', cyberbullying and Internet addiction (Donnerstein, 2012). There is clearly a need for nurses working with children, young people and families to have a fully informed evidence base with regard to the possible benefits and drawbacks of communication technology (Jones et al., 2013).

Communicating via technology occupies a unique middle ground between using spoken and written language for communication. Electronic discourse, as used in emails, text messages, etc. may in fact represent an entirely new language register and, with children and young people increasingly communicating through this new form of language, have implications for communication skills. Conversational language rules are generally adhered to online which may enhance pragmatic language skills, for example the need to provide contextual information. Users are highly aware of the social context in which they are communicating and adapt their relational tone, personal language, sentence complexity and message composition time according to the target recipients.

Ongoing advances in technology may facilitate child-centred approaches to care and establish interactive communication that may not have been possible previously. Use of smartphones and other devices may empower children to communicate directly with healthcare professionals, enabling them to be more involved in decisions regarding their care instead of relying on parents, particularly as they transition into young adulthood. Young people may be reluctant to visit a healthcare professional, so the use of text messaging can even provide an effective means of communicating regarding symptoms, appointments and other aspects of nursing care. Many children and young people turn to apps, websites and social media as a natural first solution to their need for information and to connect with others (Jones et al., 2013). Children and, in particular, young people are technologically adept and active on social media (Wysocki, 2015). The increase in the use of social media has been so rapid and their presence in children's everyday life is now so pervasive that, for some children and young people, it is the primary way they interact socially (McBride, 2011).

However, there are concerns regarding the increased use of communication technologies including social media. These include the potential to encourage social isolation, which may have a negative impact on language skills. In addition, the lack of face-to-face interaction means that many contextual and non-verbal language cues may be lost. The Internet is always available and can be easily accessed by children, often with little parental supervision. Content is often unregulated and children may be exposed to extreme forms of violence, while the sexual content of the Internet is more prevalent than on other popular media. Participation in online activities is private and anonymous, which allows children to search for materials that they would not normally access through traditional media. The opportunity to access such a range of materials plays an important role in cyberbullying and child sexual exploitation. Potential victims are readily available and the identity of the aggressor is frequently unknown.

WEBLINK:
NICE

SAFEGUARDING STOP POINT

While the use of technology in communication is clearly important, bullying and its impact on the lives of children are longstanding concerns for child healthcare professionals. Cyberbullying is a more recent phenomenon resulting from the blurring of the lines between aggressor and target as well as perceived imbalances of power in the online environment. It consists of any behaviour performed through electronic or digital media by individuals or groups that repeatedly communicate hostile or aggressive messages intended to inflict harm and includes spreading rumours about someone, making inflammatory comments about another person in public discussion areas, leaving abusive messages about the victim on social media pages and sending the victim pornography or other knowingly offensive graphic material.

Warning signs that children are experiencing cyberbullying include displaying numerous negative feelings, school grades beginning to drop, lack of eating or sleeping, all of which are very similar to those seen in other forms of bullying. Specific signs associated with cyberbullying include avoiding their computer, smartphone or tablet, appearing stressed when receiving an email or personal message and avoiding conversations about computer use. Children's nurses are well placed to observe these signs in those they care for and to report any suspicions as this is fast becoming a serious safeguarding concern for the 21st century.

VIDEO LINK 2.5:
DOS AND
DON'TS OF
SOCIAL MEDIA

You can watch the video of the dos and don'ts of social media at http://study.sagepub.com/essential childnursing

Effective communication is crucial in children's nursing. In order to be successful in communicating with children and young people, nurses must be cognisant of the child's communicative development and use appropriate verbal and non-verbal skills.

CHAPTER SUMMARY

- Children may be overshadowed by their parents or other adults in healthcare interactions, which are generally triadic in nature
- Children's nurses need to be constantly aware of the presence of the child and involve them in communication and decisions, but only to the point that that child wishes to participate Individuality in communicative style and preferences must always be respected. There is no better demonstration of the importance of effective communication than when it is utilised in difficult situations such as breaking bad news
- Play is an important means of communication with children. Although frequently seen as the domain of younger children, play can be used across the spectrum of childhood as a means of

engaging young patients, preparing them for procedures and treatments, distraction and as a means of exploring feelings and concerns

- An important member of the interprofessional team in this regard is the play specialist who can guide nurses as to the most effective way to use play in particular situations
- While many children use electronic devices for play and recreational purposes, the Internet, texting and social media have an important and continually developing role in contemporary healthcare. While there are clear advantages of using these media in this way, it is important to remember that there are risks and potential dangers, particularly in social media and texting, which can escalate into safeguarding concerns if not addressed

BUILD YOUR BIBLIOGRAPHY

Books

- Lambert, V., Long, T. and Kelleher, D. (2012) *Communication Skills for Children's Nurses*. Maidenhead: McGraw Hill.

  A comprehensive text exploring models of communication used by children and associated skills specifically aimed at children's nurses.

- Redsell, S. and Hastings, A. (eds) (2010) *Listening to Children and Young People in Healthcare Consultations*. Abingdon: Routledge.

  This book guides healthcare professionals in the best ways to engage with, and obtain the required information from, children during effective consultations.

- Shapcott, J. (2016) 'Communicating with children, young people and families', in I. Gault, J. Shapcott, A. Luthi and G. Reid (eds), *Communication in Nursing and Healthcare: A Guide for Compassionate Practice*. London: Sage.

  This chapter provides an overview of some aspects of communicating with children in the context of mindful professional communication.

Journal articles

Go to https://study.sagepub.com/essentialchildnursing for further free online journal articles related to this chapter.

FURTHER READING: ONLINE JOURNAL ARTICLES

- Lambert, V., Glacken, M. and McCarron, M. (2008) '"Visible-ness": the nature of communication for children admitted to a specialist children's hospital in the Republic of Ireland'. *Journal of Clinical Nursing*, 17, 3092-102.

  This article explores some of the challenges faced when communicating with children in hospital.

- Lambert V., Glacken M. and McCarron M. (2011) 'Communication between children and health professionals in a child hospital setting: a Child Transitional Communication Model'. *Journal of Advanced Nursing*, 67 (3), 569-82.

  This article follows on from the previous one and proposes a model to guide nurses when communicating with children.

- Coyne, I. and Gallagher, P. (2011) 'Participation in communication and decision-making: children and young people's experiences in a hospital setting'. *Journal of Clinical Nursing*, 67 (3), 2334-43.

(Continued)

(Continued)

Ensuring children are engaged in healthcare consultations and that accurate information is obtained can be challenging, so this article outlines some useful strategies that might be employed.

Weblinks

FURTHER
READING:
WEBLINKS

Go to https://study.sagepub.com/essentialchildnursing for further weblinks related to this chapter.

- UNICEF, *Communicating with Children*

  www.unicef.org/cwc

  This website provides principles and guidance for children's nurses to facilitate their ongoing development of communication skills. Child development and its importance to communication are addressed alongside the rights of children to effective communication and the influence of the media on children.

- Child Development Institute, *Communication Disorders in Children and Adolescents*

  https://childdevelopmentinfo.com/child-psychology/children_with_communication_disorders/#.WJwxpW-LTIU

  Although aimed at parents, this section of the website gives an insight into the nature and incidence of these disorders and provides useful links to other relevant sites.

- NICE, *Child Maltreatment: When to Suspect Maltreatment in under 18s*

  www.nice.org.uk/guidance/cg89/ifp/chapter/communicating-with-and-about-children-or-young-people

  This page forms part of a larger set of guidance regarding safeguarding children. It reminds children's nurses of the importance of communication with and about children and young people in such situations.

———— ACE YOUR ASSESSMENT ————

ONLINE
QUIZZES &
ACTIVITY
ANSWERS

Revise what you have learned by visiting https://study.sagepub.com/essentialchildnursing

- Test yourself with multiple-choice and short-answer questions
- Do the chapter activities in the book and check your answers online

REFERENCES

Ammentorp, J., Mainz, J. and Sabroe, S. (2005) 'Parents' priorities and satisfaction with acute pediatric care'. *Archives of Pediatrics and Adolescent Medicine*, 159: 127–31.

Beuker, K.T., Rommelse, N.N., Donders, R. and Buitelaar, J.K., (2013) 'Development of early communication skills in the first two years of life'. *Infant Behavior and Development*, 36 (1): 71–83.

Binns, F. and Hicks, P. (2012) 'Using play and technology to communicate with children and young people', in V. Lambert, T. Long and D. Kelleher (eds), *Communication Skills for Children's Nurses*. Maidenhead: McGraw-Hill.

Brown, A.B. and Elder, J.H. (2014) 'Communication in autism spectrum disorder: a guide for pediatric nurses'. *Pediatric Nursing*, 40 (5): 219–25.

Callery, P. and Milnes, L. (2012) 'Communication between nurses, children and their parents in asthma review consultations'. *Journal of Clinical Nursing*, 21 (11–12): 1641–50.

Desai, P.P. and Pandya, S.V. (2013) 'Communicating with children in healthcare settings'. *Indian Journal of Pediatrics*, 8 (12): 1028–33.

Donnerstein, E. (2012) 'Internet bullying'. *Pediatric Clinics of North America*, 59 (3): 623–33.

Fallon, D. (2012) 'Communicating with young people', in V. Lambert, T. Long and D. Kelleher (eds), *Communication Skills for Children's Nurses*. Maidenhead: McGraw-Hill.

Fisher, M.J. and Broome, M.E. (2011) 'Parent-provider communication during hospitalization'. *Journal of Pediatric Nursing*, 26 (1): 58–69.

Hayes, N. and Keogh, P. (2012) 'Communicating with children in early and middle childhood', in V. Lambert, T. Long and D. Kelleher (eds), *Communication Skills for Children's Nurses*. Maidenhead: McGraw-Hill.

Jones, R., Cleverly, L., Hammersley, S., Ashurst, E. and Pinkney, J. (2013) 'Apps and online resources for young people with diabetes: the facts'. *Journal of Diabetes Nursing*, 17 (1): 20–6.

Kopchak Sheehan, D., Burke Draucker, C., Christ, G.H., Murray Mayo, M., Heim, K. and Parish, S., (2014) 'Telling adolescents a parent is dying'. *Journal of Palliative Medicine*, 17 (5): 512–20.

Lambert, V., Glacken, M. and McCarron, M. (2008) '"Visible-ness": the nature of communication for children admitted to a specialist children's hospital in the Republic of Ireland'. *Journal of Clinical Nursing*, 17 (23): 3092–102.

Lambert, V., Glacken, M. and McCarron, M. (2010) 'Communication between children and health professionals in a child hospital setting: a Child Transitional Communication Model'. *Journal of Advanced Nursing*, 67 (3): 569–82.

McBride, D.L. (2011) 'Risks and benefits of social media for children and adolescents'. *Journal of Pediatric Nursing*, 26 (5): 498–9.

Mooney, C.G. (2013) *Theories of Childhood: An Introduction to Dewey, Montessori, Erikson, Piaget & Vygotsky*. St Paul, MN: Redleaf Press.

Price, J., McNeilly, P. and Surgenor, M. (2006) 'Breaking bad news to parents: the children's nurse's role'. *International Journal of Palliative Nursing*, 12 (3): 115–20.

Prior, M., Bavin, E.L., Cini, E., Reilly, S., Bretherton, L., Wake, M. and Eadie, P. (2008) 'Influences on communicative development at 24 months of age: child temperament, behaviour problems, and maternal factors'. *Infant Behavior and Development*, 31 (2): 270–279.

Roberts, J., Fenton, G. and Barnard, M. (2015) 'Developing effective therapeutic relationships in children, young people and their families'. *Nursing Children and Young People*, 27 (4): 30–5.

UN (1989) *Convention on the Rights of the Child*. Available at: www.unicef.org.uk/what-we-do/un-convention-child-rights (accessed 9 May 2017).

van Staa, A.L. (2011) 'Unravelling triadic communication in hospital consultations with adolescents with chronic conditions: the added value of mixed methods research'. *Patient Education and Counselling*, 82 (3): 455–64.

Wysocki, R. (2015) 'Social media for school nurses'. *NASN School Nurse*, 30 (3): 180–8.

ASSESSMENT AND MANAGEMENT OF PAIN IN CHILDREN AND YOUNG PEOPLE

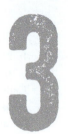

ALISON TWYCROSS AND BECKY SAUL

THIS CHAPTER COVERS

- Why is it important to assess and manage pain in children?
- Different strategies for assessing pain in children
- How to use validated pain assessment tools for children of all ages
- Pharmacological management of pain: the pharmacology of conventional analgesic drugs
- Non-pharmacological management of pain

> Access to pain management is a fundamental human right
>
> **IASP, 2015**

> I guess I would have wanted those pain medications more often, but I did not always dare to ask for them, and sometimes I was ashamed to press the call button since it made such a loud noise and my roommate was sleeping. I would have liked it if the nurses would round every hour so that I would not have to suffer from the pain because I didn't dare to use the call button. I could have told my father, but it was already eleven o'clock and he wasn't with me anymore.
>
> **Polkki et al., 2003, pp.39–40**

Visit https://study.sagepub.com/essentialchildnursing to access a wealth of online resources for this chapter – watch out for the margin icons throughout the chapter.

INTRODUCTION

The quotations above suggest that pain management in children is still not as good as it could be. This chapter starts by providing you with details of current best practice guidelines. The reasons it is important to assess and manage children's pain effectively in your practice will then be outlined. The stages of pain management are described, followed by a discussion of the different strategies that children's nurses can use to assess a child's pain. Several of the most commonly used pain assessment tools are described. Pharmacological strategies which you can use for managing a child's pain are detailed, as are several non-pharmacological methods of pain relief.

WHY IS IT IMPORTANT TO ASSESS AND MANAGE PAIN IN CHILDREN?

Unrelieved pain has several undesirable physical and psychological consequences that affect the child in the short and longer term. Pain produces a physiological stress response that includes increased heart and breathing rates to facilitate the increasing demands of oxygen and other nutrients to vital organs. Failure to relieve pain produces a prolonged stress state, which can result in harmful multisystem effects (Middleton, 2003). There is also evidence that acute (postoperative) pain can result in chronic pain in a small but significant number of children (Kristensen et al., 2012; Lauridsen et al., 2014). Given this, the need to manage children's pain effectively is clear. Pain assessment is the first step in achieving this.

WEBLINK:
MY CHILD IS
IN PAIN

Several guidelines have been developed to assist health professionals in assessing and managing children and young people's pain, including:

- Royal College of Nursing (2009) *The Recognition and Assessment of Acute Pain in Children*. Available at: www.rcn.org.uk/professional-development/publications/pub-003542 (last accessed 10 May 2017).
- Association of Paediatric Anaesthetists of Great Britain and Ireland (APA) (2012) *Pediatric Anesthesia: Good Practice in Postoperative and Procedural Pain Management*, 2nd edn. Available at: http://online library.wiley.com/doi/10.1111/j.1460-9592.2012.03838.x/epdf (last accessed 10 May 2017).
- Australian and New Zealand College of Anaesthetists and Faculty of Pain Medicine (2015) *Acute Pain Management: Scientific Evidence*, 4th edn. Available at: www.fpm.anzca.edu.au/resources/ books-and-publications/APMSE4_2015_Final.pdf (last accessed 10 May 2017).

───── SAFEGUARDING STOP POINT ─────

The Declaration of Montréal (IASP, 2015) identifies that access to pain management is a fundamental human right. However, the Healthcare Commission (2007) found that some staff are reluctant to manage children's pain adequately, leading to episodes where children were in pain some, most or all of the time. This has led to calls for paediatric services to ensure staff caring for children are adequately trained in the specialist management of children's pain (Kennedy, 2010).

WEBLINK:
DECLARATION
OF MONTRÉAL

DIFFERENT STRATEGIES FOR ASSESSING PAIN IN CHILDREN

Current best practice guidelines indicate that we should:

- Ask the child about their pain using a developmentally appropriate self-report pain tool (if possible)
- Involve the parents/carers
- Take the child's behavioural cues into account

- Note any physiological cues that may indicate that the child is in pain
- Reassess pain following the implementation of pain-relieving interventions
- Document pain assessments

Pain assessment: The basics

The stages of pain management are outlined in Figure 3.1. Pain assessment is the first step in ensuring children's pain is managed effectively. If pain is not assessed, it is difficult to evaluate the effectiveness of any interventions used and decide whether further action is needed.

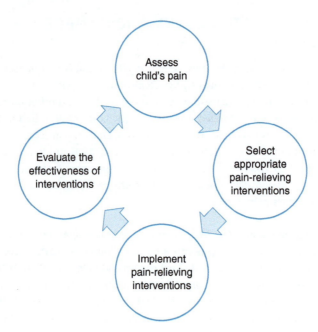

Figure 3.1   The stages of pain management (Twycross and Williams, 2014)

Self-report of pain

Self-report tools should normally be used with children who are:

- Old enough to understand and use a self-report scale (e.g. 3 years of age and older)
- Not overtly distressed
- Not cognitively impaired (Stinson et al., 2006)

With infants, toddlers, pre-verbal, cognitively impaired and sedated children, behavioural pain assessment tools should be used (von Baeyer and Spagrud, 2007). Behavioural pain assessment tools should also be used for older children if they are overtly distressed.

Behavioural indicators of pain

Children can exhibit behavioural cues indicating they are in pain. These differ and so it is important to ascertain what a child's normal behaviour is. Several researchers have provided evidence that children's self-reports of pain do not correlate strongly with their behaviour (Willis et al., 2003;

Table 3.1 Behavioural indicators of pain

Changed behaviour	Increased clinging
Irritability	Unusual quietness
Flat affect	Loss of appetite
Unusual posture	Restlessness
Screaming	Whimpering
Reluctance to move	Sobbing
Aggressiveness	Lying 'scared stiff'
Disturbed sleep pattern	Lethargic

Nilsson et al., 2008). So, if using behavioural cues to assess pain it is important to remember that they only provide an *estimate* of how much pain a child is experiencing.

Physiological indicators of pain

Physiological parameters can be used to assess whether a child is in pain.

WHAT'S THE EVIDENCE?

The evidence about how a child's physiological cues alter when they are in pain is summarised by Sweet and McGrath (1998). The main indicators are:

Table 3.2 Physiological cues

Heart rate	Increases immediately following a pain stimulus and declines as pain diminishes (whereas in infants an initial decrease is followed by a rise in heart rate) (Brummelte et al., 2014)
Respiratory rate and pattern	There is conflicting evidence about whether this increases or decreases, but there is a significant shift from baseline. Breathing may become rapid and/or shallow
Blood pressure	Increases when a child is in acute pain
Oxygen saturation	Decreases when a child is in acute pain

However, when used alone, physiological indicators are not a valid clinical measure of pain as they can be affected by other factors. Given this, a pain assessment strategy that incorporates physiological and behavioural indicators as well as self-report, it is preferred (von Baeyer and Spagrud, 2007).

VIDEO LINK **3.1:** PAIN LECTURE

HOW TO USE VALIDATED PAIN ASSESSMENT TOOLS FOR CHILDREN OF ALL AGES

Within the hospital setting it will probably be necessary to have more than one pain assessment tool on a ward to cater for all patient groups. Whenever possible, pain assessment tools should use a *common metric* – e.g. all rate pain from 0 to 10. This means that a pain score of 5 will mean the same whichever pain assessment tool is used. Information about pain assessment tools that have been developed and validated for use with children of different ages and cognitive abilities are available (Australian and New Zealand College of Anaesthetists and Faculty of Pain Medicine, 2015; Royal College of Nursing, 2009). In this chapter we will discuss the tools used most frequently.

The pain tool for neonates that has been tested most often is the Premature Infant Pain Profile (PIPP) (Stevens et al., 1996) (Table 3.3) and has evidence of reliability, validity and ability to detect change (Stevens et al., 2010). The behavioural tool used most often for pre-verbal children is the FLACC, (Face, Legs, Activity, Cry, Consolability) which has been validated for children from 2 months to 7 years (Merkel et al., 1997). The FLACC has been modified for use with children with cognitive impairment (Figure 3.2) allowing for individualised behaviours to be included. For verbal children, the use of a faces pain scale or a numerical rating scale is recommended depending on their age and developmental level (Table 3.4). Instructions on how to explain a faces pain scale to a child can be seen below in Table 3.5. Regular assessment and documentation of pain allow effective treatment and communication among members of the healthcare team as well as with the patient and family.

WEBLINK:
FLACC

Information about using the FLACC can be found at https://study.sagepub.com/essentialchildnursing

Table 3.3   The Premature Infant Pain Profile (PIPP) (Stevens et al., 1996; Stevens et al., 2014)

Indicators used	Considerations
Postmenstrual age	• Preterm and term infants (e.g. 28-40 weeks gestation)
Behavioural state	• Initially developed for procedural pain, requires further evaluation with very low birth weight neonates and with non-acute and post-surgical pain populations
Heart rate	
Oxygen saturation	• Includes contextual indicators (e.g. postmenstrual age and behavioural state)
Brow bulge	• Indicators are scored on a four-point scale (0, 1, 2, 3) for a total score of 0 to 21 based on the gestational age of the infant
Eye squeeze	
Nasolabial furrow	• A score of 6 or less generally indicates minimal or no pain, while scores greater than 12 indicate moderate to severe pain
	• Pain assessments take one minute
	• In the revised version (PIPP-R) postmenstrual age and behavioural state indicators are only applied if other variables indicate pain

Table 3.4   Pain assessment tools for verbal children

Pain assessment tool	Age range
Faces Pain Scale-Revised (FPS-R)	• Children 5-12 years old
(see Figure 3.3)	• Has been used in children aged 4-18 years (Hicks et al., 2001)
Wong-Baker FACES Pain Scale	• Children aged 3-18 years (Wong and Baker, 1988)
Numerical pain rating (NRS) scale (see Figure 3.4)	• Children aged over 8 years and adolescents for acute pain

WEBLINK:
WONG-BAKER
PAIN SCALE

Table 3.5   Instructions for using faces pain scales (Hockenberry et al., 2005)

Explain to the child that each face is for a person who feels happy because there is no pain (hurt) or sad because there is some or a lot of pain

Face 0 is very happy because there is no hurt at all

Face 1 hurts just a little bit

Face 2 hurts a little more

Face 3 hurts even more

Face 4 hurts a whole lot more

Face 5 hurts as much as you can imagine, although you do not have to be crying to feel this bad

Ask the child to choose the face that best describes how he/she is feeling

Name:	Hosp No:	Great Ormond Street **NHS**
DOB:	NHS no:	Hospital for Children

Categories	Scoring		
	0	**1**	**2**
Face	No particular expression or smile	Occasional grimace or frown, withdrawn, disinterested ***appears sad or worried***	Frequent to constant frown, clenched jaw, quivering chin ***Distressed looking face; expression of fright or panic***
Individual Behaviours			
Legs	Normal position or relaxed; ***usual tone and motion to limbs***	Uneasy, restless, tense; ***occasional tremors***	Kicking, or legs drawn up; ***marked increase in spasticity, constant tremors or jerking***
Individual Behaviours			
Activity	Lying quietly, normal position, moves easily; ***Regular, rhythmic respirations***	Squirming, shifting back and forth, ***tense or guarded movements; mildly agitated (eg. head back and forth, aggression); shallow, splinting respirations, intermittent sighs***	Arched, rigid, or jerking; ***severe agitation, head banging, shivering (not rigors); breath-holding, gasping or sharp intake of breaths; servere splinting***
Individual Behaviours			
Cry	No cry/verbalisation (awake or asleep)	Moans or whimpers, occasional complaint: ***occasional verbal outburst or grunt***	Crying steadily, screams or sobs, frequent complaints; ***repeated outbursts, constant grunting***
Individual Behaviours			
Consolability	Content, relaxed	Reassured by occasional touching, hugging, or being talked to, distractable	Difficult to console or comfort; ***pushing away caregiver, resisting care or comfort measures***
Individual Behaviours			

(Adapted from Malviya et al. 2006)

Revised FLACC-Instructions for Use

- **Individualize the tool:** The nurse should review the descriptors within each category with the child's parents or carers. Ask them if there are additional behaviours that are better indicators of pain in their child. Add these behaviours to the tool in the appropriate category.
- Each of the five categories (F) Face; (L) Legs; (A) Activity; (C) Cry; (C) Consolability is scored from 0-2, which results in a total score between zero and ten.
- **Patients who are awake:** Observe for at least 1–3 minutes. Observe legs and body uncovered. Reposition patient or observe activity, assess body for tenseness and tone. Initiate consoling interventions if needed.
- **Patients who are asleep:** Observe for at least 5 minutes. Observe body and legs uncovered. If possible reposition the patient. Touch the body and assess for tenseness and tone.

Version No: 1.0	Version date: 15/04/2010	Document development lead: Jude Middleton	I:\Pain Control Service\Assessment\Revised FLACC\Revised FLACC Paperwork.doc

Figure 3.2   Revised FLACC Scale, reproduced with permission © The Regents of the University of Michigan

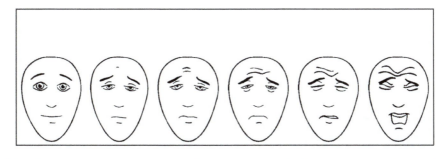

Figure 3.3   Faces Pain Scale – Revised (FPS-R; Hicks et al., 2001), reproduced with permission and available at: www.iasp-pain.org/Education/Content.aspx?ItemNumber=1519

VIDEO LINK 3.2:
MEASURING PAIN

No pain	0	1	2	3	4	5	6	7	8	9	10	Most pain

Figure 3.4   Numerical Rating Scale (NRS)

ACTIVITY 3.1: CRITICAL THINKING

Taking into account the information above, how would you assess pain in children of the following ages:

- Baby aged 6 months
- Child aged 6 years
- Adolescent aged 14 years

ACTIVITY
ANSWER 3.1

ACTIVITY 3.2: REFLECTIVE PRACTICE

- Based on your experiences on clinical placement to date, how well do you think current practices adhere to these guidelines?
- How are you going to change your practice to ensure you are practising evidence-based nursing?

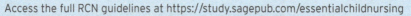

SCENARIO 3.1: JENNY

WEBLINK: RCN
GUIDELINES

Jenny is 9 years old and has been admitted via Accident and Emergency to the ward with a facial laceration. Angela is a newly qualified staff nurse and has been asked to assess Jenny's current level of pain before analgesia is prescribed. Angela accesses the online pain assessment form and finds herself presented with a bewildering array of self-report and behavioural pain assessment tools.

Access the full RCN guidelines at https://study.sagepub.com/essentialchildnursing

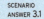

SCENARIO
ANSWER 3.1

ACTIVITY 3.3: REFLECTIVE PRACTICE

- Do you think a child's self-report of pain (using tools as mentioned above) should always be the primary consideration when assessing their pain? What other factors might you consider?
- What factors do you take into account when deciding on appropriate pain-relieving interventions?
- How well do you think pain scores are recorded in practice?

PHARMACOLOGICAL MANAGEMENT OF PAIN: THE PHARMACOLOGY OF CONVENTIONAL ANALGESIC DRUGS

Role of multimodal analgesia

Multimodal analgesia is the combined use of pharmacological techniques to achieve balanced analgesia, whereby side effects are minimised and drug efficacy is increased (Howard, 2003). It is recommended in paediatric postoperative (APA, 2012), emergency (Maurice et al., 2002), procedural (Harvey and Morton, 2007) and oncology (Raphael et al., 2010) settings. By targeting different aspects of the pain pathway, analgesics act together in a complementary manner (Howard, 2008), thus minimising the doses required and the potential side effects associated with each agent (Howard, 2014).

The World Health Organization (WHO, 2012) now advocates a *two-step strategy* for the pharmacological treatment of pain for conditions such as cancer, sickle cell disease, burns and trauma, based on the selection of analgesic drugs in relation to pain severity (WHO, 2012). The *first step* recommends the use of paracetamol and ibuprofen for mild pain; the *second step* includes the addition of low doses of strong opioids for the treatment of moderate pain, which may be increased if pain is severe (WHO, 2012).

Non-steroidal anti-inflammatory drugs

Non-steroidal anti-inflammatory drugs (NSAIDs) act both centrally and peripherally and have analgesic and antipyretic actions (Winstanley and Walley, 2002). NSAIDs work by inhibiting the action of the enzyme cyclooxygenase (COX), active during the inflammatory process, whereby arachidonic acid is the precursor to the inflammatory mediator prostaglandin (Neal, 2016) (Figure 3.5). Cyclooxygenase exists in two forms (COX-1 and COX-2) and the side effects associated with NSAIDs are related to the inhibition of the enzyme COX-1, which is responsible for homeostatic properties, such as gastric mucosa function, platelet activation and renal blood flow (Neal, 2016). The NSAIDs most commonly used in children within the UK are non-selective COX inhibitors (ibuprofen, diclofenac and mefenamic acid (Neubert et al., 2010). Ibuprofen and naproxen are thought to be weakly COX-1-selective (Dale and Haylett, 2009) and of all the non-selective NSAIDs, ibuprofen is associated with fewest side effects (Association of Paediatric Anaesthetists, 2012). Common side effects are outlined in Table 3.6.

Paracetamol

Paracetamol appears to be a selective inhibitor of the enzyme cyclooxygenase-3 (COX-3) and is thought to act centrally. This explains why it has similar properties to NSAIDs (COX-1 and COX-2 inhibitors), but lacks their peripheral anti-inflammatory action (Paul and Whibley, 2011). Paracetamol and NSAIDs used in combination produce better analgesia than either drug alone (APA, 2012). The analgesic efficacy of paracetamol is based on it reaching an optimal plasma concentration in the blood through the process of absorption which may be influenced by the route of administration (Table 3.7).

The clinical status of the child may also have a bearing on the administration of paracetamol (Table 3.8).

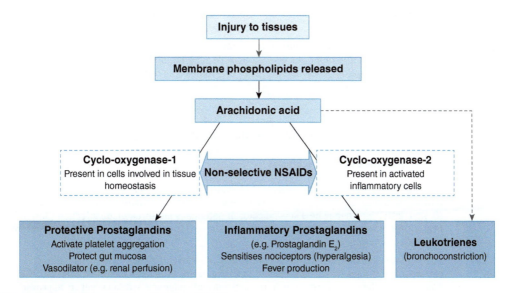

Figure 3.5 Action of non-selective NSAIDs

Adapted from: www.medscape.com

Table 3.6 Common side effects of non-selective NSAIDs (Spina, 2008; Kowalski et al., 2011; APA, 2012)

Side effect	Description and evidence
Gastric irritation	Prostaglandins protect the gut by stimulating mucous secretion and the release of bicarbonate, and by inhibiting parietal cells' gastric acid secretion NSAIDs should be avoided in children or young people with a history of peptic ulcer disease The short-term use of NSAIDs (1-3 days) is associated with low risk of gastric side effects (especially if ibuprofen is used)
Reduces renal blood flow	Prostaglandin acts on the glomerulus and cells in the renal medulla, causing vasodilation and increasing the flow of blood to the kidney Inhibition of prostaglandin by NSAIDs may reduce renal blood flow. This effect may be increased in children who are dehydrated or have renal impairment. NSAIDs should not be administered concurrently with drugs known to be nephrotoxic
Exacerbation of asthma	The inhibition of prostaglandins may increase the conversion of arachidonic acid to leukotrienes, which may potentially induce bronchospasm in asthmatic children The incidence of this is thought to be 1:1000
Disrupts platelet function	NSAIDs reduce the production of thromboxane involved in platelet aggregation (Yassin and Dawson, 2007) and should be avoided in children with coagulation disorders or those receiving anticoagulant agents

Table 3.7 Absorption of paracetamol

Route of paracetamol administration	Comments	Evidence
Oral	Dependent on gastric emptying and the transit of the drug to the duodenum, where it is rapidly absorbed	Children under 3 months may have variable rates of gastric emptying and in neonates this may be slow and erratic (Anderson, 2008). Similarly delayed gastric emptying may affect the absorption of paracetamol in the postoperative child (van der Westhuizen et al., 2011)
Rectal	Uptake may be erratic	Increased initial loading doses are recommended to achieve satisfactory analgesia (Kleiber, 2008)
Intravenous	Offers an alternative for children and young people with reduced enteral absorption (Anderson and Palmer, 2006)	Intravenous administration has been demonstrated to achieve superior analgesia to rectal (Prins et al., 2008) or oral routes (van der Westhuizen et al., 2011)

Table 3.8 Paracetamol use in children with specific clinical conditions

Condition	Evidence for the use of paracetamol
Neutropenia	Although recommended for management of acute cancer pain (Raphael et al., 2010), paracetamol may be contraindicated in the neutropenic patient because of its potential to mask pyrexia (Bryant, 2003) which may be a key indicator of potentially life-threatening infection (Barton et al., 2015). However, paracetamol may be considered if the child is receiving broad-spectrum antibiotics (Johnson, 2013)
Asthma	The proposed link between paracetamol use and later development of asthma is based on retrospective studies where confounding factors may not have been identified (ANZCA, 2015) and a causal effect of paracetamol on the incidence of childhood asthma is yet to be proved (Barr, 2008)

Opioids

Pain sensing first-order neurones (nociceptors) transmit painful stimuli to the dorsal horn of the spinal cord (Colvin and Fallon, 2012). Here a neurotransmitter (glutamate) is released, propagating the noxious signal to a second-order neurone, which transmits sensory information to the thalamus via the spinothalamic tract (Parsons and Preece, 2010). Opioid receptors are found predominantly on presynaptic nociceptors in the dorsal horn (Dale and Haylett, 2009) and respond to endogenous opioid release (Inturrisi, 2002) by supressing the release of neurotransmitter at the presynaptic membrane (Godfrey, 2005) (Figure 3.6). Opioid agents (such as morphine and tramadol) mimic the effect of endogenous opioids (Neal, 2016).

Tramadol

Tramadol is a synthetic opioid which acts as a weak opioid receptor agonist (Ozalevli et al., 2005). It also inhibits the reuptake of norepinephrine and serotonin (Bressolle et al., 2009), giving it anti-neuropathic qualities (Colvin and Fallon, 2012) and enhancing its analgesic action (Dale and Haylett, 2009). It is a medium potency analgesic that demonstrates similar efficacy to NSAIDs and one-tenth the potency of morphine (Bozkurt, 2005). Tramadol's potential side effects are outlined below (Table 3.9).

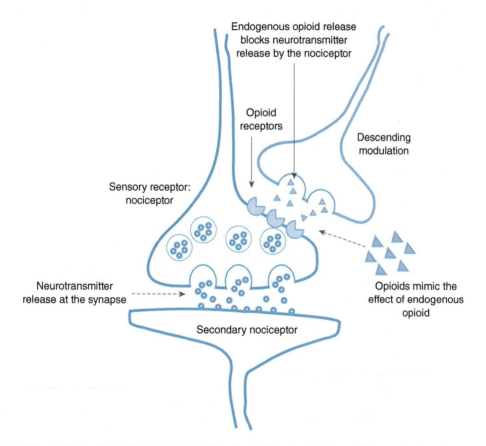

Figure 3.6 Action of opioids at presynaptic sites in the dorsal horn of the spinal cord

(Adapted from: www.biology-pages.info/D/Drugs.html)

The use of tramadol in managing children's pain

Since the withdrawal of codeine from use in children under 12 years of age (Medicines and Healthcare Products Regulatory Agency, 2013) following fatalities after codeine administration post-adenotonsillectomy to children with obstructive sleep apnoea (Kelly et al., 2012), tramadol has been identified as a potentially suitable alternative for children with mild to moderate pain (Marzuillo et al., 2014). Tramadol is cautiously recommended for reducing the postoperative rescue analgesia requirements in preschool children following minor surgery (e.g. tonsillectomy). However, its efficacy in comparison to morphine in this group is still uncertain (Schnabel, 2015). There is a lack of evidence for its use in infants (Anderson and Palmer, 2006). Tramadol causes less respiratory depression than morphine (Ozalevli et al., 2005) and has lower incidence of constipation, nausea and vomiting, and sedation (Bozkurt, 2005).

Morphine

Morphine is the opioid of first choice in children due to its efficacy, familiarity in clinical practice and affordability (Strassels, 2014). Morphine is metabolised to morphine-6-glucuronide (which has analgesic activity) and morphine-3-glucuronide (which does not). Both are excreted via the renal system (Strassels, 2014). The ability of the child to clear morphine is an important factor to consider when administering opioids. Neonates require lower morphine doses compared with older children (Bouwmeester et al., 2003) due to their immature renal function and reduced metabolism (APA, 2012). Children with impaired renal function may accumulate morphine metabolites and may require a reduced dose of opioids (Strassels, 2014). Common side effects and associated nursing care are presented in Table 3.9.

Table 3.9 Common side effects of morphine

Side effect	Comments	Nursing care
Respiratory depression	Key concern in the patient receiving intravenous opioids (Clifford, 2013) Increased risk: <ul><li>In infancy, especially for premature child (due to hepatic immaturity and decreased morphine clearance)</li><li>If obese or underweight</li><li>If there are respiratory comorbidities or the child has obstructive sleep apnoea (Chidambaran et al., 2014)</li></ul>	Close monitoring of: <ul><li>Level of consciousness, (Malviya et al., 2002)</li><li>Physiological signs, including respiratory rate and oxygen saturation (Peters, 2015)</li></ul> Use of multimodal analgesia regime to minimise opioid requirements (Chiaretti et al., 2013) Ready access to (and co-prescription of) opioid-antagonist naloxone, for use in the event of respiratory depression (McQueen et al., 2012)
Nausea and vomiting	Opioids may stimulate the vestibular apparatus or chemoreceptor trigger zone, or inhibit gut motility (Kalso, 2012)	Antiemetic therapy such as a $5\text{-}HT_3$ receptor antagonist (e.g. ondansetron) known to be effective (Gan, 2014)
Pruritus (itching)	Release of histamines from mast cells may occur following the administration of morphine (Dale and Haylett, 2009)	Antihistamines are a common choice for managing morphine-related itching; however, their sedative properties should be considered when they are administered alongside opioids (Strassels, 2014)

SEE ALSO
CHAPTER **4**

ACTIVITY 3.4: REFLECTIVE PRACTICE

Taking into account the information above how would you plan the postoperative pain management for children of the following ages?

ACTIVITY
ANSWER 3.4

- Baby aged 2 weeks
- Child aged 7 years

ACTIVITY 3.5: REFLECTIVE PRACTICE

- Based on your experiences in clinical placement to date, how well do you think current practices adhere to the WHO (2012) two-step strategy?
- How are you going to adapt your practice to ensure you are ensuring evidence-based nursing?

NON-PHARMACOLOGICAL MANAGEMENT OF PAIN

Cognitive strategies

A number of cognitive strategies can be employed to reduce pain during procedures, including methods that alter the child's perception of pain by reducing brain activity in areas associated with pain processing (Cohen et al., 2014). These are summarised in Table 3.10.

Table 3.10 Cognitive strategies for managing procedural pain

VIDEO LINK 3.3:
A PARENT'S
ROLE

Procedure	Comments	Evidence
Distraction	The child's ability to fully focus their attention on the painful experience is decreased by drawing their attention towards a distractor, thus decreasing their anxiety and pain (Koller and Goldman, 2012)	Strategies most frequently employed are: cartoons, non-procedural talk and music-distraction (DeMore and Cohen, 2005)
Hypnosis	Suggestion by the hypnotherapist, which aims to change the child's perceptions, emotions or behavioural response to a subjective experience (Richardson et al., 2006)	Changes in cerebral blood flow are higher during a hypnotic state and it is thought that hypnosis may modulate areas of the brain activated by painful stimuli (Wood and Bioy, 2008)
Guided imagery	Use of relaxation and the child's imagination to distract them from unpleasant sensations (Huth et al., 2004) such as pain and anxiety. The child is 'guided' by the health professional to explore the sights, smells and sounds of the imaginary experience in order to more fully engage them in the distraction (King, 2010)	Reduction in behavioural signs of pain in adolescents using relaxation and guided imagery during venepuncture (Forsner et al., 2014)
Virtual reality (VR)	Involves computer-generated three-dimensional environment which stimulates the auditory and visual senses (Koller and Goldman, 2012)	VR is more beneficial than passive distraction (videogames) in reducing simulated pain (holding hand in cold water). Most beneficial in adolescents aged 11-14 years (Malloy and Milling, 2010)

Behavioural strategies

Behavioural strategies include direct (e.g. swaddling) and indirect (e.g. non-nutritive sucking) strategies to reduce pain during painful procedures in neonates and are described in Table 3.11.

Table 3.11   Behavioural strategies for managing procedural pain in neonates

Strategy	Comments	Evidence
Non-nutritive sucking (NNS)	The use of a dummy to induce sucking as a form of non-pharmacological pain relief (Twycross and Stinson, 2014) Combining NNS and sucrose increases the rate of sucking, thus enhancing analgesia in pre- and term-neonates (Tsao et al., 2008).	Effective in reducing neonatal pain, (but not in preterm infants or older infants) immediately following a painful procedure (Pillai Riddell et al., 2015) Insufficient evidence to support the use in 1-3-year-old children (Meek and Huertas, 2012)
Sucrose (sugar)	Sucrose therapy is the use of sweet tasting substances for managing painful procedures. Sucrose is thought to effect endogenous opioid release through the stimulation of taste buds in the mouth (Harrison et al., 2014)	Sucrose is effective in managing single episodes of procedural pain in neonates; however, the safety and efficacy of repeated doses has not been tested (Stevens et al., 2013)
Swaddling	Swaddling is wrapping the infant in a blanket to contain their arms and legs (Twycross and Stinson, 2014)	There is low-quality evidence supporting the efficacy of swaddling in reducing pain immediately following procedures in preterm infants and neonates (Pillai Riddell et al., 2015)
Facilitated tucking (also called 'containment')	Facilitated tucking involves the infant's head and lower body being gently held in a contained supportive position (with legs flexed) during the painful procedure (Hartley et al., 2015)	There is low-quality evidence supporting the efficacy of facilitated tucking in reducing pain immediately following procedures in preterm infants and neonates (Pillai Riddell et al., 2015)

WEBLINK:
APA
GUIDELINES

PRACTICE
SCENARIO 3:
HUGO

SCENARIO 3.2: KAREN

Karen has brought her 1-year-old child George to the community health centre for his vaccinations. George has been very distressed during previous vaccinations and Karen is anxious to know what can be done to limit any pain and anxiety George may experience.

Access the full APA guidelines at https://study.sagepub.com/essentialchildnursing

Taking into account the information above, how would you plan the procedural pain management for children of the following ages?

- Baby aged 2 weeks
- Child aged 8 years
- Adolescent aged 13 years

SCENARIO
ANSWER 3.2

ACTIVITY 3.6: REFLECTIVE PRACTICE

- Based on your experiences in clinical placement to date, how consistently do you think non-pharmacological management of procedural pain is employed?
- How are you going to adapt your practice to ensure you are utilising evidence-based non-pharmacological strategies?

CHAPTER SUMMARY

- Unrelieved pain has a number of short- and longer-term consequences and so it is important to ensure children's pain is managed effectively.
- There are several validated pain assessment tools for children of all ages. These should be used to assess (and reassess) children's pain.
- There are three types of analgesic drugs used with children. If used together they have a synergistic effect.
- Non-pharmacological strategies can be used to enhance the effectiveness of analgesic drugs when managing children's pain.

BUILD YOUR BIBLIOGRAPHY

Books

- Twycross, A., Dowden, S.J. and Stinson, J. (eds) (2014) *Pain Management in Children: A Clinical Guide for Nurses and Healthcare Professionals*, 2nd edn. Oxford: Wiley-Blackwell.

  Provides an evidence-based, practical guide to care in all areas of children's pain management, and an introduction to the skills and expertise needed to manage children's pain effectively. The book starts by reviewing why it is necessary to manage pain effectively, explores the relevant anatomy and physiology of the nervous system in children, and discusses the pharmacology of analgesic drugs. The book then provides evidence for the physical and psychological methods of pain relief in children as well as a chapter outlining pain assessment tools available for children. Current evidence is summarised in relation to managing acute, chronic and procedural pain and paediatric palliative care.

- McGrath, P.J., Stevens, B., Walker, S. and Zempsky, W. (2014) (eds) *Oxford Textbook of Paediatric Pain*. Oxford: Oxford University Press.

  Brings together an international team of experts to provide an authoritative and comprehensive textbook on all aspects of pain for all ages of children. The book is divided into nine sections. Evidence-based chapters look in depth at topics ranging from the long-term effects of pain in children to complementary therapy in paediatric pain. Case examples and online materials including scales, worksheets and videos are provided to aid learning and illustrate the application of knowledge.

- McClain, B.C. and Suresh, S. (eds) (2011) *Handbook of Pediatric Chronic Pain: Current Science and Integrative Practice*. New York: Springer.

  This book presents the current knowledge base and recent advances in the management of chronic pain in neonates, children and adolescents. Chapters include the epidemiology of chronic pain and the book focuses on common peadiatric presentations including musculoskeletal and abdominal pain syndromes, sickle cell disease cancer and headaches. It also considers the role of the nurse as part of a multidisciplinary approach to the management of chronic pain.

Journal articles

Go to https://study.sagepub.com/essentialchildnursing for further free online journal articles related to this chapter.

- Idvall, E., Holm, C. and Runeson, I. (2005) 'Pain experiences and non-pharmacological strategies for pain management after tonsillectomy: a qualitative interview study of children and parents'. *Journal of Child Health Care*, 9: 196–207.

HELPFUL FOR ASSIGNMENTS!

FURTHER READING: ONLINE JOURNAL ARTICLES

(Continued)

(Continued)

This study explored children's experience of pain and the non-pharmacological strategies used to manage pain after tonsillectomy.

- Twycross, A., Williams, A., Bolland, R. and Sunderland, R. (2015) 'Parents' attitudes towards children's pain and analgesic drugs'. *Journal of Child Health Care*, 19: 402–11.

  This paper describes a study undertaken in one hospital in South West London exploring parents' (n=108) attitudes towards children's pain and the use of analgesic drugs.

- Twycross, A., Parker, R., Williams, A. and Gibson, F. (2015) 'Cancer-related pain and pain management: sources, prevalence and the experiences of children and parents'. *Journal of Paediatric Oncology Nursing*, 32: 369–84.

  This paper presents the results of a rapid review of the literature exploring children's cancer-related pain. Despite advances in pain management techniques, children with cancer regularly describe pain as the most prevalent symptom throughout the cancer trajectory.

Weblinks

FURTHER READING: WEBLINKS

Go to https://study.sagepub.com/essentialchildnursing for further weblinks related to this chapter.

- WellChild et al., *My Child Is in Pain*

  www.mychildisinpain.org.uk

  This website has been developed by researchers working with parents of children who have had day case surgery and with healthcare professionals who are experts in pain management. The information is especially useful for parents whose children are aged 2–6 years old.

- Australian Government, Department of Health, *FLACC Pain Scale*

  www.health.gov.au/internet/publications/publishing.nsf/Content/triageqrg~triageqrg-pain~triageqrg-FLACC

- RCN Guidelines on Acute Pain in Children

  The full RCN guideline at: www.rcn.org.uk/professional-development/publications/pub-003542

ONLINE QUIZZES & ACTIVITY ANSWERS

ACE YOUR ASSESSMENT

Revise what you have learned by visiting https://study.sagepub.com/essentialchildnursing

- Test yourself with multiple-choice and short-answer questions
- Do the chapter activities in the book and check your answers online

REFERENCES

Anderson, B.J. (2008) Review article: 'Paracetamol (Acetaminophen): mechanisms of action'. *Pediatric Anesthesia*, 18: 915–21.

Anderson, B.J. and Palmer G.M. (2006) 'Recent developments in the pharmacological management of pain in children'. *Current Opinion in Anaesthesiology*, 19: 285–92.

Association of Paediatric Anaesthetists (APA) (2012) 'Good practice in postoperative and procedural pain management, 2nd edition'. *Pediatric Anesthesia*, 22: 1–79.

Australian and New Zealand College of Anaesthetists and Faculty of Pain Medicine (ANZCA) (2015) *Acute Pain Management: Scientific Evidence*, 4th edn. Melbourne: Australian and New Zealand College of Anaesthetists.

Barr, R.G. (2008) 'Does paracetamol cause asthma in children? Time to remove the guesswork'. *The Lancet*, 372: 1011–12.

Barton, C.D., Waugh, L.K., Nielsen, M.J. and Paulus, S. (2015) 'Febrile neutropenia in children treated for malignancy'. *Journal of Infection*, 71: S27–S35.

Bouwmeester, N.J., van den Anker, J.N., Hop, W.C.J., Anand, K.J.S. and Tibboel, D. (2003) 'Age- and therapy-related effects on morphine requirements and plasma concentrations of morphine and its metabolites in postoperative infants'. *British Journal of Anaesthesia*, 90: 642–52.

Bozkurt, P. (2005) Review article: 'Use of tramadol in children'. *Pediatric Anesthesia*, 15: 1041–47.

Bressolle, F., Rochette, A., Khier, S., Dadure, C., Ouaki, J. and Capdevila, X. (2009) 'Population pharmacokinetics of the two enantiomers of tramadol and O-demethyl tramadol after surgery in children'. *British Journal of Anaesthesia*, 102: 390–99.

Brummelte, S., Oberlander, T.F. and Craig, K.D. (2014) 'Biomarkers of pain: physiological indices of pain reactivity in infants and children', in P.J. McGrath, B. Stevens, S.M. Walker and W.T. Zempsky (eds), *Oxford Textbook of Paediatric Pain*. Oxford: Oxford University Press.

Bryant, R. (2003) 'Managing side effects of childhood cancer treatment'. *Journal of Pediatric Nursing*, 18: 113–25.

Chiaretti, A., Pierri, F., Valentini, P., Russo, I., Gargiullo, L. and Riccardi, R. (2013) 'Current practice and recent advances in pediatric pain management'. *European Review for Medical and Pharmacological Sciences*, 17: 112–16.

Chidambaran, V., Olbrecht, V., Hossain, M., Sadhasivam, S., Rose, J. and Meyer, M.J. (2014) 'Risk predictors of opioid-induced critical respiratory events in children: naloxone use as a quality measure of opioid safety'. *Pain Medicine*, 15: 2139–49.

Clifford, T. (2013) 'Patient controlled analgesia – safe practices'. *Journal of PeriAnesthesia Nursing*, 28: 113–14.

Cohen, L.L., Cousins, L.A. and Martin, S.R. (2014) 'Procedural pain distraction', in P.J. McGrath, B. Stevens, S.M. Walker and W.T. Zempsky (eds), *Oxford Textbook of Paediatric Pain*. Oxford: Oxford University Press.

Colvin, L.A. and Fallon, M. (2012) *ABC of Pain*. Oxford: British Medical Journal Books.

Dale, M.M. and Haylett, D.G. (2009) *Pharmacology Condensed*. Edinburgh: Churchill Livingstone.

DeMore, M. and Cohen, L.L. (2005) 'Distraction for pediatric immunization pain: a critical review'. *Journal of Clinical Psychology in Medical Settings*, 12: 281–91.

Forsner, M., Norström, F., Nordyke, K., Ivarsson, A. and Lindh, V. (2014) Relaxation and guided imagery used with 12-year-olds during venipuncture in a school-based screening study'. *Journal of Child Health Care*, 18: 241–52.

Gan, T.J. (2014) 'Consensus guidelines for the management of postoperative nausea and vomiting'. *Society for Ambulatory Anesthesiology*, 118: 85–113.

Godfrey, H. (2005) 'Understanding pain, part 1: physiology of pain'. *British Journal of Nursing*, 14 (16): 846–52.

Harrison, D., Anseloni, V.C.Z., Yamada, J. and Bueno, M. (2014) 'Sucrose and sweet taste', in P.J. McGrath, B. Stevens, S.M. Walker and W.T. Zempsky (eds), *Oxford Textbook of Paediatric Pain*. Oxford: Oxford University Press.

Hartley, K.A., Miller, C.S. and Gephart, S.M. (2015) 'Facilitated Tucking to reduce pain in neonates: evidence for best practice'. *Advances in Neonatal Care*, 15(3): 201–8.

Harvey, A.J. and Morton, N.S. (2007) 'Management of procedural pain in children'. *Archives of Disease in Childhood Education and Practice Education*, 92: ep20–ep26.

Healthcare Comission (2007) *Improving Services for Children in Hospital*. London: Commission for Healthcare Audit and Inspection.

Hicks, C.L., von Baeyer, C.L., Spafford, P.A., van Korlaar, I. and Goodenough, B. (2001) 'The faces pain scale – revised: toward a common metric in pediatric pain measurement'. *Pain*, 93: 173–83.

Hockenberry, M.J., Wilson, D. and Winkelstein, M.L. (2005) *Wong's Essentials of Pediatric Nursing*, 7th edn. St Louis, MO: Mosby.

Howard, R.F. (2003) 'Current status of pain management in children'. *JAMA*, 290: 2464–9.

Howard, R.F. (2008) 'Acute pain management in children', in P. Macintyre, S.M. Walker and D.J. Rowbotham (eds), *Clinical Pain Management: Acute Pain*, 2nd edn. London: Hodder-Arnold.

Howard, R.F. (2014) 'Postoperative pain management', in P.J. McGrath, B. Stevens, S.M. Walker and W.T. Zempsky (eds), *Oxford Textbook of Paediatric Pain*. Oxford: Oxford University Press.

Huth, M.M., Broome, M.E. and Good, M. (2004) 'Imagery reduces children's post-operative pain'. *Pain*, 110: 439–48.

International Association for the Study of Pain (2015) *Declaration of Montréal – Declaration that Access to Pain Management Is a Fundamental Human Right*. Available at: www.iasp-pain.org/Declarationof Montreal?navItemNumber=582 (accessed 16 June 2017).

Inturrisi, C.E. (2002) 'Clinical pharmacology of opioids for pain'. *Clinical Journal of Pain*, 18: S3–13.

Johnson, P. (2013) 'Fever and neutropenia in the pediatric oncology patient'. *Journal of Pediatric Health Care*, 27: 66–70.

Kalso, E. (2012) 'Opioids in chronic non-malignant pain', in L.A. Colvin and M. Fallon M (eds), *ABC of Pain*. Oxford: British Medical Journal Books.

Kelly, L.E., Rieder, M., van den Anker, J., Malkin, B., Ross, C., Neely, M.N., Carleton, B., Hayden, M.R., Madadi, P. and Koren, G. (2012) 'More codeine fatalities after tonsillectomy in North American children'. *Pediatrics*, 129: e1343–47.

Kennedy, I. (2010) Getting It Right for Children and Young People: Overcoming Cultural Barriers in the NHS so as to Meet Their Needs. A review by Professor Sir Ian Kennedy. London: Department of Health.

King K, (2010) 'A review of the effects of guided imagery on cancer patients with pain'. *Complementary Health Practice Review*,15(2): 98–107.

Kleiber, C. (2008) 'Acetaminophen dosing for neonates, infants, and children'. *Journal of the Specialists in Pediatric Nursing*, 13: 48–9.

Koller, D. and Goldman, R.D. (2012) 'Distraction techniques for children undergoing procedures: a critical review of pediatric research. *Journal of Pediatric Nursing*, 27: 652–81.

Kowalski, M.L., Makowska, J.S., Blanca, M., Bavbek, S., Bochenek, G., Bousquet, J., Bousquet, P., Celik, G., Demoly, P., Gomes, E.R., Nizankowska-Mogilnicka, E., Romano, A., Sanchez-Borges, M., Sanz, M., Torres, M.J., De Weck, A., Szczeklik, A. and Brockow, K. (2011) 'Hypersensitivity to nonsteroidal anti-inflammatory drugs (NSAIDs) – classification, diagnosis and management: review of the EAACI/ENDA and GA2LEN/HANNA'. *Allergy*, 66: 818–29.

Kristensen, A.D., Ahlburg, P., Lauridsen, M.C., Jensen, T.S. and Nikolajsen, L. (2012) 'Chronic pain after inguinal hernia repair in children'. *British Journal of Anaesthesia*, 109: 603–8.

Lauridsen, M.H., Kristensen, A.D., Hjortdal, V.E., Jensen, T.S. and Nikolajsen, L. (2014) 'Chronic pain in children after cardiac surgery via sternotomy'. *Cardiology in the Young*, 24: 893–9.

Malloy, K.M. and Milling, L.S. (2010) 'The effectiveness of virtual reality distraction for pain reduction: a systematic review'. *Clinical Psychology Review*, 30: 1011–18.

Malviya, S., Voepel-Lewis, T., Tait, A.R., Merkel, S., Tremper, K. and Naughton, N. (2002) 'Depth of sedation in children undergoing computed tomography: validity and reliability of the University of Michigan Sedation Scale (UMSS)'. *British Journal of Anaesthesia*, 88: 241–5.

Marzuillo, P., Calligaris, L. and Barbi, E. (2014) 'Tramadol can selectively manage moderate pain in children following European advice limiting codeine use'. *Acta Pædiatrica*, 103: 1110–16.

Maurice, S.C., O'Donnell, J.J. and Beattie, T.F. (2002) 'Emergency analgesia in the paediatric population: Part II Pharmacological methods of pain relief'. *Emergency Medicine Journal*, 19: 101–5.

McQueen, S., Bruce, E.A. and Gibson, F. (2012) *The Great Ormond Street Hospital Manual of Children's Practices*. Chichester, West Sussex: Wiley-Blackwell.

Medicines and Healthcare Products Regulatory Agency (2013) MHRA confirms codeine not to be used in children under 12 years old. Available at: http://webarchive.nationalarchives.gov. uk/20141205150130/www.mhra.gov.uk/home/groups/comms-po/documents/news/con287049. pdf (last accessed 10 May 2017).

Meek, J. and Huertas, A. (2012) 'Cochrane review: non-nutritive sucking, kangaroo care and swaddling/facilitated tucking are observed to reduce procedural pain in infants and young children'. *Evidence-Based Nursing*, 15: 84–85.

Merkel, S.I., Shayevitz, J.R., Voepel-Lewis, T. and Malviya, S. (1997) 'The FLACC: a behavioral scale for scoring postoperative pain in young children'. *Pediatric Nursing*, 23: 293–7.

Middleton, C. (2003) 'Understanding the physiological effects of unrelieved pain'. *Nursing Times*, 99 (37): 28–31.

Neal, M.J. (2016) *Medical Pharmacology at a Glance*, 8th edn. Sussex: John Wiley & Sons

Neubert, A., Verhamme, K., Murray, M.L., Picelli, G., Hsiaa, Y., Sen, F.E., Giaquinto, C., Ceci, A., Sturkenboomb, M., Wonga, I.C.K. and on behalf of the TEDDY Network of Excellence (2010) 'The prescribing of analgesics and non-steroidal anti-inflammatory drugs in paediatric primary care in the UK, Italy and the Netherlands'. *Pharmacological Research*, 62: 243–8.

Nilsson, S., Finnstrom, B. and Kokinsky, E. (2008) 'The FLACC behavioral scale for procedural pain assessment in children aged 5–16 years'. *Pediatric Anesthesia*, 18: 767–74.

Ozalevli, M., Unlugenc, H., Tuncer, U., Gunes, Y. and Ozcengiz, D. (2005) 'Comparison of morphine and tramadol by patient-controlled analgesia for postoperative analgesia after tonsillectomy in children'. *Pediatric Anesthesia*, 15: 979–84.

Parsons, G. and Preece, W.P. (2010) *Principles and Practice of Managing Pain: A Guide for Nurses and Allied Health Professionals*. Maidenhead, Berkshire: Open University Press/McGraw Hill.

Paul, S. and Whibley, J. (2011) 'Paracetamol use in children: is it as safe as we think?' *Prescriber*, 19: 16–20.

Peters, J. (2015) *Analgesia: Patient Controlled and Nurse Controlled*. Available at: www.gosh.nhs. uk/health-professionals/clinical-guidelines/analgesia-patient-controlled-and-nurse-controlled (accessed 13 September 2017).

Pillai Riddell, R.R., Racine, N.M., Gennis, H.G., Turcotte, K., Uman, L.S., Horton, R.E., Ahola Kohut, S., Hillgrove Stuart, J., Stevens, B. and Lisi, D.M. (2015) 'Non-pharmacological management of infant and young child procedural pain'. *Cochrane Database of Systematic Reviews*, 12. Art. No.: CD006275. DOI: 10.1002/14651858.CD006275. pub 3.

Polkki T, Pietila A.-M. and Vehvilainen, K. (2003) 'Hospitalized children's descriptions of their experiences with postsurgical pain relieving methods'. *International Journal of Nursing Studies*, 40: 33–44.

Prins, S.A., Van Dijk, M., Van Leeuwen, P., Searle, S., Anderson, B.J., Tibboel, D. and Mathot, R. (2008) 'Pharmacokinetics and analgesic effects of intravenous propacetamol vs rectal paracetamol in children after major craniofacial surgery'. *Pediatric Anesthesia*, 18: 582–92.

Raphael, J., Ahmedzai, S., Hester, J., Urch, C., Barrie, J., Williams, J., Farqhuar-Smith, P., Fallon, M., Hoskin, P., Robb, K., Bennett, M.I., Haines, R., Johnson, M., Bhaskar, A., Chong, S., Duarte, R. and Sparkes, E. (2010) 'Cancer pain: part 1: pathophysiology; oncological, pharmacological, and psychological treatments: a perspective from the British Pain Society endorsed by the UK Association of Palliative Medicine and the Royal College of General Practitioners'. *Pain Medicine*, 11: 742–64.

Richardson, J., Smith, J.E., McCall, G. and Pilkington, K. (2006) 'Hypnosis for procedure-related pain and distress in pediatric cancer patients: a systematic review of effectiveness and methodology related to hypnosis interventions'. *Journal of Pain and Symptom Management*, 31: 70–84.

Royal College of Nursing (2009) The Recognition and Assessment of Acute Pain in Children – Recommendations: Revised. London: RCN Publishing.

Schnabel, A., Reichl, S.U., Meyer-Frießem, C., Zahn, P.K., Pogatzki-Zahn, E. (2015) 'Tramadol for postoperative pain treatment in children'. *Cochrane Database of Systematic Reviews*, Issue 3. Art. No.: CD009574. DOI: 10.1002/14651858.CD009574.pub2.

Spina, D. (2008) *Flesh and Bones of Medical Pharmacology*. Philadelphia, PA: Mosby.

Stevens, B., Johnston, C., Petryshen, P. and Taddio, A. (1996) 'Premature infant pain profile: development and initial validation'. *Clinical Journal of Pain*, 12: 13–22.

Stevens, B., Johnston, C., Taddio, A., Gibbins, S. and Yamada, J. (2010) 'The premature infant pain profile: evaluation 13 years after development'. *Clinical Journal of Pain*, 26: 813–30.

Stevens, B., Yamada, J., Lee, G.Y. and Ohlsson, A. (2013) 'Sucrose for analgesia in newborn infants undergoing painful procedures'. *Cochrane Database of Systematic Reviews*, 1. Art. No.: CD001069. DOI: 10.1002/14651858.CD001069.pub4.

Stevens, B.J., Gibbins, S., Yamada, J., Dionne, R., Lee, G., Johnston, C. and Taddio, A. (2014) 'The Premature Infant Pain Profile-Revised (PIPP-R): initial validation and feasibility'. *Clinical Journal of Pain*, 30: 238–243.

Stinson, J., Yamada, J., Kavanagh, T., Gill, N. and Stevens, B. (2006) 'Systematic review of the psychometric properties and feasibility of self-report pain measures for use in clinical trials in children and adolescents'. *Pain*, 125: 143–57.

Strassels, S.A. (2014) 'Opioids in clinical practice', in P.J. McGrath, B. Stevens, S.M. Walker and W.T. Zempsky (eds), *Oxford Textbook of Paediatric Pain*. Oxford: Oxford University Press.

Sweet, S.D. and McGrath, P.J. (1998) 'Physiological measures of pain', in G.A. Finley and P.J. McGrath (eds), *Measurement of Pain in Infants and Children, Progress in Pain Research Management, Vol. 10*. Seattle: IASP Press, pp. 59–81.

Tsao, J.C.I., Evans, S., Meldrum, M., Altman, T. and Zeltzer, L.K. (2008) 'A review of CAM for procedural pain in infancy: part I: sucrose and non-nutritive sucking'. *Evidence Based Complementary and Alternative Medicine*, 5: 371–81.

Twycross, A. and Stinson, J. (2014) 'Physical and psychological methods of pain-relief', in A. Twycross, S.J. Dowden and J. Stinson (eds) *Pain Management in Children: A Clinical Guide for Nurses and Healthcare Professionals*, 2nd edn. Oxford: Wiley-Blackwell.

Twycross, A. and Williams, A. (2014) 'Why managing pain in children matters', in A. Twycross, S.J. Dowden and J. Stinson (eds) *Pain Management in Children: A Clinical Guide for Nurses and Healthcare Professionals*, 2nd edn. Oxford: Wiley-Blackwell.

van der Westhuizen, F.Y., Kuo, P.W. and Holder, K. (2011) 'Randomised controlled trial comparing oral and intravenous paracetamol (acetaminophen) plasma levels when given as preoperative analgesia'. *Anaesthetic Intensive Care*, 39: 242–6.

von Baeyer, C.L. and Spagrud, L.J. (2007) 'Systematic review of observational (behavioral) measures of pain for children and adolescents aged 3 to18 years'. *Pain*, 127: 140–50.

Willis, M.H., Merkel, S.I., Voepel-Lewis, T. and Malviya, S. (2003) 'FLACC Behavioral Pain Assessment Scale: a comparison with the child's self-report'. *Pediatric Nursing*, 29: 195–8.

Winstanley, P. and Walley, T. (2002) *Medical Pharmacology: A Clinical Core Text for Integrated Curricula with Self-assessment*, 2nd edn. Edinburgh: Elsevier Science.

Wong, D. and Baker, C. (1988) 'Pain in children: a comparison of assessment scales'. *Pediatric Nursing*, 14: 9–17.

Wood, C. and Bioy, A. (2008) 'Hypnosis and pain in children'. *Journal of Pain and Symptom Management*, 35: 437–46.

World Health Organization (2012a) Persisting Pain in Children Package: WHO Guidelines on the Pharmacological Treatment of Persisting Pain in Children with Medical Illnesses. Geneva: World Health Organization.

Yassin, G. and Dawson, J.S. (2007) *Crash Course Pharmacology*, 3rd edn. Philadelphia, PA: Mosby.

MEDICATION: MANAGEMENT, ADMINISTRATION AND COMPLIANCE

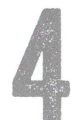

MARY BRADY AND LINDA MOORE

THIS CHAPTER COVERS

- Issues involved in administration of medication to children
- Legislation underpinning medication administration
- Errors and adverse reactions in medication administration
- Parental role in medication administration
- Drug calculation

> " Giving medicines is a large part of a nurse's role, and can seem really daunting at first. As long as you take each step at a time, follow The six R's and adhere to NMC rules, you will soon grow in confidence. There are always lots of resources available, such as the BNFc, local guidelines and your mentor, if you get stuck. Even qualified staff need to use these.
>
> **Carol, children's nurse** "

Visit https://study.sagepub.com/essentialchildnursing to access a wealth of online resources for this chapter – watch out for the margin icons throughout the chapter.

INTRODUCTION

As indicated in the quote above, drug administration is a fundamental part of the role of the children's nurse and this chapter will help to guide you towards achieving the knowledge and skills to competently address this aspect of practice within the remits of the NMC (2015) Code *Professional Standards of Practice and Behaviour for Nurses and Midwives*. As a nursing student you will be observing your mentors and other staff administer medication and also participating in drug calculations and some medication administration according to your capabilities. It is not until you are a registered nurse that you may administer medication with another children's nurse. However, to administer intravenous medication further training is required once a period of preceptorship has been undertaken.

This chapter will guide you, as a nursing student, towards the safe administration of all medication to children and young people. Current issues will be explored, so that you will have a useful overview of the knowledge required to be a safe practitioner. Current legislation will underpin the guidance regarding the ordering, storage and administration of drugs, which will be illustrated with practical examples (both here and https://study.sagepub.com/essentialchildnursing) to reinforce learning.

PRACTICE
SCENARIO **4:**
FAISAL

ACTIVITY 4.1: CRITICAL THINKING

Consider your own anxieties about drug administration to children.

ISSUES INVOLVED IN THE ADMINISTRATION OF MEDICATION TO CHILDREN

The use of 'unlicensed' and 'off label' prescribing and administration

It is not uncommon in children's nursing for 'unlicensed' or 'off label' drugs to be given to children and young people requiring specialised treatment, so it is important that the prescriber can justify the drug use and the nurse understands the rationale. Prior to this the senior Trust pharmacist would have expressed his/her approval. The use of unlicensed drugs can sometimes evoke ethical dilemmas and could potentially be dissonant to NMC guidance (NMC, 2015). Moreover, the nurse has a duty to advocate for the patient and escalate any concerns to senior staff as detailed in the Trust's 'Raising concerns' policy.

WEBLINK:
NICE

The National Institute for Health and Care Excellence (NICE) aims to provide national guidance and advice based on robust evidence. Evidence summaries (ESUOMs) are developed to guide practitioners in their decision-making regarding the use of unlicensed and 'off label' medication. These medications are only used when there is no other licensed medication available and a significant number of people require treatment. However, it is worth noting that even though an ESUOM has been developed, NICE guidance may not yet have been developed, since NICE reviews all the evidence and practical implications prior to implementing guidance.

Compliance versus concordance in medication management

The words 'compliance' and 'concordance' are sometimes used interchangeably in medication management, but each has a distinct meaning and their use will depend on the overall attitudes of the child and their family towards health and the perceived severity of the illness (Blair, 2011; Ogden, 2015).

Compliance tends to infer obedience to instructions, whereas concordance shows an appreciation that people make their own decisions about taking medicines and have the right to decline them once informed of the benefits and risks. Thus, concordance with medication is a more fitting aim for partnership working with children and their families, since as children's nurses we aim to develop a therapeutic relationship with the unique child and their family, providing care that is suitable for the individual. Working in partnership with the child and their family is an underpinning philosophy of children's nursing, where good communication and an appreciation of the diversity of family life is fundamental (Smith and Coleman, 2010).

The nurse as advocate can be instrumental in providing up-to-date relevant information to empower the child and family to make decisions. His/her approach can influence child and parental concordance with medication, so it is important that the nurse has the knowledge and skills not just to administer the medication correctly, but also to teach the parents/carers.

It is worth remembering that even when not formally teaching, the nurse is role modelling good practice that will be copied by others.

SCENARIO 4.1: JOANNA

Joanna is 16 years old and has cystic fibrosis. Recently she has had an increasing number of hospital admissions for two weeks of intravenous antibiotics and intensive physiotherapy. Over the past six months she has been prescribed high-calorie supplemental drinks between meals. Prior to this she was rarely in hospital and had managed to keep a stable weight gain appropriate to her height on the 25th centile. You have built up a good rapport with her and she reveals that this is all a waste of time; she would prefer to die than continue with a lifetime of taking drugs. She craves to be normal like her friends.

- Why is she saying this?
- What can the children's nurse do to help her manage her life and treatment schedule?

SCENARIO ANSWER 4.1

In adolescence, the experience of illness and especially chronic life-limiting conditions may have a negative effect on development and can also interfere with the young person's need for autonomy and a positive self-image within their peer group. Risk-taking behaviour is another aspect of this stage in development where boundaries are tested as the young person moves towards making more autonomous decisions regarding the management of their condition. Young people are often capable of making complex decisions but under stress their level of maturity may reduce to that of a younger child (Blair, 2011). This has increased relevance when the condition is chronic (such as with diabetes, sickle cell anaemia and cystic fibrosis) and the young person wants to be able to enjoy similar spontaneity as their peer group.

ACTIVITY 4.2: CRITICAL THINKING

For many teenagers acne is part of their adolescent years, compounding their desire to conform to a body image that appeals to their peer group. Various medical treatments exist that can reduce the severity of the problem. However, they often require medication to be given over a long period and at regular intervals.

- Why is body image of importance to this age group?
- What medication could be given?
- What are the side effects of such medication?
- How could the practice nurse or school nurse or children's nurse support the young person to be concordant with their medication?
- What other advice could be given?

ACTIVITY ANSWER 4.2

Covert administration of medication

There may be times when, for a variety of reasons, a child refuses to take medication. This situation must be discussed with the child to explore their reasons. If the healthcare professionals feel that the medication is in the best interests of the child, administration may then be disguised. This could mean that the medication is put into food to ensure the child takes it. This is not a decision made by one person but by all the healthcare professionals involved with the child and as appropriate the parents.

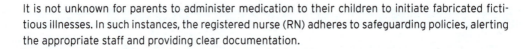

SAFEGUARDING STOP POINT

It is not unknown for parents to administer medication to their children to initiate fabricated fictitious illnesses. In such instances, the registered nurse (RN) adheres to safeguarding policies, alerting the appropriate staff and providing clear documentation.

FIND OUT
MORE!

WEBLINK:
MHRA

LEGISLATION UNDERPINNING MEDICATION ADMINISTRATION

The safe administration of medication is governed by specific legislation and the professional expectations of the Nursing and Midwifery Council (NMC) (2015).

The Medicines Act 1968 established a Medicines Commission to ensure the implementation of the Act and to advise government ministers. It also set out the regulatory controls for the manufacture and distribution of all medication. The Act was further amended in 2005 by the Medicines and Health Regulatory Agency (MHRA) and serves to advise government ministers and local authorities about medicines and to also investigate and collect information should adverse reactions occur.

Drugs are categorised under three headings:

- Those that do not require a prescription and can be sold in, for example, supermarkets under a General sales list (GSL)
- Those that can only be sold under the supervision of a pharmacist but do not require a prescription (P)
- Those that are prescription only medicines (POMs)

In the hospital environment, it is usual that two RNs check all drugs prior to administering to the child (please refer to your local policy). You will notice that medication is not left unattended; instead it is given directly to the child, thereby preventing the drug from not being administered or being taken by another child. Often parents may be present and may want to assist. It is important that they understand how to administer the drug appropriately and are aware of any potential hazards if medication is left unattended or there is a delay in administration. Any equipment used such as oral syringes, medication spoons or pots must be disposed of safely as per Trust policy.

Occasionally medication is given via injection using needles and syringes that must be disposed of promptly and safely after use in appropriate sharps receptacles as per Trust policy (RCN, 2013).

General storage of medication

In compliance with the Medicines Act 1968, all medicines are stored in locked cupboards within a hospital ward. Some medication, such as antibiotics and insulin, are sensitive to ambient temperature, so oral antibiotics are often supplied to wards in powder form to be dissolved in water for administration later. The pharmacist, or on occasions ward nurses, will dissolve the powder in the appropriate amount of sterile water. The solution then needs to be stored in a fridge. Where oral antibiotics are prescribed for use within the home, advice needs to be given to the family regarding safe storage and ensuring that the medicine is out of the reach of children and away from foods where there may be a cross-contamination risk.

Safe storage of other medication within a child's home is also important and the nurse may have to provide guidance for the family regarding safe storage that is practical and manageable within their home. Not all medicines are supplied in childproof containers, for instance those supplied in blister packs; so families need to store medication in cupboards (ideally lockable) that are out of reach of young children and at temperatures that comply with medication guidance. Prior to discharge from hospital, it is also important to watch medication being administered by the carer/parent, since sometimes incorrect techniques may be being used (for example, inhaler technique) which will render the medication less effective.

Frequently children require medication whilst at school, so the school needs to ensure that the medication is stored safely and appropriately, but accessible at all times (for example, bronchodilators for an asthmatic child). On some occasions the child may need to carry their medication with them, so the parents should liaise closely with the school to facilitate this whilst also being aware of any potential hazards to other pupils. The school nurse may be able to assist in the decision-making process.

SCENARIO 4.2: PHOEBE

You are on placement with a health visitor and have accompanied her on a new birth visit. Mandy gave birth to Joshua 12 days ago and already has a 3-year-old daughter called Phoebe. Phoebe has an ear infection and has been prescribed amoxicillin. Whilst in the house you notice that Mandy has left a packet of paracetamol and a bottle of amoxicillin on the work surface in the kitchen.

- Why might this have happened?
- What should you as a children's nurse do?
- What advice should be given to Mandy?

SCENARIO
ANSWER 4.2

Controlled drugs

The Misuse of Drugs Act 1971 controls the import, production, supply and possession of drugs. Controlled drugs are regulated under this Act since they have the potential to be harmful. These drugs have been further subdivided into three classes:

- Class A: diamorphine, cocaine, methadone
- Class B: codeine, amphetamines
- Class C: diazepam, anabolic steroids

Depending on their practice area, children's nurses can be involved in administering controlled drugs such as diamorphine, codeine, methadone and diazepam.

Nurses who are in charge of wards or areas where controlled drugs are administered to children and young people are responsible for the storage, ordering and administration of such drugs. Due to their potential for addiction, the storage of controlled drugs (CDs) is governed by various legislation; specifically the Misuse of Drugs (Safe custody) Regulations (1971, 2001 and 2007).

In hospital, the nurse in charge of the ward has responsibility for the possession, safe custody and issue of CDs. At times this might be delegated to another RN, but the nurse in charge remains responsible.

Storage of controlled drugs

CDs must be stored within a locked cabinet that is ideally made of steel fixed to a wall or the floor within another cupboard that is also lockable. The wall should be of 'suitable thickness'. The amount of CDs stored within an area or ward must be kept to a minimum, whilst also being appropriate for the potential needs of the children/young people being cared for in that area/ward.

The stock levels of CDs are checked daily by two registered nurses (RNs) on most wards and prior to the preparation for administration to a child or young person. The RNs who check the drugs must document that the amount present is in accordance with the ward controlled drug record book. When stock levels are low a requisition is completed from an ordering book with triplicate pages and sent to pharmacy. When new CDs are issued they must be carried to the area in a lockable container and immediately checked into the CD cupboard by two RNs and the CD record book updated.

SCENARIO 4.3: EMMANUEL

Your patient, Emmanuel, has been receiving a continuous infusion of morphine via an infusion pump as Patient Controlled Analgesia. The syringe is nearly empty so you have asked your mentor for a new syringe. Together with another RN your mentor prepares to draw up another syringe. On checking the CD register, there appears to be fewer morphine ampoules actually present than on the register.

- What should happen next?
- What may have happened?

SCENARIO
ANSWER 4.3

Administration of controlled drugs to a child/young person

When a child requires a controlled drug (CD), two RNs check that the prescription is appropriate and that the existing stock level correlates with the record book. The correct amount of the drug is then prepared and administered to the correct child and any unused CD is recorded as wastage in the record book. Throughout the procedure, the two RNs work together to ensure that the administration and documentation adhere to current standards.

ERRORS AND ADVERSE REACTIONS IN MEDICATION ADMINISTRATION

Medication errors do happen and are an ongoing major clinical challenge in both hospital and community settings. They can result in significant morbidity and mortality for patients (GMC, 2012). Using research findings, the phenomena will be explored and interventions that may reduce the incidence of errors and adverse reactions will be suggested whilst also emphasising the need for continued vigilance by all staff.

The Medicines and Healthcare Regulatory products Agency (MHRA) promotes the efficacy and safety of medicines and medical devices. Adverse incidents that occur in practice are reported to the MHRA via a yellow card system. This information can then be cascaded back to clinical areas as alerts to avoid further similar incidents.

Any miscalculation of the drug dose when prescribing or when administering is a potential hazard, thus numerical ability is an important requirement for all nurses. As a student your numerical ability will be tested frequently and as a registered nurse many Trusts impose mandatory annual testing to minimise the risk to patients.

WHAT'S THE EVIDENCE?

A systematic review by Sutcliffe et al. (2014) revealed that in studies conducted since 2003, the commonest errors were in prescribing and the commonest type of error was due to the omission of a prescribed drug or the administration of the wrong dose, strength or frequency, or the wrong drug.

Such errors are taken seriously. Nurses who are negligent in their medication management and have harmed patients as a result are cautioned or disciplined, and they and/or their employers will be required to take remedial action. Organisations have a responsibility to create a culture of openness where errors are reported, and to minimise and manage future risk. To reduce the incidence of error, nurses should always check that the dose correlates with guidance from the British National Formulary for Children (BNFc). This is available in hard copy as well as an online application and mobile app (see https://study.sagepub.com/essentialchildnursing).

WEBLINK: BNFC

As an advocate for children, it is imperative that the nurse is aware of correct drug dosages and checks the BNFc when unsure. Any errors in prescribing can be avoided if the nurse contacts the prescriber requesting that the appropriate amendments are made using the BNFc to support this request. Thus, drug errors such as those above are taken seriously given the risk to the patients entrusted to the nurse's care. Ultimately, nurses who are negligent in their medication management have to answer to their employer/professional body.

Watch the video from East Cheshire NHS Trust regarding safer drug management to reduce errors at https://study.sagepub.com/essentialchildnursing

The children's nurse should remember the Rights of medication administration to reduce the potential of error in this important aspect of care (Table 4.1). Since it is nurses who administer the medication in most instances, they must also ensure that they have the knowledge and skills to prepare the drug appropriately. For instance, some oral drugs need to be dissolved in water. When preparing and administering intravenous medication, the agreed Trust policy and manufacturer's guidance must be adhered to regarding adding diluents and calculating the amount of liquid to be given, taking into account displacement volumes that arise when the diluent is added to the dried preparation. In addition, some intravenous drugs need to be infused slowly whilst others can be given safely as boluses. The intravenous administration of medication requires additional knowledge and skills and is normally undertaken once the newly qualified nurse has become established in that role. It is never undertaken by a nursing student. In short, all student and registered nurses must be aware of their own sphere of competence and always work within that sphere whilst seeking the knowledge to advance their abilities.

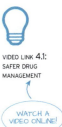
VIDEO LINK 4.1: SAFER DRUG MANAGEMENT

WATCH A VIDEO ONLINE!

Table 4.1 Six rights of medication administration

Six rights	Details
Right drug	Full generic name and strength
Right dose	Without abbreviations
Right route	Without abbreviations
Right time	Start, finish dates and frequency
Right patient	Full name of child or young person
	Age and/or date of birth
	For hospital patients:
	• Hospital number • Hospital and ward names
Right documentation completed	Child's weight in kilograms
	Allergies recorded
	Prescriber's signature
	Nurse(s) who administered the drug signature(s)

(Adapted from: Blair, 2011, p. 141)

PARENTAL ROLE IN MEDICATION ADMINISTRATION

VIDEO LINK 4.2: INTEGRATED MEDICINE MANAGEMENT

It is worth remembering that most illnesses that a child will suffer are treated at home by parents and carers. As a children's nurse, your advice and guidance may be required regarding the safe and appropriate administration and storage of medication – for instance, ensuring that medication is taken as prescribed but at realistic times that work in conjunction with family life to maximise concordance (indicated by parent voice below).

> As the parent of a child who requires administration of multiple medications every day at different times I find the process very difficult and I am only human and have forgotten one or two on many occasions. As a family we have now set alarms for each dose and put up a visual reminder for my daughter in her room so if she goes to bed and we have forgotten her inhaler she remembers when she sees the poster and we can administer. When you're a working family, juggling medications can be harder as school can be reluctant to administer medications. It can feel like a full time job just ensuring she takes everything at the right time. The GP has been very supportive and we now do electronic repeat prescriptions which go straight to the pharmacy saving time and I can request these online which is very helpful. The pharmacy has also delivered when they needed to order in medications to save us a return trip. Overall, we find the support from healthcare professionals excellent; it's the day-to-day management that can feel like a struggle.
>
> **Debbie, parent**

Safe storage within the child's home is important and the general storage advice given earlier should be adhered to (see pp. 58–9). It is also important to watch medication being administered by the carer/parent since sometimes incorrect techniques may be being used (inhaler technique) which will render the medication less effective.

DRUG CALCULATION

Doses required for children frequently require understanding of the formulation of the drug and calculation of the amount required as prescribed. This is sometimes due to the drug being designed for adult use or because the drug is available in a liquid form in a volume requiring calculation. The formula used for calculating the correct volume is:

The amount **N**eeded multiplied by the volume you **H**ave

The **S**tock amount available

You may find this mnemonic useful: $\dfrac{N \; H}{S}$

Thus if a child needed 50 milligrammes of ibuprofen and a bottle containing 100 milligrammes in 5 millilitres was available, the calculation would be:

$$\frac{50}{100} \times 5 = \frac{250}{100} = 2.5 \text{ millilitres}$$

It is also worth taking into account the size of the child and making a 'rough' estimate prior to calculating the volume to be given, so that logic is used as well as accurate calculation. Further calculations are available at https://study.sagepub.com/essentialchildnursing

REVISE: DRUG
CALCULATIONS

CHAPTER SUMMARY

- As a nursing student you will help to administer medication to children and young people.
- There is an expectation that this will be done competently and with adherence to current legislation. Thus, as a student, it is important that you witness and participate in best practice.
- Drug knowledge of the medication administered in your practice area and numerical competence are absolute requirements for nurses.

BUILD YOUR BIBLIOGRAPHY

Books

- Blair, K. (2011) *Medicines Management in Children's Nursing.* London: Sage.

  Structured around the NMC Essential Skills Clusters for medicines management, this book covers legal aspects, drugs calculations, administration, storage, record keeping, introductory pharmacology, patient communication and contextual issues in medication.

- McFadden, R. (2013) *Introducing Pharmacology for Nursing and Healthcare,* 2nd edn. Harlow: Pearson.

  This book addresses the related physiology and pathophysiology necessary to develop an understanding of how commonly used drugs work.

- Starkings, S. and Krause, L. (2015) *Passing Calculation Tests for Nursing Students,* 3rd edn. London: Sage. This book provides drug and fluid calculations that will help build your confidence with this skill.

(Continued)

(Continued)

Journal articles

Go to https://study.sagepub.com/essentialchildnursing for further free online journal articles related to this chapter.

- Roberts, R.M., Albert, A.P., Johnson, D.D. and Hicks, L.A. (2015) 'Can improving knowledge of antibiotic-associated adverse drug events reduce parent and patient demand for antibiotics?' *Health Services Research and Managerial Epidemiology*, 1–5. Available at: http://journals.sagepub.com/doi/pdf/10.1177/2333392814568345 (last accessed 11 May 2017).

  Some people believe that antibiotics are harmless, so this qualitative study was undertaken to assess the knowledge of adult patients and mothers of young patients. The findings revealed that nearly all mothers were aware that there were possible side effects with medications (including antibiotics); however, adult patients did not acknowledge this to the same extent.

- Marc, C., Vrignaud, B., Levieux, K., Robine, A., Gras Le Guen, C. and Launay, E. (2016) 'Inappropriate prescription of antibiotics in pediatric practice: analysis of the prescriptions in primary care'. *Journal of Child Health Care*, 20 (4): 530–6.

  This paper addressed the inappropriate prescription of antibiotics in primary care and highlighted that due to a lack of time GPs lacked the time to fully explain to parents why their child's infection did not warrant antibiotics and instead prescribed antibiotics that parents believed were required.

- Twycross, A.M., Williams, A.M., Bolland, R.E. and Sutherland, R. (2015) 'Parental attitudes to children's pain and analgesic drugs in the United Kingdom'. *Journal of Child Health Care*, 19 (3): 402–11.

  This study explored parental attitudes towards analgesic administration to their child. Highlighting that parents sometimes misread the amount of pain experienced by their child and their subsequent need for analgesia. Since many children will be discharged home after day surgery, this has relevance for parental advice prior to discharge so that the child's pain level is adequately managed.

Weblinks

Go to https://study.sagepub.com/essentialchildnursing for further weblinks related to this chapter.

- BNF-C, *BNF Online*

  www.bnf.org/products/bnf-online

  The formulary is regularly updated providing information about drugs that may be given to children their use, dosage, contraindications and side effects.

- Medicines & Healthcare Products Regulatory Agency

  www.gov.uk/government/organisations/medicines-and-healthcare-products-regulatory-agency

  A regularly updated resource regarding medication, devices and all aspects of drug safety.

- NICE, *Medicines management – children*

  www.nice.org.uk/guidance/ng5

ACE YOUR ASSESSMENT

Revise what you have learned by visiting https://study.sagepub.com/essentialchildnursing

- Test yourself with multiple-choice and short-answer questions
- Do the chapter activities in the book and check your answers online

REFERENCES

Blair, K. (2011) *Medicines Management in Children's Nursing*. Exeter: Learning Matters.

General Medical Council (2012) *Investigating the Prevalence and Causes of Prescribing Errors in General Practice. The PRACtICe Study*. Available at: www.gmc—uk.org/Investigating_the_prevalence_and_causes_of_ prescribing_errors_in_general_practice___The_PRACtICe_study_Report_May_2012_48605085.pdf (accessed 19 October 2017).

Nursing and Midwifery Council (NMC) (2015) *The Code: Professional Standards of Practice and Behaviour for Nurses and Midwives*. London: NMC.

Ogden, J. (2015) 'Health psychology', in J. Naidoo, J. and J. Wills, J. (eds), *Health Studies: An Introduction*, 3rd edn. London: Palgrave Macmillan Education.

Royal College of Nursing (RCN) (2013) *Sharps Safety: RCN Guidance to Support the Implementation of The Health and Safety (Sharp Instruments in Healthcare Regulations)*. London: RCN.

Smith, L. and Coleman, V. (2010) *Child and Family-centred Healthcare: Concept, Theory and Practice*, 2nd edn. Basingstoke: Palgrave Macmillan.

Sutcliffe, K., Stokes, G., O'Mara, A., Caird, J., Hinds, K., Bangpan, M., Kavanagh, J., Dickson, K., Stansfield, C., Hargreaves, K. and Thomas, J. (2014) *Paediatric Medication Error: A Systematic Review of the Extent and Nature of the Problem in the UK and International Interventions to Address It*. EPPI-Centre Social Science Research Unit, Institute of Education, University of London.

INTERPROFESSIONAL WORKING WITH CHILDREN AND YOUNG PEOPLE

5

DEBBIE MCGIRR AND SCOTT RICHARDSON-READ

THIS CHAPTER COVERS

- Core elements of interprofessional working
- Challenges and benefits of IPW
- Current IPW practices across the UK
- Health and social care integration
- IPW and team working in transition

> " Effective interprofessional working enables patients to receive an inclusive care plan which produces positive outcomes for children, young people and families. However, the biggest barriers to success are a lack of coordination, inadequate resources and poor information-sharing.
>
> **Mhairie, 3rd-year children's nursing student** "

Visit https://study.sagepub.com/essentialchildnursing to access a wealth of online resources for this chapter – watch out for the margin icons throughout the chapter.

INTRODUCTION

Interprofessional working (IPW) focuses on working relationships between various professionals from a wide variety of agencies (SCIE, 2009), and is an essential approach to meet the diverse needs of children, young people and their families. This chapter will enable you to identify some of the common principles associated with IPW working and highlight the challenges and benefits for patients and practitioners. It will also assist you to explore and understand the reasons for differing practices across the UK, highlighting the importance of the role of third sector partners in service planning and delivery. Collaboration between professionals and services is key to ensuring IPW is successful in producing individualised outcomes for children and families. However, as highlighted in the introductory quote, it is a complex process requiring clear communication, good coordination and availability of adequate resources to be effective.

CORE ELEMENTS OF INTERPROFESSIONAL WORKING

Successful IPW working relies on a number of core elements coming together. An understanding of individual roles and responsibilities across agencies is crucial in order to foster the ethos of partnership working and requires adherence to specific principles as identified above. Payne (2000) highlights the importance of communication, coordination, competence, cooperation and collaboration.

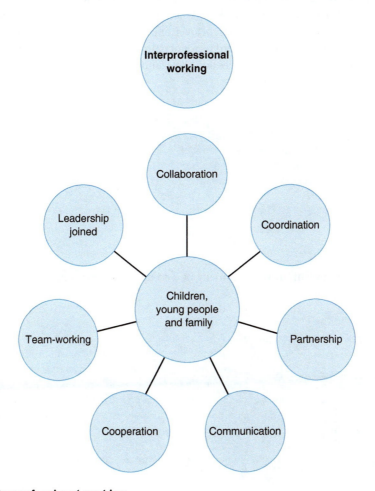

Figure 5.1 Interprofessional working

Heslop et al. (2002) indicate continuity, choice and comprehensiveness as being equally important, whilst UCSF (2014) add the attributes of team working and professionalism as key indicators to successful IPW. These principles highlight the need for joined-up working which focuses on individual needs and outcomes, placing children and families at the centre of care assessment and delivery. Thomas et al. (2014) identify it as an essential element of practice and, therefore, to work together effectively, professionals must be mindful of the influence of organisational structures, team processes and individual contribution (Mickan and Rodger, 2000). If teams are to provide both seamless and integrated care they need time to learn to work together. This requires appreciation and understanding of the theory of effective team formation. The core elements of IPW are summarised in Figure 5.1.

VIDEO LINK 5.1:
4 STAGES
OF TEAM
DEVELOPMENT

ACTIVITY 5.1: REFLECTIVE PRACTICE

Watch the short video at https://study.sagepub.com/essentialchildnursing to hear an overview of the four stages of team development identified by Tuckman and think about how you can apply them to your practice learning placement.

ACTIVITY
ANSWER 5.1

For practitioners working across statutory and third sector settings with children who have a range of long-term or complex needs, IPW working is an essential component of everyday practice. An example of this can be seen in the quotation below from the Family Support Service director of PAMIS (Promoting a More Inclusive Society), a third sector organisation that works in partnership with people with profound multiple learning disabilities and their families in Scotland:

> PAMIS worked alongside family carers and NHS Lanarkshire to develop an information booklet and DVD on postural care. This required close partnership working between family carers, PAMIS, Allied Health Professionals from the Community Learning Disability Team, and the Children and Young People Team. Effective partnership working was key to this project which resulted in the resource being successfully launched in 2016.
>
> **Michelle Morrison, Family Support Service Director, PAMIS**

However, for nursing students, IPW can initially be a complex area to understand:

> As first year nursing students we sit in a lecture theatre and learn about IPW working. We become familiar with the importance of the multidisciplinary team and how it centres care around the patient. But this didn't mean a lot to me until I saw it first-hand during a second-year hospital placement. I suddenly saw the intricate workings of the MDT and then understood how big decisions about a patient couldn't just be made by a single member of the team – all decisions needed to be considered in the light of other treatment as they may either complement patient care or potentially have a detrimental effect on it.
>
> **Linda, 2nd-year children's nursing student**

SEE ALSO
CHAPTER 8

The reality of implementation and the complexities of care delivery and partnership working between and across agencies cannot be ignored. It requires a clear purpose supported by good strategic planning and a skilled team leader, as identified by Mickan and Rodger (2000). It also requires respect for professional boundaries and responsibilities (Davis and Smith, 2012), and recognition of your professional duty of care to children and families (NMC, 2015; Gribben et al., 2016).

At an organisational level, IPW requires 'joined-up' thinking, sharing good practice and a willingness to address the realignment of roles and responsibilities. Organisations need to work within specific legal and professional frameworks to align with duties, manage budgets, meet targets, evaluate services and provide quality-based patient care which is both safe and effective in meeting shared outcomes.

ACTIVITY 5.2: CRITICAL THINKING

- Imagine you are a young person in hospital having just been diagnosed with diabetes. Why do you need professionals to work together?
- Now imagine you are a parent of a child at home with complex needs – consider and note down why you need community services to work together

ACTIVITY
ANSWER 5.2

Using an IPW approach results in traditional relationships and ways of working being challenged, which can be difficult but at times necessary. However, The King's Fund (2017) suggest there is an increasing evidence base which demonstrates that close collaboration improves care and quality of life for patients and families.

CHALLENGES AND BENEFITS OF IPW

As with any complex system, there are associated challenges and benefits. This is no different for IPW. The fact that established services, working within their own legal systems and organisations, are required to merge and identify commonalities in approaches to care delivery is in itself a complicated task. Such challenges are examined further below:

- Duplication of care, failure to provide care, clinical risk, families losing confidence in services (Doyle, 2008)
- Personal commitment, a common goal, clarity of roles, communication, institutional support (Wilson and Pirrie, 2000)
- Organisational logistics which prevent effective IPW working between agencies (Pollard et al., 2010)
- Management of resources, time management, financial resources, decision-making (Collier, 2013)

The reality of these challenges presents parents with real difficulties to overcome as evidenced below:

> We used to see a lot of professionals and I felt they were only interested in their own particular field. I always wished I could get them all in a room at the same time to discuss problems and the treatments and see how they impacted on each other. For example, the dietician wanted the feed to run slowly all day to get enough feed in but the physiotherapist wanted it stopped for an hour so that physio could be done and the neurologist prescribed medication that could not be given with food. Little things like that I felt needed a more 'joined up' approach.
>
> **Diane, carer**

In light of the above, consider the impact of fragmented communication within the team on the child and family.

For practitioners, their experiences of IPW can be equally frustrating with individual service agendas and organisational targets being seen as competing priorities which interfere with care delivery (Collins and McCray, 2012). The failure of these diverse agency agendas in communicating clearly to provide effective care and service delivery has been highlighted in a number of national inquiry reports into child abuse cases such as the Victoria Climbié Inquiry (Cm 5730, 2003), the Laming Report (DH, 2008), the Kennedy Report (DH, 2010) and more recently The Case of Ms. MN (MWC, 2016). Each report acknowledged the frustrations of children, their families and some staff in relation to poorly coordinated services and failure of organisations to share relevant information. They highlighted the need for collaborative working on a more consistent basis through shared record-keeping and consistent communication. Similar findings were also identified by the Francis Inquiry Report (Francis, 2013) into patient harm and neglect and by the Care Quality Commission (CQC) (2014) in their report *From the Pond to the Sea*.

Whilst much of the literature discusses challenges in relations between health, education and social care services (Pollard et al., 2010), additional tensions exist between statutory services and the third sector in relation to care responsibility, delivery and information sharing. For children and families, the importance of the third sector in providing essential support cannot be underestimated. However, as third sector services are not delivered or regulated by statutory services or professional bodies, it can lead to lack of trust and understanding by staff who manage and deliver services across health, education and social care.

SAFEGUARDING STOP POINT

Think about the challenges mentioned above and consider your duty of confidentiality regarding patient care. Note down what you need to be aware of during joined working in terms of data sharing processes as a children's nurse. Can you think of any legislation that might help inform this?

SAFEGUARDING
STOP POINT
ANSWER 5.1

Benefits of IPW

Despite multiple challenges, there are numerous benefits to IPW working if children and families are placed at the centre of the planning process. However, partnership working between professionals, practitioners, children and families is crucial to engender success (evidenced below).

> Working with key partners is integral to community children's nursing enabling childrens' outcomes to be met and goals achieved ensuring health potentials are attained. All successful professional relationships require investment to ensure shared respect of roles and responsibilities and also to appreciate limitations of roles and services. Effective IPW is an approach which aims to share expertise and prevent duplication of resources.
>
> **Christine, CCN team lead**

Sharing expertise means involving children and families as partners in care where possible (Anderson, 2012), acknowledging their right to be involved in decisions about their health/social care treatment. The United Nations Convention on the Rights of the Child (UNCRC), Article 12 states that all children have a right to an opinion which must be listened to and taken seriously (CYPCS, 2016). This is particularly important for children with complex and exceptional needs to enable them to have their voices heard and play a part in controlling their future life choices where possible and appropriate, as identified by CEN/Talking Mats (2015). Parents/carers who are legal guardians have a vested interest in care delivery and evaluation. They also have a legal right to be involved in decision-making using informed choice (DH, 2016). Having parents/carers involved in decision-making recognises their role as equal partners and facilitates ownership, leading to better outcomes (The King's Fund, 2011). It also offers an opportunity to maintain control, which is key for families engaged in long-term care activities due to enduring conditions.

PRACTICE SCENARIO 5: BENJAMIN

ACTIVITY 5.3: REFLECTIVE PRACTICE

Think about a recent practice learning experience involving IPW working and reflect on the various roles of the staff involved.

Successful IPW working relies on provision of holistic care which is coordinated to meet children's individual needs. This is crucial in building relationships with services, families and fellow professionals/practitioners, whilst also contributing to higher family morale by encouraging and facilitating partnership and family involvement (Doyle, 2008).

> "
> The child I foster now is mainly in the care of the respiratory team and things are much better. She was referred to the gastro-intestinal (GI) team for surgery but all the follow-up was done at the respiratory clinic. Any scans etc. are arranged for the same time as clinic appointments to avoid extra hospital visits. The dietician sees us at that clinic too and we also have appointments with a paediatrician which are held locally as part of an multidisciplinary team (MDT) clinic so the physiotherapist, occupational therapist (OT) and speech and language therapist (SALT) are there to assess her and to deal with any queries which works very well. At home we are visited by the children's community nurse who will liaise with the rest of the professionals if there is anything needed out with clinic visits. She is also closely linked to the Outreach service and the respiratory nurse specialist. They all share information and arrange training, supplies, etc.
>
> **Diane, carer**
> "

In light of the above quotation, remember that effective coordination of care is extremely important for families. Methods of delivery and coordination vary across the UK, however, although you will find commonalities in current practice in relation to key roles and responsibilities.

CURRENT IPW PRACTICE ACROSS THE UK

By now, you will appreciate how effective IPW enables support to be individualised (Thomas et al., 2014), and contributes to early identification and effective assessment where outcomes meet the healthcare needs of children and families. There are three common roles supporting key frameworks for IPW in UK-based children's nursing (outlined in Table 5.1):

Table 5.1   Key roles in IPW

Care coordinator (Greco and Sloper, 2003)	Lead professional (The Scottish Government, 2016)	Key worker (Noyes et al., 2014)
Collaborates with professionals from other services Ensures access to services, coordination and delivery of care This results in: better relationships with services higher family morale less family isolation and feelings of burden better access to services fewer unmet needs	A practitioner who is chosen in partnership with parents/carers because they have the right skills and experience Their role is to: ensure the child and parents/carers understand care delivery and involve them in decision-making ensure the child's plan is current, accurate, implemented and reviewed regularly consult and work with the child's named person (point of contact from health or education services)	Improves communication channels Makes information more accessible between families and carers Provides emotional and practical support Facilitates multiagency meetings Supports the joint assessment process Advocates for children Coordinates services around children and their families

Table 5.2   Key policies around IPW in the UK

Country	Policy/Framework	Key attributes
England, Wales	Common Assessment Framework (CAF) You can watch the CAF training video at https://study.sagepub.com/essentialchildnursing	Tool used by practitioners across agencies to standardise the assessment process and promote IPW working (Collins and McCray, 2012)
Northern Ireland	Understanding Needs of Children in Northern Ireland (UNOCINI)	Multidisciplinary tool to standardise and streamline assessment planning and implementation of child and family processes and aid communication
Scotland	Getting It Right for Every Child (GIRFEC) approach (The Scottish Government, 2015)	Embedded in the Children and Young People (Scotland) Act 2014, focusing on the health and wellbeing of children. The role of the lead professional is pivotal as part of secondary legislation within the same Act

VIDEO LINK 5.2:
CAF TRAINING

WATCH A
VIDEO ONLINE!

To meet the needs of local populations, England, Wales and Northern Ireland have adopted a specific framework to improve IPW, whereas Scotland has adopted a national approach to care delivery.

Regardless of the location, the promotion of IPW to meet the wide and varied needs of children across health, education, social care and the third sector has been endorsed by the four countries of the UK via their child health strategies and children's commissioner reports.

WHAT'S THE EVIDENCE?

WEBLINK:
CHILDREN'S
COMMISSIONERS
REPORT

Access the Report of the UK Children's Commissioners (2015) at https://study.sagepub.com/essentialchildnursing

Explore the section relating to children with disabilities and identify key recommendations in relation to service delivery, care planning and transition.

WHAT'S THE
EVIDENCE?
ANSWER 5.1

HEALTH AND SOCIAL CARE INTEGRATION

Integrated care puts the needs and experiences of people at the centre of how services are organised and delivered and is person-centred (DH, 2013). In the acute setting, the creation of integrated care pathways (ICPs) for specific conditions or specific aspects of care such as transition, has been acknowledged as an effective way for multidisciplinary care to be delivered based upon best current evidence (McNamara-Goodger, 2011).

In the community setting, integrated care refers to organisations and service models which include statutory, third sector and independent services as part of the commissioning and delivery process working together under a joint board. These models differ across localities and are dependent on the needs of the population. However, they must include the health board, social care/local authority, third sector and independent providers. Walker (2013) suggests provision of successful integrated care requires acceptance of potential conflict and disagreement amongst team members, in addition to acknowledgement of different philosophical viewpoints and service eligibility criteria, whilst at the same time acknowledging the importance of the practitioner's individual role, regardless of the service base.

The integration of care re-conceptualises service planning and delivery for children and young people. Historically, within the UK, health and social care have been involved in joint working with families whose children have enduring, complex or disabling conditions. However, although it is classed as one of the three statutory services, education has been seen as a separate field (Grek et al., 2009) rather than part of universal services alongside health and social care. This has contributed to difficulties in meeting children's needs holistically and in a person-centred way. Until recently the third sector has been seen as an 'addition' to statutory service delivery. However, for children with enduring conditions their input is part of core care provision alongside health, education and social care. Increasing expectations for integrated working through the sharing and pooling of resources to meet more complex health and social care needs sees the role of the third sector becoming recognised as a key advocate in the commissioning process (Health and Social Care Alliance, 2014).

The four countries of the UK have addressed the integration agenda with the formation of different frameworks and initiatives to meet the health and social needs of their specific populations (Table 5.3):

Table 5.3 Frameworks and initiatives addressing the integration agenda

Northern Ireland (NI)	Scotland	England	Wales
Transforming Your Care (2011) – a major health and social care reform with the creation of Integrated Care Partnerships (ICPs) across Northern Ireland providing high-quality healthcare for children A Strategy for Paediatric Healthcare Services Provided in Hospitals and in the Community (2016 – 2026) (Department of Health NI, 2016)	Strategic revision of health and social care delivery under the Public Bodies (Joint Working) (Scotland) Act 2014 with the formation of Integrated Joined Boards and production of local outcome improvements plans (LOIPs) Implementation of the Child's Plan as part of Getting It Right for Every Child (GIRFEC) and secondary legislation forming part of the Children and Young People (Scotland) Act 2014 Implementation of the Social Care (Self-directed-Support) (Scotland) Act 2013, which informs the philosophy of patient empowerment within the integration agenda	Development of a Five Year Forward View (5YFV) which proposes new models of NHS and social care to promote person-centred physical health, mental health and social care across acute and community settings	Identification of key determinants for integrated working through the development of a structural health and social care model to address primary/community and secondary healthcare interfaces (The Welsh Government, 2013)

Successful integration of statutory, third sector and independent service delivery to meet the wide variety of health and social needs of children and their families depends on a multitude of factors. The King's Fund (2013) identify one of the key drivers for success as being the need to ensure that strategic and organisational aspects are closely followed by service integration at a clinical level, using

VIDEO LINK 5.3:
SELF-DIRECTED
SUPPORT

measurable goals which assess the impact of care on patient outcomes and allow patients and families to see clear benefits of joined-up working.

IPW AND TEAM WORKING IN TRANSITION

Joined-up working relies on effective team work across services. In children's nursing, transition from child to adult services provides a clear example of the importance of effective IPW and will be utilised here to illustrate the main elements of IPW as highlighted in this chapter.

Such a transition includes health, social care, education, the third sector, welfare, housing and other areas such as transport and other local authority area placement, as young people move on from all these services at the same time. These services bridge both sides of child and adult service environments.

VIDEO LINK 5.4:
THOMAS'S
STORY

There is a range of evidence available exploring effective transitions for children with additional support needs (Forbes et al, 2002; Kelly, 2014; Richardson-Read, 2014; ANS, 2015; Jacquet, 2015; LEAD, 2015). These studies use systematic reviews, interviews and focus groups with children and their carers to explore major barriers, and in some cases solutions, to the transition process. The research identifies certain service structures and delivery processes which support continuity from children to adult services. These include the need for specialist services and skilled staff dedicated to the transition period, in addition to the need for multidisciplinary and multiagency working using a person-centred approach to care planning and delivery. The evidence highlights failure to achieve this continuity results in negative outcomes for children and those who care for them as they move through the transition process feeling unsupported and disempowered.

Principles of Good Transitions 3 (ARC Scotland, 2017) lists seven key factors all professionals need to be aware of to ensure transitions are successful.

VIDEO LINK 5.5:
THESE THINGS
TAKE TIME

1. Planning and decision-making should be carried out in a person-centred way
2. Support should be co-ordinated across all services
3. Planning should start early and continue up to age 25
4. All young people should get the support they need
5. Young people, parents and carers must have access to the information they need
6. Families and carers need support
7. A continued focus on transitions across Scotland

These principles support IPW working across all areas, and are embedded within the philosophy of child-centred care and empowerment. Additionally, they explore effective strategic, operational and professional working strategies to achieve the aims of effective integration, which in turn support positive outcomes for children and effective IPW. These results have been echoed by the findings of the Care Quality Commission in England (2014) and in the Care Act 2014 for UK social care staff and further in the NICE transitions guidelines (2016). Operationally, this approach has been laid out in the 'Talking Points' tool (Miller and Cook, 2012).

WHAT'S THE EVIDENCE?

Transition guidelines for children using health or social services (NICE, 2016) refer to the importance of using the philosophy of empowerment to embed person-centred approaches within healthcare.

Explore the benefits of empowerment for families and identify the key principles of PCP at https://study.sagepub.com/essentialchildnursing

WEBLINK:
PRINCIPLES
OF PCP

WHAT'S THE
EVIDENCE?
ANSWER 5.2

CASE STUDY 5.1: HAMISH

Hamish was 18 with a diagnosis of autism and complex physical disability, and he wanted to go to college when he left his complex needs school. He had yearly transition meetings at school with his parent/guardian, ASL teacher (and head teacher), Skills Development Scotland (SDS) representative (careers service) and duty (unallocated) social worker.

Hamish's SDS worker supported him to apply for appropriate courses, and to make his own choices. The school supported Hamish to attend various taster sessions at the college so that he could feel more secure and familiar with the environment once he'd left school. The social worker ensured the plan was appropriate and all agencies involved were meeting their obligations, whilst gathering various pieces of information to ensure the correct support could be put in place.

Hamish was then allocated a social worker from the local Transition team who would be responsible for, and oversee, his transition. Hamish's social worker completed the adult assessment form and secured funding for transport to and from college where he attended a supported course. He attended college for two years, after which he wanted to move onto day support. His social worker was again allocated to update the previous assessment and seek the funds for day support. Funding was agreed and Hamish's mum decided she would like to manage a direct payment on her son's behalf, under the principles of self-directed support.

- Think about Hamish's story and identify key areas of concern for him, his family and professionals involved. What are the challenges and benefits for Hamish? What might your role as a children's nurse be in this process?

CHECK YOUR ANSWERS ONLINE!

CASE STUDY ANSWER 5.1

An effective way to envision the transitions process as contributing to the success of IPW is as a puzzle that needs to be solved collectively, rather than individual practitioners focusing solely on their own solutions. This needs to be coupled with a clear focus from all those involved in the experience which places the wishes of the young person at the centre of the transitions process. If the young person has support in place from the third sector, it can provide invaluable input to help explore and understand the needs and outcomes of the young person in light of the assessment process. This joined-up working approach, which should start early – around the age of 14 years (Richardson-Read, 2014) – provides a focus to examine the whole life journey of the young person. Early joint planning can explore the impact of different wellbeing concerns on the young person's ability to achieve their outcomes more effectively (DfE and DH, 2014), compared to the experiences of those whose transitions happen near to the case transfer date and without adequate joint planning. Early joint planning has been enshrined within the Getting it Right for Every Child (GIRFEC) approach in Scotland as well as the approach that is taken with self-directed support (Scottish Government, 2013) and the Care Act 2014 in England. It is important for children's nurses to work flexibly alongside third sector partners. It is also important for healthcare professionals to understand the philosophy of positive outcomes rather than becoming focused on specific service provision, which tries to 'fix' the issues they are presented with. Joint working can ameliorate the impact of negative transitions on children and their families and assist them in achieving success in adult life (DfE and DH, 2014). The impact of early joint planning in partnership with the young person and their family can clearly be seen in Hamish's case study above.

Using the voices of students, practitioners and parents, and focusing on the example of transition, this chapter has presented you with 'real-life evidence' through which you can begin to link theory with practice.

CHAPTER SUMMARY

- All healthcare for children and families relies on input from a variety of organisations and people to plan and deliver streamlined care and services.
- Core components of successful IPW include collaboration, coordination, partnership, communication, cooperation, team working and leadership.
- It is important to place the children at the centre and use evidence-based practice to assess their needs using a holistic approach which ultimately delivers care which is both child focused and family centred.

BUILD YOUR BIBLIOGRAPHY

Books

- Day, J. (2013) *Interprofessional Working: An Essential Guide for Health and Social Care Professionals (Nursing and Health Care Practice)*. Andover: Cengage Learning.

  This textbook provides a range of information for nursing and healthcare students who will be working as part of an integrated and interprofessional team. It contains scenarios from practice which can be used to inform and develop critical thinking around interprofessional working in all health and social care contexts.

- Goodman B. and Clemow, R. (2011) *Nursing and Collaborative Practice: A Guide to Interprofessional Learning and Working*. UK: Dawson Books.

  This textbook provides a comprehensive overview of the roles of practitioners working in interprofessional healthcare services, covering aspects of teamwork. It also includes the voices and experiences of service users in improving care delivery.

- Kay, J. and Fitzgerald, D. (2007) *Working Together in Children's Services*. London: Taylor & Francis.

  This textbook examines a range of issues and context in multiagency working across education and health-related services. It explores key concepts such as benefits and barriers to working together, examines the policy context and discusses essential skills for interprofessional teamwork.

Journal articles

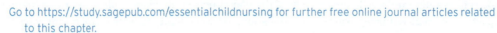
Go to https://study.sagepub.com/essentialchildnursing for further free online journal articles related to this chapter.

FURTHER
READING:
ONLINE
JOURNAL
ARTICLES

- Mackenzie, A., Craik, C., Tempest, S., Cordingley, K., Buckingham, I. and Hale, S. (2007) 'Interprofessional learning in practice: the student experience'. *British Journal of Occupational Therapy*, 70 (8): 358-61.

  This article explores the experiences of 16 occupational therapy students during a practice learning placement on an interprofessional ward. It identifies the importance of team working, development of interpersonal skills and recognition of the importance of other practitioners' roles in the clinical setting. Although the students are working in the area of older people's nursing, the core knowledge and skills they develop are transferrable across the nursing profession.

- Pullon, S., McKinlay, B., Yager, J., Duncan, B., McHugh, P. and Dowell, A. (2015) 'Developing indicators of service integration for child health: perceptions of service providers and families of young children in a region of high need in New Zealand'. *Journal of Child Health Care*, 19 (1): 18-29. Available at: http://chc.sagepub.com/content/19/1/18.full.pdf+html (last accessed 11 May 2017).

This article explores the thoughts of local parents in relation to the integration of health and social care services to provide better care outcomes for their young children. The study used individual interviews and focus groups to extrapolate data from parents and professionals. Key themes emerging from the data indicated a need for appreciation of the importance of family and child health interdependence, alongside clear acknowledgment of a lack of communication and service integration between health and social services.

- Wright, A.E., Robb, J. and Shearer, M.C. (2015) 'Transition from paediatric to adult health services in Scotland for young people with cerebral palsy'. *Journal of Child Health Care*, 20 (2): 205-13.

This study explored current service provision for young people with cerebral palsy who were transitioning from child to adult services. It used semi-structured interviews to record data from a range of consultants across 12 Scottish health boards and identified key areas for improvement including: coordination and communication within health services and coordination between health, education and social services. The study indicated the need for further research on the impact of problematic and variable transition on young people and their families.

Weblinks

FURTHER
READING:
WEBLINKS

Go to https://study.sagepub.com/essentialchildnursing for further weblinks related to this chapter.

- Scottish Transitions Forum, *Principles of Good Transitions*

  https://scottishtransitions.org.uk

  Read the Principles of Good Transitions to find out more about how effective joint working in transitions help reduce risk and contribute to child and adult safety.

- NICE, *Transition from Children's to Adults' Services for Young People Using Health or Social Care Services*

  www.nice.org.uk/guidance/ng43

  Read the NICE transitions guidelines and reflect on your role in effective joined working.

- Social Care Institute for Excellence (SCIE), *e-Learning: Interprofessional and Inter-agency Collaboration (IPIAC)*

  www.scie.org.uk/publications/elearning/ipiac/index.asp

  Undertake the exercises to further explore knowledge and understanding of the principles of IPW.

- Human Resources, *Learning & Development*

  http://hrweb.mit.edu/learning-development/learning-topics/teams/articles/stages-development

  Read more about the stages of team development.

ACE YOUR ASSESSMENT

ONLINE
QUIZZES &
ACTIVITY
ANSWERS

Revise what you have learned by visiting https://study.sagepub.com/essentialchildnursing

- Test yourself with multiple-choice and short-answer questions
- Do the chapter activities in the book and check your answers online

REFERENCES

Anderson, H. (2012) 'Collaborative practice: a way of being "with"'. *Psychotherapy and Politics International*, 10 (2): 130–45.

ARC Scotland (2017) *Principles of Good Transitions 3*. Available at: http://scottishtransitions.org.uk/summary-download (accessed 31 August 2017).

Autism Network Scotland (ANS) (2015) *Transitions Digging Deeper report*. Autism Network Scotland. Available at: www.autismnetworkscotland.org.uk/files/2015/10/Digging-Deeper-Report.pdf (accessed 31 August 2017).

Care Quality Commission (CQC) (2014) *From the Pond into the Sea. Children's Transition to Adult Health Services*. Newcastle upon Tyne: CQC.

CEN/Talking Mats (2015) *Will Anyone Listen to Us? What Matters to Young People with Complex and Exceptional Health Needs and Their Families during Health Transitions*. Edinburgh: NMCN CEN. Available at: www.talkingmats.com/wp-content/uploads/2015/11/20151027-CEN-report.pdf (last accessed 6 May 2017).

Collier, S. (2013) 'Preparation for professional practice', in C. Thurston (ed.), *Essential Nursing Care for Children and Young People: Theory, Policy and Practice*. Abingdon: Routledge.

Collins, F. and McCray, J. (2012) 'Partnership working in services for children: use of the Common Assessment Framework'. *Journal of Interprofessional Care*, 26: 134–40.

Children & Young People's Commissioner Scotland (CYPCS) (2016) 'Article 12'. Available at: www.cypcs.org.uk/rights/uncrcarticles/article-12 (last accessed 6 May 2017).

Davis J.M. and Smith, M. (2012) *Working in Multi-professional Contexts: A Practical Guide for Professionals in Children's Services*. London: Sage.

Department for Education and Department of Health (2014) *Special Educational Needs and Disability Code of Practice: 0 to 25 years*. London: Department for Education.

Cm 5730 (2003) The Victoria Climbié Inquiry: Report of an Inquiry by Lord Laming. London: TSO.

Department of Health (2010) Getting It Right for Children and Young People: Overcoming Cultural Barriers in the NHS so as to Meet Their Needs. A Review by Professor Sir Ian Kennedy. London: Department of Health.

Department of Health (2013) *Integrated Care: Our Shared Commitment*. London: Department of Health.

Department of Health (2014) *Delivering Better Integrated Care. NHS England*. Available at: www.gov.uk/guidance/enabling-integrated-care-in-the-nhs (last accessed 6 May 2017).

Department of Health (2016) *The NHS Choice Framework*. London: Department of Health.

Department of Health NI (2016) *Providing High Quality Healthcare for Children and Young People: A Strategy for Paediatric Healthcare Services Provided in Hospitals and in the Community (2016–2026)*. Belfast: Department of Health (NI).

Doyle, J. (2008) 'Barriers and facilitators of multidisciplinary team working: a review'. *Paediatric Nursing*, 20 (2): 26–9.

Forbes, A., While, A., Ullman, R., Lewis, S., Mathes, L. and Griffiths, P. (2002) *A Multi-Method Review to Identify Components of Practice Which May Promote Continuity in the Transition from Child to Adult Care for Young People with Chronic Illness or Disability*. London: NCCSDO. Available at: http://citeseerx.ist.psu.edu/viewdoc/download?doi=10.1.1.466.3915&rep=rep1&type=pdf (last accessed 6 May 2017).

Francis, R. (2013) *Report of the Mid Staffordshire NHS Foundation Trust Public Inquiry*. London: The Stationery Office.

Greco, V. and Sloper, P. (2003) 'Care co-ordination and key worker schemes for disabled children: results of a UK-wide survey'. *Child: Care, Health and Development*, 30: 13–20.

Grek, S., Ozga, J. and Lawn, M. (2009) *Integrated Children's Services in Scotland*. Edinburgh: University of Edinburgh.

Gribben, M., McLellan, S., McGirr, D. and Chenery-Morris, S. (2016) *How to Survive Your Nursing and Midwifery Course*. London: Sage.

Health and Social Care Alliance (2014) *Integration: Turning Policy into Practice*. Edinburgh: Health and Social Care Alliance. Available at: www.alliance-scotland.org.uk/what-we-do/policy-and-campaigns/current-work/health-and-social-care-integration (last accessed 6 May 2017).

Heslop, P., Mallett, R., Simons, K. and Ward, L. (2002) *Bridging the Divide at Transition. What Happens for People with Learning Difficulties and Their Families*. Glasgow: BILD.

Jaquet, S. (2015) *Evaluation of the Principles of Good Transitions 2 and Scottish Transitions Forum*. Edinburgh: ARC Scotland.

Kelly, D. (2014) 'Theory to reality: the role of the transition nurse coordinator'. *British Journal of Nursing*, 23 (16): 888–94.

Laming, The Lord (2009) The Laming Report. The Protection of Children in England: A Progress Report. London: TSO.

LEAD (2015) *LEADing Transitions*. (Research commissioned by the Education Minister). Edinburgh: HMSO. Available at: www.lead.org.uk/wp-content/uploads/2016/05/Briefing-for-Angela- Constance-on-Lead-Transition-Focus-Groups.pdf (accessed 31 August 2017).

McNamara-Goodger, K. (2011) 'Transitional care for children and young people with life-threatening or life-limiting conditions', in R. Davies and A. Davies (2011) (eds), *Children and Young People's Nursing: Principles for Practice*. London: Hodder Arnold.

Mental Welfare Commission (MWC) (2016) *The Investigation into the Death of Ms MN*. Edinburgh: Mental Welfare Commission of Scotland.

Mickan, S. and Rodger, S. (2000) 'Characteristics of effective teams: a literature review'. *Australian Health Review*, 23 (3): 201–8.

Miller, E and Cook, A. (2012) *Talking point. A personal Outcomes Approach. Practical Guide*. Joined Improvement Team. Edinburgh.

HSC NI (2011) *Transforming Your Care: A Review of Health and Social Care in Northern Ireland*. Available at: www.northerntrust.hscni.net/pdf/Transforming_Your_Care_Report.pdf (accessed 5 October 2017).

NICE (2016) Transitions from children's to adults' services for young people using health or social care services. Available at: www.nice.org.uk/guidance/indevelopment/gid-scwave0714 (last accessed 6 May 2017).

Noyes, J., Pritchard, A., Rees, S., Hastings, R., Jones, K., Mason, H., Hain, R. and Lidstone V. (2014) *Bridging the Gap: Transition from Children's to Adult Palliative Care*. Bangor University.

Nursing & Midwifery Council (NMC) (2015) *The Code: Professional Standards of Practice and Behaviour for Nurses and Midwives*. London: NMC.

Payne, M. (2000) *Teamwork in Multiprofessional Care*. Basingstoke: Palgrave.

Pollard, K., Thomas, J. and Miers, M. (2010) *Understanding Interprofessional Working in Health and Social Care: Theory and Practice*. Basingstoke: Palgrave Macmillan.

Richardson-Read, S. (2014) *Principles of Good Transitions 2*. Edinburgh: ARC Scotland.

SCIE (2009) *An Introduction to Interprofessional and Interagency Collaboration*. London: SCIE. Available at: www.scie.org.uk/assets/elearning/ipiac/ipiac01/resource/text/index.htm, (last accessed 6 May 2017).

Scottish Government (2015) *Getting It Right for Every Child (GIRFEC)*. Edinburgh: Scottish Government.

Scottish Government (2016) *GIRFEC: What is a Lead Professional?* Available at: www.gov.scot/Topics/People/Young-People/gettingitright/lead-professional (last accssed 6 May 2017).

The King's Fund (2011) *Making Shared Decision-making a Reality: No Decision about Me, without Me*. London: The King's Fund.

The King's Fund (2013) *Integrated Care in Northern Ireland, Scotland and Wales – Lessons for England*. London: The King's Fund.

The King's Fund (2017) *Improving NHS Culture.* London: The King's Fund. Available at: www.kings fund.org.uk/projects/culture (accessed 31 August 2017).

Thomas, J., Pollard, K. and Sellman, D. (2014) *Interprofessional Working in Health and Social Care: Professional Perspectives* (2nd edn). Basingstoke: Palgrave Macmillan.

UK Children's Commissioners (2015) UN Committee on the Rights of the Child: Examination of the Fifth Periodic Report of the United Kingdom of Great Britain and Northern Ireland. Available at: www.childrenscommissioner.gov.uk/sites/default/files/publications/Report%20to%20the%20 UNCRC.pdf (last accessed 6 May 2017).

University of California, San Francisco (UCSF) (2014) *Program for Interprofessional Education and Practice.* Available at: https://interprofessional.ucsf.edu/framework-competencies (last accessed 6 May 2017).

Walker, S. (2012) *Effective Social Work with Children and Families – Putting Systems Theory into Practice.* London: Sage.

Welsh Government (2013) *Health and Wellbeing Best Practice Innovations Board Integrated Care Workstream: The Determinants of Effective Integration of Health and Social Care.* Cardiff: Welsh Government. Available at: www.wales.nhs.uk/sitesplus/documents/888/The%20Determinants%20 of%20Effective%20Integration%20of%20Health%20and%20Social%20Care%20FINAL.pdf (accessed 5 October 2017).

Wilson, V. and Pirrie, A. (2000) *Multidisciplinary Teamworking: Beyond the Barriers? A Review of the Issues.* Edinburgh: The SCRE Centre.

ORGANISATION AND SETTINGS FOR CARE OF CHILDREN AND YOUNG PEOPLE

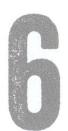

JANE HUGHES, AMANDA KELLY AND TRACEY JONES

THIS CHAPTER COVERS

- History of the nursing process
- Assessment strategies in a range of settings
- Nursing skills and patient assessment
- Identifying and planning care needs
- Implementing and evaluating care plans
- Developing technology in the organisation of care

> " Children are cared for in diverse settings and consideration of the impact, tensions and challenges is an essential component of caring for children and families.
>
> Carter et al., 2014, p.97 "

Visit https://study.sagepub.com/essentialchildnursing to access a wealth of online resources for this chapter – watch out for the margin icons throughout the chapter.

INTRODUCTION

As nurses and professionals it is important to be aware of the way in which we give nursing care to our patients or clients and in particular to children, young people and their parents and carers. As highlighted in the opening quote, CYP are cared for in a variety of settings. In this chapter we will consider assessment, planning care, implementing and evaluating care, and the handover and referral of care. In all these we will look at how we organise and deliver care and why we do this in the way we do.

In community settings, organisation and delivery of care may focus much more on who provides the services – health, social care, or education – and key strategies for promoting and protecting health. In acute clinical environments, assessment of risk and prevention of harm may be a significant issue and focus for care delivery. As Clarke and Corkin (2011) discuss, also as part of clinical governance we must be seen to practise effectively and deliver safe care, although as part of reducing costs from litigation, Clinical Negligence Schemes for Trusts (CNST) require clear risk assessment and management systems as part of the scheme (NHS Litigation Authority, 2016).

ACTIVITY 6.1: REFLECTIVE PRACTICE

Consider your current area of practice. What systems or frameworks govern the way that you work and why?

ACTIVITY
ANSWER 6.1

HISTORY OF THE NURSING PROCESS

In the past, nurses had a number of ways that care was delivered (Carter et al., 2014). Some of this was dictated by doctors, although Florence Nightingale and early nurse leaders might have argued otherwise. Some was based on tradition and the need to prevent infection and promote cleanliness. While these systems were not based on evidence and holistic patient-centred care, they had a purpose in that things were not forgotten or missed and were systematic. They reflected nursing theory of the time. McFarlane (1986) argued that there had been a need to change from this approach.

In 1967 the 'nursing process' became known through the work of Yura and Walsh. The nursing process represented a systematic approach which demonstrated a holistic basis for care and asked nurses to see the care process in a cyclical manner based on the patient's needs. This process still underpins many of the systems that we use today. This was also the basis for the development of individualised care plans.

Nursing models

Nursing models are theoretical frameworks devised to support the assessment and delivery of nursing care defined as 'abstract frameworks, linking facts and phenomena, that assist nurses to plan nursing care, investigate problems related to clinical practice, and study the outcomes of nursing actions and intervention' (McFerran, 2008). Another way of understanding this is the idea that models represent what nursing is a picture or representation of what nursing is (Pearson et al., 1996).

Nursing models were originally developed in the 1960s and were mainly North American in origin. Murphy et al. (2010) describe how a range of influences brought about their development.

Technological advances in medicine and a need to recognise the profession of nursing led to early nurse theorists' wish to demonstrate the unique body of knowledge specific to nursing, hence the development of a nursing model. In their attempts to define nursing, early theorists appeared to reflect on one of our earliest influences, Florence Nightingale, and her focus on health and the environment.

From the 1970s, and more so in the 1980s, there was a proliferation of UK-based texts demonstrating an interpretation of the initial models and their application to UK settings (Aggleton and Chalmers, 1986; Kershaw and Salvage, 1986; Walsh, 1991).

In defining the concept of a nursing model, most authors at the time described key concepts or aspects which a nursing model would incorporate. These included:

- The person – receiving nursing care
- The environment – and surroundings where the person is situated
- Health – the illness or wellness state
- Nursing actions (Kershaw and Salvage, 1986; Fawcett, 1995)

So each nursing model depends on the setting or underlying philosophy and reflects nursing from a different perspective, such as psychological or sociological principles. Nurses were encouraged to seek out the most appropriate model of nursing to their setting and patients (Walsh, 1991).

The dominance of the medical model of care based on illness-focused assessment and treatment was to some degree the political driver for nurses to develop their own framework for nursing towards a more patient-focused model which reflected what nurses actually do. However, it could be argued that the most popular models such as Roper et al.'s (1985) do reflect a systems-based approach but more closely focused on the needs of human beings. Known as the activities of daily living, these are:

- Maintaining a safe environment
- Communicating
- Breathing
- Eating and drinking
- Eliminating
- Personal cleansing and dressing
- Controlling body temperature
- Mobilising
- Working and playing
- Expressing sexuality
- Sleeping
- Dying

In acute care settings in both adult and children's settings, the activities are frequently reflected in nursing documentation today.

So it is clear that different environments and client groups require their care to be organised to reflect their needs, hence the development of models or philosophies to reflect this.

ACTIVITY 6.2: REFLECTIVE PRACTICE

Thinking about your current or most recent practice placement, what nursing model or underlying principles underpin how nursing care is delivered? If you could not identify one, why might this be important to your clients?

ACTIVITY
ANSWER 6.2

Ann Casey developed the 'Partnership model' in 1988 to represent how we work with children and families as children's nurses. Casey utilised five paradigms as in previous models: child, health, environment, family, nurse. She also demonstrates the interaction between child, family and nurse.

The principles of the model are that it demonstrates mutual respect for the child and family; it recognises the age continuum, recognises care at home and in hospital, and involves negotiation and sharing/a partnership approach. Although the model has not been further developed, the principle underlies much of how children's nursing care is delivered, and to this end it could be argued that the principle of 'family-centred care' is also a model for children's nursing practice (Smith et al., 2002; Shields et al., 2006).

Smith et al. (2002) outlined the evolving concept of family-centred care in their now key text *Family Centred Care*. Coleman reflects that changing society and policy together to reflect the wider family is such that family-centred care is a cornerstone of children's nursing practice. Their model/concept demonstrates a continuum of involvement of families, partnership with nurses to parent-led care agreed following negotiation with the parent and child. Congruent with developing knowledge and a changing approach to children and their families, the second edition of this text is entitled *Child and Family-centred Healthcare* (Smith and Coleman, 2010).

There is some debate around the validity of family-centred care in current practice (Shields et al., 2008) and recently 'child-centred nursing' has been promoted as a more appropriate term to promote the idea that children are at the centre of our thinking as active participants in their care (Carter and Ford, 2013; Carter et al., 2014). So, it could be argued that 'child-centred care' is the most current model for nursing practice.

ASSESSMENT STRATEGIES IN A RANGE OF SETTINGS

Assessment is the foundation for the provision of patient-focused care. It is key when planning the correct care process and it is integral to effective patient and family-centred care planning. Assessment is about gathering information about a patient in order to identify their needs.

Assessment usually occurs following the initial referral of care. This referral may be from a variety of sources (see below). Assessment is an essential skill that all nurses must have in order to make subsequent decisions and decide on the next step of care. This might be at delivery for resuscitation of a pre-term infant to the admission of a 15-year-old who has consumed excessive amounts of alcohol.

Nursing assessment is vital for planning safe care and a structured framework is essential. This is not a new concept but one that has evolved over time as nursing assessment tools have been developed. Nursing assessment is not deemed an easy process to complete and therefore the use of assessment tools has become an integral part of the process. These will be discussed later. An important aspect of a nurse's role in all areas where children are cared for is the ability to undertake a systematic assessment.

SCENARIO 6.1: JAKE

Jake is a four-year-old brought by his parents directly to the emergency department with wheezing. Jake has had no previous medical input or assessment. Consider the same child two hours later being admitted to a paediatric ward from the emergency department.

- You are the admitting nurse: how would the assessment process differ to that completed by the emergency department nurse? See the definitions below to help with this.

Assessment on admission requires a comprehensive nursing assessment, including patient history, general appearance, physical examination and vital signs completed at the time of admission.

The child in the above scenario, when admitted to the emergency department, would have required a complete assessment including a full history from the parents.

Assessment, when taking over patient care on a shift, differs slightly. It requires a concise nursing assessment completed at the commencement of each shift, or if the patient's condition changes at any other time during your shift. If you were the nurse taking over the care of the child in the above scenario the information received from the thorough assessment in the emergency department would reduce the need for a full assessment on the ward. You should prioritise vital signs to ensure that the condition has not changed during the time between admission and transfer to the ward. Your focus will include ensuring that the child is safe and comfortable.

A focused assessment includes a detailed nursing assessment of specific body system(s) relating to the presenting problem or current concern(s) of the patient (Royal Children's Hospital Melbourne, 2015).

A child who has received no medical input would require a more urgent assessment to alleviate any immediate concerns. This assessment may not take the same approach as that by staff working on the acute ward admitting a child who has received previous care either by the emergency department staff or by the team in theatre. There should be a structured approach. However, the priority may differ from that of immediate safety to pain control or emotional and family support.

The baseline observation and recording of clinical data forms the foundation of the process, irrelevant of the order that it takes. Accurately recording significant data such as the child's blood pressure, temperature, respiratory rate and oxygen saturations can not only form a baseline foundation to measure against but can escalate care and avoid deterioration. It is often the nurse who will have initial contact with the child and family when they enter a healthcare environment. It is the information obtained by the nursing assessment, therefore, that can direct the care provision. The respiratory rate has been identified as one of the most important clinical signs observed, especially in children, and one that can direct care to alleviate life-threatening symptoms (Breakell, 2004; Watson 2006) but also one which can has been missed in the past.

SCENARIO 6.2: JAKOB

You are taking over care of a two-day-old baby named Jakob on a children's ward. Jakob was admitted the previous day with respiratory distress. Following a clinical assessment and some oxygen therapy the child is now deemed ready for discharge. All monitoring has therefore ceased.

During your shift assessment you acknowledge that the infant now has a raised respiratory rate and subcostal recession.

- Why would this cause you concern?
- And what other assessments might you now consider?
- What would your next action be?

SCENARIO
ANSWER 6.2

Children's conditions can change rapidly and the skills of assessment to recognise these changes are fundamental to the nursing role. The reliable identification of changes in a child's condition can alleviate further deterioration or even prevent admission to intensive care areas. It has been recognised that deterioration of critically ill patients has usually been present prior to collapse (Roland, 2013).

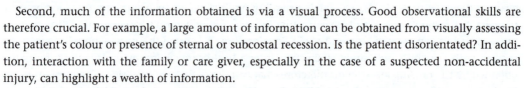

ACTIVITY 6.3: REFLECTIVE PRACTICE

Consider the assessment of a child with whom you have been recently involved during a placement. Did you utilise all of your senses when carrying out this assessment? Which sense was your most useful tool?

NURSING SKILLS AND PATIENT ASSESSMENT

SEE ALSO
CHAPTER 2

Nurses require a set of key skills to be effective in the process of patient assessment. First, they require an understanding of human physiology. In order to highlight deviations from the normal it is vital to have the ability to recognise the normal. It is important to have an understanding of why the respiratory rate in a child who has an underlying respiratory condition may be vital in the speed of escalation required. Nursing assessment of the child often requires additional skills and knowledge in addition to anatomy and physiology. The relationship between age, development and communication ability is particularly significant and it is therefore important for the nurse to have a clear understanding of developmental milestones as these may offer additional assessment information.

SEE ALSO
CHAPTER 9

Second, much of the information obtained is via a visual process. Good observational skills are therefore crucial. For example, a large amount of information can be obtained from visually assessing the patient's colour or presence of sternal or subcostal recession. Is the patient disorientated? In addition, interaction with the family or care giver, especially in the case of a suspected non-accidental injury, can highlight a wealth of information.

One of the most fundamental aspects of nursing assessment and a priority area is communication. Unlike adult patient care, where a large proportion of information is gathered directly from the patient, children's nurses work with an array of age groups some of which may not be able to communicate effectively. This is where an ability to adapt your skills is important. An understanding of child development will enable you to adapt your communication skills in order to engage effectively and gather the correct information needed for an appropriate plan of care or referral. Consider two types of questioning and how they might affect the response. Open-ended questions are more likely to elicit more detailed information. This might lead to a more probing approach to questioning should a need be perceived. Lambert et al. (2011) suggest that in practice health professionals position children as either passive bystanders or active participants in the communication process, which is a consideration when reflecting on your skills during the assessment process.

The most effective tools you can use are listening skills. The information divulged can be vital for the nursing assessment to establish the key areas of concern, both for the patient and the family.

The use of assessment tools

Assessment tools are what offer the mechanism to gather a score or referral algorithm. Because of the nature of the scoring system, all early warning systems utilise the benefits of technology in some way to aid with scoring saturation, heart rate monitoring, etc. Watson (2006) suggests that nurses have in the past been required to record but not necessarily interpret clinical observations. This, however, is not the case in many clinical areas where nurses are at the first point of patient contact and are often the gatekeepers to specific medical input. Competency is therefore paramount to safe assessment. Many acute areas now work with a triage system. Being able to interpret clinical information to direct clinical care is a skill which is required by all nurses carrying out assessment.

SBAR (Situation/background/assessment/recommendation)

Many children's observation and assessment units utilise an SBAR tool (NHS Institute, 2013). This enables the handover of care from the GP in the community to the acute paediatric area. The SBAR enables nursing coordinators not only to prepare for the child's arrival but to anticipate what has already been assessed prior to arrival. This involves communicating what treatment has already been commenced. There has been an increase in the need for nurses to assess and refer patients correctly in order to increase efficiency of care. The areas where children are cared for are constantly evolving in order to be more clinically effective and efficient. This has resulted in more responsibility being placed upon nursing assessment.

PEWS (Paediatric early warning score)

In many acute areas, the use of a PEWS is a common early warning tool. Early warning tools highlight clinical deterioration based on physiological parameters. Early warning tools were first used in adult nursing but have been adapted to suit paediatric patients. Although no early warning score for the use of children has been universally validated, many areas have adopted such a tool.

The PEWS enables clinical teams to recognise patients who are deteriorating and act accordingly. This tool can be adapted according to the patient group. It must, however, have the key areas of physiological assessment embedded, which in turn indicate a clear need for referral or escalation. Alongside the scoring tool there needs to be a recommendation flow chart, which allows the nurse to act upon the score obtained. This action may relate to an increase in clinical observations, or in more serious situations an urgent referral to the medical teams. The sequence of a clinical assessment may require some adaptation according to the age or needs of the child. Assessment often leads to referral to other professionals.

IDENTIFYING AND PLANNING CARE NEEDS

Following the underpinning approach reflected in *The Nursing Process* (Yura and Walsh, 1967) and in other developments of this cyclical process (see Figure 6.1), the second and third stages focus on the identification and planning of care needs. This follows earlier assessment of the child and family as discussed in the previous section.

Planning care needs will depend on the setting and client group, and this context may mean that different language is used to reflect the process. Early versions of the nursing process used the term 'problem' or 'patient problem', 'patient need', or 'nursing diagnosis', often in North American settings (NANDA, 2008). There is also consideration of the cause and nature of the problem – an anatomical or physiological malfunction or the inability of the person to adapt their behaviour to the situation they find themselves in. Problems or needs may be physical, social, psychological and/or spiritual, and their identification may depend on the focus of that assessment, the practitioner and the client.

Planning care can and does also take into account potential problems or assessment of risk, such as the risks of an anaesthetic or operation, or the risks to physical or mental health of certain behaviours. However, it could be argued that potential problems are not necessarily the child or family's problem, but pertain to the nurse's role in minimising risk.

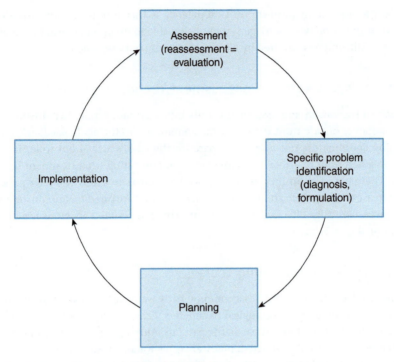

Figure 6.1 The Nursing Process (Pryjmachuk, 2011)

PRACTICE
SCENARIO 6:
CHERYL

ACTIVITY 6.4: REFLECTIVE PRACTICE

In your practice setting, when you have identified patient needs and are planning 'goals', to what degree are these goals those of the child and family or the nurse? Consider the earlier discussion in the section on nursing models about the debate around child-centred care/ family-centred care.

ACTIVITY
ANSWER 6.4

So, the focus on holistic and individualised patient care from the development of the nursing process implied that needs and goals should be patient centred and should be negotiated with the child and family (Aggleton and Chalmers, 1986). Lloyd (2010) states that in current policy it is an expectation that clients and carers are involved in all aspects of planning and that practitioners should have this philosophy at the heart of what we do. This principle has existed for many years in policy and guidance around caring for children.

Once problems and goals have been identified it is important to consider priorities in the care of children and their families. Clarke and Corkin (2011) discuss how the nurse should be able to clearly articulate and document priorities in care, communicate effectively with the child and family, and encourage and support negotiation of care planning (Corlett and Twycross, 2006).

Problems and goals may be further prioritised by considering level of need, risk and availability of resources (Lloyd, 2010). For example, for the child who is admitted to the emergency department following a head injury and is currently unconscious, although there are also safeguarding issues his immediate physical health would take priority and his level of risk of further harm would be reduced if he were admitted to hospital. The availability of access to resources such as the multidisciplinary team out of hours might be reduced at certain times, hence the need for the nurse to make competent judgements based on knowledge and experience.

Furthermore, it is recommended that goals are SMART: specific, measurable, achievable/agreed, realistic and time limited (Clarke and Corkin, 2011), which may be appropriate in some settings more than others. However, the introduction of time parameters could serve as the impetus for evaluation and reassessment of the original goal.

SCENARIO 6.3: SARAH

Sarah is 10 years old and has a diagnosis of cystic fibrosis. She was admitted to an acute paediatric ward. The hospital policy is that all medication must be administered by the nursing team. A delay in this administration caused the mother to verbalise her distress and frustration at not being given the authority to administer medication that she gives daily at home.

✓

• How could this situation have been better managed?

SCENARIO
ANSWER 6.3

Care planning in different settings may be adapted further by the use of documentation and other systems which in some cases allow standardisation of care plans. In the case of operative procedures, many trusts utilise integrated care pathways.

An integrated care pathway (ICP) is a multidisciplinary outline of anticipated care, within an appropriate timeframe, to help a patient with a specific condition or set of symptoms move progressively through a clinical experience to positive outcomes. Integrated care pathways are usually agreed within an organisation and are usually child specific. Variation from the pathway can be indicated to show individual patient need. They may also minimise risk where key actions are necessary (Clarke and Corkin, 2011).

Many acute clinical areas also use standardised care plans that can be adapted to the individual patient, which may be more time efficient. Emergency departments also incorporate clinical guidance by developing condition-related algorithms or decision trees in order to standardise treatment in fast-paced environments.

> "
> I have used ICPs and standardised care plans whilst in practice. I found that standardised care plans and pathways are a helpful tool for students who have little experience or knowledge in how to care for children with particular illnesses as they outline the care and procedures nurses need to deliver in each circumstance. I found as a student, it is a useful guide to follow which I can use to plan and implement care for the child.
>
> **Natalie, 3rd-year children's nursing student**
> "

In community settings where the focus of care is on the wider family, parenting and/or areas of other need, documents such as the Common Assessment Framework (CAF) are frequently used to identify significant areas of need to support the child in his or her environment (see the section on referrals below). The assessment of a child and family using a CAF requires the involvement of the child/family, assessing professional and any other professionals who are subsequently required to meet any identified needs of the child and/or family. There have been criticisms from professionals (head teachers, school nurses, health visitors) that the CAF is not is not very friendly to the whole family and has been too focused on assessing and meeting the needs of the child. And so the move to the use of 'Early Help Assessments' (EHAs) in places like Manchester in the north-west of

England, support the 'Think Family' approach and emphasises that any kind of early intervention assessment should be based on a conversation with the families about their needs and what they would like to get out of their involvement with agencies.

——— SAFEGUARDING STOP POINT ———

If a child is subject to a child protection plan, there is a statutory requirement for all agencies to meet as a core group with the child and parents/carers to review the plans at regular intervals as set out at the initial child protection conference. The care plans of looked after children are reviewed within 28 days of the child coming into care, then at six-monthly intervals whilst the child remains looked after. Health professionals are seen as active partners in the planning process for young people subject of CP Plans and care orders and they can request additional meetings if plans are not fulfilling the needs of the child or additional risk factors are identified.

Once care is identified and care plans are agreed practitioners are required (NMC, 2015) and the code, to communicate plans with the child and family but also the Multidisciplinary team Information sharing (HM Government, 2015b).

A number of formats and approaches may be used in different settings; this may depend on priority, risk and availability of resources as before. However, some form of written/permanent communication would normally be required to support a verbal handover via face to face or telephone, etc. The standard of documentation would be required to be in keeping with minimal Nursing & Midwifery Council (NMC) guidance (2015) and trust Caldicott guardian principles for information governance (HSCIC, 2015).

IMPLEMENTING AND EVALUATING CARE PLANS

Following on from the previous section, as care is planned and goals are agreed it is important as practitioners that we also consider the nature of the care that we deliver and how it is delivered.

The NMC (2015) asks us to ensure that care is safe and effective and that practitioners should maintain skills and knowledge for effective practice. We should also be confident that the care we implement is based on the best evidence; research and development has helped practitioners by the development of guidance, such as NICE, SIGN, clinical nursing procedures and trust guidelines for practice. However, a good deal of the care we give is not necessarily based on empirical research. McKenna et al. (2000) explore this argument in some detail. As nurses, using our clinical judgement in additional to the available evidence is key to the recognition of professional practice.

Care that is planned may not necessarily be delivered by the person who instigated the care plan; it may be handed over or delegated to another person. The NMC (2015) is very clear about the need to work cooperatively and maintain communication with others (this is explored further in the referral section of this chapter). In addition, care that is delegated should be within the competence of the person it is delegated to and the practitioner should ensure that care meets the required standard.

A qualified nurse can delegate to a student a task such as recording vital signs, but the member of staff, whether or not he or she is a mentor, must be sure the student is able to do this competently and should ascertain that the task was completed appropriately and seek assurance that this was done. He/she remains accountable.

Where care is delivered will also have an influence on how it is delivered. In acute settings there is not only local and national guidance but frequently a variety of other personnel whom practitioners can draw on for help and advice should the situation require this. In community settings, practitioners

SEE ALSO
CHAPTER 7

often work alone and the opportunity to seek advice and support is not so easily available. Hence, those working in community settings need to draw on a greater level of knowledge and experience in order to work independently (Andrews and Barnum, 2009).

Working in families' homes also brings about other considerations, in respect of the family's own environment and their family time (Sidey and Widdas, 2005).

Recording and documenting care given is also pertinent (NMC, 2015). Legal challenges have highlighted cases where care was apparently given but not documented, and decisions were given in favour of the patient where the legal point in law 'not recorded not done' was used in support of this.

The final stage of evaluation provides the end/beginning point of the cycle to allow reassessment of the situation and to assess whether the nursing intervention has been effective. Setting goals or timescales for reassessment or reassessing care on a recognised schedule allows clear pathways to evaluate and align care more closely with patient need. However, as previously discussed, the practitioner should have skills to evaluate the care and outcome with the child and family and redefine the next stage of care or decide to discharge the child from the current setting. Unfortunately, this is not always the case (see Amy's scenario).

SCENARIO 6.4: AMY

Amy is 15 years old and is being placed in foster care following child protection concerns and ongoing health issues. As a result of this move Amy has changed schools. Due to a delay in the transfer of health records the school nurse at Amy's new school has no information regarding the previous child protection concerns and therefore fails to make relevant preparations for her arrival in the school. This resulted in Amy being placed in a vulnerable situation and health needs continuing to be unmet.

- Reflect on how this situation could be avoided.

Referrals

In the community care of children where there are child protection concerns, documented evaluations of care are paramount to effective transfer of care.

The referral process often involves the transfer of clinical responsibility from one health professional to another professional. A referral is often not a simple process but a highly complex interaction involving multiple stakeholders influenced by a wide range of factors. Not all referrals are alike and research studies have put forward several typologies for distinguishing between the different types:

- Establishing diagnosis
- Treatment or operation
- Specified test/investigation
- Advice on management
- Specialist to take over management
- Reassurance/second opinion
- Reassurance for the patient and/or their family
- Other reasons

It is important to note that referrals can be emergency, routine and elective and as such will determine the differing referral processes (Foot et al., 2010).

SMART referrals in a technologically advancing healthcare environment is paramount if we want children to receive optimum healthcare that will enable them to improve their life chances.

Both commissioners and providers of healthcare need to be abreast of the health predictors affecting children today so that health organisations can employ effective strategies, systems and structures to meet the demands of increasingly complex issues ranging from acute and community care needing specialist intervention to safeguarding some of the most vulnerable groups in society.

Historically, children's health services were hosted and managed by different organisations and access to these services was often by a number of independent referral routes, differing in terms of entry, urgency criteria, who is eligible to refer and working to different geographical boundaries. Poor communication and coordination between services often led to duplication of work or confusion about who was responsible for meeting which particular part of a child and family's needs (Simpson and Stallard, 2004).

The Health and Social Care Act 2012 introduced a new ideology for health and social care services, modernising service delivery, developing new ways of working and providing integrated care. As a result, the strong focus on integration of primary, community, acute, specialist healthcare and social care should mean that services are more unified and organised around the needs of children and their families.

The multifaceted needs of children and families today mean referrers need referral pathways that readily navigate health systems so there is no delay or duplication and identify the most appropriate service. Single points of entry or single points of care (SPE, SPOC) systems and referral management schemes (RMS) aim to simplify and streamline access to children's health services, thus addressing issues of equity of access and coordination highlighted in *Improving Children and Young People's Health Outcomes: A System Wide Response* (DH, 2013a).

Many different referral pathways exist and local commissioning and resources differ from area to area depending on the needs of the local population.

Where children and young people are referred to the hospital, ambulatory assessment units (AAU) provide rapid access to care without hospital admission and, if admission is necessary, discharge patients home as soon as possible. Many conditions can be effectively managed at home with advice and support from specialist nurses and allied health professionals, so if necessary, following discharge from hospital or clinic, referrals need to be directed to appropriate services such as diabetes or asthma nurse specialists, health visitors and school nurses. These services can then work in collaboration with the multiagency team and through ongoing reassessment and evaluation, identify if referrals to other services are required, such as counselling or health weight management.

Local areas will also have good working relationships with third party and charitable organisations, and referrals can then be progressed for children who may need additional support around issues that can have health impacts. These can include services that help young people who may go missing from home or are at risk of child sexual exploitation, which can have an impact on emotional, sexual and physical wellbeing.

The National Institute for Health and Clinical Excellence also provides standards that guide health professionals in decision-making when progressing referrals for specific conditions. This too aims to improve early diagnosis and access to the most effective treatments. NICE guidelines are evidence based, and set out clear patient referral criteria and timeframes. Children have needs that are different from adults, and research does not define what a good quality referral entails but recognises it is multidimensional. If practitioners assessing these needs want to drive forward quality improvements, they need to consider the following to any referral they complete (Foot et al., 2010):

- Necessity: Are patients referred as and when necessary?
- Timeliness: Is this done without avoidable delay?
- Destination: Are patients referred to the most appropriate destination first time?

- Process: Is the process of referral a high-quality one, in the following respects:

  ○ Does the referral contain the necessary information in an accessible format?
  ○ Are children and families offered a choice of time and location, and are they supported in making this decision?
  ○ Can the referrer, patient and specialist form a shared understanding of the purpose and expectations of the referral?
  ○ Is pre-referral management adequate?

School nurses, health visitors and community nurses are well positioned to work with their multiagency partners such as education and social care to utilise the Early Help Assessment Framework (EHA) for assessing the needs of children and families. The framework allows them to identify what support is needed and, therefore, lead on progressing referrals to the appropriate services without duplication. By working with a child- and family-centred approach and consulting with other agencies they can streamline professional involvement.

The framework allows practitioners to identify where needs lie and to make a clinical judgement on the impact to the child's health using the levels of need descriptors.

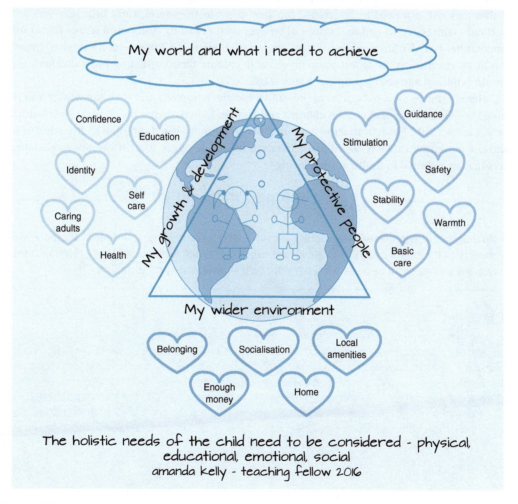

The holistic needs of the child need to be considered - physical, educational, emotional, social
amanda kelly - teaching fellow 2016

Figure 6.2 My world. Amanda Kelly, teaching fellow, University of Manchester

WHAT'S THE EVIDENCE?

Most families will at some point face an issue that requires a level of support, whether related to health, employment, poverty or other social problems. As an example, it is estimated that around 20 to 30% of children and young people will have additional needs at some point in their lives – some for a limited period, and others for longer. The human costs of reaching crisis point before services intervene and the financial costs of providing acute-level services are significantly higher than those associated with earlier interventions, leading to the logical conclusion that providing support at an earlier stage will save money over the longer term and improve individuals' quality of life (Rallings and Payne, 2016, p. 5).

Referral to treatment (RTT) within an ever-changing and technologically advancing health service is beset with potential obstacles in an effort to navigate children and families not only to the correct service but within the maximum waiting time in order to meet equality and consistency targets, and patient satisfaction and experience.

Children don't often need to be 'treated' per se; however, but they do need expert guidance from universal and specialist services in order to help them make healthier choices with a desired outcome so that they will not need to be referred for 'treatment' in the future. Early help strategies are an excellent example of this and so if universal services such as health visitors and school nurses in the communities can identify needs early, they can 'refer' children at a lower level for targeted intervention in an effort to try to deflect some preventable chronic illness afflicting the individuals today, affecting children and young people at a later stage.

Children's nurses need to be seen as preventive health champions and their knowledge and skills should be used in a way that enables children and families to make better life choices. The Health and Social Care Act 2012 has activated the move to more community-based care, and by investing in early help and preventive care it is hoped that referrals of the future can be more streamlined to health services that are essential to health and wellbeing.

SAFEGUARDING STOP POINT

Multi-agency levels of need descriptors should enable practitioners to evidence the potential impacts to the child's health from abuse and neglect. This will facilitate a SMART referral to the relevant agency and if necessary a referral for further assessment of risk/harm.

> "
> When young people are referred to the multiagency child sexual exploitation (CSE) team, they are discussed at a daily governance meeting. My role as the CSE nurse specialist is to liaise with the health professionals around that young person as they often have key information that can help inform risk assessments. My involvement enables the coordination of intervention and advice that can help to minimise further risks – i.e. referral to sexual health services or referral to healthy weight management or dental services; quite often it is issues such as low self-esteem and body confidence that can leave young people more vulnerable to exploitation.
>
> **Kathy March, senior specialist CSE nurse**
> "

DEVELOPING TECHNOLOGY IN THE ORGANISATION OF CARE

The development of a range of technology over the last 30 years has changed the way that we deliver care in a number of ways, and as technologies continue to develop, nurses need to be aware of the potential benefits to care for children and their families and considerations for professional practice.

As nurses we are generally very familiar with some of the developments of monitoring equipment and day-to-day equipment that we use. It can be difficult to consider how we would be able to function without what we now consider to be basic items of equipment, such as the bed that is adjustable in height and position, moving and handling equipment, and the increase in availability of monitoring systems for taking vital signs – even the electronic thermometer. Consider using a mercury thermometer with a wriggling child! While the benefits are clear for preventing injury, reducing risk and promoting comfort for the child, as professionals we should be mindful of the appropriate use of technology for the correct purpose, the need for training and the importance of maintenance of equipment. Some would argue that overuse of technology can lead to an overreliance on monitoring readings and a loss of key skills in assessment.

However, the availability of such equipment that is now much more portable has a direct impact on the care of children in community and home settings, such as monitoring equipment, adaptations for the home, feeding devices and other technology. Children can be cared for at home and avoid hospital admissions where community nurses, GPs and families have access to such technology.

'eHealth' is defined by the RCN (2012) as a 'means of promoting, empowering and facilitating health and wellbeing with individuals, families and communities and enhancing professional practice through the use of information management and information and communication technologies'. This can include telephone consultations, telephone or text health advice and management, submission of patient health information, remote consultation between patient and doctor – telemedicine, Internet-based social networks and support groups.

ACTIVITY 6.5: CRITICAL THINKING

Are you using any of the above aspects of eHealth with children and their families? What benefits do you see for children and their families?

Future developments projected by NHS Digital Technology (2015) for funding across a range of NHS trusts include:

- Digitally-enabled observation management
- Mobile access to digital care records across the community
- Digital capture of clinical data at point of care
- Safer clinical interventions
- Real-time digital nursing dashboards
- Smart workforce deployment

- Remote face-to-face interaction
- Digital images for nursing care (www.england.nhs.uk)

There are a number of considerations and potential drawbacks outlined in RCN guidance (2012). These include access issues, patient and staff attitudes, support for alternative language and sensory restrictions, and overuse of services.

As nurses we are both professionally and legally required to account for our actions, which involves keeping a record of assessments, conversations, care given and referrals made. We are guided by the NMC Code (2015), section 10, 'Keep clear and accurate records relevant to your practice'.

The updated guidance includes six key aspects:

- Completing records at the time
- Identifying risks and the steps taken to deal with them
- Accurate record-keeping and reporting if someone else has not done so
- Attributing records to yourself with the date and time, and no jargon or speculation
- Keeping records secure
- Treating all data and research findings appropriately

NHS trusts are required to audit the documentation of their employees on a regular basis as a part of clinical governance requirements. Trusts also have responsibilities following the Caldicott review in 1997 to appoint a Caldicott guardian (HSCIC, 2015a) who is responsible for information governance. This involves training for all employees, safe and secure systems for all records to ensure confidentiality but also appropriate access to those who need information. The move to electronic data and records brings new challenges for the NHS in developing information systems that are compatible and robust for the 21st century, particularly where health and social care professionals need to communicate and share information.

As highlighted earlier in this chapter, sharing information is key to joined-up working in healthcare practice, in particular in safeguarding information (DH, 2013b; HM Government, 2015). It is also indicated a number of times in the NMC Code (2015) in relation to working cooperatively. Considering the range of settings in which children are cared for it is understandable that there may be difficulties in accessing and sharing information, between nurses and other professions.

Community nurses may have paper-based records which they need to carry with them during visits and need to store safely between visits. In some services the records are kept in the patient's home or a duplicate version is kept with the child at home. Increasingly though, school and community nurses are using electronic records, although these systems are not always compatible. In community settings eHealth developments may include the use of specific apps and websites which support children and families with particular conditions.

In acute areas many trusts are now 'paperless', which includes electronic records, recording of vital signs on computer systems and medicines administration supported by technology. Thus it is important to recognise these are not without their limitations, such as problems with access, availability of resources, the need for training, systems and individual error.

A final consideration with regard to documentation and technology is that patients have a legal right to access to their records under the Freedom of Information Act 2000. This is also supported by the Code (NMC, 2015). As nurses we should consider how we can support children and their families in accessing their records and being partners in their care. New developments in technology may help or hinder their access to information.

CHAPTER SUMMARY

- Different environments and client groups require their care to be organised to reflect the needs of individual children and young people.
- Assessment is the foundation of care delivery and is an ongoing process which should be carried out collaboratively.
- When planning care and setting goals it is important to recognise the context and the need to work with children and families to ensure that care is delivered and evaluated in a collaborate manner.
- Looking forward, nurses need to recognise developments in technology and eHealth and utilise the benefits for children and families while being mindful of potential problems.

BUILD YOUR BIBLIOGRAPHY

Books

- Carter, B., Bray, L., Dickinson, A., Edwards, M. and Ford, K. (2014) *Child Centred Nursing: Promoting Critical Thinking*. London: Sage. Chapter 1.

  Chapter 1 introduces the history and development of family-centred care, and looks at recent development in the contexts and settings.

- Smith, L. and Coleman, V. (2010) *Child and Family-centred Healthcare: Concept, Theory and Practice*, 2nd edn. Basingstoke: Palgrave Macmillan.

  This second edition of a seminal text focusing on family-centred care includes practical demonstration of empowerment, negotiation of care and this can be demonsrated in interprofessional practice.

- Corkin, D., Clarke, S. and Liggett, L. (eds) *Care Planning in Children and Young People's Nursing*. Oxford: Wiley-Blackwell.

  This book addresses a selection of the most common issues when planning care for infants, children and young people within the hospital and community setting. See particularly Chapter 1 'Care planning and delivery', Chapter 2 'Risk assessment and management', Chapter 7 'Integrated care pathways' and Chapter 8 'Interprofessional assessment'.

Articles

Go to https://study.sagepub.com/essentialchildnursing for further free online journal articles related to this chapter.

- Coyne, I., Hallstrom, I. and Soderback M. (2016) 'Reframing the focus from a family-centred care approach for children's health care'. *Journal of Child Health Care*, 20 (4).
- Shields, L. (2015) 'Family-centred care: the "captive mother" revisited'. *Journal of the Royal Society of Medicine*, 109 (4): 137-40.

  These two articles present arguments on the changing focus around children's nursing. They present challenging philosophies to reflect current societal and practices. They also highlight

FURTHER
READING:
ONLINE
JOURNAL
ARTICLES

(Continued)

(Continued)

children's rights and current family perspectives in Western culture and challenge care givers around their own perpectives.

- Stafford, V., Hutchby, I., Karim, K. and O'Reilly, M. (2016) '"Why are you here?" Seeking children's accounts of their presentation to Child and Adolescent Mental Health Service (CAMHS)'. *Clin Child Psychol Psychiatry*, 21 (1): 3-18.
  This article explores, on referral to a Child and Adolescent Mental Health Service (CAMHS), the naturally occurring first assessments to discover the beliefs that children hold regarding their reasons for attendance and the implications this has for the trajectory of the appointment and later engagement with interventions.

- Tointon, K. and Hunt, J.A. (2016) 'How holistic nursing can enhance the quality of life of children with cystic fibrosis'. *Nursing Children and Young People*, 28 (8): 22-5.
  This article draws on a case study to demonstrate a holistic approach to providing care in both home and hospital settings for a 15-year-old girl with cystic fibrosis.

Weblinks

FURTHER
READING:
WEBLINKS

Go to https://study.sagepub.com/essentialchildnursing for further weblinks related to this chapter.

- NHS England, *NHS Digital Technology: Harnessing the Information Revolution*
  www.england.nhs.uk/digitaltechnology
  This NHS-supported website highlights developments in digital technology across the NHS.

- Nursing & Midwifery Council (NMC), *The Code for Nurses and Midwives*
  www.nmc.org.uk/standards/code
  The NMC website offers support and guidance for nurses, employers and the public around standards and expectations of all nurses. There are a number of publications including *The Code* and information about hearings.

- Action for Sick Children, *Timeline*
  www.actionforsickchildren.org.uk/timeline-2
  This website is a key charity and pressure group. Originally formed to support the care of children in hospital, they have promoted campaigns around parental accommodation and the development of children's services in the UK.

ACE YOUR ASSESSMENT

ONLINE
QUIZZES &
ACTIVITY
ANSWERS

Revise what you have learned by visiting https://study.sagepub.com/essentialchildnursing

- Test yourself with multiple-choice and short-answer questions
- Do the chapter activities in the book and check your answers online

REFERENCES

Aggleton, P. and Chalmers, H. (1986) *Nursing Models and the Nursing Process*. London: Macmillan.

Andrews, L. and Barnum, A. (2009) 'The newly qualified practitioner in acute settings', in J. Hughes and G. Lyte (eds), *Developing Nursing Practice with Children and Young People*. Oxford: Wiley.

Breakell, A. (2004) 'The Respi-check oxygen mask'. *The British Journal of Resuscitation*, 3 (2): 21.

Casey, A. (1988) 'The partnership model with child and family'. *Senior Nurse*, 4: 8–9.

Carter, B. and Ford, K. (2013) 'Researching children's health experiences: the place for participatory, child centred, arts-based approaches'. *Research in Nursing and Health*, 36 (1): 95–107.

Carter, B., Bray, L., Dickinson, A., Edwards, M. and Ford, K. (2014) *Child Centred Nursing: Promoting Critical Thinking*. London: Sage.

Clarke, S. and Corkin, D. (2011) 'Risk assessment and management', in D. Corkin, S. Clarke and L. Liggett (eds) *Care Planning in Children and Young People's Nursing*. Oxford: Wiley-Blackwell.

Corlett, J. and Twycross, A. (2006) 'Negotiation of care by children's nurses: lessons from research'. *Paediatric Nursing*, 18 (8): 34–7.

Department of Health (2013a) *Improving Children and Young People's Health Outcomes: A System Wide Response*. London: DH.

Department of Health (2013) *Information: To Share or Not to Share? The Information Governance Review*. London: DH.

Fawcett, J. (1995) *Analysis and Evaluation of Conceptual Models of Nursing*. Philadephia, PA: F.A. Davis.

Foot, C., Naylor, C. and Imison, C. (2010) *The Quality of GP Diagnosis and Referral*. London: Kings Fund. Available at: www.kingsfund.org.uk/sites/files/kf/Diagnosis%20and%20referral.pdf (accessed 28 October 2015).

Health and Social Care Information Centre (HSCIC) (2015a) *Caldicott Guardians*. Available at http://systems.hscic.gov.uk/infogov/caldicott (accessed 9 December 2015). The HSCIC is now called NHS Digital (https://digital.nhs.uk/)

Health and Social Care Information Centre (HSCIC) (2015b) *Information Governance Toolkit*. Available at www.igt.hscic.gov.uk/Caldicott2.aspx?tk=423455759240822&cb=cd0a4b06-5736-4743-bd01-8f18dd41b04d&lnv=18&clnav=YES (accessed 9 December 2015).

Holmes, L. and McDermid, S. (2014) 'The Common Assessment Framework: the impact of the lead professional on families and professionals as part of a continuum of care in England'. *Child and Family Social Work*. DOI: 10.1111/cfs.12174

HM Government (2015a) *Working Together to Safeguard Children*. London: DfE.

HM Government (2015b) *Information Sharing: Advice for Practitioners Providing Safeguarding Services to Children, Young People, Parents and Carers*. London: DfE.

Information Commissioner's Office (2015) Available at https://ico.org.uk (accessed 9 December 2015).

Kershaw, B. and Salvage, J. (1986) *Models for Nursing*. Chichester: Wiley.

Lambert, V., Glacken, M. and McCarron, M. (2011) 'Communication between children and health professionals in a child hospital setting: a child transitional communication model'. *Journal of Advanced Nursing*, 67 (3): 569–82.

Lloyd, M. (2010) *A Practical Guide to Care Planning in Health and Social Care*. Maidenhead: Open University Press.

Manchester City Council (2015) *Multi-Agency Levels of Need and Response Framework: April 2015. Delivering Effective Support for Children, Young People and Families*. Available at: www.manchester.gov.uk/download/downloads/id/21076/multi_agency_need_and_reponse_framework (accessed 31 August 2017).

McFarlane, J. (1986) in B. Kershaw and J. Salvage (eds), *Models for Nursing*. Chichester: Wiley.

McFerran, T. (2008) Fifth edition, *Oxford Dictionary of Nursing*. Oxford: Oxford University Press

McKenna, H., Cutcliffe, J. and McKenna, P. (2000) 'Evidence based practice: demolishing some myths'. *Nusing Standard*, 14 (16): 39–42.

Murphy, F., Williams, A. and Pridmore, J. (2010) 'Nursing models and contemporary nursing 1: their development, uses and limitations'. *Nursing Times*, 106: 23.

North American Nursing Diagnosis Association (NANDA) (2008) 'Appendix C 2007–2008 NANDA-approved nursing diagnoses'. Available at http://wps.prenhall.com/wps/media/objects/3918/4012970/NursingTools/koz74686_AppC.pdf (accessed 9 December 2015).

NHS England (2015) *Digital Technology*. Available at www.england.nhs.uk/digitaltechnology (accessed 9 December 2015).

NHS Institute for Innovation and Improvement (NHSIII) (2013) *SBAR – Situation Background Assessment Recommendation*. Available at: www.institute.nhs.uk/safer_care/safer_care/situation_background_assessment_recommendation.html (accessed 21 December 2015).

NHS Litigation Authority (2016) *Clinical Claims*. Available at: www.nhsla.com/Claims/Pages/Clinical.aspx (accessed 20 June 2017).

Nursing and Midwifery Council (2010) *Record Keeping: Guidance for Nurses and Midwives*. London: NMC.

Nursing and Midwifery Council (NMC) (2015) *The Code: Professional Standards of Practice and Behaviour for Nurses and Midwives*. London: NMC.

Pearson, A., Vaughan, B. and Fitzgerald, M. (1996) *Models for Nursing Practice*. Oxford: Butterworth Heinmann.

Pryjmachuk, S. (2011) *Mental Health Nursing: An Evidence-based Introduction*. London: Sage.

Rallings, J. and Payne, L. (2016) *The Case for Early Support*. London: Barnardo's. Available at: www.barnardos.org.uk/case-for-early-support-2016.pdf (accessed 30 August 2017).

Roland, D. (2013) 'Paediatric early warning scores: Holy Grail and Achilles heel'. *Postgrad Med Journal*, 89: 358–65.

Roper, N., Logan, W.W. and Tierney, A. (1985) *The Elements of Nursing*, Edinburgh: Churchill Livingston.

Royal Children's Hospital Melbourne (2015) *Clinical Guidelines (Nursing)*. Available at: www.rch.org.au/rchcpg/hospital_clinical_guideline_index/Nursing_Assessment (accessed 21 December 2015).

Royal College of Nursing (2012) *Using Technology to Complement Nursing Practice: An RCN Guide for Healthcare Practitioners*. London: RCN.

Shields, L., Pratt, J. and Hunter, J. (2006) 'Family centred care: a review of qualitative studies'. *Journal of Clinical Nursing*, 15 (10): 1317–23.

Shields, L., Pratt, J., Davis, L. and Hunter, J. (2008) 'Family-centred care for children in hospital (review)'. *The Cochrane Foundation*, 3.

Sidey, A. and Widdas, D. (2005) *Textbook of Community Nursing*, 2nd edn. Edinburgh: Elsevier.

Simpson and Stallard (2004) 'Referral and access to children's health services'. *Archives of Diseases in Childhood*, 89 (2): 109–11.

Smith, L., Coleman, V. and Bradshaw, M. (2002) *Family-centred Care: Concept, Theory and Practice*. Basingstoke: Palgrave.

Smith, L. and Coleman, V. (2010) *Child and Family-centred Healthcare: Concept, Theory and Practice*, 2nd edn. Basingstoke: Palgrave Macmillan.

Walsh, M. (1991) *Models in Clinical Nursing*. London: Bailliere Tindall.

Watson, D. (2006) 'The impact of accurate patient assessment on quality of care'. *Nursing Times*, 102 (6): 34–7.

Yura, H. and Walsh, M.B. (1967) *The Nursing Process: Assessing, Planning, Implementing, Evaluating*. Norwalk, C.T.: Appleton-Century-Crofts.

COMMUNITY CARE AND CARE IN NON-HOSPITAL SETTINGS FOR CHILDREN AND YOUNG PEOPLE

7

SARAH PRICE

THIS CHAPTER COVERS

- Context of children's community care
- Application of the nursing process to families, groups and communities
- The multiagency team and working in partnership
- Common Assessment Framework/Early Help
- Supervision within a community setting
- Home visiting and personal safety
- Health promotion and education
- School nursing: support for children and young people

> Community health services are an essential component of providing person-centred, co-ordinated care. They are a diverse sector, providing a huge range of different services, and are run by a mixed economy of types and sizes of organisation, including standalone NHS community trusts, existing acute and mental health trusts, social enterprises and independent sector providers.
>
> **Foot et al., 2014, p.2**

Visit https://study.sagepub.com/essentialchildnursing to access a wealth of online resources for this chapter – watch out for the margin icons throughout the chapter.

INTRODUCTION

The importance and value of nursing children at home has been recognised nationally and internationally for more than 50 years in a variety of channels: government policy, professional bodies, voluntary sector organisations and research evidence. The first community children's nurses (CCN) teams – in Rotherham in 1949, Birmingham and Paddington in 1954, Southampton in 1969 and Gateshead 1974 – were originally developed to care for children with acute infectious diseases or short-term conditions (Muir and Sidey, 2000, in Myers, 2005). Since the early 1990s they have evolved rapidly and most areas now have a team that cares for children in the community with a wide range of healthcare needs. Many of these teams will provide care for children with acute and chronic conditions and for children who are ventilated assisted or technology dependent.

There is increasing emphasis on community-focused nursing care with the community as the client. Community is about people, places, individuals, families, groups and organisations. Community and out-of-hospital care has therefore developed even more with the increase in walk-in centres and nurse-led clinics. New opportunities are emerging for community children's nurses to engage with children and young people and their families in the design of health services to promote safe care, clinical effectiveness and better health outcomes. It is currently an exciting time for community nursing, with more of a focus on nurses working outside of the hospital, primarily in community-based settings that focus on individuals and families and endorse their unique role, encompassing key skills and knowledge that enable children and families to be cared for at home.

In this chapter you will be developing your knowledge and understanding in relation to caring for children and families in the community setting. Inherent in this will be an examination of the roles of the community children's nursing team, and there will also be a look at the role of school nurses, identifying the crucial part they play in working with children and young people.

CONTEXT OF CHILDREN'S COMMUNITY CARE

WATCH A
VIDEO ONLINE!

VIDEO LINK 5.1:
ROLE OF THE
COMMUNITY
NURSE

Since the early 1990s community care has evolved rapidly and most areas now have a team that will care for children in the community with a wide range of healthcare needs. Some policies driving the change for children have challenged community children's nurses to ensure that government plans and national standards are translated into local standards and practice; the health and social needs of children with complex care needs are therefore jointly met. Community working is part of a flexible working environment for the benefit of patients and for the health professional to manage.

In comparison to acute care:

- The community nurse is solely responsible for decisions around the care of their patients
- Nursing care is flexible and varied, and the community nurse may visit many patients each day
- Nursing care at home builds longer-term relationships with patients (Lewis and Noyes, 2008)

ACTIVITY 7.1: REFLECTIVE PRACTICE

Consider some of the other differences between nursing children in their homes and acute care. Then reflect on what benefits there may be in nursing children at home.

ACTIVITY
ANSWER 7.1

The four pathways of community care as described in the *NHS at Home: Children's Community Nursing Service* document, (DH, 2011) include:

- Children with acute and short-term conditions – breathing difficulty, fever or diarrhoea and vomiting
- Children with long-term conditions – diabetes, asthma and epilepsy
- Children with disabilities and complex conditions, including those requiring continuing care and neonates
- Children with life-limiting and life-threatening illness, including those requiring palliative and end-of-life care

Children's community nursing not only meets patients' needs relating to personal care, it also involves thorough health assessment, care planning and delivery. This care is provided to individuals or to families and groups of children. The role of the CCN has been described by McDonald et al. (1997) as being diverse, flexible and responsive to the range of healthcare needs of children whilst also maintaining its philosophy regarding service delivery.

The future of children's community nursing

Changes to undergraduate nurse education standards (NMC, 2010) mean that in the future all nurses will receive pre-registration preparation to enable them to deliver both primary and community-based care and acquire the required additional knowledge and skills to undertake leadership and advanced clinical decision-making roles in the community (RCN, 2014).

Children's services are at the top of the government agenda in all four UK countries, resulting in significant investment to support the reform of services. The needs of children are at the centre of policy, and professional boundaries and organisational barriers to integrated working are being removed.

The role of the community children's nurse encompasses education, training, emotional support and expert clinical care requiring high order cognitive skills in relation to decision-making, problem-solving and solution-finding. *Healthy Lives, Brighter Futures* (DH and DCSF, 2009) recognised the central role that community children's nurses play in the lives of children with disabilities and those with complex health needs. Within the strategy there are clear expectations that 'commissioners will need to consider how to support the development of community children's nusing services capable of providing an all-round package, including end-of-life care, 24 hours a day, seven days a week in the location preferred by the child and family' (DH and DCSF, 2009: 72). A commitment to work with health staff to develop a 'community children's service', with nursing as a central component, was explicit within the strategy (Whiting et al., 2015).

APPLICATION OF THE NURSING PROCESS TO FAMILIES, GROUPS AND COMMUNITIES

SEE ALSO
CHAPTER 6

The nursing process is made up of four interconnecting elements and has a dynamic nature (Pearson et al., 2005).

Please see Figure 7.1, which shows the four main components to the nursing process.

But let us look at the nursing process from a community nursing perspective. Care delivery in the form of the nursing process can differ from that in hospital settings but maintains the same principles (Hackett, 2013). Assessment requires strong interviewing and listening skills which can also require going beyond collecting basic physical and psychological information and include cultural, environmental and everyday life skills. Plans of care are often broader in scope and more complex than those

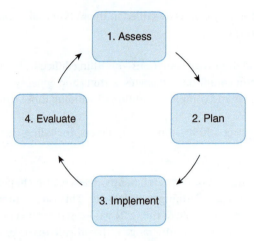

Figure 7.1 The nursing process

for hospitalised patients. The more people involved, the more extensive the plan: therefore, there is a stronger need for partnership between the nurse and client. Planned interventions need to be flexible and adapted to the client's lifestyle and the community's social and political environment. Evaluation for nurses working with large communities may be more difficult than if working with one client as this care may be measured and need more adjustments. Outcomes may not appear for a certain length of time. This means that the evaluation of care is ongoing and models and methods of cared may frequently need to be reviewed or revised.

As discussed earlier, working in the community at times needs further variation and you will face similar but different aspects of nursing care. So let us consider the nursing process more from a practical point of view when caring for children with medical needs. The example of constipation in childhood will be used here to enable you to think more critically about each element of the nursing process when applied to community care.

Constipation is the inability to pass stools regularly or empty the bowels completely (NHS Evidence, 2014). The National Institute for Health and Clinical Excellence (NICE) (2010) guideline will help all practitioners recognise their role in helping children and their families and tailoring to meet each child's individual need. Interprofessional teams will take a coordinated approach to early intervention that may reduce the incidence of constipation in children. School nurses, health visitors, children's nurses, nurses specialising in the care of children with learning disabilities and GPs have key roles in detecting and treating early symptoms of constipation.

SEE ALSO
CHAPTER 5

Throughout this section you will hear from Jamal. Jamal is aged 13 and has suffered with long-term constipation. He told me about his experiences working with the community nursing team.

Assessment

When the community nurse came to see me at home, following my operation, she came every day at first, she kept me informed of what was happening and was patient with me and didn't use big words when I was asking questions.

Jamal, child

Constipation in childhood is a problem that can cause difficulties to both the child and their family as there are a number of precipitating factors that can result in painful or infrequent bowel movements and/or soiling. It requires a thorough history and physical examination to rule out any underlying causes and exclude any other serious medical conditions, and specific symptoms need to be discussed for planning the appropriate care. A thorough assessment could prevent unnecessary admission to the ward. Specialist advice and education on an outpatient or community basis can therefore be offered.

Planning

> I know my paediatrician well and can talk to him about stuff, I always have to have my height and weight recorded and bloods taken.
>
> **Jamal, child**

It is essential for the CCN to establish a rapport with the child and family and to gain their trust, so that they feel able to share sensitive information. The CCN will share her skills with the family and empower them to make decisions about the child – independently but with support. Empowerment is a term that CCNs use consistently in their work. Allowing families to make decisions with support is something that is developed with the experience and expertise of the CCN. However, it is important to emphasise that CCNs have to exercise professional judgement and their focus is the child's safety and rights, as the child's best interests are paramount and underpin the philosophy of care. A major role of the community nursing team is to empower children together with their parents and carers to form a treatment plan that has adequate and effective use of laxative therapy, alongside possible changes to diet and lifestyle modifications, and appropriate advice and support, that can best help children to overcome this poorly understood condition.

SEE ALSO
CHAPTERS 2
AND 40

Intervention

> The nurse that visits me at home explains everything to me well, some of what I have to do is embarrassing but she makes me feel at ease and I know that it will help me.
>
> **Jamal, child**

As well as managing the day-to-day problems with constipation and soiling, parents often fear their child may be being bullied or teased. Emotional support is also critical to children suffering with constipation and soiling, and to their family, as it can cause considerable stress. There may well be an impact for some families on their social interaction, leading to feelings of isolation for the whole family. Parents may sometimes feel anger towards their child, mostly due to their frustration at being unable to find a solution to the problem. However, for most children, constipation can be successfully resolved. It can be a long journey, needing ongoing support from health professionals and much patience and encouragement from parents and carers. The quicker a child has an assessment by a health professional, the easier it will be to manage and resolve the problem.

ACTIVITY 7.2: CRITICAL THINKING

Please take a moment to think about daily activities which can help with constipation problems for children and compare them with the guidelines provided at https://study. sagepub.com/essentialchildnursing

ACTIVITY
ANSWER 7.2

Evaluation

> It has helped having the nurses visit me at home because I can still do the things I want at home rather than being stuck in the hospital or travelling to appointments all the time.
>
> **Jamal, child**

Following on from these points, evaluation is done primarily to determine whether a client is progressing. Evaluation is not always an end to the nursing process, but rather an ongoing measure. The plan of care may be modified during any phase of the nursing process when the need to do so is determined through evaluation. Client goals and expected outcomes provide the criteria for evaluation of care. The purposes of evaluation include:

- To determine the client's progress or lack of progress towards achievement of expected outcomes
- To determine the effectiveness of nursing care in helping clients achieve the expected outcomes
- To determine the overall quality of care provided

ACTIVITY 7.3: REFLECTIVE PRACTICE

Research one of the many common childhood conditions and, using the nursing process, think about your role with consideration to community working practice.

ACTIVITY
ANSWER 7.3

THE MULTIAGENCY TEAM AND WORKING IN PARTNERSHIP

Multiagency activity takes many forms and the terminology used to describe it varies, making classification and comparison between different types difficult. Community children nursing services need to be designed and developed in partnership with children and their families as well as a range of local stakeholders, organisations and sectors. Community nurses have other particular skills such as leadership, advocacy and empowerment that enable them to work in partnership with children and their families to tailor clinical and care needs within the home and within community settings. Engaging with children and families is a core component of all service delivery to ensure high-quality healthcare delivery (NHS England, 2015). The progression of Every Child Matters (HM Government, 2005) established the position of children's services in all areas. It was explicit that multiagency work should meet the needs of children and that the responsibility lies with everyone involved with the child and family. According to the philosophy of The Children Act 1989, the welfare of the child is paramount, all service delivery meets the needs of a child in need as well as at risk and their voice is heard. (Myers, 2005).

The benefits of such a model (Home Office, 2014) include:

- Early identification of any issues and intervention
- Easier or quicker access to services or expertise
- Improved achievement in education and better engagement in education
- Better support for parents
- Addressing children and family's needs more appropriately
- Better quality services
- Reduced need for longer-term or more specialist services

This highlights the importance of working together to ensure that children and families who need additional support have exactly the right professionals needed to provide support. A multiagency meeting is a group of people from different agencies that meet regularly for short periods of time to plan care for children with additional needs who may require multiagency support. Let's hear from a student nurse, her thoughts on community placements and learning about the role of the many different professionals.

> I started my nursing course with an open mind but had always been interested in community working. When we had lectures on community nursing I realised I had enjoyed learning about the different roles and wanted to work towards this – I particularly like how it incorporates the social side of nursing as well as many other aspects, which really interests me. I like how you can develop a more one-to-one relationship with children and families, over a more long-term period. I am hoping my management placement will be in a community area. Doing the course has given me some experience of community services but I haven't been shown the avenues that we can go through to this area of work. I know that I can go on to do my school nurse or health visitor training but it is nice to know I can work in the community before and gain some further experience if I needed to.
>
> **Paige, 3rd-year children's nursing student**

List of children's community health services

Take a look at some of the multiagency team of health professionals that work with children and families within the home and in community settings (Table 7.1). This is not an exhaustive list as the composition of the team very much depends on the individual needs of the child and family.

Table 7.1 Interprofessional working with children and families within the home and community settings

Team	Role
Community children's nurses (CCNs) - you can watch the videos at https://study.sagepub.com/ essentialchildnursing about how they work in the home with patients and families	CCNs provide holistic care to sick children in the community, empowering and enabling the child and family/carers to become more competent in the management of the child's condition, thereby reducing the need for hospital admissions and/or enabling early discharge. CCNs provide nursing care to children with a life-limiting condition, life-threatening condition, complex disability, long-term conditions such as asthma, eczema or allergies as well as palliative and end-of-life care

VIDEO LINK 7.2: COMMUNITY NURSING

(Continued)

Table 7.1   (Continued)

VIDEO LINK 7.3:
A COMMUNITY
NURSING TEAM

WATCH A
VIDEO ONLINE!

Team	Role
Community mental health nurses (CMHNs)	CMHNs have a wide range of expertise and offer advice and support to people with long-term mental health conditions, and administer medication. Some CMHNs specialise in treating children with emotional difficulties and in some cases drug or alcohol misuse
General practitioners (GPs)	GPs provide a complete spectrum of care within the local community, dealing with problems that often combine physical, psychological and social components
Community paediatrician	A community paediatrician is a specialist doctor who plays a key role in identifying children who may have specific or a specialised health need. This can include children with long-term disability (e.g. cerebral palsy, learning disability), children with mental health issues (e.g. autism and ADHD), special educational needs patients and children who it is feared are being abused, or children who are being fostered and adopted. They also take responsibility for advising on the health of communities
Practice nurses	Practice nurses assess, screen, treat and educate all members of the community, from babies to older people.
Health visitors	Health visitors are registered nurses or midwives who have done further training to work as vital members of the primary healthcare team, covering a specific geographical area. Their aim is to improve the health of families and children
Learning disability nurses	Learning disability nurses provide specialist healthcare and support to families of those with a range of learning disabilities. They provide support for children in schools and in their home environment
Occupational therapists	Occupational therapists work with children to help them overcome the effects of disability caused by physical or psychological illness. They provide support around fine motor and gross motor skills as well as other areas of development for children
Physiotherapists	Core skills include manual therapy and therapeutic exercise. They also have an appreciation of psychological, cultural and social factors influencing their clients. Treatment and advice for patients and carers take place in their own homes, day centres, schools and health centres
Speech and language therapists (SaLTs)	SaLTs assess and treat speech, language and communication problems. They also work with people who have eating and swallowing problems
Nurse specialists	Nurse specialists work closely with doctors and other members of the multidisciplinary team. They educate and support patients, families and carers from a variety of specialties - e.g. palliative care, diabetes and continence advisors. They play a key role in the management of patient care

School nurses are also members of the multiagency team and their role is discussed in more detail below.

COMMON ASSESSMENT FRAMEWORK/EARLY HELP

The Common Assessment Framework (CAF)/Early Help is a shared assessment and planning framework for use across all children's services. Some areas now refer to this as Early Help, whilst some remain with the CAF. The principles remain the same for both in which it aims to help early identification of children's additional needs and promote coordinated service provision to meet them.

A CAF/Early Help is a standardised approach to assessing the additional needs of children who are thought to be at risk of not achieving their potential. It is a process for gathering and recording information in a standard format about a child for whom a practitioner has concerns, identifying the needs of the child and how the needs can be met. It is a shared assessment and planning framework for use across all children's services and all local areas in the UK. It helps to identify in the early stages the child's additional needs and promote coordinated service provision to meet them.

The Common Assessment Framework/Early Help is a coordinated tool for children who have additional needs in one or more of three areas:

1. Their growth and development
2. Additional educational requirements
3. Family and environmental issues and any specific needs of the parent/carer

Its purpose is to play a key part in delivering front line services that are integrated and focused around the needs of children. Its aim is to support early intervention and improve joint working and communication between practitioners when identifying and responding to the needs of children who may not be achieving the five outcomes recognised in the Every Child Matters agenda.

SEE ALSO
CHAPTER 5

Core features of the CAF/Early Help process

Core features of the CAF/Early Help process

*   Identify the needs early: assessing whether the child may have any additional needs, gathering information and discussing the situation with the child with involvement of the parents/carers unless this is inappropriate. A child under the age of 16 can agree for a CAF/Early Help assessment as long as they have the capacity to understand. This information is recorded on the suitable forms. Considerations are then discussed as to a collaborative way forward.
*   Assess those needs: This may be through discussions with the family or liaising with other practitioners. Documentation will need to be signed, signed by the child or parent on the final version of the assessment form.
*   Deliver integrated services: determining a plan and delivering interventions to meet those identified needs. If a multiagency response is required then the practitioner must form a team around the child or family meeting.
*   Review progress: reviewing the actions and delivery plan, considering any further actions or where necessary supporting the child/young person's transitions. The CAF/Early Help is entirely voluntary, where engagement fails or is refused and concerns arise these need to be escalated to your safeguarding team. If the needs have been met, the lead professional and team may decide to close their involvement and continue with universal service as described within the healthy child programme (2009).

(CWDC, 2009)

The CAF/Early Help is a voluntary assessment and, therefore, a child or parent/carer must give their consent at the start of the process with the full knowledge of what the process will be and what will happen. Once the professional has completed the assessment, the child and or parent/carer must give their consent again for the information to be stored and shared with other services, ensuring it is accurate and up to date and therefore necessary for the purpose for which it is being shared and shared securely in accordance with local policies and procedures.

The CAF/Early Help was developed so that practitioners in all agencies working with children could communicate and work more effectively together. It is intended to provide a simple, non-bureaucratic process for a holistic assessment of a child's needs and to enable decisions to be made about how these needs should be met. The 'team around the child' is a multidisciplinary team set up on a case-by-case basis to support a child or family. The meetings are set up after a child's needs have been assessed through a thorough CAF/Early Help assessment. Professionals from different services will attend to provide tailored supporting input for the child depending on the needs that have been identified and discussed. This meeting supports the Common Assessment Framework/Early Help process. It is important that the child and their family are involved in the meetings so joint solutions and actions can be made where appropriate and promote partnership working. Multiagency meetings can maintain links with their agencies and join with other integrated services or can also be known as service hubs which are there for the community. Therefore, bringing together a range of services, usually under one roof, whose practitioners work with a multiagency approach to delivering integrated support to children and their families.

Information sharing

Information sharing differs greatly within a community setting from what happens within hospitals and can at times feel a little uncomfortable or uncertain; however, with the informed consent of the child and parents/carers you will be expected to share information about the child from your interaction and involvement with them. Information that is useful to share for the purpose of the meeting is the kind of contact you have with the child, their level of engagement in the activities your team offers and any reflections or concerns you have about the child and their family. You will not be expected to share any confidential information unless it relates to a safeguarding concern. It is good practice, where possible, to talk with the child and their family about the kind of information you will want to share at the meeting to support their participation and listen to their views about the kinds of support they would like to receive. Three areas of potential difficulty have been recognised:

- Building supportive relationships with certain families may jeopardise services to other families and increase the workload of the CCN
- Creating over-dependency on the service could inhibit families from taking control
- Ensuring that the CCN has clear professional boundaries with each family for personal protection (Pontin and Lewis, 2008)

Although such problems could arise, the experience of CCNs in relation to their awareness of family relationships and the support they receive from colleagues are some of the ways that they deal with difficult issues. In analysing the role of the CCN, it is apparent that the relationship between the CCN and their families is of a special nature (Hughes and Horsburgh, 2002).

ACTIVITY 7.4: CRITICAL THINKING

In order to prepare, look at your local authority website for information about CAF/Early Help training and resources and procedures or the equivalent in your country. How can you become part of your local team around the child?

The role of the CCN, working in partnership with other members of the interdisciplinary team, can involve the facilitation of care for children in their home or community area. This will minimise any disruption to children's lives and those of their families caused by treatments and care requirements. CCNs provide support for children's families and monitor children's health conditions. They may consider referrals to agencies for further support or liaise with other professionals for suitable care (Lewis and Noyes, 2008).

SUPERVISION WITHIN A COMMUNITY SETTING

Autonomy refers to the ability to act according to one's knowledge and judgement, providing nursing care within the full scope of practice as defined by existing professional, regulatory and organisational rules (Weston, 2008, in Weston, 2010). Working in community settings allows you to manage your own caseload and you will perform the majority of the care during the patient's treatment and take responsibility for your actions and decision-making. The NMC code requires nurses to 'gather and reflect on feedback from a variety of sources, using it to improve practice and performance' (NMC, 2015). Clinical supervision is a formal process of professional support, reflection and learning that contributes to individual development.

Common barriers to effective clinical supervision include lack of time, lack of management support, staffing resource and service inflexibility. It is therefore vital that access to supervision is both adaptable and tailored to individual staff and service needs. In practice, this is challenging but must not be a barrier to the provision of clinical supervision. Supervision is also thought to be important when building emotional resilience as, for example, safeguarding issues and caring for people in the last stages of their life can be stressful as well as rewarding.

Strengthening continued professional development (CPD) around safeguarding issues highlights the need for professionals to be equipped to identify and respond to the health and ill health needs of children and families. Clear directives in terms of safeguarding children resonate with the recommendations of the Laming Report (2009) which acknowledges the lack of high-quality specialist training on child protection across services. Regular safeguarding supervision will promote this and lead to improved outcomes for children, families, vulnerable adults, teams and individual practitioners. Supervision is also essential to help practitioners to cope with the emotional demands of work with children and their families as well as vulnerable adults, which have an impact at all levels of intervention.

SEE ALSO
CHAPTER 9

The Department of Health (HM Government, 2015) defines safeguarding and promoting the welfare of children as the process of protecting children from abuse or neglect, preventing impairment of their health and development, and determine that they are growing up in circumstances consistent with the provision of safe and effective care which is undertaken to enable children to have the best outcomes.

--- ### SAFEGUARDING STOP POINT ---

WEBLINK:
WTTSC

Take a look at the document *Working Together to Safeguard Children* (HM Government, 2015) at https://study.sagepub.com/essentialchildnursing Notice in particular the roles and responsibilities of community practitioners and the importance of supervision in practice.

HOME VISITING AND PERSONAL SAFETY

Visiting children and their families at home can be in a relaxing and calming atmosphere, but it can also become intrusive to some families at times. Community children's nurses have to be autonomous practitioners at times as well as work in teams. They therefore need to be protected by a policy concerning working alone. A lone worker policy should cover visits, communication and risk assessments. All workers are responsible for adhering to policies, safe working practices and reporting any potential risks. When working in community settings it is important to become 'streetwise' by doing your homework prior to home visits – gaining some background knowledge about the area and the family you will be visiting as you will be so closely involved with people from many different cultures, backgrounds and experiences. The following are suggested as a personal checklist (Queen's Nursing Institute, 2013):

1. Make sure that you inform others of your whereabouts at all times
2. Ensure that you have a charged mobile phone with you
3. Have a separate work mobile if possible
4. Have your car keys in an accessible place
5. Plan your access and exit route to the property
6. Do not visit known 'risk' people or areas alone
7. Adhere to your Trust policy on home visiting/lone working
8. Trust your own 'instinctive' feelings if you do not feel safe

Consideration also needs to be given to car safety – for example, where you park, what time of the day it is and where you will store your notes and equipment. Being exposed to the way people live can be a barrier or an influence to the care you provide. Remember that when visiting families you will be a guest in their home. It is not your role to make judgements and shifting the balance of the patient relationship can be difficult at first. This is where communication skills and developing trust are key. Preparing for your visit is essential so you have everything with you and the time is used effectively for you and your clients.

HEALTH PROMOTION AND EDUCATION

Government initiatives, such as the *Choosing Health* white paper (Department of Health, 2004) and *Making a Difference* (Department of Health, 1999), acknowledge the contribution that nurses need to play in the success of health promotion, by emphasising and encouraging lifestyle choices and self care. To actively promote health, you need to recognise and understand health-related behaviour. Health promotion provides the opportunity for everyone to participate and does not have to be incorporated in a lesson or classroom.

Health promotion topics include:

- Nutrition
- Exercise
- Emotional wellbeing
- Smoking prevention and cessation
- Oral health
- Prevention of infectious diseases
- Substance use and abuse
- Immunisation
- Contraception and sexual health
- Parenting

Health promotion has developed a person-centred approach. The initial prevention of disease has stretched to more education in early years and to follow the lines of *Saving Lives: Our Healthier Nation* (HM Government, 1999). Programmes that promote healthy adolescent development can help enhance a range of healthy behaviours among young people and multiple behaviour interventions may have a greater impact on public health than programmes focusing on single behaviours.

Have a look at An Implementation Guide and Toolkit for Making Every Contact Count (2014) at https://study.sagepub.com/essentialchildnursing

WEBLINK:
MAKING EVERY
CONTACT COUNT

Important topics for public health were:

- Mental health and emotional wellbeing
- Sexual health
- Substance misuse – smoking, alcohol and drugs
- Food and physical activity

ACTIVITY 7.5: CRITICAL THINKING

Have a look at the public health priorities for England from Public Health England (2014). Are these the same or have the priorities changed? Do you agree with them? Or do you feel there should be other topics?

ACTIVITY
ANSWER 7.5

WEBLINK:
PUBLIC HEALTH
ENGLAND

SCHOOL NURSING: SUPPORT FOR CHILDREN AND YOUNG PEOPLE

School nursing teams work to promote a healthy school environment and lifestyle. Support is offered for physical and emotional safety of the school community by monitoring children where there is a safeguarding concern, ensuring appropriate exclusion for infectious illnesses and reporting communicable diseases as required by law. In addition, they may also liaise with school counsellors or teaching staff in developing support plans for children with emotional difficulties – for example, self-harm, substance misuse, suicide-related issues and friendship or relationship difficulties. The school nursing team provides health promotion and education in teaching sessions and drop-ins to individuals and groups of students. The team may also be involved in health education curriculum development with schools and provide programmes for staff, families and the community.

The school nurse might liaise between school personnel, family, healthcare professionals and the community. The school nurse ensures that there is adequate communication and collaboration between families, physicians and providers of community resources for children with health needs and also those who are vulnerable or in need of support and advice. The school nurse is aware of and works with community organisations and primary care physicians to make the community a healthy place for all children and families. They have a unique position working with children. They can have one-to-one conversations or just listen to them in ways that teachers often feel unable to do. They offer greater confidentiality and a supportive link between home and school. As an advocate they can speak with or on behalf of a child, therefore ensuring that their voice is heard and listened to. School nurses and their teams use their autonomy, clinical skills and professional judgement to improve the health and wellbeing of children and reduce health inequalities. All communications should be in a style and tone that is appropriate for young people, timely and in an appropriate medium and format. The lifestyles of young people should be mapped by school nurses to ensure information and campaigns are targeted at the right time and in the right place (Independent Advisory Group on Sexual Health and HIV, 2007). Because school nurses have

VIDEO LINK 7.4:
ROLE OF THE
SCHOOL NURSE

regular contact with children who spend a significant proportion of their time in school, they can work with children in promoting, assessing and monitoring health and development (British Youth Council, 2011). This makes personal, social, health and economic education (PSHE) the best opportunity to discuss sexual health and alcohol with young people in a group format from a personal safety and public health perspective.

WHAT'S THE EVIDENCE?

In November 2010 the National Institute for Health and Care Excellence (NICE) produced evidence-based guidance on school, college and community-based PSHE education, including 'health literacy, with particular reference to sexual health behaviour and alcohol' (NICE, 2010, p.12). Substance misuse and sexual health have a powerful influence and can be affected by external factors beyond the control of an individual. Pressure from their peers is an important influence, so young people feel they have to impress their friends and have the confidence to experiment and to show maturity.

So when do you think is it a good time to start educating young people about these subjects? Consider the pros and cons for both substance misuse and sexual health.

The role of school nurses and their work with children

The role of the school nurse is integral to the health and wellbeing of children, with the increasing prevalence of public health issues such as obesity, smoking and sexual health. School nursing is a universally accessible service, acceptable to all backgrounds and communities, which has proven key to the delivery of the government's public health agenda (DH, 2012). School nurses are qualified nurses who hold an additional specialist public health qualification, which is recorded with the Nursing and Midwifery Council. School nurses, with their teams, coordinate and deliver public health interventions for school-aged children. The nature of their work requires clinical input and effective leadership, which qualified school nurses are equipped to provide with an exceptional skill mix (DH, 2012). School nurses are more important today than ever before. The care that they can provide can be for injuries and acute illness for all children as well as support and management of long-term conditions for children with specific healthcare needs.

Getting It Right for Children, Young People and Families (DH, 2012) outlines the school nursing contribution to the government white paper *Healthy Lives, Healthy People* (DH, 2011), which aimed to address inequality and social determinants of health.

Three strands to the framework in achieving its aims were identified:

- Increasing the visibility of the school nursing workforce and access to it
- Leading the delivery of the Healthy Child Programme (5–19)
- Service user participation (DH, 2012)

The school nurse has an elite role in provision of school health services for children with special health needs, including children with chronic illnesses and disabilities of various degrees of severity. An individualised healthcare plan is sometimes needed for children with chronic conditions, and where needed this could include emergency plans to manage potential significant events in the school setting (e.g. diabetes, asthma). These plans are collaboratively managed by the school nurse, the child and family, the child's paediatrician and the school. It will be regularly updated through close communication. The school nurse ensures that the individualised healthcare plan supports educational plans where appropriate. It is also the responsibility of the school nurse to provide training to educational staff where needed – e.g. epi pen training, oxygen therapy, constipation issues.

Good sources of further information can be found at: www.youngpeopleshealth.org.uk/wp-content/uploads/2016/10/AYPH_NursesToolkit_interactive.pdf and www.rcn.org.uk/professional-development/publications/pub-006316

As a leader, the school nurse will assess children's health, identifying any health problems and provide screening and referrals for a variety of health conditions. These types of screening can include health assessments, vision, hearing and BMI assessments as well as sexual health screening as determined by local policy and procedures. Health screening promotes preventative action to health and can decrease any negative effects of any health issues. Referrals to agencies and any support is therefore crucial to success and promotes appropriate use of community resources giving clear outcomes. The school nurse provides leadership for the provision of health services and is seen as the healthcare expert within schools and other education establishments. The school nurse also meets responsibilities for responding to emergencies, confidential communication and documentation of student health information.

WEBLINK: SCHOOL NURSE TOOLKIT

SCENARIO 7.1: SOPHIE

Sophie has requested to see you at your school nurse drop-in. She is requesting the morning-after pill as she had unprotected sex with her boyfriend on Saturday night. They did use a condom but it split and they didn't notice until it was too late.

Using the Royal College of Nursing (RCN) position statement 'The role of school nurses in providing emergency contraception services in education settings' (RCN, 2012), write down in a list the important questions that you need to ask Sophie in order to gather further information and provide the correct treatment and advice.

SCENARIO ANSWER 7.1

PRACTICE SCENARIO 7: YEAR 8 GIRL

WEBLINK: EMERGENCY CONTRACEPTION SERVICES

Have a look at the placement advice at https://study.sagepub.com/essentialchildnursing for tips on preparing for placements in these settings.

PLACEMENT ADVICE 7: COMMUNITY PLACEMENTS

CHAPTER SUMMARY

- The uniqueness of caring for children and their families in the community setting should not be understated
- Thorough assessment using an appropriate child-centred tool is fundamental in care, recognising that each country may have a different approach
- Interprofessional and interdisciplinary working around the child and family is crucial
- Ongoing health promotion and education must be personalised to recognise and meet the individual needs of children

BUILD YOUR BIBLIOGRAPHY

Books

- Sines, D. (2013) *Community and Public Health Nursing*, 5th edn. Chichester: Wiley-Blackwell.

  This definitive textbook covers learning disability nursing, caring for patients with mental health conditions, community children's nursing and school nursing.

- Trigg, E. and Mohammed, T.A. (2010) *Practices in Children's Nursing: Guidelines for Hospital and Community*, 3rd edn. Edinburgh: Churchill Livingstone.

  This work provides a clinical manual of common practices featuring contributions from practitioners in a variety of well-known children's hospital and community areas.

- Harris, J. and Nimmo, S. (2013) *Placement Learning in Community Nursing. A guide for students in practice*. London: Bailliere Tindall Elsevier.

  The authors bring a combination of experience, clinical practice, education and research to this pocket size guide to learning in a range of placement areas.

Journal articles

FURTHER
READING:
ONLINE
JOURNAL
ARTICLES

Go to https://study.sagepub.com/essentialchildnursing for further free online journal articles related to this chapter.

- Valentine, V. (1988) 'Using nursing process to manage the care of the child at home'. *Home Health Care Management & Practice*, 1 (2): 8-15.

  The article gives an insight into caring for children in their homes and bases this around the nursing process, as discussed in the chapter.

- Ravella, P.C. and Thompson, L.S. (2001) 'Educational model of community partnerships for health promotion'. *Policy, Politics, & Nursing Practice*, 2 (2): 161-6.

  This article discusses community aspects in nursing and their importance. Health promotion activities and models highlight collaborative working and demonstrate the need for early intervention.

- Schaffer, M.A., Anderson, L.J.W. and Rising, S. (2015) 'Public health interventions for school nursing practice'. *The Journal of School Nursing*, 32 (3). DOI: 10.1177/1059840515605361

  This paper looks at these interventions and gives thought to the realistic aspects of nursing practice.

Weblinks

FURTHER
READING:
WEBLINKS

Go to https://study.sagepub.com/essentialchildnursing for further weblinks related to this chapter.

- Department of Health, School Nursing: Public Health Services

  www.gov.uk/government/publications/school-nursing-public-health-services
  Guidance for putting in place public health services for children and young people from 5 to 19 years.

- NHS (2014) *Five Year Forward View*

  www.england.nhs.uk/wp-content/uploads/2014/10/5yfv-web.pdf
  The *Forward View* sets out some new ideas for the NHS – both in the way it delivers services to people and in the way it manages its funding.

- NHS: Health Education England, Making Every Contact Count (MECC)

  www.makingeverycontactcount.co.uk
  Supports the development, evaluation and implementation of the programme for local communities.

ACE YOUR ASSESSMENT

Revise what you have learned by visiting https://study.sagepub.com/essentialchildnursing

ONLINE
QUIZZES &
ACTIVITY
ANSWERS

- Test yourself with multiple-choice and short-answer questions
- Do the chapter activities in the book and check your answers online

REFERENCES

Association for Young People's Health (2016) *School Nurse Toolkit.* London: Association for Young People's Health.

British Youth Council (2011) *Our School Nurse.* London: British Youth Council.

Children's Workforce Development Council (CWDC) (2009) *Early Indentification, Assessment of Needs and Intervention. The Common Assessment Framework for Children and Young People. A Guide for Practitioners.* Leeds: Children's Workforce Development Council.

Department of Health (DH) and Department for Children, Schools and Families (DCSF) (2009) *Healthy Lives, Brighter Futures: The Strategy for Children and Young People's Health.* London: Department of Health.

Department of Health (1999) *Making a Difference: Strengthening the nursing, midwifery and health visiting contribution to health and healthcare.* London: Department of Health.

Department of Health (2004) *Choosing Health: Making healthy choices easier.* London: Department of Health.

Department of Health (DH) (2011) *NHS at Home: Community Children's Nursing Services.* London: DH. Available at: www.gov.uk/government/uploads/system/uploads/attachment_data/file/215708/dh_124900.pdf (last accessed 8 May 2017).

Department of Health (2012) *Getting It Right for Children, Young People and Families. Maximising the Contribution of the School Nursing Team: Vision and Call to Action.* London: Department of Health, NADH CNO Professional Leadership Team.

Foot, C., Sonola, L., Bennett, L., Fitzsimons, B., Raleigh, V. and Gregory, S. (2014) *Managing Quality in Community Health Care Services.* London: The King's Fund.

Hackett, A. (2013) 'The role of the school nurse in child protection'. *Community Practitioner,* 86 (12): 26–9.

HM Government (1999) Cm 4386. *Saving Lives: Our Healthier Nation.* London: The Stationery Office.

HM Government (2005) *Every Child Matters: Change for Children.* London: DfES. Available at: http://webarchive.nationalarchives.gov.uk/20130401151715/http://www.education.gov.uk/publications/eOrderingDownload/DfES10812004.pdf (accessed 28 June 2017).

HM Government (2015) *Working Together to Safeguard Children: A Guide to Inter-agency Working to Safeguard and Promote the Welfare of Children.* London: DfE. Available at: www.gov.uk/government/publications/working-together-to-safeguard-children--2 (last accessed 8 May 2017).

Home Office (2014) *Multi-Agency Working and Information Sharing Project Early Findings.* London: Home Office.

Hughes, J. and Horsburgh, J. (2002) 'The role of the community children's nurse: the perspective of a practitioner'. *Current Paediatrics,* 12: 425–30.

Independent Advisory Group on Sexual Health and HIV (2007) *Sex, Drugs, Alcohol and Young People Seminar Findings Independent Advisory Group on Sexual Health and HIV. A review of the impact drugs and alcohol have on young people's sexual behaviour.* Independent Advisory Group on Sexual Health and HIV. London: Department of Health.

Laming, The Lord (2009) The Laming Report. The Protection of Children in England: A Progress Report. London: TSO.

Lewis, M. and Noyes, J. (2008) 'The children's community nurse'. *Paediatrics and Child Health*, 18 (5): 227–32.

McDonald, A., Langford, I. and Boldero, N. (1997) 'The future of community nursing in the United Kingdom: district nursing, health visiting and school nursing'. *Journal of Advanced Nursing*, 26 (2): 257–65.

Myers, J. (2005) 'Community children's nursing services in the 21st century'. *Paediatric Nursing*, 17 (2): 31–4.

NHS Evidence (2014) *Constipation in Children and Young People. Evidence Update*. NHS Evidence. National Institute for Health and Clinical Excellence.

NHS (2014) *NHS Five Year Forward View*. NHS England. Available at: www.england.nhs.uk/ourwork/futurenhs/ (accessed 16 June 2015).

NHS England (2015) *A Guide to Community-centred Approaches for Health and Wellbeing*. London: Public Health England.

NICE (2010) *Constipation in Children and Young People: Diagnosis and Management*. Available at: www.nice.org.uk/guidance/cg99 (last accessed 8 May 2017).

NMC (2010) *Standards for Pre-registration Nursing Education*. Nursing and Midwifery Council. Available at: www.nmc.org.uk/standards/additional-standards/standards-for-pre-registration-nursing-education/ (accessed 28 June 2017).

Nursing and Midwifery Council (NMC) (2015) *The Code for Nurses and Midwives*. London: Nursing and Midwifery Council.

Pearson A., Vaughn, B. and Fitzgerald, M. (2005) *Nursing Models for Practice*. Oxford: Butterworth-Heinemann.

Pontin, D. and Lewis, M. (2008) 'Managing the caseload: a qualitative action research study exploring how community children's nurses deliver services to children living with life-limiting, life-threatening, and chronic conditions'. *Journal for Specialists in Pediatric Nursing*, 13 (1): 26–35.

Public Health England (2014) *From Evidence into Action: Opportunities to Protect and Improve the Nation's Health*. London: Public Health England. Available at: www.gov.uk/government/uploads/system/uploads/attachment_data/file/366852/PHE_Priorities.pdf (accessed 28 June 2017).

Queen's Nursing Institute (2013) *Transition to Community Nursing Practice*. London: The Queen's Nursing Institute.

Royal College of Nursing (RCN) (2012) *RCN position statement: The Role of School Nurses in Providing Emergency Contraception Services in Education Settings*. London: RCN. Available at: www.rcn.org.uk/professional-development/publications/pub-002772 (last accessed 8 May 2017).

Royal College of Nursing (RCN) (2014) *The Future for Community Children's Nursing: Challenges and Opportunities*. London: RCN.

Royal College of Nursing (RCN) (2017) *An RCN Toolkit for School Nurses. Supporting Your Practice to Deliver Services for Children and Young People in Educational Settings*. London: RCN.

Weston, M.J. (2010) 'Strategies for enhancing autonomy and control over nursing practice'. *OJIN: The Online Journal of Issues in Nursing*, 15, 1.

Whiting, L., Caldwell, C., Donnelly, M., Martin, D. and Whiting, M. (2015) 'Effective nursing care of children and young people outside hospital'. *Nursing Children and Young People*, 27 (5), 28–33.

LAW AND POLICY FOR CHILDREN AND YOUNG PEOPLE'S NURSING

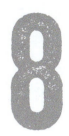

MARC CORNOCK AND ORLA McALINDEN

THIS CHAPTER COVERS

- Policy, procedure and law – what are the differences?
- How law can interact with and affect care delivery for children and young people in all settings
- Clinical scenarios and identification of key principles of care for the child
- Expert guided discussion around the professional and lawful care of children and families and their varying health and social care needs

> "
> The end of law is not to abolish or restrain, but to preserve and enlarge freedom. For in all the states of created beings capable of law, where there is no law, there is no freedom.
>
> **John Locke, 1690**
> "

Visit https://study.sagepub.com/essentialchildnursing to access a wealth of online resources for this chapter – watch out for the margin icons throughout the chapter.

INTRODUCTION

The opening quotation demonstrates succinctly what the law seeks to do in the context of nursing and healthcare – to enable and facilitate quality, to preserve what is good and restrict what is wrong. In the case of children and young people's nursing this may be seen to be enshrined in the UN Convention on the Rights of the Child. These rights are applicable in health and social care, and are relevant to the aspiring children's nurse.

The practice of nursing children in the 21st century is a complex and multifaceted set of skilled and interlinked evidence-based interventions. The contemporary children's nurse in the health and social care setting is expected to be fit for the practice of the art and science of nursing, fit for the purpose of meeting the needs of children in all health and social care settings and, last but not least, fit for the award of an academic as well as professional qualification. In a nutshell, that is what you are doing on your current academic and professional programme. If you are reading this you are most likely in year 2 or 3 of your university programme, either at undergraduate level or at continuing education/postgraduate level.

Why do you need to understand the material in this chapter, as it relates to care in children's nursing? As a registered nurse, you will be expected to be responsible and accountable for the care you assess, plan, deliver and evaluate. It is not simply about knowing the rationale or evidence base for actions; rather it is a working awareness of the often complex interactions between people, health, society, culture and organisations. This chapter provides you with the opportunity to explore these areas and gain an understanding of them now as a nursing student, in preparation for your role as a registered nurse.

WEBLINK: NMC WEBSITE

Please have a look at the *Professional Standards of Practice and Behaviour for Nurses and Midwives* (Nursing and Midwifery Council (NMC), 2015a). Remember that these are periodically updated and you should check that you are reading the current edition. You can do this by accessing the NMC website. You can access the 2017 Code of Practice at https://study.sagepub.com/essentialchildnursing

WEBLINK: 2017 CODE OF PRACTICE

FIND OUT MORE!

Children's nurses are required to safeguard the interests of children at all times, practise in a non-discriminatory manner and remain vigilant to the legal and ethical aspects of their practice. A challenging aspect of working with children is navigating the interplay of decision-making with policy, law and procedure in dealings with children, families and the multidisciplinary team (McAlinden, 2012). Interpreting and applying codes and policies and upholding the law can be a major juggling act. By year 2 most students are mastering their clinical skills fairly well, and their attention turns to the complexities of delivering 'whole care' and not just 'the bits' that involve a clinical (psychomotor) skill. This involves the policies, procedures, codes and laws associated with delivering safe and effective multidisciplinary health and social care.

> Legislation in children's nursing is everywhere and conveyed within the NMC Code, which sets out professional standards and is underpinned by the law. As a student, you will constantly refer back to the Code and reflect on your practice. The law is important to me because having heard about cases in university and viewed bad practice reports online, I want to ensure that I practise responsibly within legal frameworks.
>
> **Thomas, 2nd-year children's nursing student**

Although having to manage the various aspects of children's care – including clinical care, relationships with children and their families, decision-making, and the interplay of polices, law and ethics – all at the same time can be terrifying, it is a vital and important skill to master. You are not alone in your apprehension about being able to achieve this skill. Practice does make perfect, and your mentor and your university lecturer will help you progress towards achievement of this skill. So too will listening to the views and wishes of children and their families. Ask yourself, 'Are you acting in their best interests using the best available evidence and within your sphere of competence?'

ACTIVITY 8.1: CRITICAL THINKING

Although mastering complex skills can appear daunting at first, think back to when you first started to learn to drive. At the beginning you were probably solely 'task focused' and unable to 'look, mirror, signal, manoeuvre and read the road' all at the same time as dealing with the mechanics of actually 'driving' the car. With practice and increasing confidence you started to master the integration of the tasks, skills and knowledge – then one day you found yourself doing it with increasing ease. If you are not a driver you can probably think of other examples yourself where you had to master both cognitive and practical skills at the same time and suddenly found that they became second nature to you without you really noticing that you had mastered them.

- Reflect on recent experience in your practice where you have realised that you are completing care fairly effortlessly when previously you were worried about that same aspect of care. At what point did you realise you could complete this aspect of care without too much concern? How does this make you feel now about that aspect of care?

CHECK YOUR ANSWERS ONLINE!

ACTIVITY ANSWER 8.1

POLICY, PROCEDURE AND LAW - WHAT ARE THE DIFFERENCES?

Please read the *Oxford English Dictionary* definitions of these terms in the table below.

Table 8.1 Definitions of policy, procedure and law

Policy	Procedure	Law
A course or principle of action adopted or proposed by an organisation or individual	An established or official way of doing something	The system of rules which a particular country or community recognises as regulating the actions of its members and which it may enforce by the imposition of penalties

Source: Oxford English Dictionary

Nursing is governed by specific legislation from country to country, for example in the UK this is the Nursing and Midwifery Order 2001.

You can access the text of the legislation for regulating nurses and midwives at https://study.sage pub.com/essentialchildnursing

WEBLINK:
NMC LEGAL
FRAMEWORK

ACTIVITY 8.2: CRITICAL THINKING

Access the Nursing and Midwifery Order 2001 in the UK, or the relevant law for your country. Read and note the requirements in law of 1) a registered nurse and 2) nursing as a professional body.

HOW LAW CAN INTERACT WITH AND AFFECT CARE DELIVERY FOR CHILDREN AND YOUNG PEOPLE IN ALL SETTINGS

Nursing as a body, and within the context of health need, decides on a set of policies based on evidence and best practice from which to direct nursing activities locally and globally, for example the work of the World Health Organization (who.org.uk).

The law which governs nursing is overarching of all care interventions and the standard set in law is the minimum standard that must be achieved by all those working in health and social care. Interestingly, the professions all tend to set their professional expectations in excess of the legal standing in their codes of professional conduct. This is to make clear their emphasis on protection of the public, which is the key aspect of the professional regulator bodies such as the NMC.

It is helpful to remember that the law sets out the minimum expected standards whilst the Code sets out the best possible standards expected (McAlinden, 2012). Together these concepts can be thought of in the following way:

Law + Code = intention is to protect the public

For nurses in the UK, the NMC Code is an example in point. The NMC Code sets the standard that all registered nurses have to meet. It is the NMC Code that provides protection to the public. For nurses in other countries you should become familiar with the legislation and nursing codes and standards of your own particular jurisdiction.

The NMC Code (2015a) uses a 'principles'-based approach to the care of patients and clients; it also indicates how the law both intertwines with and informs healthcare practices. The NMC Code is a lengthy professional guidance and directive on how nurses must protect those in their care and is a combination of 'positive rules' (binding) and 'normative' rules (what a person should do). This reflects the reality and complexity of contemporary health and social care delivery.

> A lot of emphasis is put on the NMC Code in university and on placement, which really highlights how much it underpins my practice, now as a student and when I qualify as a registered nurse. I do find the NMC Code very easy to read and relate to. It is well laid out in sections, making it easy to refer to, which I often do, particularly in university work.
>
> **Amber, 3rd-year children's nursing student**
>
> I have found the NMC Code and standards very helpful in my learning as a children's nursing student, particularly with linking my theory into practice and references for assignments. It is available online, easy to understand and I like to keep updated with any revisions. I think it is important to keep referring back to the Code in everything you do as a nursing student because it has derived from the law and when working with children and their families we want to practise legally as competent practitioners.
>
> **Thomas, 2nd-year children's nursing student**

Duty of care and duty of candour

Duty of care

The legal duty of care relates to the legal obligations that one person has towards another. In the healthcare setting the legal duty of care is related to ethical and professional duties. The legal duty of care for nurses requires that nurses provide care to all those who they have a responsibility for and that the patients and clients of the nurse receive the care to a particular standard and do not come to any harm as a result of the nurse's actions or omissions (Cornock, 2014a).

VIDEO LINK 8.1:
ETHICAL AND
LEGAL ISSUES

Duty of candour

This is not a new concept as it is concerned with openness and honesty in dealing with patients and their families. However, more recently, following events at Mid-Staffordshire and subsequently serious care failings at Morecambe Bay (Kirkip, 2015), much more attention has been on what happens when failings in care occur. This led to consideration of how failings should be addressed and when. As a result, the concept of a legal duty of candour was proposed. Initially the focus was on the meaning of the term and what new regulations should be put in place for health and social care delivery. The Francis Report (2013) proposed a shift from the existing contractual duty of care to advise patients and their families of failings in care (required by employers) to a statutory (required by law) obligation on all organisations, providers and individuals.

The Duty of candour requirements are to:

- Make sure the healthcare professional acts in an open and transparent way with relevant persons in relation to care and treatment provided to people who use services in carrying on a regulated activity
- Tell the relevant person in person as soon as reasonably practicable after becoming aware that a notifiable safety incident has occurred, and provide support to them in relation to the incident, including when giving the notification
- Provide an account of the incident which, to the best of the health service body's knowledge, is true of all the facts the body knows about the incident as at the date of the notification
- Advise the relevant person what further enquiries the provider believes are appropriate
- Offer an apology
- Follow this up by giving the same information in writing, and providing an update on the enquiries
- Keep a written record of all communication with the relevant person (NMC and GMC, 2015)

CLINICAL SCENARIOS AND IDENTIFICATION OF KEY PRINCIPLES OF CARE FOR THE CHILD

ACTIVITY 8.3: REFLECTIVE PRACTICE

For all relevant reports and legislation (specific to your country) visit the appropriate websites, which you can access via https://study.sagepub.com/essentialchildnursing, and make a note of pertinent material to your practice:

WEBLINK:
GOVERNMENT
WEBSITES

- England: www.gov.uk/government/organisations/department-of-health
- Northern Ireland: www.health-ni.gov.uk

(Continued)

(Continued)

- Scotland: www.scotland.gov.uk
- Wales: http://gov.wales
- Republic of Ireland: www.gov.ie
- Irish Health Reports: www.hiqa.ie/
- World Health Organization: www.who.org
- United Nations Convention on the Rights of the Child: www.uncrc.org

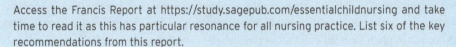

WHAT'S THE EVIDENCE?

WEBLINK:
FRANCIS
REPORT

Francis, R. (2013) The Report of the Mid Staffordshire NHS Foundation Trust Public Enquiry.

Access the Francis Report at https://study.sagepub.com/essentialchildnursing and take time to read it as this has particular resonance for all nursing practice. List six of the key recommendations from this report.

WHAT'S THE
EVIDENCE?
ANSWER 8.1

EXPERT GUIDED DISCUSSION AROUND THE PROFESSIONAL AND LAWFUL CARE OF CHILDREN AND FAMILIES AND THEIR VARYING HEALTH AND CARE NEEDS

SCENARIO 8.1: SOPHIE

PRACTICE
SCENARIO 8:
LEUAN

Sophie, a second-year nursing student, is new to the Day Surgery Unit.

She has been asked to admit a 5-year-old boy called Felix who needs dental extractions and is on the afternoon list for surgery. Her mentor is nearby and has instructed Sophie to start the admission and call for assistance with anything that she is not sure about.

Sophie introduces herself to Felix and his grandmother who has accompanied him. She takes Felix's vital signs and notes the time he last ate or drank. She records this along with his preferences and demographic details and asks both Felix and his granny if they understand why he is there.

Granny signals covertly to Sophie and takes her aside. She says that Felix doesn't know about the dental extractions; they have told him he's going for a nice sleep and when he's asleep the nurse will clean his teeth and make them all shiny and white. Sophie is not sure that this is the best way to deal with Felix but she says nothing at this point. Sophie watches as the surgeon asks Granny for her signature on the hospital consent form. Sophie is not very happy about this either but is reluctant to speak up and tell the surgeon that she is the granny and not the mummy – surely he would know? She is also not sure about telling her mentor that Felix has no idea why he's there.

- What would you do in Sophie's situation?

Compare your answers with the following discussion.

It is tempting to begin our discussion by considering whether Sophie has done anything wrong. However, a more useful starting point may be to consider the respective roles of all concerned in this scenario:

- Felix is going to have some teeth removed
- Felix's grandmother is supporting him
- Sophie has been instructed to start Felix's admission
- Sophie's mentor has to ensure that Felix is safely admitted to the Day Surgery Unit
- The surgeon is responsible for ensuring that Felix has his dental extractions safely

There is a complex interplay of legal responsibility, Trust policies and professional accountability in this scenario, as well as legal considerations regarding the operation itself. It may therefore be easiest to go through the scenario step by step to ensure that we have covered all these.

Sophie's mentor instructing her to start the admission is the first point we need to consider. Sophie's mentor is accountable for Felix's admission. He has delegated the starting of this to Sophie but this does not remove his accountability. Whilst tasks can be delegated, it is not possible to delegate accountability for that task (Cornock, 2014b). Therefore, overall accountability for Felix's admission remains with Sophie's mentor. This means that he has to check that Felix's admission has been undertaken correctly.

Sophie has responsibility for starting Felix's admission. As this has been delegated by her mentor, she is not accountable to the NMC for this as she is not on the NMC register. However, she is liable for her actions in law and has to perform her role to the necessary standard as required by law (Cornock, 2014a). This standard is known as the 'Bolam test' (Bolam v Friern Hospital Management Committee [1957] 2 All ER 118) and means that Sophie must perform her role in the same way as another second-year nursing student. Sophie must also adhere to any Trust policy regarding the admission of a child to the hospital and the Day Surgery Unit. Please go to https://study.sagepub.com/essentialchildnursing and read the document explaining the Bolam case.

WEBLINK:
BOLAM CASE

Sophie is then informed by Felix's granny that Felix does not know about the surgery but believes he is having his teeth cleaned. Sophie seems unsure whether this is the best way to deal with Felix. She is right to be concerned. All healthcare is a partnership with the patient. Felix's treatment will not end when his teeth are extracted; he will need aftercare, including pain relief and the need to rinse his mouth. He will also need to go for a check-up to ensure that everything has healed correctly. If Felix wakes up in pain and not knowing what has happened, he may be unwilling to have any further assessment or treatment for his mouth and may also be mistrustful of hospitals, nurses and doctors. On the other hand, if a child-centred care approach is taken and everything is explained to him, he will understand what is happening and why and this may be a more positive experience for him. (For further discussion on child-centred care, see Carter et al. 2014.)

At this point, Sophie's concern would seem to be that expected of a second-year nursing student.

The next point to concern us is obtaining consent. The surgeon is liable and accountable for ensuring that valid consent is obtained for Felix's operation. As a 5-year-old, Felix is not legally competent to provide his own consent. A child is able to provide their own consent if they can demonstrate to the relevant healthcare professional that they are Gillick competent (Cornock and Montgomery, 2014). This means that the child (a minor) can demonstrate they have the necessary emotional and intellectual maturity to understand the nature of the proposed procedure, as well as any possible side effects, along with the risks and possible complications, and also the risk associated with not having the treatment. The term 'Gillick competent' arises from the Gillick case (Gillick v West Norfolk and Wisbech AHA [1985] 1 All ER 533). For more information, please go to https://study.sagepub.com/essentialchildnursing and read the document on Gillick competence and Fraser guidelines.

WEBLINK:
GILLICK &
FRASER

As Felix cannot consent for himself, the law says that for a child, someone with parental responsibility can provide valid consent. Sophie notes that Felix's granny signs the consent form. However, it is not automatic that the granny has parental responsibility for Felix. Parental responsibility normally rests with the parents of a child, unless this has been changed, such as via a court order, to the contrary – for example, adoption of the child or a residence order (Cornock, 2015). Please go to https://study.sagepub.com/essentialchildnursing and watch the video on parental responsibility. It is the surgeon's responsibility to ensure that the correct person signs the consent form. However, Sophie watches this being done and has not informed the surgeon that he has been talking with Felix's granny. It may be that Felix's granny has parental responsibility for him, but Sophie has not checked this and so does not know either way.

At this point Sophie is aware that Felix does not know why he is at the Day Surgery Unit and also that it was Felix's granny who signed the consent form. We must remember that she is responsible for starting Felix's admission as it was delegated to her.

The nursing student–mentor relationship is based on trust and communication. If either of these is absent then the relationship will not work. Furthermore, Sophie was told by her mentor to ask for assistance if she is unsure of anything. Let's also not forget that Sophie is responsible for her own actions and has to meet the required standard in undertaking these.

So what should Sophie do? We need to consider what another second-year nursing student would do in Sophie's situation. This is the application of the 'Bolam test' discussed above. We do not need to consider the best second-year student, just the average one. We would expect that a second-year student unsure of something would seek the assistance of their mentor.

Therefore, to fulfil her responsibility to the required standard, Sophie needs to discuss the situation with her mentor who will become aware of Felix's lack of knowledge about his operation and be able to check whether Felix's granny has parental responsibility for him or not. The mentor can then decide how best to proceed regarding Felix's understanding of why he is at the Day Surgery Unit, and also inform the surgeon, if necessary, regarding consent.

We should note that Sophie's legal responsibility can be satisfied by Sophie informing her mentor of the relevant facts. This is not an onerous duty on Sophie. As stated above, it should be part of her relationship with her mentor. She needs to ensure that her mentor is aware of the facts before Felix undergoes his treatment. If she doesn't then she may be said to have fallen below the required standard.

If Sophie did not inform her mentor of the relevant facts, her mentor would still be expected to discuss Felix's admission with Sophie as part of the accountability in delegating the admission to Sophie. At this stage it would be hoped that the relevant facts would come to light and for the mentor to act on them as discussed above. In this situation Sophie would have breached her duty, but no harm would have occurred as her mentor would have established the facts and acted accordingly.

If Sophie does not discuss the situation with her mentor, and her mentor does not check with Sophie regarding Felix's admission, both Sophie and her mentor would have failed in their respective responsibility and accountability regarding Felix's operation.

For further information on consent, you can watch the videos available at https://study.sagepub.com/essentialchildnursing

SCENARIO 8.2: MICHAEL

Nursing student Michael loves his placement with the community children's nurse (CCN) and the health visitors; this could well be an area he would like to work in after he registers with the NMC, though it is so very different from working in an acute area. This morning he and the

CCN are planning on visiting Petra, a 9-year-old at home to check and renew a wound dressing. On arrival there is no answer for quite a while, then finally Petra opens the door. Her mum is at work, she says. When undertaking the dressing, Michael and the CCN note that Petra has a lot of fresh bruising on her arms and goes silent when asked how these bruises happened. Michael wonders how this incident and suspicions relating to safeguarding children will be managed by the CCN.

- What do you think the CCN should do regarding Petra's situation?

Compare your answers with the following discussion.

There are two issues that we need to examine in this scenario. The first is that a 9-year-old child appears to have been left alone in their house. The second is that the child has unexplained bruising on her arms, both potential safeguarding points. Let's take the issue of an unsupervised minor at home first. Michael and the CCN need to make sure that Petra is indeed alone and that there is no-one else in the house before taking any action. It could be that there is someone else in the house, perhaps another adult asleep, or that Petra's mum has gone to the shops for some food and is not at work. From a legal perspective we need to note that there is no specific age at which a child becomes old enough to be left alone on their own, or any minimum age. Rather, each child needs to be judged on their own maturity to be left alone at home. However, the National Society for the Prevention of Cruelty to Children (NSPCC) has published guidance on leaving a child at home which has links to the law on leaving children alone in England and Wales, Scotland and Northern Ireland, and this suggests that most children under 12 would not be considered mature enough to be left at home for any considerable period of time. You can read the full NSPCC guidance at https://study.sagepub.com/essentialchildnursing

WEBLINK: NSPCC GUIDANCE

Whilst the law has no specific age limit when a child can be left alone, it does make it an offence to leave a child alone if they are placed at risk, and the relevant person can be prosecuted for neglect. Therefore, if Petra has indeed been left alone for the whole time that her mother is at work, this could be seen to be an issue. The CCN would need to assess if, in her opinion, Petra is mature enough to look after herself or is at risk. We will come back to what she should do if she considers that Petra is at risk after discussing the issue of Petra's bruising. Michael and the CCN note that there is a lot of bruising on Petra's arms and that these bruises are fresh. Again, caution needs to be applied and further investigation of the bruising undertaken. The CCN should gently question Petra further to try to ascertain how the bruising occurred. The reason for this is that it is possible that Petra is an active young girl who suffers knocks and bruising in her playing. On the other hand, it could be that the bruising has been deliberately inflicted by someone else and that Petra is at further risk of being abused. The CCN has to try to determine which of these two causes is the more likely. If the CCN believes that Petra's bruising may be caused as a result of neglect or abuse she has to take action. Likewise, if she believes that Petra is at risk by being left alone she has to take action. The CCN may take the view that there are two areas of concern and this is reason to act further. It isn't necessary to be absolutely certain in these cases; suspicions or concerns should be raised so that they can be investigated by the relevant authorities. All the action that the CCN now takes has to be in Petra's best interests in order to protect and safeguard her.

All organisations that come into contact with children are required to have safeguarding policies and procedures for child protection in place. The CCN should contact her manager or the person who is responsible in her organisation for child protection issues and explain the situation, what she has found and what her concerns are. This also needs to be documented in the child's notes.

The manager or responsible person then needs to make contact with the appropriate authorities. In this instance it may be a social worker in the child protection team who is able to arrange for Petra to be either removed to a place of safety or for someone to protect Petra by staying with her. The CCN and Michael would need to stay with Petra until someone else is able to come to the house and take responsibility for Petra's safety. A key aspect of managing this situation for the CCN is communication and scrupulous record-keeping. The CCN needs to make sure that she has recorded all the relevant facts, including why her suspicions were raised, the actions she took and the names of the individuals she contacted as well as any subsequent action. It is possible that the police may be involved in this case and action taken against Petra's mother for neglect. If this does occur, Michael and the CCN may be asked to provide statements to the police regarding their involvement and actions.

SAFEGUARDING STOP POINT

WEBLINK: WTTSC

For further guidance on safeguarding children, see *Working Together to Safeguard Children* (HM Government, 2015), Chapter 1: Assessing need and providing help, available at https://study.sagepub.com/essentialchildnursing

Please also watch the videos on safeguarding available at https://study.sagepub.com/essential childnursing

VIDEO LINK 8.4: SAFEGUARDING

> " Safeguarding children is a key role of a children's nurse as often they are the first to see signs of abuse and neglect. In university we focus a lot on child protection and when I go on placement it becomes obvious why we do have so much emphasis on safeguarding. As a first-year children's nurse student I was horrified when I realised the number of safeguarding issues that were unfolding in a hospital so close to my hometown. Now, as a third-year student, I have seen many cases where children have been brought into hospital with injuries that are thought to be non-accidental and have found it very interesting working with the entire multidisciplinary team to come to conclusions about what has happened to the children and seeing social workers and other agencies becoming involved. Many of the cases are heart-breaking but it is comforting to know that as nurses, we are protecting the child and ensuring the best future for them.
>
> **Amber, 3rd-year children's nursing student** "

SCENARIO 8.3: KATHY

Whilst on lunch break in the coffee bar in the foyer, Kathy, a nursing student, has her friends enthralled as she tells them all about her morning's experiences in the A&E Department. You wouldn't believe it, she says, as she tells them all about the young person who came in with an overdose, the 13-year-old who turned out to be pregnant and the road traffic collision caused by the local school bus driver. The coffee shop is used by everyone, not just nursing staff. Some visitors are listening.

- Do you think that Kathy has done anything wrong?

Compare your answers with the following discussion.

Kathy has a duty of care to all her patients; even as a nursing student this duty exists. Part of this duty is to respect the patient's right to confidence. The right to confidence is known as confidentiality and is a fundamental principle of healthcare, encompassing law, ethics and professional regulatory principles.

To maintain a patient's confidentiality means to protect information that is obtained about or from the patient in the course of your professional practice. If you do not maintain patient confidentiality then you will have failed in your duty of care to that patient, unless there are public interest reasons to disclose the information, such as to prevent or detect serious crime or where the information needs to be disclosed to protect the patient or another person from serious harm.

So, has Kathy breached any of her patients' confidentiality?

She is in a public area discussing patients with her friends; it doesn't matter if Kathy's friends are nurses or not. The only time you should discuss patient information is when the other individual needs the information in order to care for that patient.

However, has she passed on any patient details? From the information we have it does not appear as if Kathy is actually naming her patients when she is discussing them with her friends. Does this mean that she is maintaining her patients' confidentiality?

No, Kathy may breach confidentiality even if she does not pass on the patient's name. It all depends upon the information Kathy is disclosing to her friends. If one of the visitors listening in to Kathy's conversation is able to identify one of their neighbours from the information that Kathy is sharing, such as how they were dressed and some identifiable feature such as a mole in a particular place on their face, or their job (such as school bus driver), Kathy will have breached her duty of confidentiality to those patients.

Even if Kathy does not provide identifiable features in her discussion with her friends, the question to be asked is why she is discussing her patients with her friends in a public place. Whilst this may not be breaching any law, it is unethical in that it shows a lack of respect for her patients.

So, has Kathy done anything wrong? Yes, she has. At best she has shown a lack of respect for her patients. At worst she has breached their confidentiality and the duty of care she owes to them.

Confidentiality can be a complex issue particularly with changing family dynamics. I find confidentiality is even more complex in children's nursing than it is in other areas of nursing as it can be difficult to know who you should and should not share information with. I have been involved with the care of an adolescent during my training who didn't want his parents to know about his health issue and this was a difficult situation to manage.

Amber, 3rd-year children's nursing student

Working with children is both a privilege and a challenge. This book is primarily intended for those who are studying towards their registration in this area, although it is equally applicable to the registered children's nurse and those wanting an insight into the work of children's nurses.

Working with children requires awareness and promotion of the principles of empowerment, protection of rights and respect for children and their families. Indeed, the primary role of the children's nurse is to put the children first at all times.

Nurses working with children need to understand the legal underpinning of their work, such as their duty of care to children. Through the use of specifically selected practice-focused case studies and expert commentary, this chapter has explored legislation and policy applicable to the children's nurse, such as duty of care, duty of candour, communication, accountability, consent, safeguarding and confidentiality.

Attaining registration as a children's nurse is an immense achievement but it is not the end of the journey, just the beginning of the next stage. Remaining fit for practice is the responsibility of all nurses and is a requirement of the NMC as well as a societal expectation. It is what we demonstrate in the Revalidation process (NMC, 2015b). It requires that all nurses demonstrate the required knowledge, skill and respect for those in their care.

By working through this chapter you will have had the opportunity to critically reflect, explore and discuss the implications of delivering contemporary child-centred nursing care as part of a multidisciplinary and multiagency endeavour.

CHAPTER SUMMARY

- Law + Code = the intention is always to protect the public. Each registered nurse should follow policies, procedures and the law in their individual as well as multiprofessional and multidisciplinary practice.
- You have gained awareness of the relevance of duty of care and duty of candour.
- As a children's nurse you should regularly refresh your knowledge of the Code, and general and local policies and procedures for each area in which you work.
- As a children's nurse you should refresh knowledge of child protection legislation and policy at frequent intervals.
- As a children's nurse you should deliver child-centred and relevant associated care and put the child first.
- You should always ask your mentor or seniors if unsure – do not hesitate to seek advice. Even senior nurses seek advice and check their understanding as this is a professional skill in itself.

BUILD YOUR BIBLIOGRAPHY

Books

- Carter, B., Bray, L., Dickinson, A., Edwards, M. and Ford, K. (2014) *Child-centred Nursing. Promoting Critical Thinking*. London: Sage.

  This book is an excellent resource for those wishing to better understand the imperatives underpinning contemporary child-centred nursing care.

- Smith, L. and Coleman, V. (2009) *Child and Family-centred Healthcare: Concept, Theory and Practice*. London: Palgrave Macmillan.

  This book provides a clear focus on child-centred care in interprofessional and multidisciplinary settings as well as in community care.

- Watson, G. and Rodwell, S. (2014) *Safeguarding and Protecting Children, Young People and Families: A Guide for Nurses and Midwives*. London: Sage.

  This book offers a clear explanation of the ways in which children's nurses can safeguard their patients and considers many of the challenges that a children's nurse may encounter.

Journal articles

Go to https://study.sagepub.com/essentialchildnursing for further free online journal articles related to this chapter.

FURTHER
READING:
ONLINE
JOURNAL
ARTICLES

- Cornock, M. (2010) 'Hannah Jones, Consent and the child in action: a legal commentary'. *Paediatric Nursing*, 22 (2): 14-20.

  This article explains consent relating to the child, in an accessible manner and using a real-life clinical case as the focus for contemporary discussion.

- Gilmore, S. and Herring, J. (2011) '"No" is the hardest word: consent and children's autonomy'. *Child and Family Law Quarterly*, 23 (1): 3-25.

  This article explores the difficulties associated with legal definitions of consent in children's care.

- McFarlane, A. (2011) 'Mental capacity: one standard for all ages'. *Family Law*, 41 (5): 479-85.

  This article looks at mental capacity and what it means for issues of consent.

Weblinks

Go to https://study.sagepub.com/essentialchildnursing for further weblinks related to this chapter.

FURTHER
READING:
WEBLINKS

- legislation.gov.uk, Children Act 1989

  www.legislation.gov.uk/ukpga/1989/41/contents
  An example of key legislation which you should explore in more depth is the Children Act 1989 (or the equivalent in other countries). This sets out the legal expectations and requirements around the protection and welfare of children.

- UNICEF, Convention on the Rights of the Child

  www.unicef.org.uk/what-we-do/un-convention-child-rights
  The UNCRC is important reading for the children's nurse.

- NSPCC, *Child Protection in the UK and Safeguarding Deaf and Disabled Children*

  www.nspcc.org.uk/preventing-abuse/child-protection-system
  www.nspcc.org.uk/preventing-abuse/safeguarding/deaf-disabled-children
  Useful resources on child protection in England, Northern Ireland, Scotland and Wales.

ACE YOUR ASSESSMENT

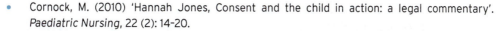

Revise what you have learned by visiting https://study.sagepub.com/essentialchildnursing

ONLINE
QUIZZES &
ACTIVITY
ANSWERS

- Test yourself with multiple-choice and short-answer questions
- Do the chapter activities in the book and check your answers online

REFERENCES

Bolam v. Friern Hospital Management Committee [1957] 2 All ER 118.

Carter, B., Bray, L., Dickinson, A., Edwards, M. and Ford, K. (2014) *Child-centred Nursing: Promoting Critical Thinking*. London: Sage.

Cornock, M. (2014a) 'Duty of care'. *Orthopaedic and Trauma Times*, (24): 14–16.

Cornock, M. (2014b) 'Legal principles of responsibility and accountability in professional healthcare'. *Orthopaedic and Trauma Times*, (23): 16–18.

Cornock, M. (2015) 'The child and consent'. *Orthopaedic and Trauma Times*, (27): 13–15.

Cornock, M. and Montgomery, H. (2014) 'Children's rights since Margaret Thatcher', in S. Wagg and J. Pilcher (eds), *Thatcher's Grandchildren*. Basingstoke: Palgrave.

Francis, R. (2013) *The Report of the Mid Staffordshire NHS Foundation Trust Public Inquiry*. London: The Stationery Office.

Gillick v. West Norfolk and Wisbech AHA [1985] 1 All ER 533.

HM Government (2015) *Working Together to Safeguard Children: A Guide to Inter-agency Working to Safeguard and Promote the Welfare of Children*. London: DfE. Available at: www.gov.uk/government/uploads/system/uploads/attachment_data/file/592101/Working_Together_to_Safeguard_Children_20170213.pdf (last accessed 8 May 2017).

Kirkip, B. (2015) *The Report of the Morecambe Bay Investigation: An Independent Investigation into the Management, Delivery and Outcomes of Care Provided by Maternity and Neonatal Services at the University Hospitals of Morecambe Bay NHS Foundation Trust from January 2004 to June 2013*. London: TSO.

Locke J. (1690) *Second Treatise of Civil Government*. Available at: www.constitution.org/jl/2ndtreat.htm. (last accessed 5 April 2017).

McAlinden, O. (2012) 'Ethical and legal implications when planning care for children and young people', in D. Corkin, S. Clarke and L. Liggett (eds), *Care Planning in Children and Young People's Nursing*. Chichester: Wiley-Blackwell.

NSPCC (2017) *Home Alone*. Available at: www.nspcc.org.uk/preventing-abuse/keeping-children-safe/leaving-child-home-alone (last accessed 8 May 2017).

Nursing and Midwifery Council (NMC) (2015a) *The Code: Professional Standards of Practice and Behaviour for Nurses and Midwives*. London: NMC. Available at: www.nmc.org.uk/globalassets/sitedocuments/nmc-publications/revised-new-nmc-code.pdf (last accessed 8 May 2017).

Nursing and Midwifery Council (NMC) (2015b) *Revalidation: What You Need to Do*. Available at: www.nmc.org.uk/standards/revalidation/how-to-revalidate (last accessed 5 April 2017).

Nursing and Midwifery Council (NMC) and General Medical Council (GMC) 2015) *Openness and Honesty When Things Go Wrong. The Professional Duty of Candour*. Available at: www.gmc-uk.org/guidance/ethical_guidance/27233.asp (last accessed 8 May 2017).

Oxford English Dictionary (2017) Available at: www.oed.com (last accessed 5 April 2017).

United Nations (1989) *UN Convention on the Rights of the Child*. Geneva: United Nations.

SAFEGUARDING CHILDREN AND YOUNG PEOPLE

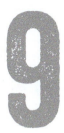

ZOE CLARK AND CAMERON COX

THIS CHAPTER COVERS

- An overview of safeguarding children, young people and families
- Multiagency working within safeguarding
- Multiagency safeguarding models
- An exploration of the issues and concerns linked to contemporary issues

> **"** I was so confused but knew what he was doing was wrong. I wanted it to stop but part of me was afraid to speak out because I didn't want to get him into trouble.
>
> **Lee, child, NSPCC** **"**

Visit https://study.sagepub.com/essentialchildnursing to access a wealth of online resources for this chapter – watch out for the margin icons throughout the chapter.

INTRODUCTION

Safeguarding children and young people is everyone's business and will form an essential part of the role of a qualified nurse. However, safeguarding remains the responsibility of any individual in contact with children and their families including nursing students. Safeguarding is far more than simply knowing the risk factors and being on alert; it's understanding what risks are posed to children in today's society, it's understanding that families are vulnerable and with this come complications with development of children and safety. This chapter aims to give you an understanding of how agencies work together to safeguard children and how to seek support from these agencies. Overall, safeguarding is a combination of knowledge including policies, research and sometimes simple 'gut instinct'. Building on the opening quote, the take-home message from this chapter is that if you have any concerns about a child or family, always raise this with someone senior, always do something and never do nothing.

AN OVERVIEW OF SAFEGUARDING CHILDREN, YOUNG PEOPLE AND FAMILIES

'Safeguarding children' and 'child protection' are terms commonly interlinked and it is clear within the guidance (RCPCH, 2014) that everybody who comes into contact with children has a responsibility to safeguard their welfare and ensure they are protected from harm. Nursing students are often drawn to this profession as they have a wish to help children.

> I got into children's nursing because I am compassionate and focused on the quality of care I feel I could give to patients in the future.
>
> **Laura, 2nd-year children's nursing student**

In recent years there has also been a movement away from children being placed on a child protection register to children having a child protection plan, suggesting a more positive action to the families involved (London Safeguarding Children Board, 2017a).

In the *Working Together to Safeguard Children* guidance (HM Government, 2015), safeguarding and promoting the welfare of children is defined as:

- Protecting children from maltreatment
- Preventing impairment of children's health or development
- Ensuring that children are growing up in circumstances consistent with the provision of safe and effective care and
- Taking action to enable all children to have the best life chances

Child protection is identified as a part of safeguarding and promoting welfare for children. However, it is focused more on the activity undertaken to protect specific children who are either suffering or are likely to suffer significant harm (HM Government, 2015). Section 47 of the Children Act 1989 provides local authorities with a duty to make enquiries into whether action is required to be taken to protect a child who is believed to be suffering or likely to suffer significant harm (London Safeguarding Children Board, 2017a). So how do we define harm?

Harm is more commonly referred to as abuse within the framework of safeguarding children. Somebody may abuse or neglect a child by inflicting harm, or by failing to act to prevent harm.

Children may be abused in a family or in an institutional or community setting by those known to them or by others (e.g. via the Internet). They may be abused by an adult or adults, or another child or children.

This can be further broken down into four main categories of abuse which children may need protecting from in relation to safeguarding children (LSCB, 2017a; Scottish Government, 2014; Welsh Government, 2017; Safeguarding Board for Northern Ireland, 2012):

1. Physical abuse

   A form of abuse which may involve hitting, shaking, throwing, poisoning, burning or scalding, drowning, suffocating or otherwise causing physical harm to a child. Physical harm may also be caused when a parent or carer fabricates the symptoms of, or deliberately induces, illness in a child (known as fabricated illness).

2. Emotional abuse

   The persistent emotional maltreatment of a child such as to cause severe and persistent adverse effects on the child's emotional development. It may involve conveying to a child that they are worthless or unloved, inadequate, or valued only insofar as they meet the needs of another person. It may include not giving the child opportunities to express their views, deliberately silencing them or 'making fun' of what they say or how they communicate. It may feature age or developmentally inappropriate expectations being imposed on children. These may include interactions that are beyond a child's developmental capability, as well as overprotection and limitation of exploration and learning, or preventing the child participating in normal social interaction. It may involve seeing or hearing the ill-treatment of another. It may involve serious bullying (including cyber bullying), causing children frequently to feel frightened or in danger, or the exploitation or corruption of children. Some level of emotional abuse is involved in all types of maltreatment of a child, though it may occur alone.

3. Sexual abuse

   Involves forcing or enticing a child or young person to take part in sexual activities, not necessarily involving a high level of violence, whether or not the child is aware of what is happening. The activities may involve physical contact, including assault by penetration (for example, rape or oral sex) or non-penetrative acts such as masturbation, kissing, rubbing and touching outside of clothing. They may also include non-contact activities, such as involving children in looking at, or in the production of, sexual images, watching sexual activities, encouraging children to behave in sexually inappropriate ways, or grooming a child in preparation for abuse (including via the Internet). Sexual abuse is not solely perpetrated by adult males. Women can also commit acts of sexual abuse, as can other children.

4. Neglect

   The persistent failure to meet a child's basic physical and/or psychological needs, likely to result in the serious impairment of the child's health or development. Neglect may occur during pregnancy as a result of maternal substance abuse. Once a child is born, neglect may involve a parent or carer failing to:

   - Provide adequate food, clothing and shelter (including exclusion from home or abandonment)
   - Protect a child from physical and emotional harm or danger
   - Ensure adequate supervision (including the use of inadequate care-givers)
   - Ensure access to appropriate medical care or treatment. It may also include neglect of, or unresponsiveness to, a child's basic emotional needs

PRACTICE SCENARIO 9: PATRICIA'S FAMILY

CASE STUDY 9.1: FRAN

Fran (30) is a mother of two children: Katlin (14) and Oisin (4 months). The family lives in a two-bedroom flat. Adam (34) the father of Oisin works as a security guard. He works night shifts and often comes back to the flat to sleep during the day. Fran is unemployed and does not like leaving the house.

Katlin is in Year 10 of the local high school. She was born prematurely at 32 weeks and has mild learning difficulties. She has an education and healthcare plan to support her to stay in mainstream education. However, she is often reported by teachers to be disengaged, tired and withdrawn in class. She doesn't have a big circle of friends and teachers have noted she is often isolated. Katlin has diabetes and was diagnosed aged 4 years. She has been having repeated admissions to hospital for poorly controlled blood sugar levels and is not compliant with her insulin regime.

Oisin is a small baby whose weight at his postnatal check was measured on the 0.4th centile. He has not been taken to any further postnatal appointments. Fran called an ambulance for Oisin two weeks ago as he was 'floppy' and 'not himself'. Oisin was admitted to the ward from Accident and Emergency due to malnutrition and dehydration. Fran is keen to get him discharged as she wants to be back at home. However, the nurses on the ward have concerns about Fran's capacity to care for Oisin.

- What are the safeguarding concerns?
- What categories of abuse are relevant to this case study?

CASE STUDY ANSWER 9.1

MULTIAGENCY WORKING WITHIN SAFEGUARDING

A wide range of health professionals including nurses, GP, health visitors, school nurses, midwives, child and adolescent mental health, drug and alcohol services and emergency care services have a critical role in safeguarding children and young people under 18 years (HM Government, 2015).

In recent years multiagency teams have been introduced to improve safeguarding approaches through better information sharing as well as high-quality and timely safeguarding approaches (HM Government, 2015). These structures of joint assessment were developed in response to children protection inquires (Cm 5730, 2003, Munro (2011), where there had been a tragic failure in services (Davis and Smith, 2012).

When safeguarding children, multiagency working is paramount. Achieving successful joint working (while safeguarding children) requires professionals to communicate effectively and recognise each other's areas of expertise (Hempton and Williams, 2011). Additionally, safeguarding is not just about protection of children; there is a broader more positive emphasis on prevention (Powell and Appleton, 2012).

Working Together to Safeguard Children (HM Government, 2015) and *National Guidance for Child Protection in Scotland*, (Scottish Government, 2014) provides statutory guidance for multiagency professionals to safeguard and promote the welfare of children (Safeguarding Board for Northern Ireland, 2012; Welsh Government, 2017). The guidance is for local agencies such as health, education, housing and police, who have a duty under section 11 of the Children Act 2004, to ensure the safeguarding needs and welfare of children are considered when carrying out their work.

Working Together to Safeguard Children (2015) also guides local safeguarding children boards (LSCBs) and local authorities to work together to safeguard children locally to provide evidence-based services to address their needs.

The following are examples of nurses that have a crucial role in multiagency arrangements to safeguard children:

- School nurses
- Health visitors
- Community children's nurses
- Specialist safeguarding midwives
- Safeguarding nurse leads and/or advisors
- Looked after children's nurses
- Accident and Emergency liaison nurses/health visitors)

SEE ALSO
CHAPTER 5

ACTIVITY 9.1: REFLECTIVE PRACTICE

Take a moment to consider the nurse's role when working as part of multiagency teams associated with safeguarding the health and wellbeing of children. The next section will discuss these models and their implications.

MULTIAGENCY SAFEGUARDING MODELS

Multiagency safeguarding hub (MASH)

There are several multiagency safeguarding models and the most common is the **Multiagency safeguarding hub (MASH)**. In some Local Authorities MASH teams are in place to screen child safeguarding referrals (LSCB, 2017a). The Home Office (2014) underlines the aims of MASH: to improve safeguarding for children through better information sharing and timely safeguarding responses. It is largely based on three common principles (see Figure 9.1) that enable effective communication across agencies and improved service delivery (Home Office, 2014). The MASH comprises five core elements (Table 9.1):

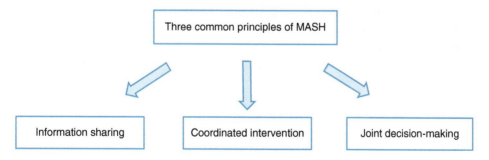

Figure 9.1 MASH

(Synthesised from Home Office, 2014 and LSCB, 2017b)

ACTIVITY 9.2: CRITICAL THINKING

Take some time to investigate your local area to establish what multiagency models are used to safeguard children. You can find out more about these in the next section.

Table 9.1 A MASH team comprises five core elements

	Core element	Procedure
1	Acts as a single point of entry	The aim is for all concerns, no matter what the level, to be routed through the MASH to enable a single route and decision-making process
2	Information sharing	A team of professionals from core agencies deliver an integrated service that will research, interpret and determine what information is proportionate and relevant to share (see Activity 9.3)
3	Confidentiality	MASH activity takes place in a confidential environment due to the sensitive nature of the information provided. The information is viewed by those who actually need to see it. It is disclosed on a strictly need-to-know basis
4	An agreed process for analysing and assessing risk	This enables the MASH to identify potential risks and have the opportunity to further address the risks through coordinated interventions
5	Early intervention	A process to identify victims, perpetrators and emerging harm through research and analysis. Early identification of these individuals and families enables services to intervene and prevent the need for more intensive interventions at a later stage

(Synthesised from: The Home Office, 2014 and LSCB, 2017b)

Multiagency risk assessment conference

Multiagency risk assessment conferencing (MARAC) is a local meeting that usually takes place monthly with a primary focus on the safety of high-risk victims of domestic abuse (10% of local cases) (LSCB, 2017a).

The main purpose of a MARAC is to:

- Reduce the risk of serious harm or even death of victims
- Share information to enhance the health safety and wellbeing of the adult victim and children
- Decide whether the alleged perpetrator poses a significant risk to either individuals and/or the general community
- Jointly construct and implement a risk management plan that provides professional support to all those at risk and reduce harm (LSCB, 2017a)

Agencies that should always be invited to a MARAC are:

- Police
- Children's social care (local authority)
- Probation services
- Health services
- Education (local authority)
- Other agencies such as the women's safety unit, youth offending teams, community mental health nurse, but it usually depends on whether they have specific involvement with the victims (LSCB, 2017b)

Collaborative working is essential in safeguarding practice as discussed here by a health visitor:

> Through collaborative working with healthcare professionals and single fathers I enabled my local NHS Trust to identify the need for a local resource specifically for single fathers, one which is available to health professionals to refer to within health promotion and its application to practice.
>
> **Shaun Lewis, children's nurse**

Multiagency sexual exploitation meeting (MASE)

Child sexual exploitation (CSE) can involve children and young people being subject to a number of exploitative situations that render them vulnerable to the risk of sexual exploitation. Commonly, the children do not see themselves as victims of sexual exploitation. Consequently, professionals, including nursing students, from all agencies should be alert to the possibility of sexual exploitation in children and report it to the appropriate child safeguarding professionals (LSCB, 2015a).

Sexual exploitation leaves a lasting imprint on children and they will often have long-term mental health concerns and/or physical illness following a period of exploitation. All children are at risk of sexual exploitation, both boys and girls and from all backgrounds and cultures. However, some risk factors have been identified to highlight children at an increased risk of sexual exploitation. These include children who have a history of running away/going missing from home, are in foster care, have special needs, are migrant children, are asylum seekers, are disengaged from education, are involved in use of drugs and alcohol or in gangs.

The overall aim for the perpetrator of sexual exploitation is to induce a power imbalance between themselves and the child. This can be in the form of threatening behaviour, violence and forced entrapment. However, encouraging sexual acts through the use of gifts, money and support may also be used. The perpetrator will form what the child feels is a safe nurturing relationship where they are spoilt with gifts and affection in return for sexual acts with them or any other person the perpetrator suggests. Often this relationship begins this way – for example, with online grooming where the child is persuaded to share sexual pictures of themselves online in return for gifts and praise. This can quickly turn and the child is then threatened into sending more and more images due to the threat of the other images being shared online, for example on social media (DCSF, 2009; Scottish Government, 2014; Welsh Government, 2016). Go to https://study.sagepub.com/essentialchildnursing to watch the educational video on how to protect personal information online.

VIDEO LINK 9.1: PROTECTING PERSONAL INFORMATION

WHAT'S THE EVIDENCE?

The Child Exploitation and Online Protection Centre (CEOP) published a thematic assessment to increase understanding of child sexual exploitation. The aim of this research was to raise awareness and knowledge to enhance prevention by understanding patterns of offenders, and the victimisation and vulnerability of children to sexual exploitation.

The full assessment can be accessed at https://study.sagepub.com/essentialchildnursing
Highlight the main findings from this evidence.

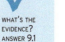
WHAT'S THE EVIDENCE? ANSWER 9.1

WEBLINK: CEOP ASSESSMENT

MASH teams (as mentioned earlier) play a vital role in identifying those at risk of CSE through the warning signs seen within referral notifications. MASH remains the first point of contact for any individual or professional who has concerns about a child or young person they feel are at risk of CSE.

Another team associated with CSE is MASE, which works in line with local safeguarding policy and procedures but unlike MASH it is not an established route for first-time referrals of CSE. Also, MASE do not work with individual cases; the prime aim is to provide a framework for regular information sharing and action planning to tackle CSE. The aim is for professionals to identify themes, patterns and trends in relation to CSE – for example, the identification of serial perpetrators, gang involvement, locations and premises associated with CSE – to discuss and address the risks and how to facilitate support that will remove the young person from the threat (LSCB,2017c). No agency should delay taking action whilst waiting for a discussion at the next meeting (LSCB, 2017a, 2017c). Each MASE should discuss and focus on all agencies working together:

- To ensure everything is being done to protect the victims and disrupt the offenders
- To ensure relevant information is being recorded on specific systems to provide appropriate agencies with access to that information
- To coordinate actions with other processes such as MARAC and MASH when required (LSCB, 2017c)

Membership of MASE is statutory for some agencies and others are encouraged to attend. It is essential they do if they have relevant information for the meeting.

Statutory agencies

- Police
- Children's social care
- Health
- Education
- Agencies that are contracted by the local authority to support victims of CSE
- Youth offending services

Other agencies

These include housing, probation, mental health services, drug/alcohol services, charities and care home providers (LSCB 2017c).

ACTIVITY 9.3: REFLECTIVE PRACTICE

Take some time to reflect on why information sharing is so important in safeguarding. You will find out more on this in the following section.

In recent years there have been several serious case reviews that have highlighted that poor information sharing has contributed to the death or serious injury of a child or children. Organisations such as health services and local authorities should have arrangements in place which set out clear guidance around the principles of information sharing (HM Government, 2015).

The LSCB (2017a), for example, bases their information-sharing principles for domestic abuse on the following:

- Professionals receiving information about domestic violence should explain that priority will be given to ensuring the safety of the mother/victim and child/ren
- If there are concerns about risk and/or significant harm to a child then it is every professional's duty to protect the child
- Professionals also have a duty to protect the mother/victim and should do so under the Crime and Disorder Act 1998. This allows accountable local authorities to share information where a crime has been committed or is going to be committed

The case study below involving Amisha helps you to further explore issues inherent in information sharing.

CASE STUDY 9.2: AMISHA

Amisha was a 19-year-old woman who had a troubled upbringing. She was first made homeless at the age of 13 and had 'sofa surfed' from then onwards. She was in and out of education and had contact with the local IAPT (Improving Access to Psychological Therapies) team for most of her adolescence. Amisha was known by two different general practitioners and she was constantly struggling to fight addiction to both alcohol and drugs. During this time she had a referral to a consultant psychiatrist to make a full mental health assessment to meet her needs. Housing were providing input to assist in her finding accommodation in privately rented accommodation. At this point Amisha attended the GP to state that she was pregnant. She also saw the drug rehabilitation team and the psychiatrist in the same week. She disclosed her housing and financial difficulties to all professionals. However, she stated that she was not taking drugs or drinking as she was happy to be pregnant. Amisha was allocated a midwife and the midwife received no history on Amisha and relied only on what was told to her.

During the later stages of her pregnancy the specialist midwife for supporting vulnerable mothers documented that a referral may be needed. However, this was never carried out. A baby was born to Amisha but died aged two days. At post-mortem, unlicensed and unprescribed drugs were found in her system. These drugs most likely passed through the placenta or breastmilk (Wonnacott, 2013).

Consider the above case study:

- What are some of the lessons learnt from this case study?
- What does the literature say in relation to information sharing?

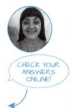

CHECK YOUR ANSWERS ONLINE!

✔

CASE STUDY ANSWER 9.2

AN EXPLORATION OF THE ISSUES AND CONCERNS LINKED TO CONTEMPORARY ISSUES

As students, it is essential for you to have an overview of contemporary safeguarding issues which include female genital mutilation and trafficking.

Female genital mutilation

Female genital mutilation (FGM) is the practice of mutilation of the outer parts of the female genitals. FGM is illegal in the UK and it is also illegal to remove a girl from the UK to another country to perform FGM (DH, 2015). Overall, there are approximately 180,000 women and children at risk of FGM in England and Wales. However, the true figures are estimated to be much higher due to the hidden nature of FGM (European Union, 2013). Estimates suggest that 20,000 girls are at risk of FGM in the UK and 66,000 women living in the UK have experienced FGM (WHO, 2017). There are four types of FGM (see Table 9.2).

Currently, FGM is mainly performed on females under the age of 15 and before puberty. However, FGM may be performed on adolescents between the ages of 15–19 years. UNICEF (2010) estimates that in some countries (e.g. Kenya and Tanzania) the numbers of adolescents undergoing FGM are falling dramatically in comparison to 30 years ago. However, in other countries, such as Somalia, numbers continue to rise and the age at which FGM is performed can be as low as infancy.

FGM has many health effects for women, varying from short-term initial effects through to longer-term effects (see Table 9.3), including depression and anxiety.

Another essential contemporary safeguarding issue for consideration is the trafficking of humans including children. You can watch the inspiring actions being taken around the world towards a future free from FGM and CEFM (child, early and forced marriage) in the UNICEF video at https://study.sagepub.com/essentialchildnursing

VIDEO LINK 9.2:
FREE FROM
FGM AND CEFM

Table 9.2   Different types of FGM

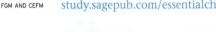

Classification	Description
Type 1	Clitoridectomy: partial or total removal of the clitoris (a small, sensitive and erectile part of the female genitals) and, in very rare cases, only the prepuce (the fold of skin surrounding the clitoris)
Type 2	Excision: partial or total removal of the clitoris and the labia minora, with or without excision of the labia majora (the labia are 'the lips' that surround the vagina)
Type 3	Infibulation: narrowing of the vaginal opening through the creation of a covering seal. The seal is formed by cutting and repositioning the inner, or outer, labia, with or without removal of the clitoris
Type 4	All other harmful procedures to the female genitalia for non-medical purposes – e.g. pricking, piercing, incising, scraping and cauterising the genital area

(WHO, 2017)

Table 9.3   Overall effects of FGM

Short-term effects	Long-term effects
Infection	Persistent urine infections
Difficulty or inability to urinate	Abnormal periods
Damage to urethra and/or bowel	Kidney impairment and possible kidney failure resulting from difficulty or inability to pass urine
Risk of contracting HIV/Hep B and Hep C	Psychological damage, including low libido, depression and anxiety (see below)
Shock/blood loss	The need for later surgery to open the lower vagina for sexual intercourse and childbirth
Pain	Complications in pregnancy and newborn deaths
	Pain from the formation of scar tissue
	Damage to the reproductive system, including infertility
	Pain during sex and lack of pleasurable sensation

(NHS Choices, 2014)

Trafficking

Human trafficking is the movement of human beings into and out of countries including the UK. Human trafficking can affect women, men and children of all ages. However, for the purpose of this chapter the focus will be on children.

Children are trafficked through the use of force, coercion, abuse or any other form of deception with the sole purpose of exploitation. This exploitation comes in many forms and is not solely linked to sexual exploitation as often is the misconception. Trafficking of children may be for labouring in big industries producing mass-produced goods through to domestic duties within a home environment. Children may also be trafficked to be forced into criminal activity including street crimes such as stealing and forced begging. Organ harvesting and forced marriage are also reasons to traffic children out of the UK (NSPCC, 2014).

Due to the difficulties in identifying these children it is hard to give exact figures to highlight the extent of the problem. However, the United Nations International Children's Emergency Fund (UNICEF) currently estimates that ten children are trafficked every week out of the UK (National Crime Agency, 2017).

Trafficking is made possible by a variety of reasons which may be affecting the country from which people are trafficked. The following is not an exhaustive list of factors contributing to the risk of trafficking but it gives an understanding of how a child may be vulnerable and therefore targeted for trafficking:

- Poverty
- Lack of education
- Discrimination
- Cultural attitudes
- Grooming
- Dysfunctional families
- Political conflict and economic transition and
- Inadequate local laws and regulations (HM Government, 2007)

Children who have been trafficked are exposed to high levels of violence and physical abuse, and sexual exploitation which may include forced sexual acts and rape. Controlling behaviour of the responsible adult is a sign that the child has been trafficked; this may include withdrawing the right to education, confiscation of passports and neglect in general of the child (Zimmerman et al., 2011).

Trafficking of children is a very serious issue of rising concern for professionals in the UK who work closely with this group. The difficulty often faced by professionals is that these children may not be aware that they have been trafficked, especially if they have come from a country outside of the European Union into the UK. These children will be fearful of the UK authorities and may lack understanding around what abuse and exploitation are. They may not disclose information, even during a visit from a health professional for example. Children trafficked out of the UK are often taken quickly and without much prior warning or signs and therefore are a difficult group to identify and protect (NSPCC, 2014).

VIDEO LINK 9.3: CHILD EXPLOITATION AWARENESS

You may have contact in your career with a child who has been the victim of trafficking. In this instance, trust your professional instinct and do not raise concerns with the adult accompanying the child. Seek support from a more experienced member of the team and attempt to assess the child without the adult present. However, consider factors such as language barriers and, if needed, make use of interpreter services. Remember that the child may be fearful of divulging information. Ensure they understand that they are safe and can talk to you. However, when responding, do not make promises you can't keep and be open about the next steps. Allow the child time to open up and never let cultural factors stand in the way of making an overall assessment (NSPCC, 2014).

Safeguarding children is everyone's responsibility and a fundamental part of children's nursing practice. In today's ever changing society it is essential to know what constitutes child abuse and how it can be addressed and prevented. Appropriate training allows professionals to recognise signs of child abuse or early indicators of concern, provide support, share information and carry out approved assessments. Joint working between agencies requires professionals to communicate effectively and respect each other's area of expertise.

Have a look at the preparing for placement advice at https://study.sagepub.com/essentialchildnursing for tips on safeguarding issues during placements.

PLACEMENT
ADVICE 9:
SAFEGUARDING
DURING
PLACEMENTS

PREP FOR
PLACEMENT!

CHAPTER SUMMARY

- Safeguarding children and young people is everyone's business and will form an essential part in the role of the qualified nurse. In addition, it remains the responsibility of any individual in contact with children and their families including nursing students.
- Child protection is part of safeguarding and promoting the welfare of children, but the main focus is to protect specific children who are suffering or likely to suffer significant harm.
- Within the framework of safeguarding children, harm is often referred to as abuse. The four main categories of abuse which children may need protecting from are physical, sexual, emotional and neglect. Understanding the definitions of child abuse is an essential aspect of safeguarding children and young people.
- Multiagency working is paramount in safeguarding practice. There are several models, the most common being the MASH and others such are MARAC and MASE, which are directed at more specific areas of safeguarding children and young people.
- It is essential to pursue help and advice if you are concerned a child has suffered or is at risk of suffering abuse.

BUILD YOUR BIBLIOGRAPHY

Books

- Cleaver, H., Cawson, P., Gorin, S. and Walker, S. (2009) *Safeguarding Children: A Shared Responsibility*. Chichester: Wiley-Blackwell.

  This book covers key areas in the principles and processes of safeguarding children, including an excellent chapter (Chapter 1) on the effectiveness of multiagency working.

- Corby, B., Shemmings, D. and Wilkins, D. (2012) *Child Abuse: An Evidence Base for Confident Practice*. 4th edn. Maidenhead: Open University Press.

  This book raises students' awareness of child abuse. See Chapter 4 on defining child abuse.

- Powell, C. (2015) *Safeguarding and Child Protection For Nurses, Midwives and Health Visitors: A Practical Guide*. 2nd edn. Maidenhead: Open University Press.

  An excellent book with an informative chapter that uses case studies to highlight importance of prevention and early help when safeguarding children and young people. See Chapter 2 on prevention and early help.

Journal articles

Go to https://study.sagepub.com/essentialchildnursing for further free online journal articles related to this chapter.

- Gonzalez-Izquierdo, A., Ward, A., Smith, P., Walford, J., Ioannou, Y. and Gilbert, R. (2014) 'Notifications for child safeguarding from an acute hospital in response to presentations to healthcare by parents'. *Child: Care, Health and Development*, 41 (2): 186–93.

  An interesting study into notifying children's social care services of safeguarding concerns when parents present at acute hospitals with drug, alcohol, mental issues and violence.

- Hempton, S. and Williams, R. (2011) 'Safeguarding children'. *Innovait*, 4 (3): 145–53.

  This is a useful article that describes important legislation and guidance if child maltreatment is suspected.

- Powell, C. and Appleton, J.V. (2012) 'Children and young people's missed health care appointments: reconceptualising "Did not attend" to "Was not brought". A review of the evidence for practice'. *Journal of Research in Nursing*, 17 (2): 181–92.

  A systematic review of relevant health policy and appropriate documentation on children's missed healthcare appointments.

- Whiting, M., Scammell, A. and Bifulco, A. (2008) 'The Health Specialist Initiative: professionals' views of a partnership initiative between health and social care for child safeguarding'. *Qualitative Social Work*, 7 (1): 99–117.

  An evaluation of multiagency working combined with building lasting partnerships between social workers and health professionals.

FURTHER READING: ONLINE JOURNAL ARTICLES

Weblinks

Go to https://study.sagepub.com/essentialchildnursing for further weblinks related to this chapter.

- NSPCC

  www.nspcc.org.uk
  The NSPCC provides a wealth of advice and support on safeguarding children.

- GOV.UK

  www.gov.uk
  A UK government website that is a useful source of the current legislation, policy and procedures in safeguarding children and young people.
  Knowledge link Chapter 8

- London Safeguarding Children Board

  www.londonscb.gov.uk
  An excellent resource for London Child Protection Procedures and Practice Guidance.

FURTHER READING: WEBLINKS

ACE YOUR ASSESSMENT

Revise what you have learned by visiting https://study.sagepub.com/essentialchildnursing

- Test yourself with multiple-choice and short-answer questions
- Do the chapter activities in the book and check your answers online

ONLINE QUIZZES & ACTIVITY ANSWERS

REFERENCES

Child Exploitation and Online Protection Centre (CEOP) (2011) *Out of Mind, Out of Sight Making Every Child Matter … Everywhere.* Executive Summary. Available at: www.ceop.police.uk/Documents/ceopdocs/ceop_thematic_assessment_executive_summary.pdf (accessed 18 July 2017).

Cm 5730 (2003) *The Victoria Climbié Inquiry: Report of an Inquiry by Lord Laming.* London: TSO.

Davis, J.M. and Smith, M. (2012) *Working in Multi-Professional Contexts: A Practical Guide for Professionals in Children's Services.* London: Sage.

Department for Children, Schools and Families (DCSF) and Home Office (2009) *Safeguarding Children and Young People from Sexual Exploitation: Supplementary Guidance to Working Together to Safeguard Children.* London: Department for Children, Schools and Families (DCSF).

Department for Education (DfE) (2015) Main tables B3 and C1 in *Characteristics of Children in Need in England, 2014–15.* London: DfE.

Department of Health (DH) (2012) *Practical Guidance on the Application of Caldicott Guradian Principles to Domestic Violence and MARACs.* London: Department of Health. Available at: www.gov.uk/government/uploads/system/uploads/attachment_data/file/215064/dh_133594.pdf (last accessed 8 May 2017).

Department of Health (DH) (2015) *Female Genital Mutilation: Help and Advice.* Available at: www.gov.uk/female-genital-mutilation-help-advice (last accessed 8 May 2017).

European Union (2013) *Communication from the Commission to the European.* Available at: http://eige.europa.eu/rdc/eige-publications/female-genital-mutilation-european-union-report (accessed 9 October 2017).

Hempton, N. and Williams, R. (2011) 'Safeguarding children'. *InnovAiT*, 4 (3): 145–53.

HM Government (2007) *Statutory Guidance on Making Arrangements to Safeguard and Promote the Welfare of Children under Section 11 of the Children Act 2004.* Available at: http://webarchive.nationalarchives.gov.uk/20130401151715/https://www.education.gov.uk/publications/eorderingdownload/dfes-0036-2007.pdf (last accessed 8 May 2017).

HM Government (2015) *Working Together to Safeguard Children: A Guide to Inter-agency Working to Safeguard and Promote the Welfare of Children.* London: DfE. Available at: www.gov.uk/government/publications/working-together-to-safeguard-children--2 (last accessed 8 May 2017).

London Safeguarding Children Board (2017a) *London Child Protection Procedures and Practice Guidance.* Available at: www.londoncp.co.uk (last accessed 8 May 2017)

London Safeguarding Children Board (2017b) *London MASH Project: The Five Core Elements.* Available at: www.londonscb.gov.uk/wp-content/uploads/2016/04/1.-Five-CORE-ELEMENTS-Final-1.pdf (last accessed 8 May 2017).

London Safeguarding Children Board (2017c) *The London Child Sexual Exploitation Operating Protocol,* 2nd edn. Available at: https://beta.met.police.uk/globalassets/downloads/child-abuse/the-london-revised-cse-operating-protocol-2nd-edition.pdf (accessed 8 May 2017).

Munro, E. (2011) *The Munro Review of Child Protection: Final Report: A Child-centred System.* London: DfE. Available at: www.gov.uk/government/uploads/system/uploads/attachment_data/file/175391/Munro-Review.pdf (last accessed 8 May 2017).

National Crime Agency (2017) *National Referral Mechanism Statistics: End of Year Summary 2016.* Available at: www.antislaverycommissioner.co.uk/media/1133/2016-nrm-end-of-year-summary.pdf (accessed 29 August 2017).

NHS Choices (2014) *Female Genital Mutilation.* Available at: www.nhs.uk/Conditions/female-genital-mutilation/Pages/Introduction.aspx (last accessed 8 May 2017).

NSPCC (2014) *Stop Child Trafficking in Its Tracks: Advice for Health Visitors*. London: NSPCC.

NSPCC (2016) *Children's Stories: Fiona's Story*. Available at: www.nspcc.org.uk/fighting-for-childhood/childrens-stories-about-abuse (last accessed 8 May 2017).

Powell, C. and Appleton, J.V. (2012) 'Children and young people's missed health care appointments: reconceptualising, "Did Not Attend" to "Was Not Brought" – a review of the evidence for practice'. *Journal of Research in Nursing*, 17 (2): 181–92.

Royal College of Paediatrics and Child Health (RCPCH) (2014) *Safeguarding Children and Young People: Roles and Competences for Health Care Staff: Intercollegiate Document*, 3rd edn. London: RCPCH.

Safeguarding Board for Northern Ireland (2012) *Role of SBNI*. Available at: www.safeguardingni.org/role-sbni (accessed 17 July 2017).

Scottish Government (2014) *National Guidance for Child Protection in Scotland*. Edinburgh: The Scottish Government. Available at: www.gov.scot/Resource/0045/00450733.pdf (last accessed 8 May 2017).

Welsh Government (2016) *National Action Plan to Tackle Child Sexual Exploitation (Wales)*. Available at: http://gov.wales/topics/health/socialcare/safeguarding/?lang=en (accessed 8 May 2017).

Welsh Government (2017) *Safeguarding*. Available at: http://gov.wales/topics/health/socialcare/safeguarding/?lang=en (last accessed 18.July 2017)

Wonnacott, J. (2013) *On Baby Z Serious Case Review*. Available at: www.westsussexscb.org.uk/wp-content/uploads/lsle-of-Wight-Baby-Z.pdf (accessed 29 August 2017).

World Health Organization (WHO) (2017) *Female Genital Mutilation: Fact Sheet*. Available at: www.who.int/mediacentre/factsheets/fs241/en/ (Last accessed 18th July 2017)

Zimmerman, C., Hossain, M. and Watts, C. (2011) 'Human trafficking and health: a conceptual model to inform policy, intervention and research'. *Social Science Medicine*, 73: 327–35.

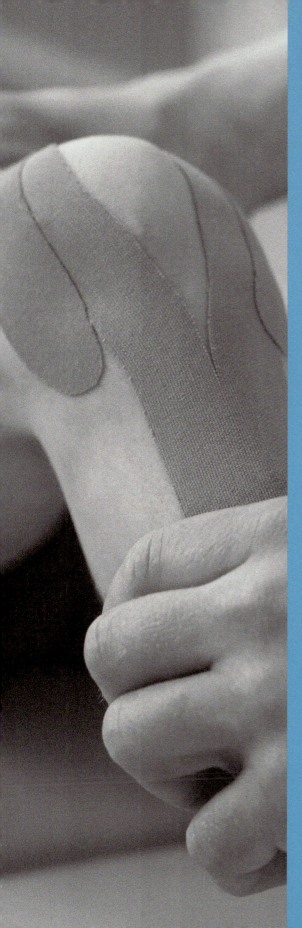

PART 2 CHILD AND INFANT WELLBEING AND DEVELOPMENT

10 Genetics and epigenetics: effects on children and young people 151

11 Infant mental wellbeing and health or 'how to grow a healthy adult' 164

12 Complexities of the developing and differing needs of children and young people 182

13 Factors influencing wellbeing and development in children and young people 194

14 Universal screening and the role of the health visitor 210

GENETICS AND EPIGENETICS: EFFECTS ON CHILDREN AND YOUNG PEOPLE

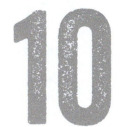

GILL LANGMACK AND ELISABETH O'BRIEN

THIS CHAPTER COVERS

- The concepts of genetics, genomics and epigenetics
- The variation in inheritance
- The concept of risk
- The essential ethical and legal implications of genomics

> " My advice to nursing students would be to look at all families with a genetic eye and don't be afraid to ask the family the difficult questions. Are there specific health problems running through a family? Understand that sometimes bad news can be good news for families, which is not something you expect as a nurse.
>
> **Marjie, genetic nurse counsellor** "

Visit https://study.sagepub.com/essentialchildnursing to access a wealth of online resources for this chapter – watch out for the margin icons throughout the chapter.

INTRODUCTION

Before starting this chapter you should know how genes pass from grandparents to parents and to children. You should understand chromosomes, genes and cell division/replication and the terms 'autosomal dominant' and 'recessive inheritance', 'monogenic' and 'mitochondrial inheritance'.

REQUIRED KNOWLEDGE

It would helpful to have an understanding of genetics and epigenetics before you start this chapter. Please read Boore (Boore et al., 2016), Chapter 3: Genetic and epigenetic control of biological systems.

Using case studies, this chapter aims to explore the basis of genetics and epigenetics through the changes that are seen when the child inherits their parents' genome. This chapter can only form an introduction but should help you start to link the child's genetic make-up to their ongoing condition. For example, it is already well known that some people respond to medications, including analgesia, differently if their genes provide the instructions to make the cytochrome P450 enzyme. The diagnosis and treatment of many conditions – for example, some types of leukaemia, asthma and solid tumours – is increasingly dependent on accurate information about an individual's genome.

CASE STUDY 10:
GENETICS
COUNSELLOR

The opening quotation from a genetic counsellor, Marjie, identifies the need for all nurses to consider the role of genetics in that everyone's health status and risk of developing diseases may be based on a genetic variation. She also indicates that there is a national move to include diagnostic testing within care pathways, which may occur before referral to genetic counselling services. The online materials available at https://study.sagepub.com/essentialchildnursing explore the role of the genetic counsellor further.

VIDEO LINK 10.1:
BEGIN BEFORE
BIRTH

It is now known that all diseases lie on a spectrum from being 100 per cent caused by genetic factors to being completely determined by the environment. During your nursing career, you will come across families and their children with symptoms, conditions and underlying syndromes that are unfamiliar to you. An understanding of the underlying principles of genetics and epigenetics can be very helpful. Watch the video 'Begin befor Birth' at https://Study.sagepub.com/essentialchildnursing

Current standards (NMC, 2010, p.18) state that 'All nurses must carry out comprehensive, systematic nursing assessments that take account of relevant ... genetic and environmental factors, in partnership with service users and others through interaction, observation and measurement'. In addition, eight competency statements were published setting out the attitudes, skills and knowledge in genetics and genomics required by all nurses in the UK at the point of registration (Kirk et al., 2011). This built on previous work by Kirk et al. (2003) outlining the situations in which those working with children need to use genetic information to:

- Provide supportive, informed communication at the time of diagnosis or receipt of definitive results
- Ensure the nurse can act as a trusted and informed carer for children growing up with genetic conditions (such as muscular dystrophy or cystic fibrosis), as they may be probing increasingly for information about the condition, its prognosis and effect on life plans
- Help parents deal with feelings of anger, guilt or blame as they acknowledge their own genetic contribution to the child's illness or consider prenatal diagnosis in a future pregnancy
- Enhance awareness of conditions which may mimic non-accidental injury or abuse, such as osteogenesis imperfecta or conditions that result in failure to thrive
- Facilitate referral to local genetic services when appropriate

ACTIVITY 10.1: REFLECTIVE PRACTICE

Children's nurses and health visitors work across a range of settings, at primary, secondary and tertiary levels of care. Think about situations in an acute or community setting when issues to do with genetics have arisen.

Look at Figure 10.1 to remind you of the typical areas you may have seen on practice placement. Consider to what extent you and your mentor were able to assess the family's genetics.

ACTIVITY
ANSWER 10.1

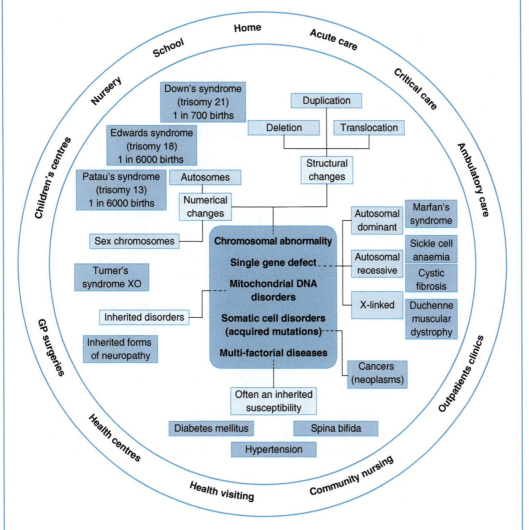

Figure 10.1 Genetic changes that can occur and the typical places where knowledge of genetics can be helpful

THE CONCEPTS OF GENETICS, GENOMICS AND EPIGENETICS

With significant advances in computing speeds and molecular techniques, our knowledge of human genetics has developed rapidly since the beginning of the Human Genome Project (HGP) in 1990. At first, the goal was to sequence the genes and produce a map of the human genome. When the full sequence of the human genome was mapped in 2003, there was an astonishing discovery that only about 1–2 per cent of the bases code for proteins. The total number of identified genes that code for proteins is approximately 30,000. This means that the role of 98 per cent of human deoxyribonucleic acid (DNA) is not known.

Genetics: Over the last 25 years it has become increasingly apparent that the concept of genes coding for proteins – the basic concept of genetics – is only a starting point for the ways DNA acts to provide 'software' for the body's development. Genes can be switched 'on 'or 'off' by various external factors and also through ribonucleic acid (RNA) which is coded by 'junk' DNA.

Genomics: This is the study of all of an individual's genes, or genome, including how they interact with other genes and the environment.

Epigenetics: This is the term used to refer to factors that influence the way our genes are expressed in the cells of our body.

Epigenetic alterations

If the following criteria are met then epigenetic alterations in DNA are likely to have occurred.

1. Two organisms have the same genotype but different phenotypes, e.g. identical twins have the same DNA (genotype) but different physical characteristics (phenotype)
2. An organism continues to be affected by an initiating event long after that event has passed, e.g. the effects of famine on the grandchildren of women who were pregnant at the time of the famine (Stein and Susser, 1975)

Epigenetic marks can change the way the DNA message is read. These changes are not permanent and can alter over time (Sharma et al., 2010). The major mechanisms by which these changes can occur include:

- Stem cell differentiation: Some processes change the way genes are expressed which changes the instructions for cells and tissues to form in the embryo

  o Methylation – adds a methyl group to the DNA. This changes how the DNA is transcribed into RNA
  o Histone modifications – DNA is packed around proteins known as histones. The tightness of the packing causes changes in the gene expression
  o RNA changes – tiny micro-RNA molecules affect the messenger RNA which makes enzymes

- De-activating an X chromosome: If a gene on one of the X chromosomes is deactivated, it prevents both chromosomes expressing the gene which may potentially affect the child.

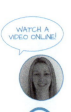

VIDEO
LINK 10.2:
EPIGENETICS

An epigenetics video (Institute of Reproductive and Developmental Biology, no date) with Professor Vivette Glover that describes how events such as stress in pregnancy and early childhood can affect the genome can be found at https://study.sagepub.com/essentialchildnursing

WHAT'S THE EVIDEMNCE?

Diabetes mellitus illustrates the different ways genes work. There are numerous causes of diabetes mellitus that prevent insulin either being created or used effectively by the body, some of which have genetic and/or epigenetic causes. In addition to type 1 diabetes mellitus (insulin stops being produced by the pancreas) and type 2 diabetes mellitus (generally seen as the result of lifestyle changes), others have been identified:

- *Maturity onset diabetes in the young (MODY)* usually develops prior to the person's 25th birthday following changes to the secretion of insulin in adolescence. Whilst there are different types of MODY, it is seen as a single gene defect which is autosomal dominant (DRDCMG, 2015)
- *Neonatal diabetes* may be a result of a gene mutation or the over-expression of a gene. This may be temporary, lasting 3–12 months, or permanent (Turnpenny and Ellard, 2012)
- *Epigenetic changes* may be triggered by changes to the DNA or activation/de-activation of a gene. There is increasing evidence that the epigenetic changes that occur in an individual's parents or even grandparents may in some cases affect the child (Bohacek and Mansuy, 2013)

Further information on the different types of diabetes can be found at the Diabetes UK (2017) website, and Diabetes Research Department and the Centre for Molecular Genetics (DRDCMG) websites, which you can access from https://study.sagepub.com/essentialchildnursing

WEBLINK:
OTHER
TYPES OF
DIABETES

THE VARIATION IN INHERITANCE

If a diagnosis is made that may have an underlying genetic cause, the question needs to be asked if there are others in the family who have a similar problem.

Identifying the family pedigree

When starting to develop a family pedigree, a family may immediately discuss a set of illnesses in one part of the family, but it's important to be specific and systematic to explore the links between family members. This needs to include the biological relationships, not the social relationships – for example, step-siblings do not have the same genetics as they are not biologically related. Family members can also be 'hidden' or 'forgotten' within families, particularly when looking at the grandparent generation, aunts, uncles and cousins.

The types of questions (National Genetics and Genomics Education Centre (NGGEC), 2011) need to include:

WEBLINK:
NGGEC

- Major medical, physical or mental health problems
- Anyone requiring hospital admission
- Serious illnesses or operations
- Age when the condition was diagnosed
- Cause of death and age at death – this should include stillborn infants
- Conditions or illnesses which seem to run on either side of the family

It is traditional to look at three generations in the family. The resulting family pedigree can help to define the risks of the condition in others in the family. Whilst it would not usually be ethical to ask about the health of others for a family, where the questions are asked for a medical purpose, as in this situation, the questions are acceptable (Royal College of Physicians, Royal College of Pathologists and British Society for Human Genetics, 2011).

Drawing the pedigree

A standard set of symbols is used to draw a family pedigree (Bennett et al., 1995; NGGEC, 2011).

When taking a history, it is essential to record the date of birth, age at death and relevant medical information. This includes symptoms or diagnosis and the age of occurrence in addition to documenting who gave the information, drew the pedigree and the completion date.

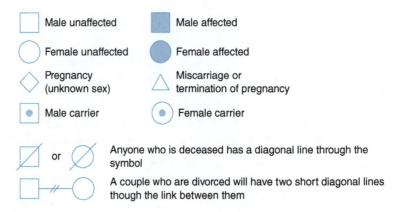

Figure 10.2 Symbols

The following two scenarios and activities should help you to develop an understanding of the complexity of assessing inheritance. Dwayne's family pedigree is more straightforward than David's. However, the techniques you develop in exploring Dwayne's pedigree need to be applied in the same way.

PRACTICE
SCENARIO 10:
LUKE

SCENARIO 10.1: DWAYNE

Dwayne is a 3-year-old who has had intermittent symptoms of feeling tired and lethargic with a racing heartbeat for the last two months. Following investigations, the doctors diagnose a conduction problem in how his heart beats, known as 'short Q-T syndrome'. His mum remembers an old discussion that a cousin of hers had a sudden heart attack as a child.

A family pedigree needs to be developed to explore the pattern of inheritance as Dwayne's condition has a genetic basis. The risk can then be determined for his parents having other children and within the wider family.

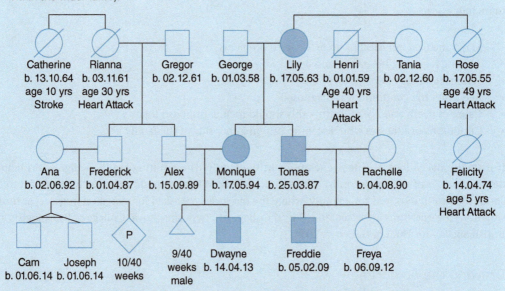

Figure 10.3 Dwayne's pedigree (showing the members of his family who have the cardiac conduction problem)

- Identify which members of Dwayne's family are affected by short Q-T syndrome.
- How would you describe the pattern of inheritance seen in Dwayne's pedigree?

SCENARIO
ANSWER 10.1

Although you may not have done this in practice, mapping a pedigree is a useful skill that enhances a thorough family history.

You can access a link at https://study.sagepub.com/essentialchildnursing which will help you explore how to undertake and record a family pedigree.

WEBLINK:
FAMILY
PEDIGREE

ACTIVITY 10.2: REFLECTIVE PRACTICE

Using the symbols in Figure 10.2, draw your own family pedigree. Try putting in three generations.

ACTIVITY
ANSWER 10.2

Dwayne's family pedigree was drawn for you, but now try David's scenario. The information a person gives can be confusing and may need clarifying before you can start to explore what is occurring.

SCENARIO 10.2: DAVID

I'm Emma. My child David who is now 5 years old was diagnosed with cystic fibrosis following the newborn screening test and then more blood tests in hospital. Although we hadn't known it, both his dad, Tony and I are carriers for the gene. David has an older brother and sister – Tom aged 12 years and Katie aged 8 years – neither has the condition but both are carriers.

Tony has one brother and two sisters. Tony's dad, David's grandfather, does not carry the gene but his mother who had died before the genetic testing took place did have a sister with a chronic lung problem who died aged 8 years old. We think this was probably cystic fibrosis too although it was never confirmed. Of Tony's mother's four children, it would appear that one girl is also a carrier for the gene, and the other two are unaffected.

On my side of the family, I'm a carrier as is my sister. She now has one child, Suzi, who is unaffected and she's very reluctant to have any more children in case they become carriers too. Her husband doesn't have the gene. My parents aren't alive to ask, but one of them must have been a carrier too.

As a genetic disease, it's not currently curable but we live in hope that gene therapy will be possible.

(Continued)

(Continued)

- Try drawing David's family pedigree. Compare your diagram with the worked example at https://study.sagepub.com/essentialchildnursing. Now try to answer the following questions:

    o Who in the family would be a carrier of cystic fibrosis?
    o What pattern of inheritance is inherited and why?

SCENARIO
ANSWER 10.2

WHAT'S THE EVIDENCE?

In relation to David, the only potential cure is currently through the use of gene therapy. If asked, what should you know about this innovative treatment in order to support the parent or sufferer who asks you?

Gene therapy is the therapeutic delivery of nucleic acid polymers into a patient's cells as a means to treat disease. The polymers are translated into proteins to interfere with or target gene expression, or to possibly correct genetic mutations.

Gene therapy is a general term to describe a range of techniques designed to tackle the root causes of genetic conditions at source. Methods currently being studied include:

- Introducing a working or healthy copy of a gene to replace a mutated gene – this is often done using a virus
- Inactivating or 'turning off' a defective gene – as in an autosomal dominant disorder
- Introducing a new gene into the body to help combat the disease

The most common form uses DNA that encodes a functional, therapeutic gene to replace a mutated gene. The polymer molecule is packaged within a 'vector' which carries the molecule inside cells.

Most gene therapy has focused on treating individuals (somatic cells) but it could be targeted towards sperm or eggs (germ cells). The idea of using germ cells for correction of genetic problems has caused ethical concerns.

- Is it appropriate to change the human genome for future generations?

WHAT'S THE
EVIDENCE?
ANSWER 10.1

SEE ALSO
CHAPTER 18

THE CONCEPT OF RISK

If a chromosomal abnormality or a single gene mutation exists, then it is possible to estimate the potential risk of a further child having the abnormality. Where one child has a condition, it does not mean the next child will not get the illness, the probability will remain the same. Predicting the potential risk of a subsequent child having a genetic condition is difficult and the family is currently offered the opportunity to be referred to a regional genetics centre to be seen by a specialist team.

Autosomal dominant patterns have an equal number of males and females affected, with each affected child having at least one affected parent, but two affected parents may have an unaffected child (see Scenario 10.1: Dwayne).

Autosomal recessive patterns are often seen in unaffected parents having an affected child (see Scenario 10.2: David).

X-linked patterns show more males affected and no male-to-male transmission. An example of this would be Fragile X inheritance.

Genetic risk

Estimating the genetic risk can be undertaken by developing a tree diagram and/or a Punnett square and assessing the probability of subsequent children having inherited the affected gene (Nichols, 2009). Both diagrams are used; however, the Punnett square is more commonly seen as being less easy to get confused.

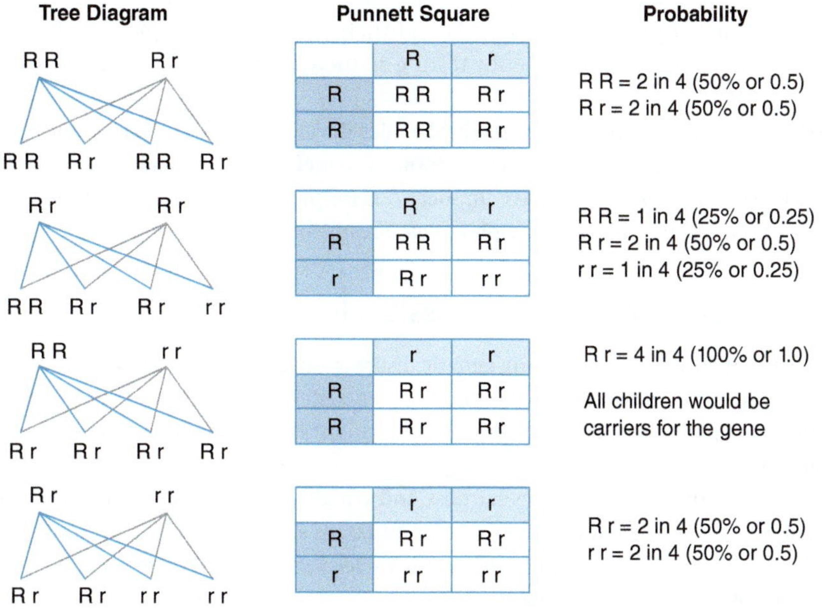

Figure 10.4 Patterns of inheritance showing dominant (R) and recessive (r) traits

The chance of having a subsequent child with a specific trait is seen in the tables and probability analysis.

For example, in David's situation (Scenario 10.2), where both parents are carriers (second table in Figure 10.4), the probability of having another child with cystic fibrosis (rr = 1 in 4 chance) would be worked out as follows:

(Child 1) 0.25 x (child 2) 0.25 = 0.0625 or 6.25%

The probability of David's parents having two further children who do not have cystic fibrosis – so having a genotype of either RR (1 in 4 chance) or Rr (1 in 2 chance) would be:

(Child 1) (0.25 + 0.5) x (Child 2) (0.25 + 0.5) = 0.75 x 0.75 = 0.5625 or 56.25%

The probability calculations become even more complex where one parent has no family history or where there are epigenetic influences. Assessing a family's understanding of risk is an integral part of genetic counselling – for example, some people will think that a 1 in 4 chance of inheritability is greater than a 25 per cent risk when in fact they are equal.

WEBLINK:
GENIE GUIDE

Please access the Genie guide from the University of Leicester via https://study.sagepub.com/essentialchildnursing It is aimed at non-specialist health professionals and explores different approaches to explain genetic risk and probability.

THE ESSENTIAL ETHICAL AND LEGAL IMPLICATIONS OF GENOMICS

Genetics is at the cutting edge of science, and therefore at the forefront of ethics and law. When planning, assessing and delivering children's care nurses should be aware of the legal, ethical and moral implications of procedures and tests and their potential consequences. This is particularly relevant to today's students as genetics testing is increasingly taking place outside mainstream genetics services.

The four fundamental principles of medical ethics developed by Beauchamp and Childress (2009) have a wide consensus. These principles of autonomy, beneficence, non-maleficence and justice might seem theoretical at first glance but have implications for practice, research and policy.

To find out more about ethical principles, please read Northway and Beech (2015).

Issues to consider for health professionals

There are many methods for diagnosing genetic disorders and abnormalities in the first two trimesters, including non-invasive testing. Prenatal diagnosis and offers of termination raise difficult questions for the individuals concerned and wider questions about the way society cares for and values those with disability.

Justice is a concept that emphasises fairness and equality. Patients in similar situations should be treated similarly, and in a broader sense, benefits and costs should be fairly distributed across a population. There is general agreement in the UK that sex selection for social preferences or family balancing is not justified as grounds for termination.

Health staff should consider the principle of *beneficence*, or acting in the child's best interests. As a general rule, the benefit should outweigh the harm and testing is best left until the child is old enough to consent, unless there are health implications which mean that treatment should begin earlier.

Testing children younger than 12 years of age is not generally justified unless there is a clear benefit. For example, if an adult has familial adenomatous polyps (FAP) then close family members will be offered screening from 12 years of age as, if any children have the altered gene, it is likely the bowel polyps, some of which may lead to cancer, will appear before the age of 20.

The principle of *non-maleficence* (or the principle of not doing harm) should be remembered. There are many issues relating to a genetic disease that a family may wish to keep private or to share. There is the difficulty of sharing results between regional genetics services when many family members are seen. Confidentiality would only be breached under extreme circumstances.

The principles underpinning genetic counselling are that it is non-directive and aims to ensure that decision-making is informed *choice*. Families should be given full information including the risks, limitations, outcomes and implications of genetic testing and the option of not participating.

The consequences of each course of action should be explored. For families to have *autonomy* they should be empowered when decisions need to be made. This means they needs accessible information but should feel free to opt out of genetic testing at any stage.

ACTIVITY 10.3: CRITICAL THINKING

On a recent insight visit, you encountered the following situations where health professionals need to consider the balance between the conflicts that inevitably arise in practice. Based on the issues you have just read about, what are the ethical, legal and societal questions that arise for each case?

- Prenatal diagnosis

Sunil and Lucy are expecting a second baby and have requested sexing of the foetus with a view to termination if it's a boy. Their first child has a condition they know is more common in boys. Overall, the risk of having another child with the same condition is 5 per cent (1 in 20)

- Children and predictive testing

Daniel and Isha have requested testing to see if their child has inherited an adult onset autosomal dominant condition that they have just found out runs in the family

- Implications for individuals, immediate and extended family

Sam is a 14-year-old boy who comes to clinic with his father after a referral from Sam's GP. Sam's dad wants him to have genetic testing for type 1 osteogenesis imperfecta but Sam is reluctant. Sam has an older sister who is due to get married and wants to start a family before her career takes her overseas

ACTIVITY
ANSWER 10.3

In complex cases the practical considerations of care management are not straightforward and there may be competing claims to ethical principles. In some cases the advice of the hospital ethics committee can be sought.

An example of this can be heard on the radio programme *Inside the Ethics Committee* (BBC, 2013) which considers genetic testing and children and which you can access from https://study.sagepub.com/essentialchildnursing This examines a real-life complex dilemma facing a woman whose husband died, in his 30s of an adult onset lung cancer linked to Li–Fraumeni syndrome which may or may not have been inherited by their four children.

Both Delves-Yates (2015), Chapter 6: 'Law' and Dimond (2008) *Legal Aspects of Nursing* provide excellent resources for those looking to explore contemporary ethical issues in healthcare.

As Marjie indicates at the very beginning of this chapter, understanding the nature of the way health problems run through succeeding generations in a family pedigree can provide the child and their family with the information they require to make informed decisions about care and future pregnancies. Please find out more about the role of the genetics counsellor at https://study.sagepub.com/essentialchildnursing

VIDEO LINK
10.3: INSIDE
THE ETHICS
COMMITTEE

SEE ALSO
CHAPTER 8

CASE STUDY 10:
GENETICS
COUNSELLOR

CHAPTER SUMMARY

- Knowledge of human genetics has developed rapidly since the beginning of the Human Genome Project (HGP) in 1990
- Understanding the nature of the way health problems run through succeeding generations in a family pedigree can provide the child and their family with information
- Genetics is at the cutting edge of science, and therefore at the forefront of ethics and law

---

BUILD YOUR BIBLIOGRAPHY

You can find references to useful books, book chapters and weblinks throughout the chapter.

Journal articles

FURTHER READING: ONLINE JOURNAL ARTICLES

Go to https://study.sagepub.com/essentialchildnursing for further free online journal articles related to this chapter.

- Barr, O. and McConkey, R. (2007) 'A different type of appointment: the experiences of parents who have children with intellectual disabilities referred for genetic investigation'. *Journal of Research in Nursing*, 12 (6): 637–52.

  This research explores the experiences of parents attending a genetics-based appointment in respect of their child with an intellectual disability.

- House, S.H. (2013) 'Transgenerational healing: educating children in genesis of healthy children, with focus on nutrition, emotion, and epigenetic effects on brain development'. *Nutrition and Health*, 22 (1): 9–45.

  This article provides an overview of epigenetic changes illustrated using historical events to show the differences between genetic inheritance and epipgenetic influences focusing on nutrition and brain development.

- Letourneau, N., Giesbrecht, G.F., Bernier, F.P. and Joschko, J. (2014) 'How do interactions between early caregiving environment and genes influence health and behavior?' *Biological Research for Nursing*, 16 (1): 83–94.

  This article explores the effects of stress on gene expression in relation to attachment and behaviour in childhood.

ACE YOUR ASSESSMENT

ONLINE QUIZZES & ACTIVITY ANSWERS

Revise what you have learned by visiting https://study.sagepub.com/essentialchildnursing

- Test yourself with multiple-choice and short-answer questions
- Do the chapter activities in the book and check your answers online

---

REFERENCES

BBC (2013) 'Genetic testing in children' (*Inside the Ethics Committee: Series 9*). Available at: www.bbc.co.uk/programmes/b038hhs7 (last accessed 15 May 2017).

Beauchamp, T.L. and Childress, J.F. (2009) *Principles of Biomedical Ethics*, 6th edn. Oxford: Oxford University Press.

Bennett, R.L., Steinhaus, K.A., Uhrich, S.B., O'Sullivan, C.K., Resta, R.G., Lochner-Doyle, D., Markel, D.S., Vincent, C. and Hamanishi, J. (1995) 'Recommendations for standardized human pedigree nomenclature'. *American Journal of Human Genetics*, 56 (3): 745–52.

Bohacek, J. and Mansuy, I.M. (2013) 'Epigenetic inheritance of disease and disease risk'. *Neuropsychopharmacology*, 38 (1): 220–36.

Boore, J. (2016) 'Genetic and epigenetic control of biological systems', in J. Boore, N. Cook and A. Shepherd (eds), *Essentials of Anatomy and Physiology for Nursing Practice*. London: Sage.

Delves-Yates, C. (2015) *Essentials of Nursing Practice*. London: Sage.

Diabetes Research Department and the Centre for Molecular Genetics (DRDCMG) (2015) *Genetic Types of Diabetes including Maturity-onset Diabetes of the Young (MODY)*. Available at: www. diabetesgenes.org (last accessed 15 May 2017).

Diabetes UK (2017) *Maturity Onset Diabetes of the Young (MODY)*. Available at: www.diabetes.org.uk/ Guide-to-diabetes/What-is-diabetes/Other-types-of-diabetes/MODY (last accessed 15 May 2017).

Dimond, B. (2008) *Legal Aspects of Nursing*, 5th edn. Harlow: Pearson Education.

Institute of Reproductive and Developmental Biology at Imperial College London (no date). *Begin before Birth*. Available at: www.beginbeforebirth.org/for-schools/films#epigenetics (last accessed 15 May 2017).

Kirk M, McDonald K, Longley M, Anstey S et al (2003) Fit for Practice in the Genetics Era: Defining what nurses, midwives and health visitors should know and be able to do in relation to genetics. Pontypridd: University of Glamorgan

Kirk, M., Tonkin, E. and Skirton, H. (2011) *Fit for Practice in the Genetics Era: A Revised Competence Based Framework with Learning Outcomes and Practice Indicators. A Guide for Nurse Education and Training*. Available at: http://genomics.research.southwales.ac.uk/media/files/ documents/2013-09-05/ffpgge-nursing-learning-outcomes.pdf (last accessed 15 May 2017).

National Genetics and Genomics Education Centre (NGGEC) (2011) *Genomics Education Programme*. Available at: www.geneticseducation.nhs.uk (last accessed 15 May 2017).

Nichols, W.M. (2009) *Genie Guide: Calculation and Communication of Genetic Risk – for Non-geneticists*. Available at: www2.le.ac.uk/departments/genetics/vgec/healthprof/resources-for-health-professionals/genie-guide-calculation-and-communication-of-genetic-risk-for-non-geneticists (last accessed 15 May 2017).

Northway, R. and Beech, I. (2015) 'Ethics', in C. Delves-Yates (ed.), *Essentials of Nursing Practice*. London: Sage.

Nursing and Midwifery Council (NMC) (2010) *Standards for Pre-registration Nursing Education*. London: NMC.

Royal College of Physicians, Royal College of Pathologists and British Society for Human Genetics (2011) *Consent and Confidentiality in Clinical Genetic Practice: Guidance on Genetic Testing and Sharing Genetic Information, 2nd edn. Report of the Joint Committee on Medical Genetics*. London: Royal College of Physicians and Royal College of Pathologists.

Sharma, S., Kelly, T.K. and Jones, P.A. (2010) 'Epigenetics in cancer'. *Carcinogenesis*, 31 (1): 27–36.

Stein, Z. and Susser, M. (1975) 'The Dutch famine, 1944–1945, and the reproductive process. I. Effects on six indices at birth', *Pediatric Research*, 9: 70–76.

Turnpenny, P. and Ellard, S. (2012) *Emery's Medical Genetics*, 14th edn. Philadelphia: Churchill Livingstone.

INFANT MENTAL WELLBEING AND HEALTH OR 'HOW TO GROW A HEALTHY ADULT'

ORLA McALINDEN

THIS CHAPTER COVERS

- What we mean by infant mental health and why is it so important?
- Strategies to improve infant mental health
- Which strategies work and how do we know this?

> "
> But the hearts of small children are delicate organs. A cruel beginning in this world can twist them into curious shapes. The heart of a hurt child can shrink so that forever afterward it is hard and pitted as the seed of a peach. Or again, the heart of such a child may fester and swell until it is a misery to carry within the body, easily chafed and hurt by the most ordinary things.
>
> Carson McCullers, 1951,
> *The Ballad of the Sad Café*
> "

Visit https://study.sagepub.com/essential childnursing to access a wealth of online resources for this chapter – watch out for the margin icons throughout the chapter.

INTRODUCTION

The concept of infant mental health (IMH) is not new. In the 1930s Sigmund Freud began examining the impact of child mental development on the later life of the adult, and this scrutiny continued with a string of interested theorists throughout the 20th century. It is now a newly resurgent topic of interest to multidisciplinary teams and a global effort of enquiry, practice and research. This is led in some part by recent advances in science and genetics, in particular the earliest stages of a child's life, before they have been born.

SEE ALSO CHAPTERS 10, 11, 13 AND 14

Whilst the science and psychological theory may be complex, the topic is an important one for you to engage with as it has a direct impact on the services that are currently offered and being developed to support wellbeing from early life onward. The quotation at the start of this chapter, for instance, aptly summarises the importance of the influences on the 'hearts of small children', and it is an important role as a children's nurse to tend to the psychological mental and physical wellbeing of your patient. This may be in early years care, or as a nurse caring for the school age or older child right into the adolescent and early years of adulthood. By association it also means considering the welfare of the parent and family as well.

Today's society has many children in need of the essential universal health services, as well as children with very particular needs (e.g. complex physical and intellectual needs, learning disability, looked after children, children leaving care, children in the custody and youth justice system, child and adolescent mental health tiers, refugees and those who are displaced and exploited for varying complex reasons). The children's nurse of today and tomorrow needs to understand what interventions are needed and the robustness of the evidence underpinning them.

SEE ALSO CHAPTERS 40 AND 41

Research clearly shows that what happens in the womb and early years can affect the development of a child into adulthood and beyond. This is why the topic is so important to all health and social care professionals: the best start in life is needed for a good finishing chance – this is part of what a 'good outcome' looks like for children.

This chapter will first explore definitions of infant mental wellbeing and health as a touchstone for measuring the success of identified interventions, and explore why it is so important, giving a summary of seminal and recent scientific and psychological research. It will then look at how services and interventions address emotional and mental wellbeing for all, not just those at risk, how the services are developing and the evidence behind them. Finally, it will examine one of the main recent developments in the UK and USA – the Family Nurse Partnership (FNP).

WHAT DO WE MEAN BY INFANT MENTAL HEALTH AND WHY IS IT SO IMPORTANT?

Zero to Three's (2009) definition of infant mental health is:

WATCH A VIDEO ONLINE!

VIDEO LINK 11.1: BEGIN BEFORE BIRTH

> the young child's capacity to experience, regulate and express emotions, form close and secure relationships, and explore the environment and learn. All of these capacities will be best acknowledged within the context of the caregiving environment which includes family, community and cultural expectations for young children. Developing these capacities is synonomous with healthy social and emotional development.

There are varying definitions and some criticism that the above timeframes start too early and end too soon. Barlow and Svanberg (2009) prefer broader timeframes which include the important pre- and perinatal periods. They and others (Institute of Reproductive and Developmental Biology, n.d.; O'Donnell et al., 2009) place great importance on the role of the placenta in the early influences on the developing foetus and strongly support the idea that early intervention should start ideally in the pre-conceptual and antenatal/perinatal periods if an improvement in children's life and health chances is sought.

SEE ALSO CHAPTER 10

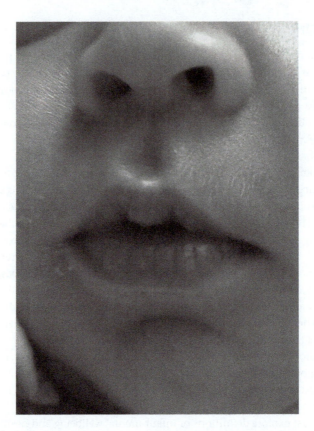

Figure 11.1 Baby face

There is now much more research and enquiry into these periods, which is enhanced by the increased contemporary scientific and research technology capability available. There is also growing recognition that IMH is influenced both by parenting and the environment, which includes the placenta as an 'environment' with a hitherto under-recognised role (O'Donnell et al., 2009).

VIDEO LINK 11.2:
CHARLIE'S
STORY

There is greater will to provide a good start in life for infants and children, one which will optimise their life chances and improve their resilience to multiple adverse childhood events (ACEs); in other words, help them cope better with life and family stresses and go on to be a young adult who is better equipped to deal with negative life events.

Emotional wellbeing

WEBLINK:
INFANT MENTAL
HEALTH

Emotional wellbeing is important for all children. It should not be left until problems with emotional, psychological and mental health surface in later years and is an excellent reason why knowledge of this area should be reflected in all health, social care and education interventions. For an example, see the children's strategy for your country by visiting the appropriate goverment website.

There is strong evidence to support preventing mental and emotional ill health rather than trying to deal with the negative outcomes in later years. Remember that as a children's nurse you have a social, professional and employment imperative to do the best for your children and their families.

SEE ALSO
CHAPTER 37

Recent developments in psychology indicate a shift in orientation from a deficit (the skills you do not have) to a strengths perspective (the skills you do have). This is known as 'positive psychology'

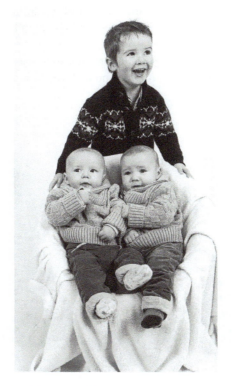

Figure 11.2 Darragh with twins Cathal and Conor

and aims to promote adaptation and recovery to a stage where there is a limited dysfunction of life experiences, giving a better quality of life for the individual.

It is generally becoming better recognised in the literature that what happens in early childhood will shape the later stages of childhood and adulthood (Minnis et al., 2007; Barlow and Svanberg, 2009; Ball et al., 2012), and there is growing awareness of the potential for shaping positive outcomes in the emerging areas of epigenetics and neurobiology (Barlow and Svanberg, 2009, 2013). These biogenetic elements appear to shape infant and children's future development and adjustments in life.

SEE ALSO
CHAPTER 10

This understanding of good IMH is crucial because the message is clear that early intervention is important in order to ensure that infants and children have the best possible start in life. This also involves multiprofessional learning and working, at all levels and across agencies, skills which a children's nurse should be both familiar with and competent in demonstrating.

SEE ALSO
CHAPTERS 2
AND 5

There is a growing acknowledgement that those first early years of a child's life are absolutely crucial. Getting it right as parents with professional help and public resource to support where needed has the potential to make a huge difference to how that child will grow into an adult contributing to society. Putting this approach at the heart of what Government does, across all party divides, has the potential to be life-changing literally which makes the work of the APPG (All Party Coalition Government) so important.

(Tim Loughton MP for East Worthing & Shoreham and Co-chair of the All Party Parliamentary Group Conception to Age 2: first 1001 days. Available at: www.1001criticaldays.co.uk/ (accessed 26 September 2017))

This has major implications for parenting and shaping of global health and social policy and for strategies for teaching and educating parents, families and communities as well as current and future students of health and social care.

All children's and mental health nurses are particularly well placed to influence positive parenting and promote emotional wellbeing in infants and children in order to stabilise and promote the foundations of resilience.

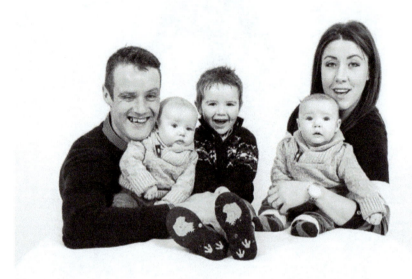

Figure 11.3 Peter and Diedre and their children

WEBLINK:
SAFEGUARDING

It is also true that adult nurses, and indeed anyone who comes into contact with infants, children and families, can make an impact on the future development of that individual. This development is also inextricably linked with the issue of safeguarding. Please go to https://study.sagepub.com/ essentialchildnursing to read more about this.

SEE ALSO
CHAPTER 9

STRATEGIES TO IMPROVE INFANT MENTAL HEALTH

Public health strategies from all four UK countries, the Republic of Ireland and further afield recognise the importance of the findings discussed above, as well as the role of the nurse (in all four fields of practice) in enhancing the path from the prenatal period, through to childbirth and early years and on towards adolescence and adulthood.

There have been numerous initiatives and programmes designed to support the improvement of infant mental health. They include:

- Infant massage techniques
- Brazelton Neonatal Behavioural Assessment Scale
- First Steps Parenting Programme
- Family Partnership Model of intervention and support
- The Parental Couple in Parenting
- PEEP Model – Learning together
- Early screening and intervention re. secure attachment

- Black and Ethnic Minorities (BEM)
- Mellow Babies
- Mellow Bumps
- Solihull Approach
- Solihull Plus
- Ounce of Prevention
- Working with mothers who have mental health needs
- Parenting with support for parents who have learning difficulties
- Breastfeeding initiatives and WHO 'Baby Friendly' policies (see https://study.sagepub.com/essential childnursing for more information and resources on the 'Baby Friendly Initiative')
- Developing infant-centred services
- Sure Start programmes from 2000 onwards
- Child and family centres

WEBLINK:
BABY FRIENDLY
INITIATIVE

There are also many US programmes including the Abecedarian Project, High Scope/Perry Preschool, Chicago Child–Parent Centers, Early Head Start, HomeVisiting, and the Doula Program (theounce.org) amongst others.

WEBLINK:
THE OUNCE

These interventions cannot effectively work alone but must be part of a broader drive and focus on research education practice and policy in order to succeed. There needs to be ongoing consistent evidence to show that the gains will be worth the initial early investment. This is particularly important in times of global austerity when there must be compelling evidence to show that investment works (the 'invest-to-save' principle).

The expected return (gain) period on IMH investment is estimated to be in the region of seven years of no return, or actual loss, before any material gains can be seen in monetary terms (Marmot, 2010; Munro, 2011; Tickell 2011). This means that IMH is particularly vulnerable to underfunding or inconsistent investment unless a strong approach is taken by all countries.

Approaches and interventions should ideally mean seamless access for all families. This includes midwives, health visitors, GPs and children's centres, and services should engage with families as soon as possible, not waiting for dysfunction or a crisis to occur. Ideally the approach should be during or before pregnancy. All contact that parents have with services before and after the birth of their child provides a unique opportunity to work with them at the stage which is an essential precursor to the healthy development of our children.

SEE ALSO
CHAPTERS 13
AND 14

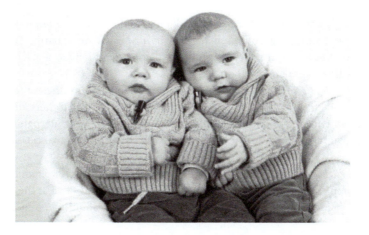

Figure 11.4 Cathal and Conor

The first few years of a child's life are fundamentally important. Evidence tells us that they shape children's future development, and influence how well children do at school, their ongoing health and wellbeing and their achievements later in life. The Government is clear that all young children, whatever their background or current circumstances, deserve the best possible start in life and must be given the opportunity to fulfil their potential.

But this is not just about doing the best for individual children and families. A strong focus on the first few years of children's lives leads to huge economic, social and emotional benefits later on, both for individuals and for society as a whole. (DfE and DH, 2011, p.2)

WHICH STRATEGIES WORK AND HOW DO WE KNOW THIS?

Central to any decision about introducing new policy or strategy is the question 'What works and what evidence is there?' In recent times this has been gaining more interest and importance as governments and policy makers aim to raise the topic higher on the health, social care and justice agenda (DH, 2011; Galloway, 2014; Leadsom et al., 2013).

WEBLINK: CHILD
PSYCHOTHERAPY
TRUST

The Child Psychotherapy Trust document *An Infant Mental Health Service* (2012) and the Ounce of Prevention website are good starting places for an overview of the experiences of the early years and the importance of evidence informing early years intervention. You can access both via https://study.sagepub.com/essentialchildnursing

The UK Cross Party Manifesto (Leadsom et al., 2013) called *The 1001 Critical Days*, the first of its kind, stressed that the approach should be one of agency rather than passive engagement and in the foreword states:

as our understanding of the science of development improves, it becomes clearer and clearer how the events that happen to children and babies lead to the structural changes that have life-long ramifications...

...we know too that not intervening now will affect not just this generation of children and young people but also the next. Those who suffer multiple adverse childhood events achieve less educationally, earn less, and are less healthy, making it more likely that the cycle of harm is perpetuated into the following generation...

This publication sets out key areas for attention as:

- *The importance of the foundation years*: All children should be able to enjoy their childhood, in a supportive and nurturing environment, and be protected from harm. The United Nations Convention on the Rights of the Child also sets the precedent here to make clear that children's needs are a right and not an afterthought.
- *Parents and families at the heart of services*: There has often been insufficient focus on the central role of families in children's earliest years, which has meant that mothers and fathers have not always received enough, or sufficiently timely, advice and support. Recognition and inclusion of fathers as parenting partners and positive role models is another goal (RCM, 2014; Widarsson et al., 2015).

WEBLINK:
CHILD &
MATERNAL
HEALTH
NETWORK

- *Focusing on child development and intervening early*: The 'Healthy Child Programme' can be fully and consistently implemented. This programme, from pregnancy to age five, is the overarching frame-work for NHS foundation years provision for all children, with additional early help for vulnerable families needing support using tools such as those at the National Child and Maternal Health Network (http://webarchive.nationalarchives.gov.uk/20170302100842/http://www.chimat.org.uk/preview).

- *Skilled professionals*: There has not been a sufficiently coherent framework to date for professional development and progression, highlighting the critical importance of continuing to improve the skills and qualification levels of workforces.
- *A strong relationship with the sector*: Children's centres in the community will be developed to provide access to a range of integrated universal and targeted services to meet locally defined need.

Please go to https://study.sagepub.com/essentialchildnursing to read more about *The 1001 Critical Days*.

FIND OUT MORE!

FURTHER INFO 11.1: THE 1001 CRITICAL DAYS

Evidence for interventions

Good quality evidence which underpins practice is a key concern, especially in times of austerity. It is required for ethical, professional, accountable practice and justification for the spending of public money. It is also a key election driver and can be used to influence health and social care policy at each term of government.

SEE ALSO CHAPTER 41

There is a wide range of early years interventions employed UK-wide in order to improve and empower parenting capability and bolster infant mental health practices. The evidence is not readily available for some, and for others the evidence suggests that there may be ways of better managing interventions, either because of cost or because of outcome (Little et al., 2013; Neville et al., 2013).

Other research over the years suggests that early intervention can work well (Heckman, 2000; Center on the Developing Child, undated; Galloway, 2012; Eurochild, 2012; Svanberg and Barlow, 2013).

Eurochild (2012) states that intervention can range from low-threshold advice and support to every parent, to very targeted, specialised services for the most vulnerable parents. All services aimed at family and parenting support must be non-stigmatising, empowering, have a participatory and strengths-based orientation, be accessible to all and must be underpinned by a child-rights approach, and be readily accessible.

VIDEO LINK 11.3: DEVELOPING CHILD

Moulin et al. (2014) conducted research into parenting and providing a secure attachment for children, and this work yields some interesting evidence. The report clearly identifies how secure attachment can also narrow the 'school readiness' gap and improve children's life chances. This study suggests that more support from health visitors, children's centres and local authorities in helping parents bond with young children could play a role in narrowing the education gap. The report also found that securely attached children are more resilient to poverty, family instability, parental stress and depression. For example, boys growing up in poverty are two and a half times less likely to display behaviour problems at school if they formed secure attachments with parents in their early years.

In cases where mothers have poor bonds with their babies, research suggests their children are also more likely to be obese as they enter adolescence. Parents who were insecurely attached themselves, who are living in poverty or who have poor mental health find it hardest to provide sensitive parenting and bond with their babies.

Secure attachment develops through sensitive and responsive parenting in the first years of life and parenting plays a causal role in attachment: an improvement in parental sensitivity is necessary for an improvement in attachment security (DfE and DH, 2011; Svanberg and Barlow, 2013).

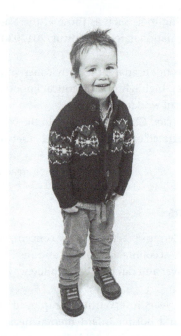

Figure 11.5   Darragh aged two-and-a-half years

WHAT'S THE EVIDENCE?

In the research discussed above Moulin et al. (2014, pp.22-7) looked at several programmes (summarised below) promoting parenting, attachment and socio-emotional development for under-3s, identifying each model's elements:

- Evaluation
- Benefits to child and family
- Approximate cost of the intervention

Table 11.1   Baby bonds

Family Nurse Partnership	Intense one-to-one home-visiting Relationship building with first-time teenage mothers	Randomised control trial (Memphis, USA) with low-income, first-time, young mothers	FNP children had better emotional development at age 4, amongst other positive, lasting gains	£3,000 per family, per year
	Nurses	15-year follow up		
	From early pregnancy to age 2	Trialled in the UK and elsewhere		
Circle of Security	Parent education, therapy and peer support in small groups of 5-7	Pre-test/post-test, 65 parents recruited through Head Start and Early Head Start Federal programmes for low-income families in the USA	The number of children securely attached rose from 20% to 54% after treatment Number with highest risk (disorganised) attachment fell from 60% to 25%	£1,200 for training per head
	Therapists			
	Weekly 75-minute sessions over 20 weeks			

Minding the Baby	Home-visiting supports reflective parenting	A randomised control trial (RCT) in Connecticut, USA is a work in progress	RCTs still underway	Not yet available
	Specialist social workers and nurses working together		Early US findings show improved reflective functioning and more secure attachment	
	From the third trimester of pregnancy weekly until age 1, fortnightly until age 2	An independent RCT in the UK with 320 first-time mothers under 25 began in spring 2014		
Child–Parent Psychotherapy	Child–Parent Psychotherapy and Parenting	RCT with high-risk families in New York State, USA	At age 2, 61% formed a secure attachment, compared to 2% of the control in the control group of standard community services	£1,900 a head for training
	Educational therapists			
	Sessions over 10 to 12 months			
Incredible Years	Social-learning model using video, role-play, peer support	Parent Training for 4-8 year olds has undergone multiple	Benefits for other programmes include improved positive	£850 for the programme materials
	Masters-level group leaders and parenting practitioners	randomised control trials in the USA	affect, emotional regulation and behaviour	
	8-10 sessions for babies under 1 and toddlers 1-3			
Parents Early Education Partnership (PEEP)	Home-visiting and group sessions, based on reflective functioning for first-time parents	An evaluation by Warwick Medical School began in 2014	The aim is to impact on secure attachment through increased parental reflective functioning	£450 to train a practitioner; £450 per family for 8 sessions
	Level-3 qualified parenting practitioners	It is a controlled realist evaluation with 25 families and 25 in the control		
	One prenatal home visit, 3 group sessions and 4 postnatal group sessions			
Oxford Parent Infant Project (OXPIP)	One-to-one support, video-feedback	Small, internal pre-test, post-test evaluation in Oxford, UK	The proportion of infants who were rated 'adapted' or 'well adapted' rose from 3% to 29% after the intervention	£800 per family on average
	Therapists			£4,000 a head for training
	Average of 10 sessions, from conception to age 2			

Source: Adapted with permission from Moulin, S., Waldfogel, J. and Washbrook, E. (2014) *Baby Bonds: Parenting, Attachment and a Secure Base for Children.* London, UK: The Sutton Trust.

This study by Moulin concludes that:

1. Early interventions can work with all, especially with very high-risk or troubled families with children under 3 years of age
2. Early interventions can promote secure attachment and development, especially when skilled practitioners support parents

(Continued)

(Continued)

3. For both national and local policy makers, this would represent a sound preventative investment

- Consider what you know so far about attachment and write a definition in your own words. Read the report by Moulin et al. (2014) and consider their definition of attachment. Does this match or exceed your own definition?

ACTIVITY 11.1: CRITICAL THINKING

- Which political parties have a consistent track record of promoting infant and child welfare?
- What specific services to promote infant and child welfare are there in your area or country? (Refer to your local jurisdiction websites)

A rapid health review (PHE, 2015) provided compelling evidence updates in relation to key areas affecting IMH, including: parental mental health; smoking; alcohol/drug misuse; intimate partner violence; preparation and support for childbirth and the transition to parenthood; attachment; parenting support; unintentional injury in the home; safety from abuse and neglect; nutrition and obesity prevention; and speech, language and communication. The Children and Young People's Mental Health Taskforce has produced key reports (DH, 2015a, 2015b), which recognise that:

> Our childhood has a profound effect on our adult lives. Many mental health conditions in adulthood show their first signs in childhood and, if left untreated, can develop into conditions which need regular care. (DH, 2015b, p.5)

The Family Nurse Partnership (FNP)

The FNP programme was originally developed in the USA by Professor David Olds (Olds et al., 1986, 2010; Olds et al., 2010). It is an intensive 'nurse' home visiting programme designed to improve the health, wellbeing and self-sufficiency of first-time parents and their children. FNP visits start early in pregnancy and continue until the child reaches 24 months. The specially trained nurse home-visitor's attention is focused on the social, emotional and economic context of the client's life, and activities are based on understanding human interactions.

At the time of writing the FNP is widely used in the UK and is led by the Family Nurse Partnership National Unit which heads the national delivery of the FNP programme and supports local organisations with implementation as commissioned by the Department of Health, which holds the licence in England. The National Unit also works closely with NHS England to assure the quality of local programme delivery and to support preparation in new areas. Their role includes:

- Providing strategic direction and working with national partners
- Overseeing research and development
- Providing the Family Nurse Partnership learning programme for family nurses and supervisors
- Providing clinical guidance to supervisors and family nurses
- Advising on programme set-up in local areas and sub-licensing organisations to provide the programme

- Supporting local and national quality improvement and providing technical advice and guidance to local areas
- Leading adaptations to the programme so it remains relevant to the UK social context and developing knowledge
- Developing related models and products that support children's development in pregnancy and the early years

The FNP programme has been evaluated mostly positively to date (Ball et al., 2012) with further reviews and evaluations expected from both UK and US data as the programme is further refined and developed.

The pivotal element of the home visits and one of the distinguishing characteristics of the Nurse Family Partnership (NFP) model, as it is known in the USA, is building a therapeutic relationship between the nurse and the client. The aim is to build and empower clients' skills, confidence and hope in a manner that values the clients' ability to determine their own futures. The programme in England has been renamed the Family Nurse Partnership to better reflect the UK method of working but practitioners also made a collective decision to call themselves family nurses (FNs) to distinguish their role from previous posts such as health visitor or community health nurse. It remains essentially the same as the original US Nurse Family Partnership (NFP). It is an evidence-based, manualised, preventive intervention and according to FNP this is one of the main reasons that it was selected rather than any alternative UK interventions with weak or no evidence (Ball et al., 2012).

Evidence for the FNP programme is of higher quality than many other early intervention programmes and it is commonly named when examples of programmes with good evidence for success are sought (Ball et al., 2012). Whether this evidence-based US intervention can be applied in a different cultural and institutional context has been considered. It is also relevant that some 'competing' interventions developed within the UK context may feel that their programmes are as effective, but have not as yet been able to conduct the necessary randomised trials with long-term follow-up that the NFP/FNP has achieved to date.

Initial UK results in the Ball et al. (2012) study showed that the parents involved liked FNP in comparison with other services, particularly the different way they were perceived by FNP staff, not judged and undermined but supported and strengthened. Most participants found the programme better than they had expected, particularly some of the young men interviewed as they felt more involved as 'fathers to be'. These appear to be significant measures of the success of the FNP in the UK, with research and evaluation data still being collected. This was further augmented by the Department of Health initiative in the context of the Healthy Child Programme to increase the health visiting workforce by 4,200 by 2015 (DH, 2015a; 2015b; Public Health, 2015). Importantly, the role of the FNP family nurse is seen as a separate, specialist role, different from that of a health visitor or community nurse. You can read more about FNP at https://study.sagepub.com/essentialchildnursing

WEBLINK:
FNP

Two of the three theories upon which FNP is based – *attachment theory* (Bowlby, 1969) and *ecological systems theory* (Bronfenbrenner, 1979) are widely understood and used to plan interventions and guide interactions.

SCENARIO 11.1: BERNEICE AND ZARA

Berneice was pregnant at 17 and her boyfriend did not stay with her. Berneice felt abandoned and afraid. She knew she could not rely on her mother, also a single parent, as Berneice's own upbringing had been chaotic and complicated, with several episodes of social work involvement due to concerns

(Continued)

PRACTICE
SCENARIO 11:
ISSAQ &
SHAFIQUE

(Continued)

about Berneice's growth and development. Her boyfriend had been her only constant companion for the previous year, and now he had abandoned her. Berneice lived at home with her mother. Initially she was not at all sure about the FNP nurse and was reluctant to engage but with time and patience she grew in confidence over her pregnancy, had a successful birth of Zara, and was supported by her mother. Over the first months and years Berneice developed her communication skills, insight and awareness of her own strengths and limitations. She worked hard with her FNP nurse to maximize her strengths and practical parenting skills, and her mother seemed to benefit from the support also. Gradually, Berneice was able to start to think about her future with Zara and started a part-time animal welfare course at the local college. The college had a crèche which helped with childcare and enabled Berneice to concentrate on her studies.

- Make notes on Berneice's story and critically reflect on the main negative and positive issues in her story
- Critically reflect upon whether it is a children's nurse's role to to facilitate successful attachment bonding and development of parenting skills
- Cross-reference your notes with:

  o   the UN Convention on the Rights of the Child
  o   the NMC Code (use the most current edition)
  o   your own country's current children's welfare policy (e.g. DH 2015a or 2015b)

SCENARIO
ANSWER 11.1

WEBLINK:
CHILDREN'S
VIEWS

ACTIVITY 11.2: CRITICAL THINKING

How good are our children's lives? What do they say?
   Read and reflect upon the information given by children in Jacobs Foundation (2015), which you can access via https://study.sagepub.com/essentialchildnursing

- Take some time out to reflect on the various elements of this study
- Make notes on where you might like to grow up if you had a choice, and why
- Do these findings in any way surprise you?

ACTIVITY
ANSWER 11.2

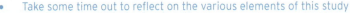

The research and case studies above demonstrate some of the ways the relationship between the family nurse and the family can, with consent and motivation, be strengthened to increase capacity and improve outcomes for the child and family.

- Start a media or social media 'watch' to capture any coverage of campaigns or interventions on the topic of IMH. This will help you focus on what is happening locally and nationally (e.g. Sure Start programmes, early years iniatiatives, Baby Friendly services, breast feeding friendly organisations and places, baby massage sessions, parenting skills – including for fathers)
- Shadow a public health nurse, health visitor or FNP nurse to enhance your understanding and evidence base. This will help you see very clearly the ways in which public health strategies and services can marry up. You can see policy in action and also see gaps in services. You can use this

as reflection for revalidation or for lobbying for better local services. You can also gain valuable experience from role-modelling opportunities

- Access websites for health and social care for your country and check what is available locally for children and maternity care services. You may also develop your literature search skills and knowledge of your locality. This information may prove very useful to you later in your practice. You can access the websites and literature via https://study.sagepub.com/essentialchildnursing

WEBLINK:
HEALTH &
SOCIAL
CARE

The following section is a reflective exercise considering the negative effects of poor infant mental health or parenting.

ACTIVITY 11.3: CRITICAL THINKING

In every nursery there are ghosts. They are the visitors from the unremembered pasts of the parents, the uninvited guests at the christening... These intruders from the past have taken up residence in the nursery, claiming tradition and rights of ownership. They have been present at the christening for two or more generations. While no one has issued an invitation, the ghosts take up residence and conduct the rehearsal of the family tragedy from a tattered script... The baby in these families is burdened by the oppressive past of his parents from the moment he enters the world. The parent, it seems, is condemned to repeat the tragedy of his own childhood with his own baby in terrible and exacting detail. (Fraiberg et al., 1975, p. 164-5)

- What do you *feel* when you read this representation of the intergenerational effects of disrupted attachment, bonding and parenting upon the child?
- What are your *thoughts* on the apparent inevitability of 'repeating the tragedy'? Is this only applicable in 'extreme' cases?
- Find out what the *specific provision* is in your local area for enhancing attachment, bonding and parenting skills in the early years of a child's life

ACTIVITY
ANSWER 11.3

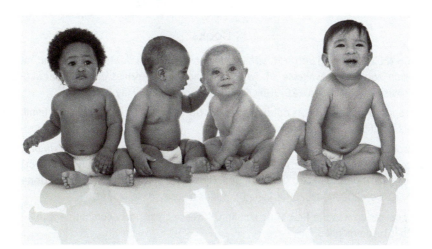

Figure 11.6 Baby group

Overall, the main focus of debate in recent years on health and social care has been biased towards an ageing population, with less regard evident for the outcomes for children (DH, 2015a).

This appears to be a false economy and furthermore is a shocking indictment of how we as a group of nations view and value our youngest citizens.

This must change and is the basis for the ongoing professional argument for the introduction of a national child and young persons health strategy – this should include early as well as ongoing mental and emotional health action and outcomes fulfilment.

Building capacity, improving life chances and resilience to deal better with adverse situations and events and achieve better emotional and mental health is key to building a healthy adult. Finding the best strategies, through good quality research and evidence, and working in an effective interdisciplinary and interagency manner, in accordance with the wishes and needs of the child and family is the ongoing 'Holy Grail'. Our children and families need you to recognise and support them as part of your professional duty of care.

HEALTH
PROMOTION
11: INFANT
MH &
WELLBEING

Have a look at the health promotion advice at https://study.sagepub.com/essentialchildnursing for more on health promotion issues related to this chapter.

CHAPTER SUMMARY

- Infant mental health and wellbeing is a resurgent and evidenced-based topic which can positively impact on the whole development of the child
- There are several examples of evidence-based theoretical models used in the UK. Perhaps the most well-known is the Family Nurse Partnership
- Ongoing and long-term follow up research is required to continue to test theories of 'what works' in the area of Infant mental health
- There should be an interdisciplinary approach involving statutory and voluntary services across care settings to promote and share good examples of IMH

BUILD YOUR BIBLIOGRAPHY

Books

- RCPCH (2016) *Securing Better Health for Northern Ireland's Infants, Children and Young People: A vision for 2016*. Available at: www.rcpch.ac.uk/system/files/protected/news/RCPCH%20 NI%20vision_Embargoed%2019Nov_0.pdf (last accessed 16 May 2017).

  This report from RCPCH sets out the vision for Northern Ireland's children and families in terms of best practice aspirations.

- Leadsom, A., Field, F., Burstow, P. and Lucas, C. (2013) *The 1001 Critical Days: The Importance of the Conception to Age Two Period*. Available at: www.wavetrust.org/sites/default/files/reports/1001%20 Critical%20Days%20-%20The%20Importance%20of%20the%20Conception%20to%20 Age%20Two%20Period%20Refreshed_0.pdf (last accessed 16 May 2017).

  This publication was the first of its kind in UK where cross party commitment to infant mental health is recommended.

Journal articles

Go to https://study.sagepub.com/essentialchildnursing for further free online journal articles related to this chapter.

FURTHER READING: ONLINE JOURNAL ARTICLES

- Mountain, G., Cahill, J. and Thorpe, H. (2017) 'Sensitivity and attention interventions in early childhood: A systematic review and meta analysis'. *Infant Behaviour and Development*, 46: 14-32.

  This article looks at the effects on infant behaviour of parental input such as increased handling, cuddling, speaking to the infant and other nurturing interventions.

- De Pascalis, L. et al. (2017) 'Maternal gaze to the infant face: Effects of infant age and facial configuration during mother-infant engagement in the first nine weeks'. *Infant Behavior and Development*, 46: 91-9.

  This article similarly looks at the matenal-child gaze and recognition of same by infant in the first few weeks of life.

- Newland, R., Parade, S., Dickstein, S. and Seifer, R. (2016) 'The association between maternal depression and sensitivity: Child-directed effects on parenting during infancy'. *Infant Behaviour and Development*, 45: 47-50.

  This paper explores how maternal sensitivity in general and in particular towards the infant can be blunted during a period of maternal depression

Weblinks

Go to https://study.sagepub.com/essentialchildnursing for further weblinks related to this chapter.

FURTHER READING: WEBLINKS

- The Association for Infant Mental Health (AIMH)

  www.aimh.org.uk
  AIMH provides discussion, comment and resources on the topic as well as evidence-based reports and information on conferences.

- Family Nurse Partnership

  http://fnp.nhs.uk
  The Family Nurse Partnership website sets out the evidence for the programmes and provides valuable resources and links for supporting infants and parents in the early years.

- Institute of Health Visiting (IHV)

  http://ihv.org.uk
  The IHV website contains many excellent resources and signposts to relevant materials relevant to early years wellbeing.

 ## ACE YOUR ASSESSMENT

Revise what you have learned by visiting https://study.sagepub.com/essentialchildnursing

ONLINE QUIZZES & ACTIVITY ANSWERS

- Test yourself with multiple-choice and short-answer questions
- Do the chapter activities in the book and check your answers online

REFERENCES

Ball, M., Barnes, J. and Meadows, P. (2012) *Issues Emerging from the First 10 Pilot Sites Implementing the Nurse–Family Partnership Home-visiting Programme in England.* London: DH.

Barlow, J. and Svanberg, P.O. (2009) *Keeping the Baby in Mind: Infant Mental Health in Practice.* London: Routledge.

Bowlby, J. (1969) *Attachment and Loss. Vol. 1. Attachment.* New York: Basic Books.

Brazelton, T. and Kramer, B. (1991) *The Earliest Relationship.* Reading, MA: Perseus Books.

Bronfenbrenner, U. (1979) *The Ecology of Human Development.* Cambridge, MA: Harvard University Press.

Center on the Developing Child (n.d.) Available at: https://developingchild.harvard.edu/ (accessed 13 September 2017).

Child Psychotherapy Trust (2012) *An Infant Mental Health Service: The Importance of the Early Years and Evidence-based Practice.* London: CPT.

Children and Young People's Mental Health Taskforce (2015) *Future in Mind: Promoting, Protecting and Improving Our Children and Young People's Mental Health and Wellbeing.* London: Department of Health. Available at: www.gov.uk/government/uploads/system/uploads/attachment_data/file/414024/Childrens_Mental_Health.pdf (last accessed 16 May 2017).

Department for Education (DfE) and Department of Health (DH) (2011) *Supporting Families in the Foundation Years.* London: DfE. Available at: www.gov.uk/government/publications/supporting-families-in-the-foundation-years (last accessed 16 May 2017).

Department of Health (DH) (2011) *Health Visitor Implementation Plan 2011–15: A Call to Action.* London: DH.

Department of Health (DH) (2015a) *Children and Young People's Health Outcomes Forum: 2014 to 2015.* London: DH.

Department of Health (2015b) *Future in Mind: Promoting, Protecting and Improving Our Children and Young People's Mental Health and Wellbeing.* London: DH.

Eurochild (2012) *Compendium of Inspiring Practices on Early Intervention and Prevention in Family and Parenting Support.* Available at: http://ec.europa.eu/social/main.jsp?langId=en&catId=89&newsId=1693&furtherNews=yes (last accessed 16 May 2017).

Fraiberg, S., Adelson, E. and Shapiro, V. (1975) 'Ghosts in the nursery. A psychoanalytic approach to the problems of impaired infant-mother relationships'. *Journal of the American Academy of Child & Adolescent Psychiatry,*14(3): 387–421.

Galloway, S. (2014) *Infant Mental Health: The Scottish Context.* NSPCC: Scotland.

Heckman, J.J. (2000) *Invest in the Very Young.* Chicago, IL: Ounce of Prevention Fund and University of Chicago Harris School of Public Policy Studies.

Institute of Reproductive and Developmental Biology at Imperial College London (no date). *Begin before Birth.* Available at: www.beginbeforebirth.org/for-schools/films#epigenetics (last accessed 15 May 2017).

Jacobs Foundation (2015) *Children's Views on Their Lives and Well-being in 15 countries: A Report on the Children's Worlds Survey, 2013–14.* York: Children's Worlds Project. Available at: www.isciweb.org/_Uploads/dbsAttachedFiles/ChildrensWorlds2015-FullReport-Final.pdf (last accessed 16 May 2017)

Leadsom, A., Field, F., Burstow, P. and Lucas, C. (2013) *The 1001 Critical Days: The Importance of the Conception to Age Two Period.* Available at: www.wavetrust.org/sites/default/files/reports/1001%20Critical%20Days%20-%20The%20Importance%20of%20the%20Conception%20to%20Age%20Two%20Period%20Refreshed_0.pdf (last accessed 16 May 2017).

Little, M., Berry, V., Morpeth, L., Blower, S., Axford, N., Taylor, R., Bywater, T., Lehtonen, M. and Tobin, K. (2013) 'Evidence-based programmes delivered in public systems'. *International Journal of Conflict and Violence*, 6 (2): 260–72.

Marmot, M. (2010) *Fair Society, Healthy Lives: The Marmot Review: Strategic Review of Health Inequalities in England post-2010*. London: Department for International Development.

McCullers, C. (1951) *The Ballad of the Sad Café*. Boston, MA: Houghton Mifflin.

Minnis, H., Reekie, J., Young, D., O'Connor, T., Ronald, A., Grayand, A. and Plomin, R. (2007) 'Genetic, environmental and gender influences on attachment disorder behaviours'. *British Journal of Psychiatry*, 190: 490–5.

Moulin, S., Waldfogel, J. and Washbrook, E. (2014) *Baby Bonds: Parenting, Attachment and a Secure Base for Children*. London: The Sutton Trust.

Munro, E. (2011) *The Munro Review of Child Protection: Final Report – A Child-centred System*. London: TSO.

Neville, H.J., Stevens, C., Pakulak, E., Bell, T.A, Fanning, J., Kleina, S. and Isbell, E. (2013) 'Family-based training program improves brain function, cognition, and behavior in lower socioeconomic status preschoolers'. *PNAS*, 110 (29): 12138–43.

O'Donnell, K., O'Connor, T.G. and Glover, V. (2009) 'Prenatal stress and neurodevelopment of the child: focus on the HPA axis and role of the placenta'. *Developmental Neuroscience*, 31(4): 285–92.

Olds, D.L.(2006) 'The nurse–family partnership: an evidence-based preventive intervention'. *Infant Mental Health J.*, 27: 5–25.

Olds, D.L., Henderson, C.R., Tatelbaum, R. and Chamberlin, R. (1986) 'Improving the delivery of prenatal care and outcomes of pregnancy: a randomized trial of nurse home visitation. *Pediatrics*, 77, 16–28.

Olds, D.L., Kitzman, H.J., Cole, R.E., et al. (2010) 'Enduring effects of prenatal and infancy home visiting by nurses on maternal life course and government spending'. *Arch. Pediatric Adolescent Medicine*, 164 (5), 419–24.

Public Health England (2015) *Rapid Review to Update Evidence for the Healthy Child Programme 0–5*. Available at: www.gov.uk/government/uploads/system/uploads/attachment_data/file/429741/150520_RapidReviewHealthyChildProg_UPDATE_poisons_summary.pdf (accessed 3 July 2017).

Royal College of Midwives (RCM) (2014) *Making the Most of Fathers to Improve Maternal and Infant Health* [leaflet]. London: RCM.

Svanberg, P.O. and Barlow, J. (2013) 'The effectiveness of training in the Parent–Infant Interaction Observation Scale for health visitors'. *Journal of Health Visiting*, 1 (3): 162–6.

Tickell, C. (2011) *The Early Years: Foundations for Life, Health and Learning. An Independent Report on the Early Years Foundation Stage to Her Majesty's Government*. London: DfE.

Widarsson, W., Engström, G. ,Tydén, T., Lundberg, P. and Hammar, L.M. (2015) 'Paddling upstream': fathers' involvement during pregnancy as described by expectant fathers and mothers'. *Journal of Clinical Nursing*, 24 (7–8): 1059–68.

Zero to Three (2009) *Definition of Infant Mental Health*. Washington, DC: Infant Mental Health Steering Committee.

COMPLEXITIES OF THE DEVELOPING AND DIFFERING NEEDS OF CHILDREN AND YOUNG PEOPLE

TIM McDOUGALL

THIS CHAPTER COVERS

- Key development stages of childhood and adolescence
- Therapeutic child-centred relationship when working with children and their parents
- Decision-making with and for children
- The importance of health information and education
- Issues of privacy and confidentiality

> " Grown-ups never understand anything by themselves, and it is tiresome for children to be always and forever explaining things to them.
>
> **Antoine de Saint-Exupéry,**
> *The Little Prince* "

Visit https://study.sagepub.com/essentialchildnursing to access a wealth of online resources for this chapter – watch out for the margin icons throughout the chapter.

INTRODUCTION

Additional complexities exist when caring for infants, children and young people. This is due to the variance in deveopmental and intellectual/cognitive presentations at different stages of the age and developmental continuum. Where children and young people (or indeed their parents) are on this continuum will have major implications for the communication, understanding, consent and engagement in care delivery. The child and young person's nurse should be in a unique position to care effectively, compassionately and inclusively across the interfaces of age, development, disability and distress.

The opening quote illustrates the differences in how children and adults perceive the world, and the importance of taking a developmentally appropriate approach to nursing care with children. This chapter focuses on the specific needs of children and explores how children's nurses can address these. Attachment theory and child and adolescent developmental psychology are applied to help you understand some of the important principles and practice implications when nursing children. Reflection points and the voice of the child encourage you to pause and think about your day-to- day practice as a children's nurse.

As childhood and adolescence are evolving life phases, this chapter will demonstrate the importance of keeping nursing interventions with children both appropriate and under regular review. This is because the beliefs that children hold about health and mortality change over time, just as their attitude to care and treatment or that of their parents or carers may also shift. Ultimately it is our responsibility as registered child nurses to ensure that all needs are met, physically, emotionally and psychologically. This approach of mastering the complexities of presentation, assessment and management is best managed by listening to the voice and wishes of the child or young person.

Finally, this chapter illustrates that nursing children who may have experienced trauma or suffering is an emotionally challenging experience for all concerned. The importance and value of regular support and supervision is discussed, and the need for you to remain a resilient and compassionate care giver is critical.

WHAT'S THE EVIDENCE?

The field of children's health and their specific needs has been extensively researched. Readers are encouraged to consult a number of well-known texts for a summary of the evidence base. These include *Child-Centred Nursing* by Bernie Carter and colleagues (2014) and *Ethical and Philosophical Aspects of Nursing* by Gosia Brykczynska and Joan Simons (2011). So how can you make sense of the literature related to children's health? One way is to rely on evidence-based sources or summaries such as those published by the National Institute for Health and Care Excellence (NICE) or Cochrane Reviews which are systematic reviews of primary research in human healthcare and health policy.

WEBLINK:
COCHRANE
REVIEWS

KEY DEVELOPMENTAL STAGES OF CHILDHOOD AND ADOLESCENCE

For you to provide appropriate holistic, child-centred care you must have a broad but general understanding of child development, communication needs and engagement strategies. You must also consider the views and wishes of the child and their parents or carers, and the available evidence base to guide best practice.

Al Aynsley-Green, a former National clinical director for children, once famously announced that there was no such thing as a child. What he actually meant by this was that there are many developmental stages between birth and adulthood. The needs of neonates, infants and adolescents are all different and thus describing children as a whole may give an impression that all children have the same needs.

It will be obvious to most nurses and other professionals that the way in which one communicates with a toddler is profoundly different from how one behaves towards a teenager. However, how best to take the most appropriate approach with an older child or younger adolescent may be less clear for most of us. This is further complicated by the difference between the chronological age of a child, which is usually clear, and their developmental age, which is less obviously defined.

Nathan, a staff nurse in CAMHS explains how important it is to take a child-focused approach:

> Coming from adult services I knew there would be differences but nothing prepared me for how different working with children and young people actually is. We have to use different language, explain things in terms that children and young people understand and make sure parents are involved too. Sometimes we get this wrong, particularly with teenagers. Some want to be treated like adults, but sometimes it is obvious that they are emotionally immature and can't cope with the technical details. Others seem young for their age but are more independent and expect all the information an adult would. I've learned that the best way is to check this out with them and have an open conversation about what they understand and how I should involve their parents. This isn't always an easy conversation and we don't always agree, but it is better than not asking at all.
>
> **Nathan, staff nurse**

ACTIVITY 12.1: REFLECTIVE PRACTICE

Think about the nursing environment in which you work. How appropriate is it for the children you care for? How could you change the environment to help improve engagement and the child's experience of care? Is your service information material suitable for all children?

ACTIVITY
ANSWER 12.1

What are the different stages?

Broadly speaking, the major developmental periods that take place between birth and adulthood occur during infancy, the preschool period, the primary school years and adolescence. Throughout these stages the child experiences significant cognitive, emotional and social growth. It is important that you as a nurse have a basic overview of the key milestones involved.

Infancy

In infancy, the toddler begins to walk and talk, interacts with others and actively explores the world around them. They begin the process of emotional regulation and move away from instant gratification or the desire to experience pleasure or fulfilment without delay.

Childhood

As a child, regulation is provided by parents and carers through the process of attachment and the provision of a secure base. Discipline and boundaries, rewards and punishments and limit-setting enable children to internalise the ability to self-regulate. Over time, children develop skills of self-regulation. These include self-soothing and self-distracting techniques to avoid aversive experiences, and the ability to talk with others and negotiate ways to resolve difficulties and challenges.

Throughout the time children are at school their physical growth occurs at a steady pace. A final growth spurt begins at the start of puberty, usually when the child is between ages 9 and 15. During the pre-school phase, emotional and psychological development is faster than physical growth and motor development. Starting school involves separation and independence. Some children cope with this transition well, whereas others find it anxiety provoking and stressful. They may regress to pre-school behaviours and be clingy with a parent. It is a time of problem-solving and social development.

Adolescence

Adolescence is often described as a tumultuous period during which the bodies and minds of teenagers undergo many simultaneous changes. Eating habits commonly change, and as adolescents enter puberty their hygiene needs become more important. This will be obvious to any parent of a teenager, and it is important that nurses have some understanding of this developmental stage in order to help and support young people.

Research suggests that teenage behaviour tends to be governed less by parental rules or standards and more by perceptions of what other young people may think (Overseas Development Institute, 2015). This is important to keep in mind when you are planning health promotion or delivering interventions. Adolescence is a time when young people engage in sexual behaviour or experiment with drugs and alcohol. Whilst this behaviour can be relatively harmless it can also be associated with significant harm and death. It is therefore important that you are aware of how risk-taking behaviours may affect family relationships as well as physical health and emotional wellbeing. Practical child- and person-centred strategies to minimise risk of harm include the provision of age-appropriate health promotion information and access to credible sources of advice and support in complex situations such as those provided by Young Minds.

WEBLINK:
YOUNG
MINDS

SAFEGUARDING STOP POINT

Are you concerned that the behaviour of a child places them or others at immediate risk? If so, you have a duty to report your concerns to statutory agencies in order to help keep people safe. It is good practice to inform the child you are doing this and explain why, as well as inform their parents or carers unless to do so would increase the risk.

ACTIVITY 12.2: CRITICAL THINKING

CHECK YOUR
ANSWERS
ONLINE!

Think about the developmental needs of the child in your care. Are they old enough to understand concepts such as self-esteem, confidence or stress? Do they have particular needs which mean that you need to adapt your health promotion or illness intervention strategies? To what extent can the child you are nursing self-soothe and manage their own care needs? To what extent do you need to involve their parents or carers? How will you get the right balance?

ACTIVITY
ANSWER 12.2

THERAPEUTIC CHILD-CENTRED RELATIONSHIP WHEN WORKING WITH CHILDREN AND THEIR PARENTS

Friedman (1989) suggests that the promotion of health, the prevention of problems, and their treatment and rehabilitation when they arise can best be accomplished with the active cooperation and engagement of young people in an atmosphere of trust and cooperation. Ryan and McDougall (2009) suggest that the therapeutic relationship is the bedrock on which successful care and treatment is based. Through their holistic approach, children's nurses have a long tradition and history of creating strong therapeutic partnerships with children and families. Some argue that this is the very essence of nursing regardless of the nature of the illness or disability.

ACTIVITY 12.3: CRITICAL THINKING

Imagine the child or young person arriving at the Accident and Emergency (A&E) department following self-harm or coming into hospital for surgery. They may be distressed, confused or frightened, and the way in which you engage and respond to them will influence their engagement and experience of healthcare for better or worse. What can you do to help ensure that the child or young person in your care experiences you as compassionate and caring?

ACTIVITY
ANSWER 12.3

Research has shown that a young person who presents at A&E with self-harm may experience a range of responses from staff of disgust or blame through to compassion and understanding (Palmer et al., 2007). There has been extensive research on the voice of the child in this situation. The children and young people talk about feeling 'dirty' or 'worthless' as they present for help, and the way in which nurses sometimes respond leaves them feeling 'blamed' or 'attention seeking' (McDougall et al., 2010). Part of forming a therapeutic relationship involves making those involved feel at ease. Talking to children and young people about general issues can help engage them and help set the conditions for the therapeutic relationship. Asking what they like and dislike is a way of connecting in a genuine, warm and compassionate way. According to Lewer (2006), this experience of feeling accepted and understood assists with the process of care, treatment and recovery.

ACTIVITY 12.4: CRITICAL THINKING

There is evidence that children's subjective experience of events may differ significantly from those of adults (Livesley and Long, 2013). Try stepping into the child's shoes. How might they be feeling and what might they be thinking? What can you say, do or give them to read that might put their mind at ease? What support might their parents need?

ACTIVITY
ANSWER 12.4

VIDEO LINK 12.1:
COMMUNICATING
WITH PARENTS

Go to https://study.sagepub.com/essentialchildnursing and watch the video on communicating with parents.

Children experience uncertainty or fear in different ways. How they cope with a planned or unplanned hospital admission will depend on their age, knowledge and understanding of what is entailed and how significant others cope and react to the process. A child who sees that their parent is highly anxious about the admission is not likely to feel contained and reassured, and may experience fear, anxiety and stress themselves. A young person who is supported sensitively and in a skilled way to ask questions to help understand the risks and benefits of their admission may feel reassured by the information they are given and more able to engage in complex situations particularly where emotions and mental health are their main concern. So what does this mean for you as a nurse?

The importance of attachment theory

Fans of Winnie the Pooh will be familiar with the following excerpt from *House at Pooh Corner* by A.A. Milne, which was first published in 1928 and epitomises the phenomenon of attachment:

> Piglet sidled up to Pooh from behind.
>
> 'Pooh!' he whispered.
>
> 'Yes, Piglet?'
>
> 'Nothing,' said Piglet, taking Pooh's paw. 'I just wanted to be sure of you.'

Attachment theory emphasises the importance and biological function of intimate relationships between individuals, the central role of caregivers on a child's development and the persistence of attachment styles throughout life (Cotgrove, 2013). Attachment theory has had a profound influence on the helping professions, including children's and young people's nurses in particular. Nurses should understand the essential principles of attachment to understand related issues of engagement, bonding and to respond to children whose health needs may be related to, or worsened by, attachment difficulties. Miles (2011) illustrates the value of attachment theory as a way of understanding the complex bond between children and the people with whom they have emotional ties – usually caregivers.

Concepts of health and illness

It is generally accepted that beliefs about health and illness affect how one copes, for better or worse (Bower et al., 2009; Kirk et al., 2010). The knowledge, belief and attitudes that children and young people hold about health and illness are important for you to understand. Without this insight you will struggle to provide effective health promotion, illness prevention or compassionate management strategies. Nor are you likely to be able to evaluate how motivated the child may be to self-manage their condition.

Children and young people especially tend to be less concerned about their health and wellbeing than we are as adults. To some extent this is understandable because health generally declines with age, and the sense of immortality that children and young people enjoy wears off as we get older. However, this is not to say that they do not have health beliefs or that their beliefs stay the same. Indeed, the Children's Society (2015) point out that health is one of the top ten concerns for children growing up in the UK.

Different coping styles

We have heard that children and young people all cope with illness in different ways. This is as much about health and illness beliefs as age, predisposition and temperament. The health beliefs of their parents or carers as well as their peer support opinions also play a role in mediating the process of coping and adjustment.

So what does this mean for you as a child or young person's nurse? The important principle to remember is that there is no standardised way of supporting and responding to children's health needs. However, there are some basic things that you can address which may make the process less stressful for children and young people. For example, the unfamiliar hospital or assessment surroundings may bring uncertainty and a change of routine. Whilst this may bypass the busy nurse whose work environment has become second nature, to every child admitted it is a new and uncertain experience. For those who rely more on familiarity or routines, such as younger children or those with learning disabilities, this may be additionally stressful. Simply going through how the hospital day works or what the sounds on the ward are about may help alleviate anxiety and uncertainty.

Coping with health changes

Children today are surviving at much higher rates than they did 50 years ago (Office for National Statistics, 2016). Better survival rates following low birth weight and advances in care and treatment mean that many more are living with complex health conditions and disabilities (Halfon and Newacheck, 2010). For example, Canadian researchers found that a child born with cystic fibrosis during the 1980s could expect to live approximately 14 years. By 2000, that life expectancy had increased to 18 years. A child born today with cystic fibrosis can expect to live well into his or her 30s, 40s and beyond (OACCAC, 2013). Childhood diseases that were once fatal are now preventable or curable and can be successfully treated and managed through modern healthcare. There is an extensive evidence base relating to how children cope with chronic illness and much of this is rich and invaluable qualitative information that can inform your work as a nurse. It is important to remember that not just the healthcare need may be complex; so too is the exchange of information, understanding and perspective.

DECISION-MAKING WITH AND FOR CHILDREN

There are a number of guiding principles that you as a children or young person's nurse must always take into account in your day-to-day practice. One is to always consider the best interests and views of the child. Another is that decisions in relation to and involving children and young people must be made in a way which is consistent with their evolving developmental capacities.

As children and young people grow up and mature towards independence, their views and wishes should be given increasing weight and importance, as much as those of their parents in the decision-making process. Children's competence is determined by their maturity and understanding rather than their fixed chronological age. The legal status of a child is determined by age boundaries and does not represent the level of maturity and understanding that an individual may hold (Spencer, 2000). Keating (2004) suggests that one of the most important developmental tasks of adolescence is the process of achieving a stable, positive adult identity whilst giving up parental dependence. However, there is a consensus that a child's identity is less firmly formed than an adult's, and that the values, wishes and intentions on which they base their decisions may be less secure (Dickenson and Jones, 1996).

SEE ALSO
CHAPTER 40

So what does this mean in practice? You need to regularly review the child's views and wishes about their care and treatment and consider how these may influence decision-making.

Working with parents or carers

Children's law dictates that regardless of their age, children are entitled to be involved in planning and reviewing their own nursing care and treatment. The Children Act 1989 requires that the involvement of parents or carers should also be encouraged unless there are particular reasons why this should not happen or the child who is competent to decide does not wish this to happen. The Children Act 1989 defines parental responsibility as 'all the rights, duties, powers, responsibilities and authority which by law a parent has in relation to a child and his property'. It is important for you to remember that having a child with a health problem can be an anxiety provoking experience for parents or carers. They too have support needs, and this is regardless of their child's age or wishes about information sharing.

SEE ALSO
CHAPTER 41

THE IMPORTANCE OF HEALTH INFORMATION AND EDUCATION

Whatever the age of the child or young peoson, you should always keep them as fully informed and involved as possible. They should receive clear and detailed information in a format that is appropriate to their age and developmental understanding. The ability to self-manage an illness or condition depends on access to information and skills to support positive behaviour change. For instance, the successful self-management of a young person's insulin regime depends on understanding diabetes and the interventions that may be required when blood sugars are unstable. This will obviously be different for young children and teenagers, and the language you use and the supporting literature you provide will be different.

Written information can be helpful for you to provide when engaging and involving children as well as parents and carers. For example, leaflets can be designed which provide information about the service they expect to receive and the care and treatment involved. Written information can also set out the choices available to children and young people, including those related to the gender of the nurse and the location of treatment.

For older children and adolescents 'e-health' methods are becoming increasingly popular and are an effective and appropriate means of providing social networking or self-management support (Treadgold and Grant, 2014).

Healthy lifestyle choices

Children and young people need a range of health information and education if they are to make healthy lifestyle choices. Whether you are a school nurse, practice nurse or A&E nurse, you are well placed to help them choose healthy lifestyles. This can be in relation to diet and exercise, personal health and hygiene, healthy sexual behaviour and the harmful effects of drugs and alcohol. You also play an important role in helping them access appropriate, evidence-based health promotion literature specifically geared to their needs.

NICE guidelines and quality standards are also an important source of information that you can utilise to inform health education interventions. These include those related to physical activity for children (NICE, 2009); lifestyle and weight management programmes for obesity (NICE, 2015); and school-based interventions for smoking prevention (NICE, 2010) and alcohol (NICE, 2007). It is also important to give children and young people information about the treatments they may be receiving. The information provided should be culturally competent, gender sensitive and at a level that is appropriate to their age, developmental status and understanding.

WEBLINK:
NICE
GUIDELINES

ISSUES OF PRIVACY AND CONFIDENTIALITY

PRACTICE
SCENARIO 12:
LEILA

SCENARIO 12.1: LEANNE

You are a school nurse and Leanne (age 10) has sent you a note saying that something is making her unhappy. You are aware that Leanne is a private girl and is rarely seen around school without Kirsty who is an equally quiet and reserved girl. You have also noticed that Leanne appears to have lost some weight and is generally looking tired and preoccupied.

- How should you prepare for meeting Leanne? What happens if you try to discuss her note but she refuses to open up? What are your professional obligations as a nurse? Are you concerned about Leanne's safety or welfare or can you help her feel better by talking things through or accessing further help for her? Can you keep the discussion private or should you inform Leanne's parents? Should you suggest that she might want to bring Kirsty with her?

✓

SCENARIO
ANSWER 12.1

Just as adults have the right to privacy, dignity and respect, so too do children and young people. Despite this, young people sometimes tell us that they do not feel involved in decisions and have their privacy, dignity and confidentiality compromised (McDougall et al., 2010). When engaging with young people you should discuss the limits of confidentiality and explain your duties in relation to safeguarding the welfare of children.

Supervision and support for children's nurses

Nursing children can be an emotionally complex experience. Many in their care are in pain or dying; others survive treatment with life-changing conditions. Most make full recoveries and return to or reach good health. This ever-changing context in which nurses practise is a rollercoaster of emotions, and it is important that you can access regular supervision in order to remain compassionate and resilient. Without this, children and young people's nurses risk becoming overwhelmed.

ACTIVITY 12.5: REFLECTIVE PRACTICE

Think about the work you do and the effect it has on you. Do you have time and space to talk about the emotional impact on you as a person? How can you create time and space to ensure you remain emotionally resilient and in touch with the human effects of nursing care?

Reflection in nursing can enable creative, innovative and inspirational nursing practice which is safe, accountable and up to date. It is also a requirement for revalidation. It is important to remember that nurses, like all people, have emotional limits. Awareness of our own strengths, vulnerabilities and weaknesses affects the way in which we intervene and support children, young people and their families. Working with children with a range of difficulties may evoke strong feelings in us. It is therefore essential that you have access to support and supervision in relation to what can often be highly emotive work. A good source of information on the value and importance of reflection in nursing has been published by Bulman and Schutz (2013).

CHAPTER SUMMARY

- Nursing children and young people involves holistic care and practice. Children exist as whole people and their needs, as well as those of their family, are broad and varied
- When planning and delivering care, you must always take into consideration issues such as age of the child, their developmental understanding and the views of their parents or carers. This is not always a straightforward process and you may sometimes require guidance and the support of your multidisciplinary colleagues or nurse managers
- It is important that nurses recognise that they do not practise in isolation. After all, it is the combined breadth of skills and expertise in the wider children's workforce which makes the whole greater than the sum of its parts
- It is important to remember that young people and children have rights (see UN Convention on the Rights of the Child)

BUILD YOUR BIBLIOGRAPHY

Books

- Carter, B., Bray, L., Dickenson, A., Edwards, M. and Ford, K. (2014) *Child-Centred Nursing: Promoting Critical Thinking.* London: Sage.

  This book contains lots of useful information about children's health and their nursing care. It encourages you to think about children in the context of their family and offers guidance on a range of nursing practice issues.

- Brykczynska, G. and Simons, J. (2011) *Ethical and Philosophical Aspects of Nursing Children and Young People.* London: Wiley-Blackwell.

  This book focuses on ethical and philosophical dilemmas when providing nursing care for children. It complements this chapter by providing additional theory on child psychology and development.

- Delves-Yates, C. (2015) *Essentials of Nursing Practice.* London: Sage.

  This book encourages nurses to take a person-centred approach to care and describes a range of therapeutic interventions which are relevant to the care of children.

Journal articles

Go to https://study.sagepub.com/essentialchildnursing for further free online journal articles related to this chapter.

- Taylor, R., Gibson, F. and Franck, L. (2008). 'A concept analysis of health-related quality of life in young people with chronic illness'. *Journal of Clinical Nursing*, 17 (14): 1823-33.

  This paper provides a clear definition of quality of life from the health perspective, which is helpful for use with children to guide practice and research.

- Coyne, I. (2005) 'Consultation with children in hospital: children, parents' and nurses' perspectives'. *Journal of Clinical Nursing*, 15 (1), 61-71.

  Facilitating children's involvement in decisions about their care is often a complex process for nurses. This article encourages nurses to examine the basis of their decisions and use more explicit criteria for making decisions about the involvement of children.

FURTHER READING: ONLINE JOURNAL ARTICLES

(Continued)

(Continued)

- Soanes, C. and Timmons, S. (2004) 'Improving transition: a qualitative study examining the attitudes of young people with chronic illness transferring to adult care'. *Journal of Child Health Care*, doi: 10.1177/1367493504041868

  This paper examines the attitudes of young people with chronic illness who were facing transition, considering what young people wanted from a transition service and the ways in which provision could be improved from their perspective. It highlights the importance of taking an individualised approach to care of young people and actively involving them.

Weblinks

FURTHER
READING:
WEBLINKS

Go to https://study.sagepub.com/essentialchildnursing for further weblinks related to this chapter.

- YoungMinds

  www.youngminds.org.uk
  YoungMinds is the UK's leading charity committed to improving children's emotional wellbeing and mental health. It actively campaigns, researches and influences policy and practice.

- mymind.org.uk

  www.mymind.org.uk
  This is an excellent resource which has been created by children with the support of professionals. The site has been developed for everyone interested in the mental health and wellbeing of children across Cheshire and Wirral but it is relevant to children, nurses and other professionals from all over the UK.

- National Institute for Health and Care Excellence (NICE)

  www.nice.org.uk
  NICE provides guidance, advice and quality standards to improve health and social care and helps nurses and other professionals to maximise use of evidence and guidance.

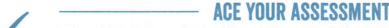

ACE YOUR ASSESSMENT

ONLINE
QUIZZES &
ACTIVITY
ANSWERS

Revise what you have learned by visiting https://study.sagepub.com/essentialchildnursing

- Test yourself with multiple-choice and short-answer questions
- Do the chapter activities in the book and check your answers online

REFERENCES

Bower, P., Blakeman, T., Kennedy, A., Protheroe, J., Richardson, G., Rogers, A. and Sanders, C. (2009) *What Influences People to Self-care?* Manchester: National Primary Care Research and Development Centre, University of Manchester.

Brykczynska, G. and Simons, J. (2011) *Ethical and Philosophical Aspects of Nursing Children and Young People*. Chichester: Wiley-Blackwell.

Bulman, C. and Schutz, S. (2013) *Reflective Practice in Nursing*. London: Blackwell Publishing.

Carter, B., Bray, L., Dickinson, A., Edwards, M. and Ford, K. (2014) *Child-Centred Nursing*. London: Sage.

Children's Society (2015) *The Good Childhood Report*. London: Children's Society.

Cotgrove, A. (2013) 'Inpatient care', in T. McDougall and A. Cotgrove (eds) *Specialist Mental Health Care for Children and Adolescents: Hospital, Intensive Community and Home Based Services*. London: Routledge.

Dickenson, D. and Jones, D. (1996) 'True wishes: the philosophy and developmental psychology of children's informed consent'. *Philosophy, Psychiatry and Psychology*, 2 (4): 287–303.

Friedman, H. (1989) 'The health of adolescents: beliefs and behaviour'. *Social Sciences and Medicine*, 29 (3): 309–15.

Halfon, N. and Newacheck, P. 'Evolving notions of childhood chronic illness'. *Journal of the American Medical Association*, 303 (7): 665–6.

Keating, D.P. (2004) 'Cognitive and brain development', in R.M. Lerner and L. Steinberg (eds) *Handbook of Adolescent Psychology*, 2nd edn. New Jersey: John Wiley and Sons.

Kirk, S., Beatty, S., Callery, P., Milnes, L. and Pryjmachuk, S. (2010) *Evaluating Self-care Support for Children and Young People with Long-term Conditions: Report for the National Institute for Health Research Service Delivery and Organisation Programme*. London: NIHR.

Lewer, L. (2006) 'Nursing Children and Young People with Eating Disorders', in McDougall, T. (Ed.), *Child and Adolescent Mental Health Nursing*. London: Blackwell.

Livesley, J. and Long, T. (2013) 'Children's experiences as hospital in-patients: voice, competence and work: messages for nursing from a critical ethnographic study'. *International Journal of Nursing Studies*, 50 (10): 1292–303.

McDougall, T., Armstrong, G. and Trainor, G. (2010) *Helping Children and Young People Who Self Harm: An Introduction to Self-harming and Suicidal Behaviours for Health Professionals*. London: Routledge.

Miles, K. (2011) 'Using attachment theory in mentoring'. *Nursing Times*, 107 (38): 23–5.

Milne, AA. (1928) *The House at Pooh Corner*. London: Methuen.

National Institute for Health and Care Excellence (2007) *Alcohol: School-based Interventions*. London: NICE.

National Institute for Health and Care Excellence (2009) *Physical Activity for Children and Young People*. London: NICE.

National Institute for Care Excellence (2010) *Smoking Prevention in Schools*. London: NICE.

National Institute for Health and Care Excellence (2015) *Obesity in Children and Young People: Prevention and Lifestyle Weight Management Programmes*. London: NICE.

Office for National Statistics (2016) *Childhood Mortality in England and Wales: 2014*. Available at: www.ons.gov.uk/peoplepopulationandcommunity/birthsdeathsandmarriages/deaths/bulletins/ childhoodinfantandperinatalmortalityinenglandandwales/2014 (last accessed 31 May 2017).

Ontario Association of Community Care Access Centers (OACCAC) (2013) *Health Comes Home: A Conversation about Children with Complex Health Needs*. Ontario: OACCAC.

Overseas Development Institute (2015) *Social Norms, Gender Norms and Adolescent Girls: A Brief Guide*. London: ODI.

Palmer, L. Blackwell, M. and Stevens, P. (2007) *Service Users' Experiences of Emergency Services Following Self-harm: A National Survey of 509 Patients*. London: Royal College of Psychiatrists' Centre for Quality Improvement.

Ryan, N. and McDougall, T. (2009) *Nursing Children and Young People with ADHD*. London: Routledge.

Spencer, G. (2000) 'Children's competency to consent: an ethical dilemma'. *Journal of Child Health Care*, 4 (3): 117–22.

Treadgold, P. and Grant, C. (2014). *Evidence Review: what does good health information look like? Report commissioned by the Patient Information Forum*. Available at: www.pifonline.org.uk/wp-content/ uploads/2015/03/What-does-good-health-information-look-like-October-2014.pdf (last accessed 6 June 2017).

FACTORS INFLUENCING WELLBEING AND DEVELOPMENT IN CHILDREN AND YOUNG PEOPLE

13

MELANIE ROBBINS AND CILLA SANDERS

THIS CHAPTER COVERS

- What are health and wellbeing?
- Parenting capacity
- Family and environmental factors

> " Relationships are at the heart of children's well-being. When children talk about what is important in their lives, they highlight their need for love, support, respect, fairness, freedom and safety ... Children acknowledge that material items are important, but they see them as secondary to relationships.
>
> **The Children's Society, 2015, pp.14–15** "

Visit https://study.sagepub.com/essentialchildnursing to access a wealth of online resources for this chapter – watch out for the margin icons throughout the chapter.

INTRODUCTION

It is acknowledged that children's development and wellbeing are influenced by many factors and that these begin before the child is born. Once the child is born, these factors can support or sabotage the child in meeting their full potential physically, emotionally and cognitively, and as the quote above acknowledges, children identify these aspects, somewhat surprisingly, as more important than material aspects. Your role as a children's nurse requires you to be aware of these factors so that you can assess, plan and implement a holistic approach to care, which can support or mitigate these factors and ensure that the child and family voice is heard at policy level.

Most of the documentation used in a clinical setting directs us towards assessing the physiological systems – for example, the cardiovascular system – before eventually assessing the child and family situation, and wider influences. However, the trend for shorter stays in acute care may limit the effectiveness of that holistic assessment. If you truly want to improve the health and wellbeing of children, an understanding of the wider influences needs to become a cornerstone of your care alongside assessment of physiological status.

WHAT ARE HEALTH AND WELLBEING?

Health is a complex issue and many authors have tried to define it. The World Health Organization's (WHO) seminal definition (1948) stated that 'Health is a complete state of physical, mental and social wellbeing not merely the absence of disease or infirmity'. This is considered an idealised view that few would recognise as being related to everyday life. The WHO developed their definition, stating that

> a conception of health is the extent to which an individual or group is able, on the one hand, to realise aspirations and satisfy needs, and, on the other hand, to change or cope with the environment. Health is, therefore, seen as a resource for everyday life, not just the object of living. (WHO, 1986)

ACTIVITY 13.1: CRITICAL THINKING

Is it possible for the children below to achieve a state of health?

- A child with a congenital condition - for example, talipes
- A child who has learning disabilities
- A child who has a long-term condition - for example, type 1 diabetes

ACTIVITY
ANSWER 13.1

Develop your understanding of the factors which influence health by accessing the video on the *Social Determinants of Health* or read *Health Inequalities and the Social Determinants of Health* (RCN, 2012) via https://study.sagepub.com/essentialchildnursing and discuss with your mentors and peers.

You need to consider how children may define health, which is closely linked to cognitive and emotional development and life experiences. This will enable you to provide care that incorporates the child's perspective. However, life experiences may accelerate their understanding of health and illness – for example, a young child with a life-threatening illness as a brief experience verses a child who has to manage a chronic life-limiting disease.

VIDEO LINK
13.1: SOCIAL
DETERMINANTS
OF HEALTH

WEBLINK:
HEALTH
INEQUALITIES

ACTIVITY 13.2: CRITICAL THINKING

Watch the video entitled *We asked London children – What does being healthy mean to you?* via https://study.sagepub.com/essentialchildnursing Make notes on what you think about the children's views and if they surprise you or not. Would these views be different in another country or part of the world?

A number of studies have linked a child's understanding of illness to Piaget's stages of development, but this approach has been criticised on the grounds that Piaget's stages underestimate a child's development and development is not always linear. It has been shown that a child's understanding of health is separate from illness. Myant and Williams's (2005) work shows that children can hold separate concepts of what it means to be healthy and what it means to be ill. They explored this in different age ranges and for different illnesses, those which are contagious (common cold, chicken pox) and those which are not (asthma). As the child grows, a more complex understanding develops which includes aspects of health-promoting behaviours – that is: eating well, wearing appropriate clothing against the cold – rather than just an absence of illness.

You can see that when establishing what health means, you need to consider the biological *and* the psychosocial and emotional influences.

WHAT'S THE EVIDENCE?

Our understanding of how children process information and develop their understating is evolving. Toyama (2016) extends the work of Myant and Williams (2005) and demonstrates that even young children recognise that illness is not the result of a misdemeanour and that children actually obtain information from a wider source than parents and teachers and suggests television and other media as additional sources. Katz et al. (2015) explore the use of the Internet in teenagers in assisting with homework, health information and development of self and found that parents are poor at assessing how frequently their children use this source for these activities.

- How can you use this information to aid a child's understanding of an illness? Think about how we explain signs, symptoms and disease process to children
- We should acknowledge that children are accessing online information but should we also take account the quality of the information and assess the accuracy of their understanding?

SCENARIO 13.1: SAMIRA

Samira is 7 years old and has suffered repeated urinary tract infections since she was 2. She takes prophylactic antibiotics and has regular scans to monitor renal functioning. Samira lives in privately rented accommodation with her mum and brother aged 3 years. Mum, Jamila, does not work at the moment and suffers with depression and anxiety and relies on child benefit and Jobseeker's Allowance to financially support the family.

Their house does not provide the best living conditions – the children share a bedroom whilst Jamila sleeps in the lounge. The kitchen is basic; the fridge is old and only two rings on the cooker work. Samira hates the cold, damp bathroom and delays using the toilet. As a consequence she occasionally wets herself.

Samira attends school, which she enjoys but she has made few friends and one of her peers has called her smelly.

Jamila does her best to look after her children on her own but sometimes she wishes she could just stay in bed. She knows she needs to encourage Samira to empty her bladder regularly but her brother demands so much of her attention that Samira doesn't get a look in. Jamila feels guilty as she sometimes forgets to give Samira her medicine.

- What do you think Samira's definition of health would be?
- List the influences, both positive and negative, on Samira's health and wellbeing
- Do you think Samira's definition of health would be the same as Jamila's?

SCENARIO
ANSWERS 13.1

These concepts have been summarised in *Working Together to Safeguard Children* (HM Government, 2015).

SEE ALSO
CHAPTERS 11
AND 14

Assessment Framework

Health
Education
Emotional &
Behavioural Development
Identity
Family & Social
Relationships
Selfcare Skills

CHILD'S DEVELOPMENTAL NEEDS

PARENTING CAPACITY

Basic Care
Ensuring Safety
Emotional Warmth
Stimulation
Guidance &
Boundaries
Stability

CHILD
Safeguarding &
promoting
welfare

FAMILY & ENVIRONMENTAL FACTORS

Community Resources · Family's Social Integration · Income · Employment · Housing · Wider Family · Family History & Functioning

Figure 13.1   The Assessment Framework (HM Government, 2015, p.22) © Crown copyright

It is not by chance that a child's developmental needs, parenting capacity and family and environmental factors are portrayed as sides of a triangle. Each contributes uniquely to the hoped-for outcome, a healthy and well child. A child needs the fundamental aspects to be met: nutrition to grow physically and also to be stimulated and nurtured and educated, including learning how to get along with others so that they grow cognitively and emotionally. The environment they live in influences positively or negatively the carer's ability to provide these aspects but also the child's ability to utilise these to the fullest.

VIDEO LINK
13.3: CHILD
HEALTH AND
NUTRITION

You now need to consider these aspects, reviewing the evidence and degree of influence in more depth.

PARENTING CAPACITY

When exploring the effects of parenting on child health and illness, many studies review what happens when aspects of parenting capacity are absent or negative. We know that where parents provide

SEE ALSO
CHAPTER 37

SEE ALSO
CHAPTERS 10
AND 11

warmth and love this mitigates, to some degree, other aspects such as poverty. However, even in the warmest of environments, poverty limits opportunity and life experiences, which can hinder the child's cognitive and emotional growth, impacting on their choice of career, earning capacity and so adversely affects subsequent generations. You will have explored the importance of genetics and the health of the mother before conception and during pregnancy in previous chapters. Genetic primacy has long held to be true that we are what we inherit, but there is now growing evidence that the environment also influences how those genes work. A key component of providing basic care is nutrition. There is a wealth of evidence that demonstrates that breastfeeding has many immediate and longer-lasting benefits for the child and mother.

Basic care and nutrition

The UNICEF breastfeeding initiative (2013) summarises a number of studies which outline the benefits, which include:

- Reduced risk of admission of the newborn for respiratory conditions and gastroenteritis
- A correlation between higher rates of breastfeeding prevalence and lower rates of inpatient admissions among infants under one year old for a number of conditions
- Lower rates of inpatient admissions among infants under one year old for a number of conditions
- Evidence from America also suggests that babies who have not been breastfed have a higher risk of obesity, hypertension and type 2 diabetes

Petherick (2010) suggests that the current debate between breast versus formula feeding is polarised, with both groups exaggerating their position that one is better than the other. However, the more we know about the micro-constituents of breast milk the more we realise formula cannot replicate breast milk. The Promotion of Breastfeeding Intervention Trial (PROBIT), a study conducted in Belarus, divided centres into those which:

- Delivered the WHO Baby-Friendly Hospital Initiative (BFHI) (where healthcare professionals received specific training and education in breastfeeding support)
- Offered normal care, which did not include any specific breastfeeding initiatives or support

They found differences in weight and reduction of illnesses in the PROBIT group up to the age of one year. Ongoing reviews found that by the age of six, weight and height were similar but in the 'exclusively breastfed for six months' group, teachers rated the children's IQ scores as being higher. However, Martens (2012) suggests caution because the study groups did not include non-breastfed children, and that non-breastfed children or other influencing factors need to be considered. In Belarus it is normal for mothers to be with their children for the first three years of life, so other factors cannot be excluded. Nevertheless, the findings led to a change of policy for the WHO as it now advocates exclusive breastfeeding for the first six months of life and the continuation of breastfeeding, alongside solid foods, for two years (WHO, 2003). Indeed, understanding confounding issues are key when reviewing an issue such as breastfeeding, as women who breastfeed are more likely to be of a higher social group, better educated and have the income to enable them to take maternity leave. However, Iacovou and Sevilla-Sanz (2010, p.2) reviewed the evidence assessing the benefits of breastfeeding on the impact of cognitive development for children in England and concluded that in English, maths and science there is a statistical significance in improved scores which continues to the age of 14 and they suggest this effect grows over time.

Nutrition is important throughout life. We know we have an obesity problem in the Western world. Data is collected differently across the UK, making comparisons between nations difficult. However, all surveys show higher rates of obesity where deprivation is also highest.

Table 13.1 Percentage of children classified as obese in the UK

	Age 4-5		Age 2-6		Age range - see within box		Gender differences
	Over-weight	Obese	Over-weight	Obese	Over-weight	Obese	
England*	13%	9%			10-11 year old 14.3%	10-11 year old 19.8%	Aged 4-5, more boys are overweight or obese compared to girls, 22.7% vs 21.5%. This increases significantly by ages 10-11 when the rates are 36% (boys) and 32.3% (girls)
Wales**	14.5%	11.5%					In 4-5 age slightly more boys are overweight or obese compared to girls 11.9% vs 11.5%
Scotland⁺			14%	13%			In the 12-15 age range, girls are recorded as being more at risk of excess weight than boys 43% vs 32%
Northern Ireland⁺⁺					Age 2-15 16%	Age 2-15 9%	Girls more likely to be overweight or obese than boys

Source: Adapted from House of Common Library briefing paper Number 3336, 20 January 2017. Available at: http://researchbriefings.parliament.uk/ResearchBriefing/Summary/SN03336
* National Child Measurement Programme England, 2015/16 school year ** The Child Measurement Programme for Wales 2015/16, ⁺Scottish Health Survey (2014) term the rates as 'risk of obesity' rather an obese, ⁺⁺ Health Survey N. Ireland (2015/16)

Public Health England (PHE Obesity, 2017) review the evidence on the effects of obesity in childhood and suggest that children are more likely to miss schooling and have other health-related illnesses such as asthma, type 2 diabetes, cardiovascular disease and muscular skeletal disease, and that whilst the evidence is not conclusive that obesity impacts on a child's self-esteem; adolescents who are obese are more at risk of low self-regard and impaired quality of life. PHE states clearly that an obese or overweight child is more likely to become an obese adult with all the potential health risks.

Social interaction and emotional warmth

Social interaction and emotional warmth are also important factors in promoting a child's health development. This is a difficult area to research because we cannot deliberately put a child in an environment which does not meet their needs, and so the focus of research tends to be at the extremes, where there are clear anti-social behaviours demonstrated by the child, or where there is extreme deprivation or abuse. Much of the work exploring emotional warmth has been around attachment, attachment theory and the study of children where attachment has been adversely affected, such as mothers with postnatal depression (PND). However, this is a difficult area to study because of many interlinked themes, such as:

VIDEO LINK 13.4: ATTACHMENT

- Parenting styles (high or low warmth, consistent parenting approach)
- Poverty
- Availability and type of social support

These factors can worsen or mitigate the effects of a lack of emotional warmth, consistent boundaries or meeting basic physical needs. The Department of Health have highlighted characteristics of good parenting:

> Good parenting involves caring for children's basic needs, keeping them safe, showing them warmth and love, and providing the stimulation needed for their development and to help them achieve their potential, within a stable environment where they experience consistent guidance. (DCSF, 2010, p.2)

These characteristics of good parenting are reflected in the Assessment Framework (HM Government, 2015) above.

A child needs stability and an environment demonstrating love and security to be able to grow, develop and take advantage of experiences offered to them. A child who lacks a secure attachment is less likely to be able to form secure and meaningful relationships in later life. They also need to feel secure to be able to explore their environment and to try new experiences, as exploration develops a child's imagination, their inquisitiveness and ability to assess and manage risks (McCluskey and Robbins, 2009). McManus and Poehlmann's (2011) study explored the effect of maternal PND on the cognitive development of pre-term infants and found that infants's cognitive development was influenced in those whose mothers showed PND symptoms. The presence of PND symptoms at nine months post-birth was associated with lower cognitive functioning at 16 months of age. Their study supports other studies that socioeconomic factors and maternal social support can mitigate the effects of PND.

Resilience

The concept of resilience explores whether building resilience within the child and/or family, by providing them with strategies or resources, could help them manage adverse life events. However, resilience is recognised as difficult to define. Joslyn (2015) suggests that it could be described as either a group of positive characteristics that individuals display even if they have experienced negative situations earlier in their life, or a level of competence gained and utilised even in times of great stress. Factors which can help resilience develop or not, include:

* Being secure – a physical (safe environment) and emotional feeling of safety
* The ability to develop and sustain social relationships which involves being able to negotiate and demonstrate empathy with others
* A positive view of themselves, feeling they have worth and can contribute to society

Promoting effective parenting programmes (1)

Furlong and McGilloway (2014) reviewed a parenting programme of children aged 3–8 years where the child was demonstrating 'anti-social behaviour' (though not defined) and how long its effects could be seen in families. For 14 weeks the parents attended sessions where trained facilitators worked with them to develop positive child–parent relationships through actions such as:

* Play
* Positive reinforcement – for example, praise and rewards
* Ignoring negative behaviours
* Operating 'time out' strategies

In these ways they provided a consistent approach for the child. The families were followed up at 6, 12, and 18 months post-intervention. They found that 18 months after the intervention the majority of parents were still able to use the interventions with good effect. Interestingly, the parents also reported positive outcomes around self-efficacy and self-empathy. They viewed themselves more positively, recognising that they could bring about a change in their child's behaviour, sometimes seeking appropriate help to do so – for example, contacting the school when the issue involved a teacher. However, many of the families did report relapses lasting between two and four months, linked to families not continuing with the parenting practices at stressful times – for example, pressures of work or family, bereavement and other negative factors relating to school, neighbourhood or having an uncooperative partner. Parents who then re-implemented the positive parenting plan reported an improvement in the child's behaviour. This study has limitations, particularly because the study group was small and may not have been representative or generalisable to older children.

Promoting effective parenting programmes (2)

Minding the Baby is a study conducted by the NSPCC in three locations in Scotland and the north of England. It utilises work undertaken in the USA and is based on attachment theory, that fostering good attachments will provide for the emotional and cognitive development of the child.

By providing additional support from health and social care workers to young first-time mothers, it is hoped mothers will develop a good attachment that is beneficial to both their baby and to the mother.

ACTIVITY 13.3: REFLECTIVE PRACTICE

Review the video *Saving Brains, A Grand Challenge* which explores how all these factors affect brain development. You can access the video at https://study.sagepub.com/essentialchildnursing

How can you:

- Ensure you maintain stimulation for children in hospital?
- Encourage parents to engage in stimulating their child?

ACTIVITY ANSWER 13.3

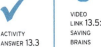

VIDEO LINK 13.5: SAVING BRAINS

Gertler et al. (2014) followed up the Saving Brains study 20 years later and found, significantly, that the earnings of the children in the stimulation group and nutritional and stimulation group were 25 per cent higher than the control group and that they had caught up with the children in the comparison group, that of well-fed children.

SAFEGUARDING STOP POINT

A lack of parenting capacity must always be assessed by considering safeguarding issues. Neglect is a form of abuse whether it is by deliberately withholding basic needs, warmth and love or where circumstances, such as lack of finance or knowledge, make it difficult to provide for these needs. However, that does raise the question, 'Who is the abuser, parents or society?'

ACTIVITY 13.4: CRITICAL THINKING

Review Samira's story. What are the positive and negative factors that are influencing Jamila's ability to parent Samira?

ACTIVITY
ANSWER 13.4

FAMILY AND ENVIRONMENTAL FACTORS

The discussion above focuses on the relationship between parents and children, and the capacity of parents to nurture and respond to their child's developmental needs. We must acknowledge that children (and indeed their parents) do not exist within a softly cushioned vacuum. The Assessment Framework (HM Government, 2015) urges us to consider the impact that family, environment and society can have on parents, and consequently their child's development and wellbeing.

Family functioning

The role of the family in promoting a child's development and wellbeing is an important one. Non-statutory guidance for local authorities on parenting and family support makes the point that 'Family is of life-long importance but for children its significance cannot be overstated: what happens within the family has more impact on children's wellbeing and development than any other single factor'. The guidance goes on to say, 'Family influence remains a potent influence through childhood and adolescence and indeed beyond' (DCSF, 2010, pp.16–17).

Extensive research demonstrates that the quality of relationships between parents can have a positive effect on parenting, and directly results in improved outcomes for children (O'Connor and Scott, 2007). Coleman and Glenn (2009) found that parents who experienced a happy and loving relationship together, promoted mental and physical health for all members of the family. Parents are role models and in a loving home, children learn how to relate to others, share, be kind, say sorry and manage conflict (DCSF, 2010). Conversely, children experiencing high levels of parental conflict can become anxious, aggressive or withdrawn (Harold and Murch, 2005). Close relationships with other family members can help children cope with family stress. Being able to talk about their feelings and knowing they are loved can help children deal with stressful family situations, with the added benefit building resilience; giving them strategies to deal with stressful situations in the future.

SAFEGUARDING STOP POINT

Conflict is frequently hidden from the outside world, even from the family. The Crime Survey of England and Wales 2013/14 (Office of National Statistics, 2014) noted that one in four women will experience domestic violence in their lifetime. Wolfe et al.'s (2003) meta-analysis of 41 studies found that children's developmental outcomes, including social, emotional, behavioural, cognitive and general health functioning, are significantly compromised when exposed to domestic violence. Further reading to raise your awareness of the signs and symptoms of domestic violence or intimate partner violence (IPV) is recommended (see the Weblinks on p. 207).

When children are admitted to hospital, diagnosed with a health problem or are living with a chronic and complex health need, this can often lead to acute and ongoing psychological stress for parents and other family members. In our nursing assessment of children and their families, we need to consider how parents are coping with their child's illness and their additional health needs.

The wider family

Parents and their children are influenced by members of their wider family. In today's society, it can be difficult to define exactly who 'the wider family' are – for example, grandparents, aunts, uncles, step-parents, half siblings, neighbours, childminders and babysitters can all be thought of as part of the wider family. Each person, with their own family history and upbringing, can subsequently have positive and negative influences on parenting style, and on the decisions parents make about their child's health and wellbeing.

ACTIVITY 13.5: REFLECTIVE PRACTICE

Reflect and discuss with a mentor or peers what influences:

- A parent's decision to immunise their child
- How a parent disciplines their child
- A parent's attitude towards their teenagers drinking alcohol

ACTIVITY
ANSWER 13.5

We cannot discount the influence of education, money, society and the media on parenting. However, each parent's personal family history, their upbringing and relationships may override our attempts to provide parents with the knowledge and skills they require to meet their child's needs. By developing our knowledge and skills in forming therapeutic relationships with families we can begin to work in partnership to promote a parent's understanding about child development and wellbeing.

Housing

It has been long recognised that poor housing has a detrimental effect on health. The UK housing charity Shelter (2013) highlights that poor housing can have an impact on a child's physical and mental health, education and opportunities in adulthood. Overcrowded and poor housing can:

- Increase the spread of infection, increasing susceptibility to respiratory problems, tuberculosis and meningitis
- Increase symptoms such as coughing and wheezing, leading to poor sleep, and slow growth
- Increase the risk of accidents
- Decrease school attendance due to increased illness and infections, leading to delays in cognitive developmental and communication skills

When visiting one mother and child it was obvious this mother knew exactly what this child needed to be safe, e.g. baby gates on the stairs and locked kitchen cupboards so the child couldn't access them. However, every time the health visitor attended the house the mother hadn't put these in place. It then became apparent she couldn't afford to purchase these items and therefore was provided with help from the local children centre who helped her get all the necessary safety equipment for her child.

> On a hospital placement after this, I saw multiple children who attended hospital with preventable falls and consumption of liquids/tablets they should not have taken. I then saw the importance of good education to children and parents as well as contacting health visitors to continue with the support and also sign-posting parents to other agencies who could the help them keep their children safe.
>
> **Sarah-Louise, 3rd-year nursing student**

In our assessment of where a child and family live, we should use our knowledge of the geographical area, areas of wealth or deprivation, the location of social housing and available local services and amenities. Each local authority, clinical care group or NHS commissioning board now has the responsibility of carrying out a Joint Strategic Needs Assessment. This involves an assessment of the current and future health and social care needs of the local community, including wider factors that impact on their community's health and wellbeing, and local assets that can help to improve services and reduce inequalities (DH, 2013). This information is of value to both acute and community-based children's nurses, enabling accurate assessment of the issues that may affect a child and family, and providing insight into local services that may offer support. Your local CCG will carry out an assessment, but remember England, Scotland, Wales and Northern Ireland will have an individual strategy.

Income and employment

The choice to have children without doubt has financial implications; most parents hope they can provide for and meet the needs of their child. For some, this equates to buying beautiful clothes, costly travel systems and fancy toys that claim to nurture the inner Einstein in their offspring. For other parents, however, ensuring the basic needs of food, warmth and shelter can be a daily struggle.

The Joseph Rowntree Foundation (JRF, 2015) found that 3.7 million children in the UK live in poverty, (figures from 2013–14). A more tangible analogy by the Child Poverty Action Group (2016) equates this to nine children, in a classroom of 30, living in poverty.

What is poverty?

There are numerous definitions of and opinions about the concept of poverty. Townsend provided a useful definition in the 1970s, which is still relevant:

VIDEO LINK
13.6: CHILD
POVERTY

> Individuals, families and groups in the population can be said to be in poverty when they lack resources to obtain the type of diet, participate in the activities and have the living conditions and amenities which are customary, or at least widely encouraged and approved, in the societies in which they belong. (Townsend, 1979, p.31)

In the UK, the concept of 'relative poverty' is used. A household is in relative poverty (also called relative low income) if their income is below 60 per cent of the median household income. Because the government is measuring quality of living rather than earning power, incomes are measured after taxes and benefits (Full Fact, 2015). When reading reports and government papers, check carefully the type of poverty being discussed.

It is disconcerting that employment is not a guaranteed route out of poverty. The Department of Work and Pensions (DWP, 2015) states that nearly two-thirds (64%) of children growing up in poverty live in a family where at least one member works, as families may lose benefits and have to pay taxes. Barnardo's (2012), in its review of work, childcare and poverty, highlights the increased burden for lone parents (and second earners) who have the added costs of childcare to consider. Although the numbers of lone parents in employment have risen over the past decade, we are reminded that forms of work have changed to include zero-hour contracts and unsociable working hours. These forms of employment do not guarantee a regular income and can push a family into 'in-work poverty' (Philpott, 2014) with families using food banks to ensure children are fed. In addition, rising fuel costs are also pushing families into a phenomenon known as 'fuel poverty'. This is where a family's fuels costs exceed the national average, meaning their remaining income leaves families in relative poverty (Department of Energy and Climate Change (DECC), 2015). Living in a low-income family affects parents' ability to meet the basic needs of food and warmth, quality of housing and access to health and education.

The impact of poverty on child development and wellbeing is far-reaching and poverty affects many aspects of family life. Children living in poverty are:

- More likely to be born prematurely, have low birth weight and die in their first year of life (HM Treasury, 2004)
- More likely to report long-standing illness and less likely to report good or very good general health (HM Treasury, 2004)
- More likely to have a mental disorder – in families from unskilled, working-class backgrounds they are three times as likely to have a mental disorder; in families where the parents have never worked the rate is 20% (DCSF, 2007)
- Significantly more likely to be obese (HM Treasury, 2008)
- More vulnerable to accidents – 13 times more likely to die from unintentional injury and 37 times more likely to die as a result of exposure to smoke, fire or flames (Audit Commission, 2007)
- Experience an increase in inter-parental conflict which negatively affects individual family members' health and wellbeing (EIF, 2017)

Social integration, availability and access to community resources

Today, integration is most often linked with immigration and discussion of how individuals from other countries become part of the UK. However, whether the family is settling in the UK for the first time or moving from one part of the UK to another, Ferragina et al. (2013) identify participation in society to be about belonging. They highlight that one measure of family social integration and participation is through the nature of their relationships with neighbours, and engagement with formal organisations in society. Akin to the positive effects that strong relationships within the wider family can bring, being part of, and contributing to, society has benefits for children and their families and can give both families and individuals a sense of identity and purpose, and increase their self-esteem. Joslyn (2015) recognises that without a strong sense of belonging and clear connections, a feeling of detachment limits the child and family's sense of control, and reduces their sense of self-worth. However, once again cost and availability need to be considered; it costs money to be a Brownie or part of the football team, if they exist in the local area, and can become a further drain on family resources. Therefore, should we as children's nurses argue for free access to such valuable resources?

To conclude, the factors influencing children's health and wellbeing fall under three distinct headings:

- Children's growth and development
- Parenting capacity
- Social and environmental factors

However, these headings mask the complexity of the issues. Whilst for ease of reading these have been separated within the chapter, in truth they are interlinked and interdependent. As a children's nurse you must understand how these can impact on a family and tailor your care and advice to ensure these factors are taken into account. You need to be aware of how social policy decisions and service provision may help or hinder a child and family's health and wellbeing.

CHAPTER SUMMARY

- There are various definitions of health which are complex and ever changing
- There are many factors that affect parenting which can impact on the health and wellbeing of a child and family due to the complex interaction of social factors
- Identifying positive coping strategies and protective factors can influence the development of children and families

BUILD YOUR BIBLIOGRAPHY

Books

- Green, L. (2016) *Understanding the Life Course: Sociological and Psychological Perspectives*. Cambridge: Polity Press.

  The book discusses traditional theories surrounding child development and offers insight into the social and psychological issues that can impact upon the life course.

- Joslyn, E. (2016) *Resilience in Childhood: Perspective, Promise and Practice*. London: Palgrave.

  The book analyses the concept of resilience and uses vignettes to give practice examples.

- Warwick-Booth, L. (2012) *Contemporary Health Studies: An Introduction*. Cambridge: Polity Press.

  Discussion of the complexities and determinants of health and the need for nurses to understand and engage with health policy.

Journal articles

Go to https://study.sagepub.com/essentialchildnursing for further free online journal articles related to this chapter.

FURTHER READING: ONLINE JOURNAL ARTICLES

- Masten, A. and Monn, A. (2014) 'Child and family resilience: a call for integrated science, practice and professional training'. *Family Relations*, 64: 5–21.

  This article summarises the development of risk and resilience theory to date and what it offers to our understanding of how families manage the complex nature of their lives.

- Crawford. D.A. (2002) 'Keep the focus on the family'. *Journal of Child Healthcare*, 6 (2): 133–46.

  The article highlights many of the theories that seek to discover how the family unit works, factors affecting family functioning (including socio-economic inequalities), and how child health and development can be supported by the family.

Weblinks

Go to https://study.sagepub.com/essentialchildnursing for further weblinks related to this chapter.

FURTHER
READING:
WEBLINKS

- The Children's Society, *The Good Childhood Report 2015*

  www.childrenssociety.org.uk/sites/default/files/TheGoodChildhoodReport2015.pdf
  Children identify what are important influences in their lives. We need to understand what are key worries for the children in our care, so we can ensure we tailor care packages that meet these needs.

- HM Government (2009) *Together We Can End Violence Against Women and Girls: A Strategy.* Available at: www.homeoffice.gov.uk/crime/violence-against-women-girls/

  Extend your knowledge on the effects of domestic abuse on children and families by reviewing some of the available government literature.

- HM Government (2009) *Tackling Violence Against Women and Girls: A guide to good practice communication.* www.equalities.gov.uk/news/vaw_guidance.aspx

- NSPCC, Assessing parenting capacity factsheet (2014)

  This factsheet outlines some of the areas you need to consider in your assessment of parenting capacity.
  www.nspcc.org.uk/globalassets/documents/information-service/factsheet-assessing-parenting-capacity.pdf

- The Poverty Site, *Relative Poverty, Absolute Poverty and Social Exclusion*

  www.poverty.org.uk/summary/social%20exclusion.shtml
  Read the definitions of poverty.

ACE YOUR ASSESSMENT

Revise what you have learned by visiting https://study.sagepub.com/essentialchildnursing

ONLINE
QUIZZES &
ACTIVITY
ANSWERS

GREAT FOR
REVISION!

- Test yourself with multiple-choice and short-answer questions
- Do the chapter activities in the book and check your answers online

REFERENCES

Audit Commission (2007) *Better Safe than Sorry*. London: Audit Commission.

Barnardo's (2012) *Paying to Work: Childcare and Poverty*. Ilford: Barnardo's.

Child Poverty Action Group (2016) *Child Poverty Facts and Figures*. Available at: www.cpag.org.uk/child-poverty-facts-and-figures (accessed 21 June 2017).

Coleman, L. and Glenn, G. (2009) *When Couples Part: Understanding the Consequences for Adults and Children*. London: One Plus One.

Department for Children, Schools and Families (DCSF) (2007) *Children and Young People Today: Evidence to Support the Development of the Children's Plan*. London: DCSF.

Department for Children, Schools and Families (DCSF) (2010) *Parenting and Family Support: Guidance for Local Authorities in England*. London: DCSF.

Department of Energy and Climate Change (DECC) (2015) *Fuel Poverty Statistics*. Available at: www.gov.uk/government/collections/fuel-poverty-statistics (accessed 11 December 2015).

Department of Health (DH) (2013) *Statutory Guidance on Joint Strategic Needs Assessments and Joint Health and Wellbeing Strategies.* London: DH.

Department of Work and Pensions (DWP) (2015) *Households below Average Income: An Analysis of the Income Distribution 1994/95–2013/14*, Table 4.5db. London: DWP.

Early Intervention Foundation (EIF) (2017) *Interparental Conflict and Outcomes for Children in the Contexts of Poverty and Economic Pressure.* Available at: www.eif.org.uk/publication/inter-parental-conflict-and-outcomes-for-children-in-the-contexts-of-poverty-and-economic-pressure (accessed 28 June 2017).

Ferragina, E., Tomlinson, M. and Walker, R. (2013) *Poverty, Participation and Choice.* York: Joseph Rowntree Foundation. Available at: www.jrf.org.uk/report/poverty-participation-and-choice (last accessed 17 May 2017).

Full Fact (2015) *Poverty in the UK: A Guide to the Facts and Figures.* Available at: https://fullfact.org/economy/whats_happened_to_poverty_parliament-39908 (last accessed 17 May 2017).

Furlong M. and McGilloway (2014) 'The longer term experiences of parent training: a qualitative analysis'. *Child Care Health Dev,* 41 (5): 687–96.

Gertler, P., Heckman, J., Pinto, R., Zanolini, A., Vermeersch, C., Walker, S., Chang, S.M. and McGregor S.G. (2014) 'Labor market returns to an early childhood stimulation intervention in Jamaica'. *Science,* 344 (6187): 998–1001.

Harold, G.T. and Murch, M.A. (2005) 'Inter-parental conflict and children's adaptation to separation and divorce: theory, research and implications for family law, practice and policy'. *Child and Family Law Quarterly,* 17 (2): 185–205.

HM Government (2009) *Working Together to Safeguard Children: A Guide to Inter-agency Working to Safeguard and Promote the Welfare of Children.* London: DCSF.

HM Government (2010) *Support for All: The Families and Relationships Green Paper.* London: TSO.

HM Government (2015) *Working Together to Safeguard Children: A Guide to Inter-agency Working to Safeguard and Promote the Welfare of Children.* London: DfE. Available at: www.gov.uk/government/publications/working-together-to-safeguard-children--2#history (last accessed 17 May 2017).

HM Treasury (2004) *Child Poverty Review.* London: HM Treasury.

HM Treasury (2008) *Ending Child Poverty: Everybody's business.* [online] Available from: http://webarchive.nationalarchives.gov.uk/20100403012101/www.hm-treasury.gov.uk/bud_bud08_child.htm (accessed 13 December 2015).

Iacovou M. and Sevilla-Sanz A. (2010) *The Effect of Breastfeeding on Children's Cognitive Development.* Colchester: Institute for Social and Economic Research. Available at: www.iser.essex.ac.uk/research/publications/working-papers/iser/2010-40 (last accessed 17 May 2017).

Joseph Rowntree Foundation (JRF) (2015) *Monitoring Poverty and Social Exclusion 2015.* York: JRF. Available at: www.jrf.org.uk/mpse-2015 (last accessed 17 May 2017).

Joslyn, E. (2015) *Resilience in Childhood: Perspective, Promise and Practice.* London: Palgrave.

Katz, S., Lee, T. and Byrne, S. (2015) 'Predicting parent–child differences in perceptions of how children use the Internet for help with homework, identity development, and health information'. *Journal Of Broadcasting and Electronic Media,* 59 (4): 574–602.

Martens, P.J. (2012) 'What do Kramer's Baby-Friendly Hospital Initiative PROBIT studies tell us? A review of a decade of research'. *J Hum Lact,* 28 (3): 335–42.

McCluskey, H. and Robbins M. (2009) 'Safeguarding children', in A. Glasper, G. McEwing and J. Richardson (eds), *Foundation Studies for Caring.* Basingstoke: Palgrave Macmillan.

McManus, B.M. and Poehlmann, J. (2011) 'Maternal depression and perceived social support as predictors of cognitive function trajectories during the first 3 years of life for preterm infants in Wisconsin'. *Child: Care, Health and Development,* 38 (3): 425–34.

Myant, K.A. and Williams, J.M. (2005) 'Children's concepts of health and illness: understanding of contagious illnesses, non-contagious illnesses and injuries'. *Journal of Health Psychology*, 10 (6): 805–19.

O'Connor, T. and Scott, S. (2007) *Parenting and Outcomes for Children*. York: Joseph Rowntree Foundation.

Office of National Statistics (2014) *Statistical Bulletin: Crime in England and Wales, Year Ending December 2014*. Available at: www.ons.gov.uk/ons/rel/crime-stats/crime-statistics/year-ending-december-2014/crime-in-england-and-wales--year-ending-december-2014.html (accessed 4 December 2015).

Petherick, A. (2010) 'Development: mother's milk: a rich opportunity'. *Nature*, 468, S5–7.

Philpott, J. (2014) *Rewarding Work for Low-paid Workers*. York: The Joseph Rowntree Foundation.

Public Health England Obesity (2017) Available at: http://webarchive.nationalarchives.gov.uk/20170210161227/http://www.noo.org.index.php (accessed 26 September 2017).

Royal College of Nursing (RCN) (2012) *Health Inequalities and the Social Determinants of Health*. London: RCN.

Shelter (2013) *NatCen Social Research that works for society. People living in bad housing, numbers and health impacts*. Available at: http://england.shelter.org.uk/__data/assets/pdf_file/0010/726166/People_living_in_bad_housing.pdf (last accessed 28 June 2017).

The Children's Society (2015) *The Good Childhood Report*. Available at: www.childrenssociety.org.uk/sites/default/files/TheGoodChildhoodReport2015.pdf (last accessed 17 May 2017).

The Information Centre for Health and Social Care (2008). *National Child Measurement Programme: 2006/07 School Year, Headline Results*. Available at http://content.digital.nhs.uk/catalogue/PUB02302/nati-chil-meas-prog-resu-2006-2007-rep.pdf (last accessed 17 May 2017).

Townsend, P. (1979) *Poverty in the United Kingdom*. London: Allen Lane.

Toyama. N. (2016) 'Adults' explanations and children's understanding of contagious illnesses, non-contagious illnesses, and injuries'. *Early Child Development and Care*, 186 (4): 526–43.

UNICEF (2013) *The Evidence and Rationale for the UNICEF UK Baby Friendly Initiative Standards*. Available at: www.unicef.org.uk/wp-content/uploads/sites/2/2013/09/baby_friendly_evidence_rationale.pdf (last accessed 17 May 2017).

Wolfe, D.A., Crookes, C.V., Lee, V., McIntyre-Smith, A. and Jaffe, P.G. (2003) 'The effects of children's exposure to domestic violence: a meta-analysis and critique'. *Clinical Child and Family Psychology Review*, 6 (3): 171–87.

World Health Organization (WHO) (1948) *Preamble to the Constitution of the World Health Organization as adopted by the International Health Conference*, New York, 19–22 June 1946.

World Health Organization (WHO) (1986) *The Ottawa Charter for Health Promotion*. First International Conference on Health Promotion, Ottawa, 21 November 1986. Available at: www.who.int/healthpromotion/conferences/previous/ottawa/en (last accessed 17 May 2017).

World Health Organization (WHO) (2003) *Global Strategy for Infant and Young Child Feeding*. Available at: www.who.int/nutrition/topics/global_strategy/en (last accessed 17 May 2017).

UNIVERSAL SCREENING AND THE ROLE OF THE HEALTH VISITOR

14

MANDY BRIMBLE AND SARAH REDDINGTON-BOWES

THIS CHAPTER COVERS

- The role of the health visitor
- The value of universal screening and the evidence that underpins practice
- Universal screening programmes in the UK
- How screening activities are used to monitor development and promote health

> "
> A popular perception is that health visitors drink cups of tea and weigh babies. That's certainly all I knew about the service.
>
> **Terry, 2nd-year children's nursing student**
> "

INTRODUCTION

Many children's nursing students undertake a health visitor placement, so understanding their role is important for improving your own practice and gaining an appreciation of the difference they make to children and families. The quotation above from a 2nd-year nursing student is typical, not only of nursing students but also the general public. Health visiting is so much more than this and is a highly skilled role. This chapter will outline how health visitors carry out universal screening programmes in the UK, together with the evidence that underpins them. Scenarios are used to bring practice to life and to highlight typical issues and interventions. Working in partnership with parents is essential for successful relationships which benefit the child and family.

SEE ALSO
CHAPTER 7

THE ROLE OF THE HEALTH VISITOR

The work of health visitors is embedded in public health and reflects its history, which began in 1862 when the Manchester and Salford Ladies Sanitary Reform Association decided to employ 'sanitary visitors' to offer practical help, advice and health education in people's homes (Adams, 2012). This primary focus on public health makes it unique among the caring professions (Malone et al., 2003 in Baldwin, 2012) and, in fact, the formal title of a health visitor is 'specialist community public health nurse' (SCPHN). The principles of health visiting underpin the work of the profession and are:

- The search for health needs
- The stimulation of an awareness of health needs
- The influence on policies affecting health
- The facilitation of health enhancing activities (Cowley and Frost, 2006, p.1)

The first two points mean that health visitors carry out assessments to determine the health needs of children and families and in some cases highlight that a need exists – some families may be unaware that they have a health need if their upbringing, culture or outlook normalises something which is detrimental to their health. The third principle applies to all nurses. However, health visitors are autonomous and closely linked to communities so they have first-hand, detailed knowledge of the needs of local populations. They have, therefore, a key role in responding to government consultation documents and may be involved in lobbying for change which promotes health. The final principle involves instigating activities which promote health – for example, baby massage classes which promote parent–child attachment, parenting groups and postnatal depression support groups (CPHVA, 2007).

To qualify as a health visitor, registered nurses undertake an intensive and rigorously assessed year-long programme of academic study and practice placement (NMC, 2004). They are knowledgeable in all aspects of child and maternal health and are skilled communicators with excellent interpersonal skills (Robinson, 2012). Their role requires tact and diplomacy whilst being assertive and upholding the primary principle of the Children Act (1989) – that is, the welfare of the child is paramount. Whilst health visiting practice is highly autonomous, health visitors are an integral part of the primary care multidisciplinary team, and partnership working with colleagues across health and social care is essential (Cousins, 2010).

Health visiting is a universal service (offered to all). Universalistic services are effective in reaching those who do not identify their own needs or are reluctant/unable to take up services. This is especially important as these sections of the population are usually those in most need (Black Report, 1980). Most health visitors work with families who have children aged 0–5 years, although there are roles that cover specific conditions like diabetes and population groups such as travelling families. Health visitors often work with families for a long time, sometimes over a decade depending on the spacing between births and circumstances. The strength of this relationship is indicated by Terry's thoughts below.

> The relationships that the health visitor had built over the years in
> the community were formidable.
>
> **Terry, 2nd-year children's nursing student**

The service is highly valued by parents and a real lifeline in times of crisis, as shown by the quotation below. This was a mother's response when asked, 'What is a health visitor?'

> I was lost and in a scary place and my health visitor was the rock
> I needed to help guide me …
>
> **Child, Unite/CPHVA Twitter feed, 12 July 2016**

THE VALUE OF UNIVERSAL SCREENING AND THE EVIDENCE THAT UNDERPINS PRACTICE

SEE ALSO
CHAPTER 13

Universal screening is the main way in which health visitors fulfil many of the principles outlined above. The purpose of screening is to monitor children's health and development and detect early on deviations from normal development or physical abnormalities. The regular contact with children and families provided by screening programmes is also used to promote health and wellbeing (Hall and Elliman, 2003). There is evidence that these activities significantly improve long-term health, social and educational outcomes for the individual child, communities and the nation (Marmot, 2010).

Much of the knowledge underpinning screening activities has been provided by David Hall and David Elliman in their series of publications (1989–2003), commonly referred to as 'The Hall Report'. The last of these, 'Hall 4' (Hall and Elliman, 2003) was controversial because it suggested a more targeted approach. Health visitors felt that this went against the principles of universal provision and that it would be difficult to target those most in need without first screening all children. There was much debate about this in 2003, and more recently the impact of this change has been researched (see 'What's the evidence?' below). The lessons learned from this approach are likely to have led to the graded levels of service set out in the Healthy Child Programme (see 'Theory stop point' below). The level of need is identified at the start of the child's life and regularly reviewed via the Family Health Needs Assessment, discussed in more depth later.

WHAT'S THE EVIDENCE?

King (2015) examined health visitors' accounts of the impact of 'Hall 4' on their practice and profession. The trigger for the study was health visitors' strong reaction to the major change in service delivery. This was a qualitative study which used interviews to collect data. Sixteen health visitors with between 8 and 30 years' experience took part in the study, which found that the implementation of 'Hall 4' had impacted negatively on health visiting practice and morale. The researcher concluded that health visitors play a crucial role in policy implementation and their feelings can shape how families experience the service. Recommendations were made to engage health visitors in consultations about changes to policy.

- What do you think may be the consequences of targeted rather than universal health visiting practice?

WHAT'S THE EVIDENCE? ANSWER 14.1

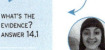

CHECK YOUR ANSWERS ONLINE!

UNIVERSAL SCREENING PROGRAMMES IN THE UK

Universal screening activities are delivered via a variety of frameworks across the UK. These differ slightly due to devolved government in Wales, Scotland and Northern Ireland. In England, the Healthy Child Programme sets out the screening activities and developmental checks undertaken by the health visitor (DH, 2009) and the Healthy Child Wales Programme (Welsh Government, 2012) is similarly configured. The significant challenges of child poverty in some areas of Wales have been recognised by the Welsh Government which has invested in Flying Start programmes (Welsh Government, 2012) that aim to enhance life chances for children living in deprived circumstances. In Scotland, the framework is The Scottish Child Health Programme (NHS National Services Scotland, 2015). In 2014 the Scottish Government pledged an additional 500 health visiting posts by 2018, demonstrating their recognition of the importance of the universal services health visitors provide. This was also increased by a further 180 posts in 2016 (Scottish Government, 2016). Northern Ireland also has its own version of the Healthy Child Programme, called Healthy Child, Healthy Future (DHSSPSNI, 2010). All four of these frameworks include fundamental visits such as the new birth visit (10–14 days post-delivery) and development checks (at ages predetermined by each framework). The scenarios used in this chapter relate to universal screening activities carried out as part of these frameworks. These (fictitious) scenarios are not framed within any particular country of the UK, as the principles of health visiting are central to practice, whichever framework is used. This chapter is structured around these scenarios in order to show universal screening in action. The 12-month review is covered in most depth as this is considered the end of infancy, the period in which the most dramatic trajectories of growth and development occur (Sharma and Cockerill, 2014). Many aspects of this assessment apply to other developmental checks.

ACTIVITY 14.1: EVIDENCE-BASED PRACTICE

Access the 'Foundation Years – Great early years and childcare' website via https://study.sagepub.com/essentialchildnursing
   Click on the link to the Marmot Review *Fair Society, Healthy Lives* (2010) and write a brief summary of the report and how it will impact on your practice.

SCENARIO ANSWER 14.1

WEBLINK: FOUNDATION YEARS

Family Health Needs Assessment

As part of the Healthy Child Programme, health visitors complete a robust Family Health Needs Assessment (FHNA) with each family for each new birth. This occurs sometime between the 28th and 36th weeks of the antenatal period and the New Birth Visit, which is conducted 10–14 days post-delivery.

VIDEO LINK 14.1:
SUPPORTING NEW
PARENTS

A needs assessment by health visitors is a continuing process and is essential to home visiting and the professional–client relationship. The main skills and knowledge required for making these assessments and professional judgements are observation, empathy, application of knowledge and highly developed interpersonal skills (Cowley et al., 2015). The FHNA should therefore be reviewed by the health visiting team at every contact and/or change in family dynamics. The contact is face to face and in the new parent's home. The health visitor promotes sensitive parenting to include sustaining good emotional care and good mother–father–infant relationships, relationship development with the practitioner and a thorough assessment of growth and development in the infant. The family situation is assessed in order to decide the most appropriate service provision – the categories are fully explained in the Theory stop point below and represent a combination of universal and targeted services once the level of need has been assessed.

WEBLINK:
FNP

FOUR LEVELS OF HEALTH VISITING SERVICE

Health visiting teams offer four levels of service to families with children under five:

Your community offers a range of services, including children's centre services and the services families and communities provide for themselves. Health visitors work to develop these and make sure local families know about them.

Universal services from the health visitor team working with GPs to ensure that families can access the Healthy Child Programme, that parents are supported at key times and have access to a range of community services.

Universal plus offers a rapid response from the local health visiting team when specific expert help is needed – for example, because of postnatal depression, a sleepless baby, weaning or concerns about parenting.

Universal partnership plus provides ongoing support from the health visiting team and a range of local services to deal with more complex issues over a period of time. These include services from children's centres, other community services including charities and, where appropriate, the Family Nurse Partnership.

Source: Adapted from *Health Visitor Implementation Plan 2011-15* (DH, 2011)

Table 14.1 shows the 4, 5, 6 health visiting model (DH, 2015) which includes the 4-level service model outlined above, the 5 mandated visits within the Healthy Child Programme, England, and the 6 high-impact areas of the model together with the underpinning aims of this approach.

Table 14.1   4, 5, 6 health visiting model (DH, 2015)

4-level service model	5 mandated elements	6 high-impact areas
• Your community • Universal • Universal Plus • Partnership Plus	• Antenatal health-promoting visits • New baby review • 6–8-week assessment • 1-year assessment • 2–2½ year review	• Transition to parenthood and the early weeks • Maternal (perinatal) mental health • Breastfeeding • Healthy weight • Managing minor illness and reducing accidents • Health, wellbeing of child aged 2 and support to be 'ready for school'

Improved access

Improved experience

Improved outcomes

Reduced health inequalities

VIDEO LINK 14.2:
HEALTH VISITOR
SERVICES

Used with permission under the terms of the Open Government Licence http://webarchive.nationalarchives.gov.uk/+/http://www.nationalarchives.gov.uk/doc/open-government-licence

HOW SCREENING ACTIVITIES ARE USED TO MONITOR DEVELOPMENT AND PROMOTE HEALTH

The 12-month review

Health visitors in England and Scotland conduct developmental assessments at 12 months and 2–2½ years (these are two of the five 'core' contacts in England and two of the 11 'core' contacts in Scotland). These contacts give the practitioner an opportunity to further explore the dynamics within a family, revisit the FHNA, assess the growth and development of the child against evidence-based assessment tools – for example, Mary Sheridan (Sharma and Cockerill, 2014), Denver Developmental Screening Test (Frankenburg and Dodds, 1967), Ages and Stages Questionnaire [ASQ] (Brookes, 2015) and Schedule of Growing Skills [SOGS] (GL Assessment, 2015). During these visits, routine assessments of parental mental health and wellbeing are also made.

The 12-month review should take place in a mutually agreed venue such as a clinic, children's centre, nursery or the child's home. Both parents are encouraged to attend and participate in the review, giving them time to discuss their concerns and aspirations for their child. If the parents do not accept the invitation, a second appointment will be sent. If the family fail to attend a second time, where there are concerns regarding the child's social or medical development or evidence of poor engagement with services, the health visitor is responsible for contacting the family to decide future action. This may be in liaison with members of the team or other relevant agencies.

The 12-month review is a face-to-face contact with a child to systematically assess growth, social and emotional development and detect possible abnormalities while reviewing the family's strengths, needs and risks. This will include actions to address any needs identified and agreeing future contact with the service.

This review aims to:

- Improve emotional and social wellbeing
- Improve learning, speech and language development
- Ensure early detection of and action to address developmental delay or abnormalities, ill health and growth impairments

- Maximise protection against communicable disease
- Prevent obesity and promote healthy behaviours
- Reduce the adverse impact on the child of poor parenting, disruptive family relationships, domestic violence, mental health issues and substance abuse
- Address parental concerns
- Review immunisation status
- Raise awareness of dental health and prevention, and give advice about healthy weaning, portion sizes, types of food and meal-time routines, feeding cups, Healthy Start and vitamin supplements, obesity risk factors and iron deficiency
- Give practical advice about sensitive parenting, healthy sleep practices and managing crying
- Promote age-appropriate local activities
- Raise awareness of injury and accident prevention, including car safety
- Review the health needs of the family, give advice about smoking cessation and preventing inhalation of second-hand smoke
- Promote interaction between parent and child via reading through the Bookstart scheme (see www.bookstart.org.uk)
- Raise awareness of skin cancer prevention
- Discuss as appropriate referral of families whose first language is not English to relevant local services

There are many competencies required to undertake this and other developmental and family assessments. Practitioners are expected to be trained in and have an understanding of child development and of factors that influence health and wellbeing. This knowledge needs to be applied so that health visitors can recognise the range of normal development and identify deviations from it, together with possible causes. Practical skills such as being adept at using scales, measuring length and head circumference and completing growth charts are essential for the accurate recording of measurements. In addition, practitioners need consultation skills, purposeful listening skills and an ability to use guiding questions (motivational interviewing skills) in order to interact and gain maximum benefit from the contact for the parents of the child. Knowledge of care pathways, the Common Assessment Framework, safeguarding, child protection procedures and an awareness of domestic abuse/intimate partner violence risks are also key to the role as this will enable identification of major stressors and risks in a timely manner.

VIDEO LINK 14.3:
BEING A HEALTH
VISITOR

PRACTICE
SCENARIO 14:
CHANELLE

SCENARIO 14.1: BEAU

Teenage parents Jade and John are invited to an appointment for Beau's 12-month review at the local children's centre. The appointment is sent well in advance. The health visitor, Sally, sent a reminder text to Jade's mobile phone the day before. There was no response. On the morning of the appointment neither Jade nor John attend with their daughter Beau.

Sally decided to complete an opportunistic home visit rather than invite them to another appointment because the parents had not brought Beau to the clinic or been seen for some time. When Sally visited, she found Jade to be at home with Beau. Jade let Sally in and disclosed that her relationship with John had broken down. She was in debt and felt very low. Sally was able to actively listen to Jade, complete a mood assessment and signpost Jade to the local Depression and Anxiety service. Sally offered weekly listening visits whilst Jade awaited the appointment. Jade was encouraged to access the children's centre to support her in managing debt and to socialise with other mums. Beau was assessed as meeting her developmental milestones and her growth was satisfactory. Sally offered visits by the community nursery nurse to support the relationship between Jade and Beau. Sally decided to defer some of the health promotion activities usually carried out during the 12-month review until future visits because she wanted to prioritise Jade's mental health and her relationship with Beau.

- How is health promotion defined by the World Health Organization?
- List the health promotion activities usually carried out at the 12-month review

✓ SCENARIO ANSWER **14.1**

SEE ALSO CHAPTER **11**

Being flexible: Being truly needs led

There may be many occasions when health visitors need to defer matters until another visit. In some instances this may be to prioritise another health need as described in the scenario above. It could also be that the main purpose for the visit – for example, a developmental check – is temporarily put on hold if there is a crisis occurring at the time of the visit. There would be little point in pressing on with a development check if the parents/carers are experiencing a highly stressful situation such as eviction or disconnection of utility services. Similarly, efforts to promote health by encouraging smoking cessation may fall on deaf ears if the parent is using smoking as a stress reliever. Decisions to delay activities which are a key part of a screening activity must be taken carefully and not suspended indefinitely; otherwise the welfare of the child may be compromised. However, even when universal screening is carried out in line with local frameworks, issues can arise. The section below describes such an instance.

The three-year review

Many developmental review frameworks include an assessment at around the age of 3 years. Since many children start school soon after this time the term 'school readiness' is often used (UNICEF, 2012) to describe what is being assessed. This is an area where early years practitioners can have a significantly positive effect on outcomes for children who are vulnerable and living in disadvantaged circumstances (Ofsted, 2014). There is no national definition of school readiness but in the Ofsted (2014) document *Are You Ready?* a primary school teacher suggests that the child should:

- Be able to separate from their parent/carer
- Demonstrate listening skills – that is, show interest and pay attention
- Have sufficient language to express their needs
- Say their name, age and something about their family
- Be able to interact with an adult
- Be able to interact with their peers – for example, take turns in play
- Take responsibility for their actions
- Show interest in what is around them
- Notice things and ask questions
- Hold a book
- Understand the narrative of an age-appropriate book
- Respond to boundary setting

The scenario below outlines issues identified during a 3-year developmental check.

SCENARIO 14.2: ANGHARAD

Angharad is 3. She lives in a deprived area with her mother Sian and her sibling Tom, aged 9. Angharad was last reviewed by the health visitor, Jane, when she was aged 18 months. At that time her development was satisfactory. At the 3-year check Angharad's development is significantly delayed. She says very few words. She grunts and points to make herself understood but she appears to understand what is asked of her. Her fine motor skills development is delayed; she is unable to hold a pen and is still using a 'palmar grasp' to pick up small objects, rather than the 'pincer grasp' expected at age 3 (Sharma and Cockerill, 2014). Her gross motor skills are also delayed; she is unable to ride a tricycle or kick a ball. The health visitor discusses her concerns with Sian. She is mindful of using a non-judgmental and supportive approach. Sian is unconcerned, stating that Angharad is lazy. However, she agrees to referrals to the community paediatrician and the speech and language therapist (SALT). Jane discusses ways in which Sian and Tom can encourage Angharad's speech development in the meantime.

The community paediatrician advises Jane that her assessment identified global developmental delay due to insufficient stimulation.

Sian does not take Angharad to the SALT appointment. The SALT offers another appointment but they do not attend this either. Sian tells Jane that she doesn't see the point as she is not worried about Angharad's speech.

- Explain the value of universal services in this scenario
- Why is a non-judgemental and supportive approach essential when working with families who have failed to meet their child's needs?

SCENARIO
ANSWER **14.2**

This scenario shows that parents are not always willing to work in partnership with the health visitor, even when a need has been clearly identified. In some cases this may be a minor issue. In others it may present a real cause for concern about the wellbeing of the child.

SAFEGUARDING STOP POINT

SEE ALSO
CHAPTER **9**

Physical, sexual and emotional abuse together with neglect and fabricated illness are categories of abuse (HM Government, 2015).

Based on the circumstances outlined above it could be argued that Sian has neglected Angharad and continues to do so by not attending appointments. Neglect is defined by the NSPCC (2016) as 'the ongoing failure to meet a child's basic needs'. Although Angharad has her food, shelter and clothing needs met, other basic needs identified in the UN Convention on the Rights of the Child (UN, 1989) are lacking. Keeping in mind the primary principle of the Children Act (1989) that the welfare of the child is paramount, if this situation continues or deteriorates, the health visitor may need to escalate the matter so that further support can be provided.

PLACEMENT
ADVICE **14:**
HEALTH
VISITING

Have a look at the placement advice at https://study.sagepub.com/essentialchildnursing for tips on preparing for health visiting placements.

CHAPTER SUMMARY

- Evidence exists to underpin the universal screening activities for the under 5s and the role of the health visitor in implementing evidence-based frameworks
- Universal screening provision in the UK is wide ranging and these activities are used to monitor development and promote health
- The role and responsibilities of the health visitor are diverse and are much more than drinking tea and weighing babies
- Health visitors work in collaboration with other professionals and services to ensure health and wellbeing for children and families

BUILD YOUR BIBLIOGRAPHY

Books

- Luker, K.A., Orr, J. and McHugh, G. (2012) *Health Visiting: A Rediscovery*, 3rd edn. Chichester: Wiley-Blackwell.

  A critical exploration of health visiting practice in the current social and policy context.

- Sharma, A. and Cockerill, H. (2014) *From Birth to Five Years: Practical Developmental Examination*. London: Routledge.

  A key text in guiding practitioners through early-years assessments.

- Watkins, D. and Cousins, J. (2010) *Public Health and Community Nursing*, 3rd edn. London: Bailliere Tindall Elsevier.

  This book places health visiting and other community health and social care professions in the public health context. It provides an excellent insight into the professions themselves and how they work in partnership for the best outcomes.

Journal articles

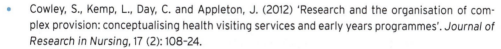

Go to https://study.sagepub.com/essentialchildnursing for further free online journal articles related to this chapter.

FURTHER READING: ONLINE JOURNAL ARTICLES

- Cowley, S., Kemp, L., Day, C. and Appleton, J. (2012) 'Research and the organisation of complex provision: conceptualising health visiting services and early years programmes'. *Journal of Research in Nursing*, 17 (2): 108-24.

  This article discusses universal and more targeted provision so it links with the article outlined in the 'What's the evidence?' section and to the format of the Healthy Child Programme.

- Kemp, L. and Harris, E. (2012) 'The challenges of establishing and researching a sustained nurse home visiting programme within the universal child and family health service system'. *Journal of Research in Nursing*, 17 (2): 127: 38.

  Useful in gaining an understanding of the challenges of implementing changes in practice.

- Aston, M., Price, S., Etowa, J., Vukic, A., Young, L., Hart, C., MacLeod, E. and Randel, P. (2015) 'The power of relationships: exploring how public health nurses support mothers and families during postpartum home visits'. *Journal of Family Nursing*, 2 (1): 11-34.

  An insight into one of the key areas of health visiting practice.

Weblinks

FURTHER
READING:
WEBLINKS

Go to https://study.sagepub.com/essentialchildnursing for further weblinks related to this chapter.

- Community Practitioner and Health Visitors Association (CPHVA) www.unitetheunion.org/how-we-help/list-of-sectors/healthsector/healthsectoryourprofession/cphva/cphvaaboutus

  Unite/CPHVA is the leading professional body and union representing health visitors, school nurses and community nursery nurses.

- Institute of Health Visiting (iHV)

  http://ihv.org.uk
  The Institute of Health Visiting is a new professional body. It provides many educational resources and professional development opportunities.

- Healthy Child Programme

  www.gov.uk/government/uploads/system/uploads/attachment_data/file/167998/Health_Child_Programme.pdf
  Different countries of the UK have their own version of the Healthy Child Programme. The link above is to the one produced by the Department of Health for England.

- BMJ Blogs, Anna's student nursing experience

  http://blogs.bmj.com/ebn/2015/08/26/annas-student-nursing-experience
  A children's nursing student perspective on the health visitor placement.

ONLINE
QUIZZES &
ACTIVITY
ANSWERS

——— ACE YOUR ASSESSMENT ———

Revise what you have learned by visiting https://study.sagepub.com/essentialchildnursing

- Test yourself with multiple-choice and short-answer questions
- Do the chapter activities in the book and check your answers online

REFERENCES

Adams, C. (2012) 'The history of health visiting'. *Nursing in Practice*, 68. Available at: www.nursinginpractice.com/article/history-health-visiting (last accessed 18 May 2017).

Anonymous (2016) Community Practitioner and Health Visitors Association/Unite the Union Twitter feed 12 July 2016 at https://twitter.com/Unite_CPHVA?lang=en-gb

Baldwin, S. (2012) 'Exploring the professional identity of health visitors'. *Nursing Times*, 108 (25): 12–15.

Black, D. (1980) *Inequalities in Health: Report of a Research Working Group*. London: DHSS.

Brookes, P. (2015) *Ages and Stages Questionnaires*. Available at: http://agesandstages.com (last accessed 8 November 2017).

Cousins, J. (2010) 'Partnership working in health and social care', in D. Watkins and J. Cousins, *Public Health and Community Nursing*, 3rd edn. London: Bailliere Tindall Elsevier.

Cowley, S. and Frost, M. (2006) *The Principles of Health Visiting: Opening the Door to Public Health Practice in the 21st Century*. London: CPHVA.

Cowley, S., Whittaker, K., Malone, M., Donetto, S., Grigulis, A. and. Maben, J. (2015) 'Why health visiting? Examining the potential public health benefits from health visiting practice within a universal service: a narrative review of the literature'. *International Journal of Nursing Studies*, 52: 465–80.

CPHVA (2007) *The Distinctive Contribution of Health Visiting to Public Health and Wellbeing: Addressing Public Health Priorities Using the Principles of Health Visiting*. London: CPHVA.

Department of Health (DH) (2009) *Healthy Child Programme: Pregnancy and the First Five Years of Life*. London: DH.

Department of Health (DH) (2011) *Health Visitor Implementation Plan 2011–15: A Call to Action*. London: DH.

Department of Health (DH) (2015) *Universal Health Visitor Reviews: Advice for Local Authorities in Delivery of the Mandated Universal Health Visitor Reviews from 1 October 2015*. London: DH.

Department of Health, Social Services and Patient Safety Northern Ireland (DHSSPSNI) (2010) *Healthy Child, Healthy Future: A Framework for the Universal Child Health Promotion Programme in Northern Ireland*. Available at: www.health-ni.gov.uk/publications/healthy-child-healthy-future (last accessed 18 May 2017).

Frankenburg, W.K. and Dodds, J.B. (1967) 'The Denver Developmental Screening Test'. *The Journal of Paediatrics*, 77: 181.

GL Assessment (2015) *Schedule of Growing Skills*. Available at: www.gl-assessment.co.uk/products/schedule-growing-skills (accessed 9 October 2017).

Hall, D.M.B. and Elliman, D. (2003) *Health for All Children*, 4th edn. Oxford: Oxford University Press.

HM Government (2015) *Working Together to Safeguard Children: A Guide to Inter-agency Working to Safeguard and Promote the Welfare of Children*. London: DfE. Available at: www.gov.uk/government/publications/working-together-to-safeguard-children--2 (last accessed 8 May 2017).

King, C. (2015) 'Health visitors' account of the impacts of "Hall 4" on their practice and profession: a qualitative study'. *Community Practitioner*, 88 (2): 24–7.

Marmot, M. (2010) *Fair Society, Healthy Lives: Strategic Review of Health Inequalities in England Post 2010*. London: Department for International Development. Available at: www.institute ofhealthequity.org/resources-reports/fair-society-healthy-lives-the-marmot-review (last accessed 18 May 2017).

NHS National Services Scotland (2015) *Child Health Programme: Child Health Systems Programme Pre-School (CHSP Pre-School)*. Available at: www.isdscotland.org/Health-Topics/Child-Health/Child-Health-Programme/Child-Health-Systems-Programme-Pre-School.asp (last accessed 18 May 2017).

NSPCC (2016) *Neglect: What Is Neglect?* Available at: www.nspcc.org.uk/preventing-abuse/child-abuse-and-neglect/neglect (last accessed 18 May 2017).

Nursing and Midwifery Council (NMC) (2004) *Standards of Proficiency for Specialist Community Public Health Nurses*. London: NMC.

Ofsted (2014) *Are You Ready? Good Practice in School Readiness*. Manchester: Ofsted.

Robinson, K. (2012) 'Managing knowledge in health visiting', in K.A. Luker, J. Orr and G. McHugh (eds) (2012) *Health Visiting: A Rediscovery*, 3rd edn. Chichester: Wiley-Blackwell.

Scottish Government (2016) *A Plan for Scotland: The Scottish Government's Programme for Scotland 2016-17: 3 Transforming Public Services – Nurturing our NHS, Working for a Healthier Scotland, and Making Scotland Safer*. Available at: www.gov.scot/Publications/2016/09/2860/6 (last accessed 29 June 2017).

Sharma, A. and Cockerill, H. (2014) *Mary Sheridan's From Birth to Five Years: Children's Developmental Progress*, 4th edn. London: Routledge.

UNICEF (2012) *School Readiness: A Conceptual Framework*. New York: UNICEF.

United Nations (1989) *United Nations Convention on the Rights of the Child* (UNCRC). Geneva: United Nations.

Welsh Government (2012) *A Vision for Health Visiting in Wales*. Cardiff: Welsh Government.

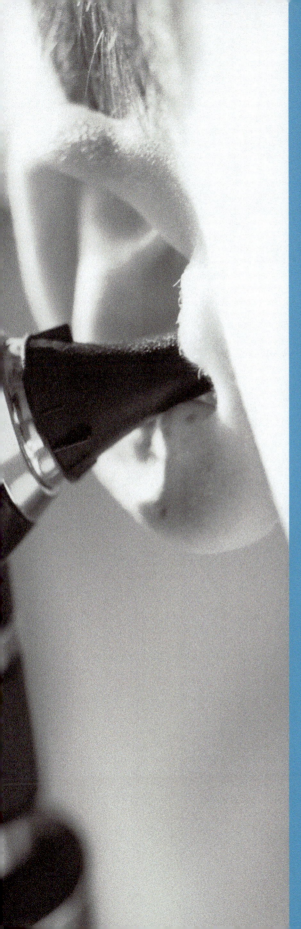

PART 3 CARING FOR CHILDREN AND YOUNG PEOPLE WITH ACUTE HEALTHCARE NEEDS AND INJURY

15 Assessment and care of children and young people with acute needs 225

16 Preparing children and young people for hospitalisation 247

17 Care of children and young people in the peri- and postoperative recovery period 257

18 Care of children and young people with respiratory problems 270

19 Care of children and young people with cardiovascular problems 285

20 Care of children and young people with neurological problems 301

21 Care of children and young people with urinary and renal problems 318

22 Care of children and young people with endocrine problems 330

23 Care of children and young people with immunological problems 350

24 Care of children and young people with musculoskeletal problems 361

25 Care of children and young people with haematological problems 386

26 Care of children and young people with dermatological problems 397

27 Care of children and young people with a thermal injury 409

28 Care of children and young people with fluid and electrolyte imbalance 426

29 Care of children and young people with gastrointestinal problems 438

30 Discharge planning and transfer for children and young people 456

ASSESSMENT AND CARE OF CHILDREN AND YOUNG PEOPLE WITH ACUTE NEEDS

RACHAEL BOLLAND

15

THIS CHAPTER COVERS

- Assessment and treatment of a child with a fever
- Assessment and care of a child with a gastrointestinal disturbance
- Assessment and care of a child having a seizure
- Assessment and care of a child with sepsis
- Unintentional injury in children

> " William Mead was born on the 27th November 2013. He died on the 14th December 2014. The coroner's inquest identified missed opportunities in relation to earlier diagnosis and escalation which could probably have prevented William's death.
>
> NHS England, 2016 "

INTRODUCTION

Children become ill. This is a predictable and normal occurrence. In most instances the child's illness will be self-limiting and resolve in a couple of days. However, there are a number of illnesses and injuries that can have devastating consequences for the child and their family. William Mead died of sepsis in December 2014 when he was only 12 months old. In this chapter we will look at some of the most common illnesses and injuries and how you can assess which children are acutely unwell and need urgent care and treatment.

It is important that all children who present with an acute care need are thoroughly assessed. Poor assessment contributes to avoidable deaths (Hogan, 2014). A child's physiological parameters often deviate from the normal in the hours before they collapse. Serious case reviews have highlighted that critical conditions are not always recognised by healthcare professionals and this leads to children being only partially treated or not treated at all (Roland, 2015).

**SEE ALSO
CHAPTER 6**

Assessment needs to take into account the age and developmental level of the child and any underlying health need. You need to observe the child, record vital signs but most important of all you need to listen to the child and their parent/carer. What are they worried about? What changes have they noted in their child? Parents often feel that their concerns are not heeded or they may lack the confidence to raise their fears (Roland, 2015). Parents and carers generally know and understand their child best.

Do not be lulled into a false sense of security. Just because a child is talking doesn't mean that they aren't sick.

> "
> In a younger child I would have been concerned about their observations if they were scoring red on the early warning scoring system. But she was a teenager and she was talking. I was really shocked when I heard she had died.
>
> **Aaravshah, Children's nurse**
> "

**WATCH A
VIDEO ONLINE!**

**VIDEO LINK
15.1:** IMPROVING
COMMUNICATION

ACTIVITY 15.1: CRITICAL THINKING

In the case of William Mead his parents contacted healthcare professionals on numerous occasions but the professionals did not hear and react appropriately to his parents' concerns (NHS England, 2016). NHS England has developed the ReACT tool to encourage a collaborative approach between healthcare professionals and parents/cares and to empower parents to speak up.

- Listen to the talks accessible via https://study.sagepub.com/essentialchildnursing on Improving Communication with Families on the ReACT - the Respond to Ailing Children tool (NHS England, 2015)

Reflect on how you communicate and engage with parents and carers. How good are you at listening to families? How could you improve your skills?

**ACTIVITY
ANSWER 15.1**

Various assessment frameworks have been developed to help you assess and recognise the child with an acute care need and guide you in their care management. We will look now at how you can apply these in practice.

ASSESSMENT AND TREATMENT OF A CHILD WITH A FEVER

As a children's nurse you will see many children who present with a fever. Feverish illness is one of the most common reasons for a child to be taken to see a healthcare professional and is the second most common reason for a child to be admitted to hospital (NICE, 2013). Fever can distress a child and cause anxiety in their parent/carer (Purssell, 2009, 2014) because although the cause is usually a viral infection that is self-limiting, it can also be a sign of more serious illness such as bacterial meningitis (see Table 15.1). NICE (2013) has developed guidance on the assessment and initial management of children younger than 5 years. You should follow this guidance until a clinical diagnosis of the underlying condition has been made.

Table 15.1 Summary of symptoms and signs suggestive of specific diseases (NICE, 2013)

Diagnosis to be considered	Symptoms and signs in conjunction with fever
Meningococcal disease	Non-blanching rash, particularly with one or more of the following:
	☐ an ill-looking child
	☐ lesions larger than 2 mm in diameter (purpura)
	☐ capillary refill time of ≥3 seconds
	☐ neck stiffness
Bacterial meningitis	Neck stiffness
	Bulging fontanelle
	Decreased level of consciousness
	Convulsive status epilepticus
Herpes simplex encephalitis	Focal neurological signs
	Focal seizures
	Decreased level of consciousness
Pneumonia	Tachypnoea (RR >60 breaths/minute, age 0–5 months; RR >50 breaths/minute, age 6–12 months; RR >40 breaths/minute, age >12 months)
	Crackles in the chest
	Nasal flaring
	Chest indrawing
	Cyanosis
	Oxygen saturation ≤ 95%
Urinary tract infection	Vomiting
	Poor feeding
	Lethargy
	Irritability
	Abdominal pain or tenderness
	Urinary frequency or dysuria
Septic arthritis	Swelling of a limb or joint
	Not using an extremity
	Non-weight bearing

VIDEO
LINK 15.2:
NEUROLOGICAL
OBSERVATIONS

(Continued)

Table 15.1 (Continued)

Diagnosis to be considered	Symptoms and signs in conjunction with fever
Kawasaki disease	Fever for more than five days and at least four of the following: ☐ bilateral conjunctival injection ☐ change in mucous membranes ☐ change in the extremities ☐ polymorphous rash ☐ cervical lymphadenopathy

RR= respiratory rate

NICE (2013) defines fever as 'an elevation of temperature above the normal daily variation'.

The normal daily variation or normal child range is 36.6–37.7°C.

Measuring fever in children

As part of your assessment it is important that you accurately measure body temperature using the most appropriate route and device (Table 15.2). Forehead chemical thermometers are unreliable and should not be used by healthcare professionals (NICE, 2013; Foley, 2015). Parental perception of fever must be taken seriously by healthcare professionals (NHS England, 2015).

Table 15.2 Sites and devices to be used when measuring body temperature in infants and children

Age	Site and device
< 4 weeks	Electronic thermometer in the axilla
	The oral and rectal route must not be routinely used
4 weeks to 5 years	Electronic thermometer in the axilla
	Chemical dot thermometer in the axilla
	Infra-red tympanic thermometer
	The oral and rectal route should not be routinely used
5 years upwards	Electronic thermometer in the axilla or mouth
	Chemical dot thermometer in the axilla or mouth
	Infra-red tympanic thermometer

Assessing children with feverish illness

It is important that you identify any immediately life-threatening features. Use the ABCDE approach.

A: Is the airway patent? Do you need to support the airway?

B: Is the child breathing? – Look, listen and feel

C: Check circulation. Measure pulse: rate, rhythm, strength

D: Check temperature, blood glucose (if possible), ascertain if they are on any regular medications, have a history of seizures or could have had access to any drugs/poisons

E: Whilst respecting the child's dignity carry out an examination to see if the child has any rashes, bruises or visible injuries

Once you have completed your ABCDE assessment look for the presence or absence of any signs and symptoms that could predict the risk of serious illness. NICE (2013) has developed a traffic-light system to help identify the risk factors. For children with a learning disability, you must take account of the child's learning disability when interpreting the traffic-light table.

WEBLINK:
TRAFFIC LIGHT
SYSTEM

FIND OUT
MORE!

Caring for the child according to risk of serious illness

Once you have assessed the child using the traffic-light system your actions should be guided by the level of risk of serious illness (Table 15.3).

Table 15.3 Management according to risk of serious illness (NICE, 2013)

Risk	Management
Life-threatening signs and symptoms	If outside the hospital setting, refer for immediate medical care by the most appropriate means of transport (usually 999 ambulance)
Red features but not considered immediately life threatening	Referred urgently to paediatrician
Amber features with no diagnosis	Can either be cared for at home by parents/carers or referred to a paediatrician for further assessment. If the child is cared for at home, the parents should be given a 'safety net'. This should include verbal and written information on warning symptoms and how further healthcare can be accessed. They should be advised: • To offer cool oral fluids regularly and continue breastfeeding if the child is breastfed • To encourage the child to drink more fluids • Not to underdress or overwrap the child • Not to use tepid sponging to cool the child
Green features only	Can be cared for at home with appropriate advice (see advice under amber features) including when to seek further help

Antipyretic interventions

Due to parental anxiety leading to 'fever phobia', parents/carers tend to treat fever in children aggressively and use over-the-counter medication inappropriately (Purssell, 2009, 2014; Purssell and While, 2013). When assessing the child's temperature, it is important to check with their parents/carers what medication they have given and when they last gave it. Antipyretic measures do not prevent febrile convulsions and so should not be used specifically for this purpose (NICE, 2013).

Physical interventions

It is important not to over-cool a child with fever as this can cause the child to shiver and raise the set point. *Tepid sponging is contra-indicated*. The environment should be kept cool by opening a window and *not* pointing a fan directly onto the child.

Pharmacological interventions

Ibuprofen and paracetamol should only be used if the feverish child is distressed. They should not be used simultaneously unless the child's distress continues or recurs before the next dose of the chosen medication is due.

ACTIVITY 15.2: CRITICAL THINKING

- Are there any potential benefits for a child having a fever?

Think about what effect a temperature has on a child's immune system and tissue repair. Does a temperature increase or decrease the rate of pathogen replication?

ACTIVITY
ANSWER 15.2

SCENARIO 15.1: ZAHRA

PRACTICE
SCENARIO 15:
JAY

Zahra is 3 years old. Her nursery contacted her mother earlier today as she was irritable and had a fever of 37.8°C per axilla. The nursery had given her a dose of paracetamol and were encouraging her to drink, although she was reluctant to do so.

Her parents collected her from nursery and took her to their local urgent care centre as they were anxious about the temperature as Zahra had previously had a febrile convulsion.

At the urgent care centre she was found to have a temperature of 38.2°C per axilla, heart rate of 142 beats/minute, respiratory rate of 28 breaths per minute and oxygen saturations of 96 per cent. Zahra appeared pale, was sleepy and not smiling at her parents, she was reluctant to drink and had not had a wet nappy since the morning. There is no obvious source of infection.

- Using the traffic-light system (NICE, 2013) for identifying risk of serious illness, describe what level of risk Zahra is displaying
- What actions would you take and why?
- Zahra is seen in the rapid assessment clinic at the local hospital and the decision is made to admit her. With reference to the NICE guidelines what further investigations would need to be performed?
- How often would you record Zahra's observations (vital signs in hospital)?
- What anti-pyretic interventions will Zahra require?

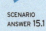

SCENARIO
ANSWER 15.1

ASSESSMENT AND CARE OF A CHILD WITH A GASTROINTESTINAL DISTURBANCE

SEE ALSO
CHAPTER 28

Diarrhoea and vomiting are common symptoms in children, especially in children under 5 years of age. Ten per cent of all children under the age of 5 will present to healthcare services each year with diarrhoea and vomiting (NICE, 2009). The child develops loose or watery stools and/or a sudden onset of vomiting usually as a result of gastroenteritis. The vomiting usually resolves after one to two days whilst the diarrhoea usually resolves after five to seven days. Whilst the majority of children can be cared for at home some children will need admission to hospital because of the risk of dehydration and shock.

Which children are most at risk of dehydration?

Infants under 6 months of age or with a low birth rate are especially at risk. The signs of dehydration may be less obvious in this age group, leading to a risk of rapid and severe deterioration (BNFc, 2015).

Children are also at risk of hypernatraemic dehydration – a life-threatening condition requiring immediate treatment (Powers, 2015). You should suspect hypernatraemia in any child who presents with jittery movements, increased muscle tone, hyperreflexia, convulsions or drowsiness.

To help you identify which children are most at risk of dehydration it is important that you assess the child fully to identify any specific risk factors such as:

- passing six or more stools in the previous 24 hours
- vomiting three or more times in the previous 24 hours
- not tolerating supplementary feeds
- infants who have stopped breastfeeding during this illness
- children showing signs of malnutrition (assess using a validated tool such as STAMP, PYMS, UK-WHO Growth Chart (RCPCH, 2016))

You can access the screening tools via https://study.sagepub.com/essentialchildnursing

To help you gain this information you need to ask the parent/carer the following questions:

WEBLINK: SCREENING TOOLS

- How long has your child had diarrhoea and vomiting?
- How frequent is their diarrhoea and/or vomiting?
- What does their stool look like – for example, colour, smell, consistency? Did it contain any blood, mucus, pus or undigested food?
- Does your child have any other symptoms such as abdominal pain, vomiting or bloating?
- Has your child had/got a fever? (Assess using NICE (2013) traffic-light table)
- Has your child had any recent infections?
- Has your child lost weight recently? (This could be an indication of gut dysfunction alongside failure to thrive and symptoms of anaemia)
- Has your child travelled abroad recently?
- Are any other family members or other contacts unwell at the moment?

SEE ALSO CHAPTER 30

NICE (2009) recommends that in children under 5 you use the table below (Table 15.4) to assess the severity of dehydration.

Table 15.4 Assessing dehydration in children under 5 years (NICE, 2009)

Increasing severity of dehydration

	No clinically detectable dehydration	Clinical dehydration	Clinical shock
Symptoms (remote and face-to-face assessments)	Appears well	**Red flag** Appears to be unwell or deteriorating	–
	Alert and responsive	**Red flag** Altered responsiveness (e.g. irritable, lethargic)	Decreased level of consciousness
	Normal urine output	Decreased urine output	–
	Skin colour unchanged	Skin colour unchanged	Pale or mottled skin
	Warm extremities	Warm extremities	Cold extremities
Signs (face-to-face assessments)	Alert and responsive	**Red flag** Altered responsiveness (for example, irritable, lethargic)	Decreased level of consciousness
	Skin colour unchanged	Skin colour unchanged	Pale or mottled skin

(Continued)

Table 15.4 (Continued)

Increasing severity of dehydration

	No clinically detectable dehydration	Clinical dehydration	Clinical shock
	Warm extremities	Warm extremities	Cold extremities
	Eyes not sunken	**Red flag** Sunken eyes	-
	Moist mucous membranes (except after a drink)	Dry mucous membranes (except for 'mouth breather')	-
	Normal heart rate	**Red flag** Tachycardia	Tachycardia
	Normal breathing pattern	**Red flag** Tachypnoea	Tachypnoea
	Normal peripheral pulses	Normal peripheral pulses	Weak peripheral pulses
	Normal capillary refill time	Normal capillary refill time	Prolonged capillary refill time
	Normal skin turgor	**Red flag** Reduced skin turgor	-
	Normal blood pressure	Normal blood pressure	Hypotension (decompensated shock)

When should you take a stool specimen from a child with diarrhoea and vomiting?

Financial constraints in the NHS have led us to question which investigations are necessary. You need to ask – how will the results of the investigation influence the child's care and treatment? For the majority of children, stool culture is unnecessary and will not influence the child's care and treatment. A stool specimen should only be obtained if the child meets one of the following criteria:

- There is a suspicion that the child may have septicaemia
- The child has blood and/or mucous in the stool
- The child is immuno-compromised
- The child has recently travelled abroad
- The child's diarrhoea has not improved by day 7
- There is uncertainty about the diagnosis of gastroenteritis

ACTIVITY 15.3: EVIDENCE-BASED PRACTICE

Do all children with diarrhoea and vomiting need intravenous fluids? You will remember that we said earlier that most children can be cared for at home. Most children who are not displaying signs of dehydration can be cared for at home – therefore the answer is no, not all children need intravenous fluids. Parents caring for their child at home will need advice on what food and fluids their child can have, infection control measures and when a child can go back to school/nursery.

- What advice regarding food and fluids would you give to a parent caring for their child at home?

ACTIVITY ANSWER 15.3

What fluids would you give to child who has diarrhoea and vomiting and is dehydrated?

These children also do not need intravenous therapy as first-line treatment unless they have any red flag symptoms (Table 15.4). They should be given a low osmolarity oral rehydration salt (ORS) solution. It should be given frequently and in small amounts (see BNFc, 2015 for formulations and dosage). The ORS can be supplemented with the child's normal fluids including milk feeds and water but not fruit juices or fizzy drinks (including those that have been allowed to go 'flat'). If the child is unable to drink the ORS or persistently vomits you will need to consider passing a naso-gastric tube through which to give the ORS.

You must maintain an accurate record of the child's input and output. It is important that you regularly reassess the child and look for signs of improvement or deterioration.

When should intravenous therapy be commenced?

You should commence intravenous fluids if the child has any red flag symptoms (Table 15.4), shows signs of clinical deterioration (despite ORS rehydration therapy) or shock (suspected or confirmed) or if the child persistently vomits the ORS solution via the oral or naso-gastric route.

It is vital that the most appropriate intravenous fluids are used (NPSA, 2007; NICE, 2015). An isotonic solution such as 0.9 per cent sodium chloride or 0.9 per cent sodium chloride with 5 per cent glucose should be prescribed both for fluid replacement and maintenance (see NICE, 2009 and BNFc, 2015 for dosing guidelines). To ensure that each child receives the most appropriate fluids you must monitor their blood plasma regularly and ensure that the medical team adjusts their fluids accordingly.

Once a child has been rehydrated they can start back on full-strength milk straight away and their usual solid food. It is a myth that they must have half-strength milk or a light diet only. The only fluids that they need to avoid until their diarrhoea stops are fruit juices and fizzy drinks (including carbonated drinks that have been allowed to go 'flat').

Any child whose diarrhoea lasts for longer than two weeks needs to be further investigated. There are a number of reasons that the child could have prolonged diarrhoea. Non-specific toddler diarrhoea is the commonest cause of loose stools in children. Parents and carers may report that the child has undigested vegetables in their stool. Non-specific toddler diarrhoea is thought to be due to the immaturity of the toddler's GI tract with rapid intestinal motility. The toddler appears well and thrives, showing no other signs of gut dysfunction.

Prolonged diarrhoea may be due to infections such as rota virus and adenovirus. It can also occur after a child has had a bout of gastroenteritis and is known as post-gastroenteritis syndrome. Prolonged diarrhoea may also indicate a more serious underlying condition leading to malabsorption such as coeliac disease, cystic fibrosis, cow's milk protein intolerance or irritable bowel disease (IBD).

ASSESSMENT AND CARE OF THE CHILD HAVING A SEIZURE

SEE ALSO
CHAPTER 20

Seizures may also be referred to as convulsions and fits. Most seizures are generalised, usually last two to three minutes and stop by themselves. Epilepsy is a term used when fits recur and is usually diagnosed by a neurologist.

The commonest cause of seizures in children is a high temperature. Febrile convulsions are most common in toddlers. Other causes include:

- Epilepsy
- CNS infection
- Aspiration/gastro-oesophageal reflux disease

- Metabolic – hypoglycaemia, hyperglycaemia, hyponatraemia, hypernatraemia or hypomagnesaemia
- Vitamin D deficiency (RCPCH, 2013a)
- Cerebral hypoxia
- Head trauma/non-accidental injury
- Toxins/poisoning

Immediate assessment and care in the community setting

Seizures can appear frightening to parents and bystanders so it is important that you remain calm. Call 999 to request an ambulance/assistance. Children should be assessed and managed using the ABCDE approach we discussed earlier in the chapter.

Assessment and care in the emergency department.

The more detailed ABCDE approach is suitable for the emergency department setting and should be used to assess the child and direct their management (see Table 15.5).

Table 15.5 Assessment and management of the fitting child/status epilepticus

AIRWAY
Apply oxygen via a non-rebreathe mask
Support airway
Consider naso-pharyngeal airway
Monitor oxygen saturations
BREATHING
Assess effort and efficacy of breathing
Support breathing as required
CIRCULATION
Secure IV/IO access
Monitor heart rate and blood pressure
Check venous blood gas, U&E, bone profile, magnesium, blood glucose, anticonvulsant levels (if appropriate)
DISABILITY
Correct hypoglycaemia 2mL/kg of 10% dextrose
Correct electrolyte abnormalities slowly
If seizure > than 5 minutes give:
Lorazepam IV/IO 0.1mg/kg Max dose 4mg **or**
Diazepam IV/IO 0.25mg/kg Max dose 10mg **or**
Rectal diazepam 0.5mg/kg Max dose 10mg **or**
Buccal midazolam 0.5mg/kg Max dose 10mg
If seizure lasts for a further ten minutes
give a second dose of benzodiazepine
Check if the child received a dose of benzodiazepine before coming to the hospital. Do not give more than two doses.
Start to prepare the phenytoin

Senior review

Reconfirm that it is an epileptic seizure

Phenytoin 20mg/kg IV or IO over 20 minutes. Max dose 2g.

Caution: risk of thrombophlebitis with peripheral infusion. Give via large vein.

Phenytoin can cause dysrhythmias and hypotension: monitor ECG and BP

If already on phenytoin give:

Phenobarbitone 20mg/kg (max dose 1g) IV or IO over five minutes

---

20 minutes from start of infusion:

Rapid sequence induction

Inform Paediatric Care Unit (PICU)

ASSESSMENT AND CARE OF A CHILD WITH SEPSIS

SCENARIO 15.2: TOBIAS (1)

Tobias is 7 years old. He is usually fit and healthy. However, for the last two days he has been feeling too unwell to go to school. He looks pale and is very lethargic, wanting to sleep all the time. Earlier today he had a temperature but when his mum felt him just now he felt very cold.

Initially his mum thought that he just had a virus and would be better in a couple of days. Now she is very concerned about him as she recently saw a poster about sepsis at the GP's and thinks he has some of the signs. She decides to take him straight to the emergency department at her local hospital. At the emergency department she tells the receptionist that she thinks he has sepsis and needs to be seen straight away.

Goldstein et al. (2005) define sepsis as systemic inflammatory response syndrome (SIRS). SIRS is a generalised response which presents with two or more of the following:

- An abnormal core temperature of < 36°C or > 38.5°C
- Abnormal heart rate for age – either tachycardia or bradycardia
- Raised respiratory rate for age
- Abnormal white cell count (WCC) in circulating blood – above or below normal range for age, >10% immature white cells

(Abnormal temperature or abnormal WCC must be one of the criteria)

Sepsis affects 10,000 children each year in the UK (UK Sepsis Trust, 2015; Plunkett and Tong, 2015). It can be hard to diagnose because the signs and symptoms can mimic other childhood illnesses. Not all children will present with a fever and children are able to compensate during the early stages.

Globally, 60 per cent of deaths in children under 5 are attributable to infection. It is therefore important to recognise sepsis early and treat aggressively to decrease the number of preventable deaths from sepsis.

As discussed earlier in the chapter, William Mead died of sepsis aged 12 months in December 2014. At the inquest into William's death the coroner identified missed opportunities for an earlier diagnosis and escalation that might have prevented his death (NHS England, 2016). To aid early recognition and treatment of sepsis, NICE published a guideline in July 2016 (NICE, 2016a), as shown in Table 15.6 below.

Table 15.6 Risk stratification tool for a 7-year-old with suspected sepsis (Adapted from NICE, 2016a)

	High risk criteria	Moderate to high risk criteria	Low risk criteria
Behaviour	Evidence of altered behaviour or mental state (assessing using AVPU or age-appropriate GCS) Appears ill to a healthcare professional Does not wake or if roused does not stay awake	Not behaving normally Decreased activity Parent or carer concern that the child is behaving differently from usual	Behaving normally
Respiratory	Raised respiratory rate: 27 breaths per minute or more	Raised respiratory rate: 24-26 breaths per minute	No high risk or moderate to high risk criteria met
Circulation and hydration	Raised heart rate: 120 beats per minute or more	Raised heart rate: 110-119 beats per minute	No high risk or moderate to high risk criteria met
Skin	Mottled or ashen appearance Cyanosis of skin, lips or tongue Non-blanching rash of skin		
Other		Leg pain Cold hands or feet	

SCENARIO 15.2: TOBIAS (2)

Tobias is seen by the triage nurse in the emergency department. He listens to Tobias's mother's concerns and assesses Tobias using the age-appropriate risk stratification tool for children with suspected sepsis guideline and algorithm (NICE, 2016a) (Table 15.6).

Tobias is found to have a core temperature of 38.6°C, a heart rate of 140 beats per minute, a respiratory rate of 18 per minute, oxygen saturations of 92 per cent in air, capillary refil>3 seconds and systolic blood pressure of 100/75. He is sleeping but responds to his mother's voice. However, he falls straight back to sleep. He appears pale.

Tobias is graded as having a high risk of sepsis. The nurse fast bleeps the paediatric registrar.

- You are the nurse who has assessed Tobias. Outline the conversation you would have with the registrar using the SBAR tool.

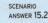
SCENARIO
ANSWER 15.2

SEE ALSO
CHAPTER 6

Screening for Red Flag Sepsis

The table below outlines the next steps to take in screening for Red Flag Sepsis, which in our scenario is performed by the registrar.

Table 15.7 Emergency department Red Flag Sepsis criteria for children aged 5-11 years

- Objective change in behaviour or mental state
- Doesn't wake if roused or won't stay awake
- Looks very ill to health professional
- SpO2 < 90% / new need for oxygen
- Severe tachypnoea
- Severe tachycardia
- Bradycardia (< 60 per minute)
- Not passed urine in last 18h
- Non-blanching rash/mottled/ashen/blue
- Temperature <36°C

Source: UK Sepsis Trust (2016)

SCENARIO 15.2: TOBIAS (3)

The registrar comes straight to the emergency department to review Tobias. She assesses Tobias using the emergency department Red Flag Sepsis Criteria for Children aged 5-11 years (Table 15.7).

Tobias has several red flags (review his observations against the criteria) and urgent intervention is required. The registrar informs her consultant and paediatric intensive care unit (PICU).

Management: Urgent intervention

In cases which need urgent intervention, the emergency department team will normally implement the Paediatric Sepsis 6 procedures (as in Table 15.8). All elements must be completed within one hour.

Table 15.8 Example of Paediatric Sepsis 6 chart: Complete all elements within one hour (UK Sepsis Trust, 2016)

	Date/Time Sign
1. Give high flow oxygen:	
2. Obtain IV / IO access & take blood tests:	

a. Blood cultures
   b. Blood glucose - treat low blood glucose
   c. Blood gas (+ FBC, lactate / CRP as able)	

3. Give IV or IO antibiotics:	
– Broad spectrum cover as per local policy	
4. Consider fluid resuscitation:	

– Aim to restore normal circulating volume and physiological parameters
   – Titrate 20 ml/kg Isotonic Fluid over 5 - 10 min and repeat if necessary
   – Caution with fluid overload: Examine for crepitations & hepatomegaly	

5. Involve senior clinicians / specialists early:	
6. Consider inotropic support early:	
– If normal physiological parameters are not restored after ≥ 40 ml/kg fluids – NB adrenaline or dopamine may be given via peripheral IV or IO access	

SCENARIO 15.2: TOBIAS (4)

After the emergency department team have implemented Paediatric Sepsis 6 procedures, Tobias is moved to the paediatric intensive care unit for further observation and treatment.

VIDEO LINK 15.3: SPOTTING SEPSIS

VIDEO LINK 15.4: TALKING ABOUT SEPSIS

You can find further information on sepsis at https://study.sagepub.com/essentialchildnursing There you will also be able to listen to Melissa Mead, William Mead's mother, talk about William and the failings in his care.

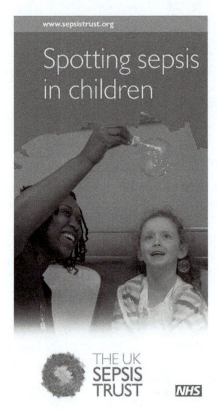

Figure 15.1 Poster from the UK Sepsis Trust who provide support and advice to healthcare professionals and families

UNINTENTIONAL INJURY IN CHILDREN

The term 'unintentional injury' is the term we now use to describe 'accidents' to recognise that these injuries are the result of events that can be prevented.

Unintentional injuries to children under the age of 15 account for 108,000 hospital admissions and around two million attendances at the emergency department each year (Child Accident Prevention Trust, 2013). NICE (2016b) calculates that this costs the NHS over £277 million each year. The Audit Commission (2007) and the Royal College of Paediatrics and Child Health (RCPCH, 2013b) found that unintentional injury is the most frequent cause of death in children. Between 1980 and 2010, 31 per cent of deaths in children aged 1–4 years were from unintentional injuries (RCPCH, 2013b).

Which children are most at risk of unintentional injury?

Risk is affected by a number of factors:

- Age
- Developmental level
- Underlying medical condition(s)

- Behaviour – for example, risk taking
- Environment – for example, poor quality housing

NICE (2010) reports that:

- Children under 5 years old are more vulnerable to unintentional injuries in the home
- Children over the age of 11 years are more vulnerable to unintentional injuries on the road

In this chapter we will focus on falls, fractures and head injury.

PROMOTING HEALTH

How can we prevent unintentional injury in children?
The following publications outline how we might prevent unintentional injury in children. The key messages are:

- Preventing unintentional injury is an important factor in improving public health outcomes. It is important that healthcare professionals and the NHS work with local government and the voluntary sector
- Parents need advice on maintaining safety in the home. Simple measures can significantly reduce risk. For example, stairgates can reduce the number of children falling downstairs when fitted securely at the top and bottom of stairs. The introduction of window restrictors saw a 96 per cent reduction in fall from windows admissions to emergency departments
- Information leaflets on prevention and safety in the home should be available in all healthcare settings. They need to be engaging and colourful to appeal to parents and carers. See the examples on child accidents at https://study.sagepub.com/essentialchildnursing

WEBLINK:
CAPT

  o Audit Commission (2007) *Better Safe than Sorry*
  o Child Accident Prevention Trust (2017) *Keeping Children Safe From a Serious Fall*
  o NHS Choices (2016) *Baby and Toddler Safety*
  o NICE (2016b) *Preventing Unintentional Injury in Under 15s*
  o Public Health England (2014) *Reducing Unintentional Injuries in and around the Home among Children under five Years*
  o WHO (2008) *Children and Falls*

Assessment and care of a child or young person following a fall

Children under 5 are most at risk of being admitted to hospital for treatment of injuries following a fall (Public Health England, 2014). They fall over and get knocks and bruises while learning to walk, but serious injuries can be avoided. The World Health Organization (WHO) (2008) defines a fall as 'an event which results in a person coming to rest inadvertently on the ground or floor or other lower level'.

Most cuts and grazes are minor and can be treated at home. The parent/carer should be advised to clean the cut or graze thoroughly and cover with a plaster or dressing. However, parents/carers should be advised to dial 999 to request an ambulance if their child:

- Stops breathing or is struggling to breathe
- Is unconscious or seems unaware of what is happening around them
- Won't wake up
- Has a fit for the first time, even if they seem to recover

They should be advised to take their child to the emergency department if their child has:

- A leg or arm injury and can't use the limb
- A cut that may have something in it such as a piece of glass

SEE ALSO
CHAPTER 9

SAFEGUARDING STOP POINT

All children who present following a fall out of windows or from buildings should be assessed under your safeguarding children processes.

SEE ALSO
CHAPTER 24

Assessment and care of a child or young person with a fracture

A fracture is a partial or complete break in the bone. It can be an open (compound) fracture where the bone breaks through the skin. Or it can be a closed (simple) fracture where the bone is broken but the skin is still intact.

Although fractures are common in children (approximately 66 per cent of boys and 40 per cent of girls will sustain a fracture by the age of 15) we should still try to reduce the rate of unintentional injuries. In children over 5 years, 85 per cent of fractures are due to unintentional injuries.

SAFEGUARDING STOP POINT

WEBLINK:
NSPCC
BRUISES &
FRACTURES

Fractures can also be an indication of child abuse and indicate a serious assault on a child (NSPCC, 2012a).

When should you be concerned that a child may have been abused?

Look up your local safeguarding guidelines including those on the management of bruises or marks in non-ambulant babies/children, and the following leaflets by the NSPCC which are available via https://study.sagepub.com/essentialchildnursing

NSPCC (2012a) *Core-Info: Fractures in Children*

NSPCC (2012b) *Core-Info: Bruises on Children*

SEE ALSO
CHAPTER 9

If you see any of the following signs or symptoms you should suspect that the child may have a fracture:

- Pain or swelling in the injured area
- Obvious deformity in the injured area
- Difficulty using or moving the injured area in a normal manner
- Warmth, bruising or redness in the injured area

First aid

Parents/carers should be advised to seek medical care immediately. If the child has an open fracture or a neck or spinal injury they should not be moved because unnecessary movement can cause paralysis. For other fractures, if a parent/carer can't easily move the child without causing them pain, they should be advised to call an ambulance. If it is possible for them to move their child, they should do so gently, putting one hand above the injury and the other below it to stabilise the fracture. Blankets or clothing can be used to support it. They should also be advised to give their child some pain killers, following the instructions on the label, comfort the child and take them to the emergency department.

How are fractures in children treated?

On arrival at the emergency department the nurse practitioner or doctor will examine the injured area(s) for tenderness, redness and swelling, and order diagnostic imaging tests.

WEBLINK: CARING FOR PLASTERCASTS

Specific treatment for a fracture depends on the type of fracture, its severity and the child's age. In the majority of cases they can be treated with a splint or cast. These immobilise the injured bone, promoting healing and reducing pain and swelling (see NHS Choices (2015) How should I care for my plaster cast?).

Some children will require surgery and the insertion of metal rods or pins. Neurovascular observations should be performed examining colour, warmth, sensation and movement of the affected limb.

SEE ALSO CHAPTERS 16 AND 17

The child's pain should be assessed and appropriate analgesia administered. Some doctors have expressed concerns about the use of NSAIDs (non-steroidal anti-inflammatories) as they believe that they may inhibit new bone growth following surgery. There are no studies to support this view (APA, 2012). If it is a fracture to a lower limb then the nursing team should liaise with the orthopaedic surgeon to ascertain whether the child can weight bear and along with the physiotherapists support the child to learn to use crutches and be able to walk up and down stairs.

SEE ALSO CHAPTER 3

The assessment and early management of a child with a head injury

A head injury is any trauma to the head other than superficial injuries to the face (NICE, 2014). Head injury is the commonest cause of death and disability of people aged 1–40 years in the UK. The majority of people attending the emergency department will have minor or mild head injuries but we need to ensure that all patients are assessed to identify those who will develop serious acute intracranial complications (Mulryan, 2015).

SEE ALSO CHAPTER 20

—————————— SAFEGUARDING STOP POINT ——————————

WEBLINK:
NSPCC HEAD
INJUIRY

It is estimated that 25–30 per cent of children under the age of 2 who are admitted to hospital will have an abusive head injury (NICE, 2014). Those who survive the injury may have significant long-term disabilities such as cerebral palsy, visual impairment, epilepsy, learning and behavioural problems (NSPCC, 2014).

A clinician who has been trained in safeguarding children should be involved in the assessment of any child presenting in the emergency department with a head injury. It is important to examine them for other injuries such as retinal haemorrhages, bruises, burns, bites, oral injuries or fractures. Any concerns should be identified and documented and local safeguarding procedures followed (NICE, 2014).

SEE ALSO
CHAPTER 9

Assessment and treatment of head injuries

The NICE guidelines *Head Injury: Assessment and Early Management* (2014) should be followed. These cover:

- Pre-hospital assessment, advice and referral to hospital
- Immediate management at the scene and transport to hospital
- Assessment in the emergency department
- Investigating clinically important brain injuries
- Investigating injuries to the cervical spine
- Information and support for families and carers
- Transfer from hospital to a neuroscience unit
- Admission and observation
- Discharge and follow-up

———————————— WHAT'S THE EVIDENCE? ————————————

NICE first produced a head injury guideline in 2003. It was updated in 2007 and most recently in 2014. Each update is based on up-to-date evidence and key NHS changes such as the introduction of regional trauma networks with major trauma triage tools within NHS England. The guidelines have resulted in CT scanning replacing skull radiography and have led to an increase in the proportion of people being cared for in specialist centres. This has been associated with a decline in fatality among patients with a severe head injury.

- Read the NICE guidelines and think about what you have seen in practice. Does the Trust follow these guidelines? How are policies developed in the Trust to ensure they are based on the best available evidence?

CHAPTER SUMMARY

- When assessing children with acute needs it is crucial to remember to select an appropriate assessment tool and to adopt an ABCDE approach
- It is essential that as a children's nurse you should listen to and involve parents in the assessment of children
- You should use a child-centred approach when assessing and managing a child with acute health needs
- Particular vigilance is required to ensure signs of sepsis are spotted early and acted upon immediately

BUILD YOUR BIBLIOGRAPHY

Books

- Carter, B., Bray, L., Dickinson, A., Edwards, M. and Ford, K. (2014) *Child-centred Nursing: Promoting Critical Thinking.* London: Sage.

  Read Chapter 6 on 'Understanding children's and young people's experience of illness'. This will help you to gain further insight into the impact that illness and hospitalisation has on a child.

- Standing, M. (2017) *Clinical Judgement and Decision Making in Nursing.* London: Learning Matters.

  Read Chapters 3 and 4 on 'Using observations to inform decisions' and Systematic clinical decision-making'. These reinforce key messages from this chapter.

Journal articles

Go to https://study.sagepub.com/essentialchildnursing for further free online journal articles related to this chapter.

FURTHER READING: ONLINE JOURNAL ARTICLES

- Richard, M. and Purssell, E. (2015) 'Who's afraid of fever?' *Archives of Disease in Childhood*, 100 (9): 818-20.

  Read this article to see how research and evidence-based practice are incorporated into national fever guidelines.

- Power, K. (2015) 'Dehydration: isonatremic, hyponatremic and hypernatremic recognition and management'. *Pediatrics in Review*, 36 (7): 274-85.

  The article links with the section of the chapter entitled 'How do we assess and care for a child with a gastrointestinal disturbance?' and looks at the different types of dehydration a child is susceptible to.

Websites

FURTHER
READING:
WEBLINKS

Go to https://study.sagepub.com/essentialchildnursing for further weblinks related to this chapter.

- BMJ Learning, *Sepsis in Children*

  http://learning.bmj.com/learning/module-intro/.html?moduleId=10053348&searchTerm="sepsis"&page=1&locale=en_GB

  Access this module on Sepsis in Children developed by Plunkett and Tong (2015). It covers the epidemiology of sepsis in children, causes and ways in which it can be prevented, and how to recognise the clinical signs of sepsis.

- The Triangulation of Thought, *Learning from a Child's Death: Turning the Rhetoric into Reality*

  http://thetriangulationofthought.blogspot.co.uk

  This is a blog written by Zoe Picton-Howell. Her son Adam was blind and had cerebral palsy but loved to tweet and write poetry. Sadly he died of sepsis in 2015, aged 15. Read the entries where his mother details the challenges she and Adam faced in being heard when Adam was unwell.

- Spotting the Sick Child

  www.spottingthesickchild.com/registration

  Register for an account on the Spotting the Sick Child website. This is an interactive tool commissioned by the Department of Health and Health Education England to support healthcare professionals in the assessment of acutely unwell children.

ONLINE
QUIZZES &
ACTIVITY
ANSWERS

ACE YOUR ASSESSMENT

Revise what you have learned by visiting https://study.sagepub.com/essentialchildnursing

- Test yourself with multiple-choice and short-answer questions
- Do the chapter activities in the book and check your answers online

REFERENCES

Association of Paediatric Anaesthetists of Great Britain and Ireland (APA) (2012) 'Good practice in postoperative and procedural pain management 2nd edition'. *Paediatric Anaesthesia*, 22, Supplement 1, 1–79.

Audit Commission (2007) *Better Safe than Sorry: Preventing Unintentional Injury to Children.* Available at: www.bipsolutions.com/docstore/pdf/15817.pdf (last accessed 18 May 2017).

BNFc (2015) *BNF for Children 2015–2016.* London: Pharmaceutical Press and RCPCH Publications Ltd.

Child Accident Prevention Trust (2013) *Tackling Inequalities in Childhood Accidents.* Available at: www.makingthelink.net/sites/default/files/resources/PHE-external-tackling-inequalities-factsheet.pdf (last accessed 18 May 2017).

Child Accident Prevention Trust (2017) *Safety Advice: Falls.* London: Child Accident Precvention Trust. Available at: www.capt.org.uk/falls (last accessed 28 June 2017).

Foley, V. (2015) 'Clinical measurement', in C. Delves-Yates (ed.), *Essentials of Nursing Practice*. London: Sage.

Goldstein, B., Girior, B. and Randolph, A. (2005) 'International pediatric sepsis consensus conference: definitions for sepsis and organ dysfunction in pediatrics'. *Pediatric Critical Care Medicine*, 6 (1): 2–8.

Hogan, H. (2014) The Scale and Scope of Preventable Hospital Deaths. PhD dissertation, London School of Hygiene and Tropical Medicine. Available at: http://researchonline.lshtm. ac.uk/1776586/1/2014_PHP_PhD_Hogan_H.pdf (last accessed 18 May 2017).

Mulryan, C. (2015) 'First Aid', in C. Delves-Yeates (ed.) *Essentials of Nursing Practice*. London: Sage.

NHS Choices (2015) *How Should I Care for my Plaster Cast?* Available at: www.nhs.uk/chq/Pages/2543. aspx?CategoryID=72&SubCategoryID=721 (last accessed 18 May 2017).

NHS Choices (2016) *Baby and Toddler Safety*. Available at: www.nhs.uk/Conditions/pregnancy-and-baby/pages/baby-safety-tips.aspx (last accessed 28 June 2017)

NHS England (2016) Root Cause Analysis Investigation Report 2014/41975. Available at: www. england.nhs.uk/south/wp-content/uploads/sites/6/2015/03/root-cause-analysis-wm-report.pdf (last accessed 18 May 2017).

NICE (2009) *Diarrhoea and Vomiting in children. Diarrhoea and Vomiting Caused by Gastroenteritis: diagnosis, assessment and management in children younger than 5 years*. Available at: www.nice.org. uk/guidance/CG84 (last accessed 28 June 2017).

NICE (2010) Public Health Guidance 29, 30, 31: *Strategies to Prevent Unintentional Injuries among Children and Young People Aged under 15*. London. NICE.

NICE (2013) *Fever in under 5s. Assessment and inititial management*. Available at: www.nice.org.uk/ guidance/cg160/chapter/1-recommendations (last accessed 28 June 2017)

NICE (2014) *Head Injury: Assessment and Early Management*. Available at: www.nice.org.uk/guidance/ cg176/resources/head-injury-assessment-and-early-management-35109755592901 (last accessed 18 May 2017).

NICE (2015) *Intravenous Fluid Therapy in Children and Young People in Hospital*. Available at: www. nice.org.uk/guidance/ng29/resources/intravenous-fluid-therapy-in-children-and-young-people-in-hospital-1837340295109 (last accessed 18 May 2017).

NICE (2016a) *Sepsis: Recognition, Diagnosis and Early Management*. Available at: www.nice.org.uk/ guidance/ng51/resources/sepsis-recognition-diagnosis-and-early-management-1837508256709 (last accessed 18 May 2017).

NICE (2016b) *Preventing Unintentional Injuries in under 15s*. NICE quality standard (QS107). Available at: www.nice.org.uk/guidance/qs107/resources/preventing-unintentional-injury-in-under-15s-75545242682821 (last accessed 18 May 2017).

NPSA (2007) *Reducing the Risk of Hyponatraemia when Administering Intravenous Infusions to Children*. Available at: www.nrls.npsa.nhs.uk/alerts/?entryid45=59809&p=3 (last accessed 18 May 2017).

NSPCC (2012a) *Core-Info: Fractures in Children*. Available at: www.nspcc.org.uk/globalassets/ documents/advice-and-info/core-info-fractures-children.pdf (last accessed 18 May 2017).

NSPCC (2012b) *Core-Info: Bruises on Children*. Available at: www.nspcc.org.uk/globalassets/ documents/advice-and-info/core-info-bruises-children.pdf (last accesed 18 May 2017).

NSPCC (2014) *Core-Info: Head and Spinal Injuries in Children*. Available at: www.nspcc.org.uk/services-and-resources/research-and-resources/2014/head-spinal-injuries-core-info (last accessed 18 May 2017.

Plunkett, A. and Tong, J. (2015) 'Sepsis in children'. *BMJ*, 351: h3704.

Powers, K. (2015) 'Dehydration: isonatremic, hyponatremic and hypernatremic recognition and management'. *Pediatrics in Review*, 36 (7): 274–85.

Public Health England (2014) *Reducing Unintentional Injuries in and around the Home among Children under Five Years*. Available at: www.gov.uk/government/uploads/system/uploads/attachment_data/ file/322210/Reducing_unintentional_injuries_in_and_around_the_home_among_children_under_ five_years.pdf (last accessed 18 May 2017).

Purssell, E. (2009) 'Parental fever phobia and its evolutionary correlates'. *Journal of Clinical Nursing*, 18: 210–18.

Purssell, E. (2014) 'Fever in children – a concept analysis'. *Journal of Clinical Nursing*, 23: 3575–82.

Purssell, E. and While, A. (2013) 'Does the use of anti-pyretics in children who have acute infections prolong febrile illness? A systematic review and meta-analysis'. *The Journal of Paediatrics*, 163: 822–7.

RCPCH (2013a) *Guide for Vitamin D in Childhood*. Available at: www.rcpch.ac.uk/system/files/protected/page/vitdguidancedraftspreads%20FINAL%20for%20website.pdf (last accessed 28 June 2017).

RCPCH (2013b) *Overview of Child Deaths in the Four UK Countries*. Available at: www.hqip.org.uk/resources/overview-of-child-deaths-in-the-four-uk-countries (last accessed 18 May 2017).

RCPCH (2016) *UK-WHO Growth Charts, 0–18 years*. Available at: www.rcpch.ac.uk/growthcharts (last accessed 28 June 2017).

Roland, D. (2015) *Re-ACT – the Respond to Ailing Children Tool*. NHS England. Available at: www.england.nhs.uk/patientsafety/re-act/ (last accessed 11 October 2017).

UK Sepsis Trust (2015) *Clinical Toolkit 6: Emergency Department Management of Paediatric Sepsis*. Available at: http://sepsistrust.org/wp-content/uploads/2015/08/sepsis-toolkit-FINAL-09151.pdf (last accessed 18 May 2017).

UK Sepsis Trust (2016) *ED/AMU Paediatric Sepsis Screening & Action Tool*. Available at: http://sepsistrust.org/wp-content/uploads/2016/07/ED-5-11-NICE-Final-1107–1.pdf (last accessed 18 May 2017).

WHO (2008) *Children and Falls*. Available at: www.who.int/violence_injury_prevention/child/injury/world_report/Falls_english.pdf (last accessed 18 May 2017).

PREPARING CHILDREN AND YOUNG PEOPLE FOR HOSPITALISATION

16

LORNA ASHBROOKE AND JIM RICHARDSON

THIS CHAPTER COVERS

- The needs of children and young people (up to age 18) coming to hospital
- Evidence of how children experience healthcare environments
- Strategies to keep children safe and comfortable during the hospitalisation period

> " It may seem a strange principle to enunciate as the very first requirement in a hospital that it should do the sick no harm.
>
> **Florence Nightingale** "

Visit https://study.sagepub.com/essentialchildnursing to access a wealth of online resources for this chapter – watch out for the margin icons throughout the chapter.

INTRODUCTION

Being admitted to hospital, even as a day case patient, is an experience that many children will experience and which many will experience as challenging and difficult. The opening quotation makes clear the importance from a historical perspective of safety within the hospital environment. This is still relevant today. Thus, in this chapter we will reflect on what factors make hospital a potentially less than pleasant encounter and what steps we can take to make the whole experience better for children. In order to do this, we will use the United Nations Convention on the Rights of the Child (United Nations, 1989) as a values framework. This gives us a clear guide of what children are entitled to expect and what, if these rights are satisfied, will make healthcare visits a less scary experience (Richardson, 2011).

THE NEEDS OF CHILDREN AND YOUNG PEOPLE (UP TO AGE 18) COMING TO HOSPITAL

This section will look at the needs of children coming to hospital by understanding the legislation around it and relating it to examples in practice through a conversation between a 12-year-old and a nursing student.

The United Nations Convention on the Rights of the Child

The United Nations Convention on the Rights of the Child was launched in 1989 and ratified by the United Kingdom in 1991. The Convention is a statement of the rights that any child, that is a person under the age of 18, can expect to ensure their wellbeing. These rights can be conveniently classified into three areas:

SEE ALSO
CHAPTER 8

- Protection – these are the rights that protect the child from harm
- Promotion – under this banner are a set of rights aimed at improving children's situation
- Participation – this category of rights aims at ensuring that the child is involved in decisions which will have an impact on his/her life and that her/his voice is heard

---

ACTIVITY 16.1: CRITICAL THINKING

Access a copy of the UN Convention on the Rights of the Child (UN, 1989). You can do this easily via the UNICEF website. Looking at the document, try to decide to which of the three categories the following articles belong:

- Article 9
- Article 28
- Article 12

Once you have done this, make some notes on how each of these articles might have an impact on your everyday work. It would really help with your understanding of the Convention if you could continue this activity by working through the other articles and thinking about how you could ensure they should guide the work of the children's nurse.

WEBLINK:
RIGHTS OF
THE CHILD

Now consider the following conversation between Chloe, a 12-year-old who was admitted as an emergency having fractured her humerus in an accident, and Jac, a nursing student. Chloe underwent surgery and is struggling to make sense of what has happened to her. Jac is orientating to a new ward placement and is keen to learn from Chloe's perspective what it is like to be in hospital as a patient.

SCENARIO 16.1: JAC AND CHLOE

Jac: Good morning, Chloe, how are you feeling now?

Chloe: Oh, hi, Jac. Yeah, I'm OK, my arm's still a bit sore but I feel more awake now and I enjoyed my breakfast.

Jac: You were quite disturbed yesterday evening by everything that was happening to you. How do you feel now?

Chloe: A bit more steady now but it was all a bit of a shocker really. I just didn't see the cyclist at all when she came up behind me – I just stepped into her path. Are cyclists supposed to ride on the pavement? Then everything happened so fast – the ambulance, the paramedics, the X-rays, the splint, the pain. Lots of it all seems like a bit of a blur now – and things were happening that I didn't really understand – then or now.

Jac: I'm interested in hearing about your experience of being cared for. When you feel up to it, would you like to tell me about your impressions at each stage of this experience? Perhaps talking it through will help you to make sense of it. In addition, it helps me in becoming a children's nurse to understand the whole healthcare experience from the point of view of the young person. Would you like to do that?

Chloe: I think that's a great idea.

- When Jac listens to Chloe's account of her perceptions of what has happened to her since she has had her accident, it seems clear that she just does not have all the information she needs to be able to understand and make sense of what has happened and what might happen during the next few days. Which articles of the Convention could you use to help rectify this situation if they were applied?

EVIDENCE OF HOW CHILDREN EXPERIENCE HEALTHCARE ENVIRONMENTS

The particular challenges posed by healthcare as well as the anxieties they can cause will be identified further.

Understanding the impact on the child and family of hospital admission

WHAT'S THE EVIDENCE?

James Robertson produced films about how being admitted to hospital in the 1950s helped to revolutionise the way we care for children in hospital (Lindsay, 2003). It is worth bearing in mind that right into the 1970s it was common practice to restrict parents' or carers' visits to a child in hospital and there were no facilities for them to stay overnight with the child. At the extreme, the child was dropped off at hospital and there was no contact with the parent until the child was picked up to go home. Although this might seem like ancient history, it is worth looking at some of the footage in this film. It will give you a clear sense of the factors in the hospital environment which are most disturbing, challenging and potentially damaging for children. Once we have identified these we can then formulate a plan of action to help to prevent these factors exerting a negative impact.

(Continued)

VIDEO
LINK 16.1:
2-YEAR-
OLD IN
HOSPITAL

(Continued)

- Look for articles in journals which provide further evidence for the perspective presented by James Robertson. You could start by looking at the work of Philip Darbyshire and Imelda Coyne.

Access the clip of James Robertson's *A Two Year Old Goes to Hospital*. It is available on YouTube. While you are watching this short film make notes about the factors which the little girl seems to find most upsetting. Take care as you might find this film a bit upsetting yourself.

Separation anxiety

One factor which may be involved in the reactions that the little girl in the video clip displays might be separation anxiety. Separation anxiety can be described as the discomfort experienced by a child when separated from a caregiver, such as their mother, to whom they are strongly attached. The toddler from 18 months to 3 years is most at risk from this form of anxiety. To an extent, this is simply a normal reaction to an undesirable situation. However, if the separation is prolonged, the anxiety may become abnormally severe (McCann and Kain, 2001). This anxiety has been noted to cause a series of reactions. In the first the child *protests* by becoming angry and uncooperative with strangers such as nurses who try to offer care and comfort. This stage is characterised by loud crying and protest. This phase may be followed by one of *despair* if the child's anxiety is not relieved by being reunited with their primary attachment figure. At this stage, the child is disinterested, passive and withdrawn and, significantly, quiet. Typically, they look as if they have lost hope. At this point the child may return to the protest phase when the mother returns in that they become angry and cry noisily. If separation anxiety is allowed to continue the child passes to a state of *denial* when they appear to have got over their anxiety; they are happy to receive attention from any stranger who approaches them. Since the child appears happy and relaxed it is easy to assume that they have got over the anxiety and there is no longer a problem. Sadly, this is not the case since the child in this state is sustaining significant psychological damage from which recovery can be prolonged and difficult. Indeed, there is some suggestion that unrelieved separation anxiety in early childhood can lead to continuing psychological problems in adulthood (Lewinsohn et al., 2008).

It is easy to see how healthcare professionals at that time could have concluded that the child in the denial phase was quiet and contented. Equally, when the child reverted to protest and cried when the mother or other carer came to visit, it must have seemed that the parent visiting was disrupting and upsetting the child. These false beliefs were, for a long time, the justification for restricting parental visiting times.

ACTIVITY 16.2: CRITICAL THINKING

Return to James Robertson's video clip. In the light of the information above about separation anxiety, at what stage of anxiety would you say the little girl is? Take a moment to reflect on the factors which led you to this conclusion.

Shock of the unfamiliar

Even for a young person or adult the environment of healthcare settings can be unsettling and disorientating (Livesley and Long, 2013). It is unfamiliar and vaguely threatening. If the hospital visit relates to a need for a surgical operation this can be compounded as, without preparation, it involves confronting an experience about which most of us know little. This raises the sensation of threat and risk. Overall, in the midst of unfamiliar surroundings and events, the child struggles to make sense of what is happening and what it all means. The hospital staff also have a special language or jargon which is very difficult for patients and their family to understand (Lambert et al., 2012). It is difficult to come to terms with what is happening if they are unable to interpret what it all means for them and how to cope with it. It is important that the children's nurse appreciates this and uses strategies to reduce the negative consequences of such an experience. These will be explored later in the chapter.

Dislocation

A hospital admission has the potential to be very disruptive, and the sense of disruption is all the greater the younger the child is as the young child is very sensitive to disturbances in their daily routine. It may feel like the social fabric of their life is thrown into confusion with the potential loss of contact with siblings, friends, pets, etc. In addition, most children have a range of little daily routines such as having a story read to them after an evening bath and before settling down to sleep. It can really unsettle the child if this routine does not happen and it is, again, a challenge for the children's nurse to try to reduce the impact of this. This is an area where the use of the philosophy of child-centred care within a family context can be very useful indeed (Li et al., 2007). If parents/carers are encouraged and supported to care for their child as far as possible in line with the child's familiar routine then the disturbance experienced by the child might be reduced to a minimum. In achieving this goal, close partnership between the family and the children's nurse is vitally important.

Frightening

The sights and sounds of healthcare settings can be very frightening (Wilson et al., 2010) as there may be people suffering and expressing distress and other strong emotions. The bustle and busyness of the staff can convey a sense of urgency and heightened threat. It can be very disturbing if healthcare professionals tend to 'take over' and the parents' and carers' input is reduced (RCN, 2013). This is compounded if the child senses that their parent is upset by what is happening which is, of course, likely to be so in an emergency situation such as sudden illness or an accident. Another factor which may be of importance for the older child or young adult is the perception of loss of control and powerlessness. This can be the unintentional consequence if nurses do things *for* rather than *with* the child. It can be heightened if the child feels that they are not being informed about what needs to happen and why and they have no sense of having a say in what happens or a measure of control.

ACTIVITY 16.3: CRITICAL THINKING

- Read the relevant chapter in another children's nursing textbook and make notes on the extent to which the two sources agree on the principal points in relation to this issue. It would be helpful to access the evidence presented in the other chapter and think about the quality of the evidence presented in these sources. Make notes for yourself on why you believe that this is good quality evidence.
- Which articles of the United Nations Convention on the Rights of the Child are relevant in this situation and which might ensure a better outcome from the child's point of view if they are observed? (Think in particular about the articles concerned with participation.)

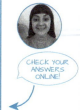

CHECK YOUR
ANSWERS
ONLINE!

ACTIVITY
ANSWER 16.3

STRATEGIES TO KEEP CHILDREN SAFE AND COMFORTABLE DURING THE HOSPITALISATION PERIOD

Children can be very sensitive to the threat of unwanted attention from strangers. Healthcare professionals may intend to be kind, comforting and helpful but in the child's eyes they are simply a stranger. This is especially relevant since children today are taught early on about 'stranger danger'. It is important that the nurse should take this into account when they first meet the child and tailor their approach in accordance with the child's reactions.

Context and timing

Ideally, many of the negative consequences and reactions to an admission to hospital can be reduced or avoided through preparation which involves giving information and answering questions. This is most easily achieved when the child's admission is planned (Gordon et al., 2010), but even when the child is admitted on an emergency basis this can be achieved. Information giving is most successful when it is relevant to the child's concerns, so a dialogue which explores what the child feels and might be worried about is vital for successful and effective information giving (Coyne and Kirwan, 2012). Play is a marvellous vehicle for giving information to children (Li et al., 2014) since play is fun and part of every child's daily life. Every children's ward will have a collection of soft toys sporting a range of dressings and plaster casts (Ullan et al., 2014)! Even complex procedures such as organ transplantation can be demonstrated using anatomically correct dolls. Many play specialists have developed this form of information giving (Perry et al., 2012).

PRACTICE
SCENARIO 16:
PETER

SCENARIO 16.2: MAREK

Marek is a 7-year-old boy who was admitted overnight with prolonged vomiting and dehydration. He was being treated with intravenous fluids. He and his mother were both visibly upset; on gentle probing, it emerged that placing the intravenous cannula in a vein in his left arm had been very difficult and painful, and entailed several attempts before a more senior clinician had been called to complete the procedure. The little boy was holding his arm rigid and slightly off the surface of the bed. His mother was upset and angry with the way the situation had been handled and expressed the wish to make a formal complaint. On exploring the situation a little further it seemed that both boy and mother were concerned about his having a needle in his arm. It was clear that they both needed further information. A nurse demonstrated to them using another cannula that the device contained a needle only for the period of its being placed and what now remained in the child's arm was just a soft plastic tube which was flexible and would allow him to move his arm with no risk of further discomfort. Both mother and child were enormously relieved by this explanation and demonstration and were able to relax.

- What were the principal care needs of this little boy and his mother?
- In what way could communication strategies be used to improve this situation?
- What are the clear consequences of not getting the necessary information for child and parent?

This example demonstrates that simply trying to see a situation from the perspective of the child and family helps us to address the issues that really matter to the child.

Whole-family education

In terms of providing information to reduce anxiety, it is important to take a whole- family approach (Shields et al., 2008; Chorney and Kain, 2010). This is in line with a philosophy of child-centred care within a family context (Smith and Coleman, 2010). If the parent or carer has a full and detailed understanding of what is happening and what is likely to happen, they are able to prepare their child for what is happening and what to expect (He et al., 2015). This is very empowering and helps the parent to achieve a sense that they are able to make an important contribution to their child's feeling comfortable and secure (Healy, 2013). Whole-family education is a process rather than a one-off event as it must respond to a dynamic and evolving situation.

In the activity below some of the principles offered in this chapter can be explored and applied. In light of the factors discussed in this chapter, you can also consider the potential benefits of Chloe and Jac's chat exploring Chloe's experience.

ACTIVITY 16.4: REFLECTIVE PRACTICE

Consider the planned admission of a 7-year-old for an ENT procedure.

- How can this child's admission be made as comfortable and constructive as possible?

Now consider the emergency admission of a 12-year-old who has dislocated her patella trying to escape from bullies.

- What are the special considerations in this case to help ensure this child's safety and wellbeing?

Consider the return admission of an 18-year-old who has had inequality of leg length treated with an external fixator which now needs to be removed following successful treatment.

- What are the factors in making this admission as comfortable as possible in the light of this young person's age and previous experience?

ACTIVITY
ANSWER 16.4

SAFEGUARDING STOP POINT

Since safeguarding is a significant part of this activity, it would be useful to thoroughly review the actions which should be undertaken in accordance with your local child protection procedures. Focus particularly on what needs to be done to protect the 12-year-old girl from harm. Consider whether the bullies might require safeguarding protection.

PROMOTING HEALTH

Every healthcare encounter is an opportunity to improve the child and family's knowledge, skills and insights into their own health and how to maintain and improve this. Family education should there-fore be an important component of any hospital admission. Make notes for yourself on the ways that you could propose taking action to promote child and family health. You might find this easier if you refer back to the case studies, reviewing the principal points of the chapter.

ACTIVITY 16.5: CRITICAL THINKING

Once you have read the chapter through and made notes on the key points, address the following questions:

- What is it that children find disturbing about the experience of being cared for in hospital?
- Which factors might reduce the negative impacts on hospital admission for children?
- How will an awareness of children's rights help to improve the overall hospital experience for children?
- In what ways might effective family care make the hospital experience more productive for the child?
- Consider how you might make use of the points you have identified to help you prepare for your next acute hospital practice placement
- Make notes summarising your conclusions. These will be helpful in the future when you are preparing for NMC revalidation

CHAPTER SUMMARY

- Admission to hospital is sometimes necessary to ensure the child's health and wellbeing. However, this experience has the potential to be unnerving or even distressing for the child and family
- It is clear from practice experience and the literature that there are steps which the children's nurse can take to reduce the negative consequences of admission
- A commitment to upholding the rights of the child as expressed in the United Nations Convention on the Rights of the Child can help to ensure that the child's voice is heard and that the child is encouraged to be a full participant in her/his own care. This also helps to ensure that the child is always treated in a respectful manner
- Receiving appropriate information in a timely fashion can also defuse some of the anxieties the child and family might feel
- Parent and child should come away from the healthcare encounter with the feeling that their ability to cope with health issues has been strengthened

BUILD YOUR BIBLIOGRAPHY

Books

- Carter, B., Bray, L., Dickinson, A., Edwards, E. and Ford, K. (2014) *Child-Centred Nursing*. London: Sage.

  A thought-provoking book which at its core describes how children's experience of health care can be improved.

- Lambert, V., Long, T. and Kelleher, D. (2012) *Communication Skills for Children's Nurses*. London: Open University Press.

  A thorough exploration of the central skill set underpinning effective and satisfactory children's nursing care.

- Long, T. (2016) *Children's Nursing Case Book*. London: Open University Press.

  This scenario-based book covers the range and implications of encounters in healthcare settings.

Journal articles

Go to https://study.sagepub.com/essentialchildnursing for further free online journal articles related to this chapter.

FURTHER
READING:
ONLINE
JOURNAL
ARTICLES

- Lambert, V., Glacken, M. and McCarron, M. (2013) 'Meeting the information needs of children in hospital'. *Journal of Child Health Care*, 17 (4): 338–53.

  The article considers the opinions of 49 children aged from 6 to 16 regarding their information needs and the optimal timing for information giving.

- Lewis, P., Kerridge, I. and Jorden, C.F.C. (2009) 'Creating space: hospital bedside displays as facilitators of communication between children and nurses'. *Journal of Child Health Care*, 13 (2): 93–100.

  This article investigates a novel way of enhancing communication between children and nurses in hospital.

- Leonhardt, C., Margraf-Stiksrud, L.B., Szerenci, A. and Maier, R.F. (2014) 'Does the "Teddy Bear Hospital" enhance pre-school children's knowledge? A pilot study with a pre/post-case control design in Germany'. *Journal of Health Psychology*, 33 (1): 51–5.

  An investigation illustrating how a Teddy Bear Hospital engages the interest of children in kindergarten and facilitates effective information giving.

Weblinks

Go to https://study.sagepub.com/essentialchildnursing for further weblinks related to this chapter.

FURTHER
READING:
WEBLINKS

- What? Why? Children hospital, *Preparing for Hospital*

  www.whatwhychildreninhospital.org.uk
  A range of interesting video clips designed to help parents prepare their child for a hospital admission or visit.

- www.whatwhychildreninhospital.org.uk/video-prepare-for-hospital

  A general introduction to hospital admission to help parents give information to their children to prepare them for this experience.

- www.whatwhychildreninhospital.org.uk/video-prepare-for-cannula

  An information video for parents to give an understanding of what happens when an intravenous cannula is sited. This aims to relieve anxiety and help pass information to the children.

- www.whatwhychildreninhospital.org.uk/video-prepare-for-general-anaesthetic

  A video giving full information about a common hospital procedure which is anxiety-provoking for parents and children. The resource aims to reduce this anxiety.

ACE YOUR ASSESSMENT

Revise what you have learned by visiting https://study.sagepub.com/essentialchildnursing

ONLINE
QUIZZES &
ACTIVITY
ANSWERS

- Test yourself with multiple-choice and short-answer questions
- Do the chapter activities in the book and check your answers online

REFERENCES

Chorney, J.M. and Kain, M.D. (2010) 'Family-centred pediatric perioperative care'. *Anesthesiology*, 112 (3): 751–5.

Coyne, I. and Kirwan, L. (2012) 'Ascertaining children's wishes and feelings about hospital life'. *Journal of Child Health Care*, 16 (3): 293–304.

Gordon, B.K., Jaaniste, T., Bartlett, K., Perrin, M., Jackson, A., Sandstrom, A., Charleston, R. and Sheehan, S. (2010) 'Child and parental surveys about pre-hospitalisation information provision'. *Child: Care, Health and Development*, 37 (5): 727–33.

He, H-G., Zhu, L-X., Chan, W-C.S., Liam, J.L.W., Ko, S.S., Li, H.C.W., Wang, W. and Yobas, P. (2015) 'A mixed-method study of effects of a therapeutic play intervention for children on parental anxiety and parents' perceptions of the intervention'. *Journal of Advanced Nursing*, 71 (7): 1539–51.

Healy, K. (2013) 'A descriptive survey of the information needs of parents of children admitted for same day surgery'. *Journal of Pediatric Nursing*, 28: 179–85.

Lambert, V, Long, T. and Kelleher, D. (2012) *Communication Skills for Children's Nurses*. Maidenhead: Open University Press/McGraw-Hill Education.

Lewinsohn, P.M., Holm-Denoma, J.M., Small, J.W. and Seely, J.R. (2008) 'Separation anxiety disorder in childhood as a risk factor for future mental illness'. *Journal of the American Academy of Child and Adolescent Psychiatry*, 47 (5): 548–55.

Li, W.H.C., Lopez, V. and Tin, L.I.L. (2007) 'Psychoeducational preparation of children for surgery: the importance of parental involvement'. *Patient Education and Counseling*, 65: 34–41.

Li, W.H.C., Chan, S.S.C., Wong, E.M.L., Kwok, M.C. and Lee, I.T.L. (2014) 'Effect of therapeutic play on pre- and post-operative anxiety and emotional responses in Hong Kong Chinese children: a randomised controlled trial'. *Hong Kong Medical Journal*, 20 (6): 36–9.

Lindsay, B. (2003) 'A 2-year-old goes to hospital': a 50th anniversary reappraisal of the impact of James Robertson's film'. *Journal of Child Health Care*, 7 (1): 17–26.

Livesley, J. and Long, T. (2013) 'Children's experiences as hospital in-patients: voice, competence and work. Messages for nursing from a critical ethnographic study'. *International Journal of Nursing Studies*, 50: 1292–1303.

McCann, M.E. and Kain, Z.N. (2001) 'The management of preoperative anxiety in children: an update'. *Anaesthesia and Analgesia*, 93: 98–105.

Perry, J.N., Hooper, V.D. and Masiongale, J. (2012) 'Reduction of preoperative anxiety in pediatric surgery patients using age-appropriate teaching interventions'. *Journal of PeriOperative Nursing*, 27 (2): 69–81.

Richardson, J. (2011) 'A review of children's rights as applied to paediatric nursing', in G.M. Brykczynska and J. Simons (2011) *Ethical and Philosophical Aspects of Nursing Children and Young People*. Chichester: Wiley-Blackwell.

Royal College of Nursing (RCN) (2013) *Children and Young People in Day Surgery (Guideline 3)*. London: RCN.

Shields, L., Pratt, J., Davis, L. and Hunter, J. (2008) 'Family-centred care for children in hospital' (Review). *The Cochrane Library*, 1. Available at: www.thecochranelibrary.com (last accessed 5 January 2016).

Smith, L. and Coleman, V. (2010) *Child and Family-centred Healthcare: Concept, Theory and Practice*, 2nd edn. Basingstoke: Palgrave Macmillan.

Ullan, A.M., Belver, M.H., Fernandez, E., Lorente, F., Badia, M. and Fernandez, B. (2014) 'The effect of a program to promote play to reduce children's post-surgical pain: with plush toys it hurts less'. *Pain Management Nursing*, 15 (1): 273–82.

United Nations (1989) *United Nations Convention on the Rights of the Child*. United Nations: Geneva. Available at: www.unicef.org.uk/what-we-do/un-convention-child-rights (last accessed 18 May 2017).

Wilson, M.E., Megel, M.E., Enenbach, L. and Carlson, K.L. (2010) 'The voices of children: stories about hospitalisation'. *Journal of Pediatric Health Care*, 24 (2): 95–102.

CARE OF CHILDREN AND YOUNG PEOPLE IN THE PERI- AND POSTOPERATIVE RECOVERY PERIOD

17

DAWN JAMES

THIS CHAPTER COVERS

- Different children's surgical conditions requiring surgery/a procedure
- The specific care needs of children in the peri- and postoperative period
- The role of the children's nurse perioperatively
- The collaborative approach required for effective peri- and postoperative care of children
- The role of the children's nurse in promoting recovery in the postoperative period

> " The worst thing about being in hospital is not knowing what is going to happen … if nurses and doctors can just relate more to how the child feels, it would make them feel a lot more comfortable and homely whilst they're in hospital.
>
> **Madi, child** "

Visit https://study.sagepub.com/essentialchildnursing to access a wealth of online resources for this chapter – watch out for the margin icons throughout the chapter.

INTRODUCTION

It is widely recognised that children have unique healthcare needs and care should therefore be adapted to reflect this. Hospital admissions can be a stressful experience for any patient; however, potentially more so for children and their families. Unfamiliar surroundings and people, separation anxiety, along with a disruption in routine can add to the fear, pain and discomfort associated with a surgical condition and its required treatment. This stress can be exacerbated if a general anaesthetic is required or other potential surgical risks are identified. Effective preparation of the child and their family to recognise these potential stressors may help them to develop coping strategies, promote postoperative recovery and improve their hospital experience overall. As a children's nurse working in this setting, you will need the knowledge and skills to support patients' and families' specific needs during surgical treatment. This chapter will discuss issues surrounding peri- and postoperative care of children and will guide you to develop the knowledge you require to care for this group's particular needs.

DIFFERENT CHILDREN'S SURGICAL CONDITIONS REQUIRING SURGERY/A PROCEDURE

SEE ALSO
CHAPTER 3

VIDEO LINK 17.1:
TALKING ABOUT
GASTROSCHISIS

Surgical conditions may present at different ages, with different symptoms, and will require investigation to confirm diagnosis and guide treatment (Table 17.1). Whilst there may be some specific care issues required for different conditions, there are also general peri- and postoperative surgical principles that apply to all conditions. Through the use of age-specific communication, nurses work as part of the multidisciplinary team to explain the condition, the need for surgery and what children and their families will experience whilst in hospital. An essential part of the nurse's role is to ensure that the child and family understand the information that they are given, answer any of their questions and support them through investigations undertaken to aid diagnosis. In this way, the feeling of uncertainty that Madi described in the opening quotation can be overcome.

THE SPECIFIC CARE NEEDS OF CHILDREN IN THE PERI- AND POSTOPERATIVE PERIOD

SEE ALSO
CHAPTER 16

Children and young people are distinct patient groups with specific developmental needs. Hospitalisation can create anxiety and fear for children, and inadequate preparation for hospitalisation/surgery can have long-term psychological effects on the child. Pre-admission preparation programmes designed for children requiring planned surgery aim to improve their hospital experience.

Some pre-admission programmes allow children and their families to visit the ward and operating theatres, to familiarise themselves with the environment and reduce the fear of the unknown. Furthermore, research has demonstrated that pre-operative family-focused preparation can reduce the anxiety of the child and family during anaesthesia induction, improve recovery times and reduce the need for analgesia postoperatively (Kain et al., 2007; Chorney and Kain, 2010). Ideally, all children would have the opportunity to attend pre-admission days. However, there will always be children who require emergency surgery and so this preparation will not be possible. Children requiring emergency surgery will look to the nurse to provide adequate preoperative information, support and answers to their questions. It is for this reason that children's nurses need the knowledge and skills to adapt their practice to children's particular needs. Think about this in relation to Scenario 17.1.

Table 17.1 Some children's conditions that may require surgery

	Description	Incidence: Live births	Presentation	Diagnosis	Associated conditions	Specific preoperative care
Diaphragmatic hernia	Failure of diaphragm to close allowing the gut to migrate into the chest	1:4–5000	Usually early infancy but smaller defects can present later in childhood	– Antenatal USS – X-ray	– Cardiovascular – Pulmonary hypotension	– ECHO – Pre-/post-ductal saturations – NG free drainage – Sedation +/– paralysis
Trach-oesophageal fistula (TOF)	A blind ended oesophagus (OA) +/– TOF – abnormal communication between the trachea and oesophagus	1:3000	Early in infancy	– Polyhydramnios on antenatal USS – Difficulty passing NG tube – Chest X-ray – will identify NG tube curled up in oesophagus: air in stomach = TOF; no air in stomach OA only	– VACTERL: see case study	– Replogle tube on low grade suction – Avoid respiratory support such as CPAP with suspected TOF
Gastroschisis	Failure of abdominal wall to close	1:6000	Congenital	– Antenatal – Visual	– Bowel atresias	– Cover bowel – NG tube on free drainage – Fluid replacement
Duodenal atresia	Abnormal closure of the duodenum which prevents food and fluid from passing from the stomach into the intestines	1:10,000	Usually early infancy	– Polyhydramnios – 'Double bubble' on X-ray – Barium swallow confirms atresia	– T21	– NG tube on free drainage – Chromosome testing and ECHO if T21 suspected
Malrotation	Failure of the bowel to coil up in the correct position and fix properly into the abdominal cavity	1:2500–3000	Usually early infancy – but can present later in childhood	– Abdominal X-ray may be similar to duodenal atresia but a contrast study will show abnormal rotation	– Volvulous	– NG tube on free drainage

(Continued)

Table 17.1 (Continued)

	Description	Incidence: Live births	Presentation	Diagnosis	Associated conditions	Specific preoperative care
Hirschprung's	Absence of ganglion cells in the submucosa of the distal bowel	1:5000 (>% in boys)	Usually in early infancy	– Barium enema will indicate narrowing of bowel – Rectal biopsy will confirm aganglionic cells	– Central apnoea	– NG tube on free drainage – Rectal washouts
Pyloric stenosis	Narrowing in the opening (pylorus) between the stomach and small intestine	2–4:1000 (>% – boys)	Usually around week 6	– Thickened muscle can be felt – Usually confirmed with USS	– Nil	– NG tube on free drainage
Intussusception	Telescoping of a bowel segment into itself	>boys	6 months to 3 years	– Abdominal X-ray will indicate soft tissue mass – Confirmed with barium enema	Associated with cystic fibrosis	– NG tube on free drainage
Posterior urethral valves	Abnormal formation of the urethral valves near the bladder, causing a blockage and prevention of normal elimination	1:8000 Only in boys	Usually early infancy	– Bladder and kidney USS – may be picked up antenatally – Micturating cystogram to identify urinary reflux	Associated with hydronephrosis	– Urinary catheter – Prophylactic antibiotics
Scoliosis	Abnormal twisting and curvature of the spine	3–4:1000	Can develop at any age, but most common 10–15 years	– Visually detected; confirmation with X-ray	May be associated with cerebral palsy and muscular dystrophy	– Back brace prior to surgery
Hydrocephalus	Excess fluid on the brain	1:1000	Congenital or acquired	– A/N USS, visual, cranial USS after birth, MRI, CT scan	Cysts, brain haemorrhage, tumour, neural tube defects	– Temporary reservoir, prior to shunt insertion
Neural tube defect	Incomplete formation of the spinal, leaving an opening in the spine	0.8:1000	Congenital	– A/N USS, visual, cranial USS, MRI, CT	Hydrocephalus	– Dressing over lesion to prevent fluid loss

SCENARIO 17.1: JOHN

John, a 12-year-old boy, has been admitted to the ward via the children's emergency department. John is complaining of abdominal pain, has been vomiting and has a high temperature. The surgical registrar believes that John has appendicitis and needs to go to theatre for removal of his appendix urgently.

- How will preparing John for theatre differ from a routine theatre admission?
- What can the children's nurse do to support John through this admission?

✔

SCENARIO
ANSWER 17.1

The children's nurse may provide surgical nursing care to patients across a wide age range and she/ he needs to recognise the different needs of each patient. One element of care that applies to all age groups is the provision of play. Play is an important element of children's lives and can be essential when preparing them for both admission and surgery. Age-specific play can help a child to come to terms with fears, develop coping strategies and relieve anxiety. Children can also use play as a distraction, to maintain control of the situation they find themselves in and to develop an understanding of the options available to them. Many children's wards have play therapists within the team that are trained specifically to use play therapy to support children whilst in hospital and in preparation for surgery. However, when this service is not available, the children's nurse must endeavour to use their knowledge of play to support children before and after surgery.

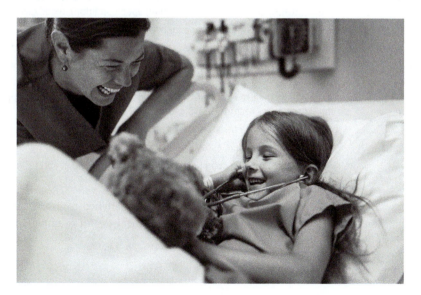

Figure 17.1 Preoperative play

THE ROLE OF THE CHILDREN'S NURSE PERIOPERATIVELY

As outlined above, perioperatively the children's nurse has the important role of ensuring that children and their families are physically and psychologically prepared for surgical investigation and intervention. Implementation of family-centred care (FCC) (care that takes into account the

SEE ALSO
CHAPTER 1

preferences of the family and child) allows the children's nurse to work in partnership with children and their families.

Providing children with the opportunity to vocalise any concerns/fears is important and advocating their right to be heard is a crucial part of the role of the children's nurse's (NMC, 2015). There will also be times when the children's nurse will need to negotiate with children and their families to ensure procedures, such as clinical investigations, occur. This can be challenging – for example, insertion of intravenous access – but by using effective age-appropriate communication, the children's nurse can develop a trusting, therapeutic relationship that will help with this negotiation. The children's nurse can utilise specialist knowledge of child development and cognition to develop strategies that will encourage children to partake in preoperative assessments and activities.

Preparation for theatre

The children's nurse has an essential role to play in supporting children and their families through stabilisation and preparation for theatre, as outlined in Table 17.2.

Table 17.2 Preparation for theatre

	Investigations/readings/interventions
Baseline observations	HR, RR, BP, oxygen saturation monitoring (SaO2), capillary refill time (CRT)
Ventilation requirements	Air, oxygen, CPAP, ventilation
Thermoregulation	Temperature, thermal care
Baseline bloods	Full blood count (FBC), group matching, urea and electrolytes (U&E), C-reactive protein (CRP), blood cultures (depending upon condition), blood gas, blood sugar
Intravenous access	Peripheral cannulas, arterial line (depending upon condition)
Fluid therapy/balance	Fluids containing dextrose and electrolytes, if required monitoring of fluid balance
Nil by mouth	4-6 hours prior to the operation (age dependent); NG tube on free drainage (condition specific)
Identification and documentation	Wrist bands, theatre checklist, anaesthetic chart, consent form, care plans, nursing/multidisciplinary records, PEWS chart, SBAR document
Consent	Informed consent to be gained and consent form signed
Pain assessment	Use of appropriate pain assessment tool and documentation
Medications	Antibiotics, pain relief, condition-specific medications - e.g. anti-reflux

The children's nurse will use their specialist knowledge and experience to assess the child's pre-operative condition and identify any special requirements for theatre – for example, blood products that need to be ordered in preparation for theatre.

ACTIVITY 17.1: CRITICAL THINKING

What are the challenges when caring for a family who are Jehovah's Witnesses? What considerations need to be taken into account when discussing the potential need for blood products in theatre?

ACTIVITY
ANSWER 17.1

Anaesthesia

Recognising instability in children and acting upon this is essential if potential risks associated with anaesthesia and surgery are to be avoided. The effect of anaesthesia in children is distinctly different from adults. The different size, physiology and behaviour of children, all of which have an impact on response to anaesthesia, will change substantially with age. Generally, healthy young children often need more anaesthesia due to their increased ability to eliminate the anaesthetic drugs. However, if oxygen levels are low (hypoxia) prior to receiving anaesthesia, perfusion to kidneys and liver will be reduced, which may prolong the effects of anaesthesia in children. This may be exacerbated if there is also acid in the blood (acidosis). Conversely, if the blood pressure or circulating blood volume is low (hypotension/hypovolemia) then blood will flow preferentially to the brain, which will increase the effects of anaesthesia. This highlights why preoperative assessment of cardiorespiratory status is essential. In addition, if children have a low temperature (hypothermia) prior to surgery, then this may affect the body's ability to form blood clots (essential for wound healing) and cause an increase in metabolic rate and oxygen consumption during surgery. Whilst responding to the thermoregulatory needs of children is an essential part of the role of the children's nurse, it is a priority prior to surgery.

VIDEO LINK 17.2: MY GENERAL ANAESTHETIC

VIDEO LINK 17.3: PREPARING CHILD FOR ANAESTHESIA

WATCH A VIDEO ONLINE!

A&P LINK

To remind yourself of the relevant anatomy and physiology, please read the A&P link: 'Thermoregulatory needs' at https://study.sagepub.com/essentialchildnursing

A&P LINK 17.1: THERMOREGULATORY NEEDS

Fasting

Appropriate fasting is required to reduce the risk of aspiration pneumonitis. Depending upon the age of the child and food intake they will need to go nil by mouth (NBM) four to six hours prior to the operation. Infants may have a feeding tube in situ and those at risk of developing hypoglycaemia will be placed on IV fluids. Urea and electrolytes need to be checked to allow the team to respond to any electrolyte imbalances prior to theatre. The children's nurse will need to support children and families to overcome the discomfort/clinical manifestations associated with prolonged fasting.

Consent

Gaining informed consent is a complex process and one that you must understand the principles of.

The process of gaining consent begins with the healthcare worker giving information about a surgical procedure and then checking that the patient and family have understood. Those gaining consent must have the ability to explain all the issues clearly (including the side effects of having or not having the procedure), resolve misunderstandings, encourage children and parents in their reasoned decision-making (without putting pressure on them) and respect their decisions. Research has demonstrated that most children want to partake and share the decision-making with their doctors and parents when consent is being obtained (Chorney and Kain, 2010). Whilst some competent children may wish to sign consent for treatment, the reality of this happening in practice appears to be limited.

SEE ALSO CHAPTER 8

THE COLLABORATIVE APPROACH REQUIRED FOR EFFECTIVE PERI- AND POSTOPERATIVE CARE OF CHILDREN

Completion of the pre-theatre checklist creates an opportunity for the multidisciplinary team to work together to reduce the risks associated with surgery. Identifying any potential risks, ensuring premedications are prescribed (if needed) and assessing IV access and preoperative bloods prior to theatre can help to minimise any delays in the patient's surgery. Children's nurses will work closely with all team members (e.g. surgeons, anaesthetists, surgical nurse practitioners and play therapists) to ensure thorough preparation of the child and family for surgery. By working with others, children's nurses can utilise their specialist knowledge and skills to support children and their families during this stressful time, vastly improving their hospital experience.

Transfer to theatre

The safe transfer of children to theatre is crucial if stability is to be maintained. Considerations of how children will be transferred to surgery (incubator, cot or bed), is essential and will depend on age and condition. Parents are encouraged to accompany the child to theatre and will have the opportunity to remain in the anaesthetic room until the child is prepped. Handover of care is usually given to the operating department practitioner (ODP). Their role is to:

- Ensure a thorough handover is obtained from ward staff
- Develop a rapport with the family and child
- Assess the child and parents' understanding of the procedure
- Reassure the child and family, and
- Use effective communication to maintain the child's safety

By reviewing the pre-theatre checklist, consent form and medication chart, the ODP can promote safe practice – for example, by identifying any allergies. The ODP will identify the child's wishes and engage with the child and family whilst anaesthesia is being administered.

WEBLINK:
SBAR

ACTIVITY 17.2 REFLECTIVE PRACTICE

Think about the last time you witnessed a good handover between two members of staff. What was good about that handover? Was a structured handover tool such as SBAR (Situation, Background, Assessment, Recommendation) used?

ACTIVITY
ANSWER 17.2

Patient safety during theatre has been improved with the implementation of the WHO *Surgical Safety Checklist* (2009). By following a few critical steps, healthcare professionals can minimise the most common and avoidable risks endangering the lives and wellbeing of surgical patients. Care during theatre should be a continuation of the nursing/medical care received preoperatively. In addition, as there is the potential for pressure injuries, regular pressure area relief and assessment of skin is required during surgery. To maintain thermoregulatory needs, theatre staff (typically consisting of nurses, anaesthetists and surgeons) should minimise heat loss and utilise heating devices effectively. Children require continuous assessment during surgery to ensure airway management/ventilation is maintained and to assess for complications and pain. As blood loss is possible, an accurate fluid balance is required. Parents may wish for regular updates through the surgery and then an overall update once surgery is complete. Where possible parents should be present when the child wakes in recovery, to reduce anxiety. The following patient voice excerpt clearly notes this:

> When I woke up the nurse was in the ward sat right by me. About ten minutes later they called my mum to come – I felt a lot better then.
>
> **Madi, child**

WHAT'S THE EVIDENCE?

The Royal College of Nursing (2011) has developed a good practice guidance in relation to the safe transfer of children to and from theatre.

WEBLINK:
SAFE
TRANSFER OF
CHILDREN

- At what age can children provide informed consent? How would you safely transfer a child from theatre to the ward?

THE ROLE OF THE CHILDREN'S NURSE IN PROMOTING RECOVERY IN THE POSTOPERATIVE PERIOD

For seamless postoperative care to occur, a comprehensive handover is required. The children's nurse has the crucial role of reviewing the notes and postoperative care plan, assessing the child and promoting recovery in the postoperative period (Table 17.3).

Table 17.3 Postoperative care

	Investigations/readings/interventions
Baseline observations	HR, RR, BP, SaO2, CRT
Ventilation requirements	Air, oxygen, CPAP, ventilation
Thermoregulation	Temperature, thermal care
Baseline bloods	FBC, U&E, CRP, blood cultures (condition/symptom dependent), blood gas, blood sugar
Intravenous access	Peripheral cannulas, arterial line (condition dependent), central line (condition dependent)
Fluid therapy/balance	Continue IV fluids as required. Monitoring of fluid balance - ensure adequate urine output, monitor for oedema
Nutrition	Dependent upon age and condition, the child may start feeds once effects of anaesthetic have worn off. Adequate nutrition is required for good wound healing
Documentation	Review of operation sheet instructions: ensure procedure, any complications and specific postoperative care are documented in notes; PEWS chart; SBAR document
Wound care	Wound care to be assessed regularly, and if sutures are not dissolvable note the date for removal

(Continued)

Table 17.3   (Continued)

	Investigations/readings/interventions
Stoma care (condition dependent)	Care of stoma: stoma appearance and activity, measurement of output, skin integrity, bag adherence, education for parents
Pain assessment	Use of appropriate pain assessment tool and documentation
Medications	Antibiotics, pain relief, condition-specific medications – e.g. anti-reflux

If wound care management is to be optimal, the children's nurse needs to understand the principles of wound healing. The wound healing process goes through four phases (Figure 17.2).

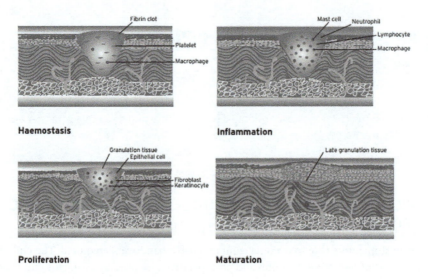

Figure 17.2   Wound healing process

A warm, moist and clean environment is best for the natural wound healing process. It is therefore essential that the child's thermoregulatory needs are maintained, the wound is kept moist and wound cleansing follows aseptic principles.

A&P LINK

A&P LINK 17.2: SKIN & WOUND HEALING

To remind yourself of the relevant anatomy and physiology, please read the A&P links: 'Skin' and 'Wound healing' at https://study.sagepub.com/essentialchildnursing

---

SCENARIO 17.2: JESSICA

Jessica is 3 years old and is being discharged home following surgery for intussusception. Jessica has not been eating well and her wound is slow to heal.

PRACTICE SCENARIO 17: MATTHEW

- What information/documentation is required to ensure seamless transition of care?

SCENARIO ANSWER 17.2

Emotional wellbeing is as important as physical wellbeing in the child's recovery. Children undergoing surgical procedures will experience pain. It is imperative that pain is pre-empted and steps taken to prevent/manage pain effectively. Non-pharmacological strategies such as reducing noise and light, minimal handling, containment, distraction, imagery and relaxation can all be used to reduce pain. Children's cognition and experiences of illness/hospitalisation may affect their ability to perceive, cope with and report pain. The aim of postoperative pain management in children is to implement individualised pain management strategies that facilitate postoperative recovery and minimise pain and discomfort.

SEE ALSO
CHAPTER 3

When assessing a child's pain, the level of cognitive development and method of pain assessment must be identified. A valid and reliable pain assessment tool should be used. A number of tools are available and are often age specific. Once pain is assessed, the pain score should be recorded, initial appropriate management implemented and the child's pain should be re-evaluated in a timely manner.

VIDEO LINK
17.4: PAIN
RELIEF

Oral or IV medications (paracetamol, non-steroidal anti-inflammatories, opioids) can be utilised effectively for mild to moderate pain in children's post- surgery. Depending on age/cognition, different pain management strategies can be implemented.

Patient and nurse controlled opioid analgesia can be effective pain relief with the former being found to be effective in children over 5 years old. The use of epidural pain relief for surgery is becoming more common within the child population for the benefits noted in Table 17.4.

Table 17.4   Benefits and drawbacks of epidural pain relief

Benefits	Drawbacks
– Excellent intra-/postoperative analgesia – Avoid side effects of IV opioids – Avoid prolonged postoperative ventilation – No breakthrough pain – Quicker recovery	– Cannot be used if patient has coagulation abnormalities or anatomical abnormalities – Risk of local/systemic sepsis – Requires a skilled practitioner to place one

Regular assessment of the child is required to ensure pain is managed effectively. Unrelieved pain has both physical and psychological consequences and parents will worry about this. Promoting child-centred care that ensures effective pain relief will promote wellbeing and aid the child's recovery from surgery.

CHAPTER SUMMARY

- The children's nurse has the essential role of supporting children and their families through the peri- and postoperative period
- Children have specific care needs whilst admitted for surgery and a collaborative family-centred approach to care is required
- Comprehensive preoperative assessment and stabilisation is essential if side effects of surgery and anaesthesia are to be minimised
- Effective handover of care during the peri- and postoperative periods is essential if safety is to be maintained
- Wound care and effective pain management are integral to the role of the children's nurse

BUILD YOUR BIBLIOGRAPHY

Books

Delves Yates, C. (2015) *Essentials of Nursing Practice*. London: Sage.
Chapter 28 provides an introductory overview of pain management principles and skin integrity.
Chambers, M.A. and Jones, S. (2007) *The Surgical Nursing of Children*. Oxford: Butterworth-Heinemann.
This book provides practical guidance, covering general surgical child nursing and more specialised areas of practice, as well as day-care patients.

Journal articles

FURTHER
READING:
ONLINE
JOURNAL
ARTICLES

FIND OUT
MORE!

Go to https://study.sagepub.com/essentialchildnursing for further free online journal articles related to this chapter.

These articles will help you to explore some of the key concepts covered in this chapter in more detail.

- Ford, K., Courtney-Pratt, H. and FitzGerald, M. (2012) 'Post-discharge experiences of children and their families following children's surgery'. *Journal of Child Health Care*, 16 (4): 320–30.
- Mattsson, J.Y., Forsner, M. and Arman, M. (2011) 'Uncovering pain in critically ill non-verbal children: nurses' clinical experiences in the paediatric intensive care unit'. *Journal of Child Health Care*, 15 (3): 187–98.
- Unsworth, V., Franck, L.S. and Choonara, I. (2007) 'Parental assessment and management of children's postoperative pain: a randomized clinical trial'. *Journal of Child Health Care*, 11 (3):186–94.
- Wilson-Smith, E.M. (2011) 'Procedural pain management in neonates, infants and children'. *British Journal of Pain*, 5 (3): 4–12.

Weblinks

FURTHER
READING:
WEBLINKS

Go to https://study.sagepub.com/essentialchildnursing for further weblinks related to this chapter.

- Royal College Nursing (RCN), *Transferring Children to and from Theatre*
  www.rcn.org.uk/professional-development/publications/pub-004127
  Position statement and good practice guidance in relation to the safe transfer of children to and from theatre.
- UW Health, *Easing Kids' Fears in the Operating Room*
  www.youtube.com/watch?v=TvTReVA3ZTY
  Preparing the child and family for anaesthesia.
- One Born Every Minute, *Complications at Birth – Gastrosschisis*
  www.youtube.com/watch?v=gNPm-kccGtl
  Mother talking about gastroschisis.

ACE YOUR ASSESSMENT

ONLINE
QUIZZES &
ACTIVITY
ANSWERS

Revise what you have learned by visiting https://study.sagepub.com/essentialchildnursing

- Test yourself with multiple-choice and short-answer questions
- Do the chapter activities in the book and check your answers online

REFERENCES

Chorney, J.M. and Kain, Z.N. (2010) 'Family-centered pediatric perioperative care'. *Anesthesiology*, 112: 751–5.

Kain, Z.N., Calderswell-Andrews, L.C., Mayes, L.C., Weinberg, M.E., Wang, S. Maclaren, J.E. and Ronald, L. (2007) 'Family-centred preparation for surgery improves perioperative outcomes in children: a randomised control study'. *Anesthesiology*, 106 (1): 65–74.

Nursing and Midwifery Council (NMC) (2015) *The Code: Professional Standards of Practice and Behaviour for Nurses and Midwives*. London: NMC.

Royal College of Nursing (RCN) (2011) *Transferring Children to and from Theatre: RCN Position Statement and Guideline for Good Practice*. London: RCN.

World Health Organization (2009) *Surgical Safety Checklist*. Available at: www.who.int/patientsafety/safesurgery/en (last accessed 19 May 2017).

CARE OF CHILDREN AND YOUNG PEOPLE WITH RESPIRATORY PROBLEMS

18

ZOE VEAL, ORLA McACLINDEN AND DOREEN CRAWFORD

THIS CHAPTER COVERS

- Respiratory assessment
- Common respiratory conditions
- Nursing care and management
- Discharge planning and continuing care in the community

REQUIRED KNOWLEDGE

A&P LINK 18.1: RESPIRATORY SYSTEM

It would be helpful to have an understanding of the anatomy and physiology of the respiratory system before you start this chapter. Go to the A&P link: 'Respiratory system' at https://study.sagepub.com/essentialchildnursing

> " A lot of nurses describe respiratory support and oxygen administration as the bread and butter of children's nursing. I have begun to understand this since my placement on a general medical ward. Most children on the ward require some sort of respiratory support.
>
> **Sarah, children's nursing student** "

Visit https://study.sagepub.com/essentialchildnursing to access a wealth of online resources for this chapter – watch out for the margin icons throughout the chapter.

INTRODUCTION

The respiratory system is vital for life, supplying oxygen to the body and removing carbon dioxide. Respiratory illnesses such as coughs and colds and other upper respiratory tract infections are very common, especially in young children (Harding, 2016). Respiratory conditions can, however, be life limiting and life threatening, with a major impact on lifestyle, affecting both the child and their family. As a nursing student, you are highly likely to provide care to children with respiratory conditions, both in hospital and in the community.

A&P LINK

To remind yourself of the relevant anatomy and physiology, please read 'Respiratory embryology' at https://study.sagepub.com/essentialchildnursing

---

A&P LINK
18.2:
RESPIRATORY
EMBRYOLOGY

RESPIRATORY ASSESSMENT

Respiratory assessment is a key aspect in identifying the child's physical status (Fergusson, 2008) and although respiratory distress usually occurs due to respiratory illness, it can also be seen in other conditions where the child is acutely unwell (ALSG, 2016). Respiratory assessment involves more than counting the rate of respiration, although frequently that is all that is indicated in the respiratory section of a vital signs observation chart.

Table 18.1 Normal respiratory rates

Age	Respiratory rate at rest (breaths per minute)
Birth	25-50
3 months	25-45
6-12 months	20-40
18 months	20-35
2-7 years	20-30
8-11 years	15-25
12 years and over	12-24

(Adapted from Advanced Life Support Group, 2016)

Respiratory assessment involves assessment of rate, depth, effort, sounds and physical appearance (see Table 18.2). By carrying out a thorough respiratory assessment, you will be able to identify children who are at risk of further deterioration and respiratory failure. Although cardiorespiratory arrest is uncommon in children, the primary cause is respiratory failure (Resuscitation Council (UK), 2015) and the outcome is often poor (ALSG, 2016). Early recognition through observation and assessment is therefore vital.

SEE ALSO
CHAPTER 15

Assessment should follow a structured approach in the unwell child, assessing ABCDE – Airway, Breathing, Circulation, Disability and Exposure in that order. Patency of the airway is of primary importance. Talking and crying provide an indication that the airway is patent, but this may be compromised in the child who is snoring, has stridor, is drooling or showing signs of reduced responsiveness.

Table 18.2 Respiratory assessment and signs of respiratory distress

Respiratory assessment	Rationale and associated signs of respiratory distress
Rate	Varies according to age. Indicates if breathing is too fast/slow or within normal range. For accuracy, assess over a full minute, without the child's knowledge to avoid subconscious rate changes
Depth and expansion	Shallow, moderate or deep? Gives an indication of breathing efficacy. The chest should expand equally on both sides
Regularity	Each breath should be equally spaced and rhythmical, (infants may have a mildly irregular pattern). Observe for paradoxical 'seesaw' breathing where the chest and abdomen move opposite to each other
Effort (work of breathing)	Respiration should be effortless. Recession or the use of accessory muscles to improve gas exchange indicates that the child is working hard to breathe. Intercostal recession, head bobbing and/or nasal flaring involve accessory muscle use and indicate respiratory distress, resulting in tiredness and potential collapse
Sounds	Breathing should be quiet. Noises include stridor, a high-pitched noise on inspiration, or grunting and wheezing on expiration. Grunting is a sign of severe respiratory distress. Sounds heard on auscultation (listening with a stethoscope) include crackles, crepitations, wheezes, rhonchi and friction rub and may be of use in diagnosis. A silent chest is a pre-terminal sign and requires immediate attention
Physical appearance	
• Position	Sitting forward with neck extended indicates respiratory difficulty
• Skin colour	Observe skin for pallor, which indicates low oxygenation
	If central cyanosis is present, respiratory arrest is close
• Level of consciousness	Inappropriate drowsiness/reduced responsiveness may indicate tiredness and deterioration. Agitation may indicate hypoxia
• Facial expression	Respiratory distress can cause children to appear tense and anxious
Oxygen saturation (pulse oximetry)	Normal oxygen saturation is above 97%, but can be lower in children with congenital heart disease. Provides a good indication of breathing efficacy

As a nursing student, you should learn the medical terminology related to normal and abnormal respiration so that you are able to understand nursing handover, medical/nursing notes and treatment instructions. Some of the common terminology is listed below, but you may also find the use of a medical/nursing dictionary helpful.

Table 18.3 Common terminology and descriptors

Term used	Description
Inspiration	The act of breathing in
Expiration	The act of breathing out
Tachypnoea	Faster respiratory rate than expected for the child's age

Term used	Description
Bradypnoea	Slower respiratory rate than expected for the child's age
Apnoea	Absence of respiration
Hyperpnoea	Rapid, deep breathing
Dyspnoea	Difficulty in breathing
Hypoventilation	Slow, shallow breathing
Air trapping	Usually associated with the presence of a wheeze, this is difficulty in breathing out
Hypoxia	Deficiency of oxygen in the tissues
Hypoxaemia	Deficiency of oxygen in the blood
Cyanosis	Bluish discolouration of the skin and mucous membranes caused by an increase in deoxygenated haemoglobin
Silent chest	Absence of breath sounds, indicating a lack of airflow in and out of the lungs. *This is a pre-terminal sign*
Compensation	The body's ability to cope with functional deficiency. Children frequently compensate when unwell
Decompensation	Occurs when the body is no longer able to cope with functional deficiency. When a child tires, they lose the ability to compensate and rapidly deteriorate
Grunting	Occurs by exhaling against a partially closed glottis in an attempt to prevent airways from collapsing at the end of expiration. Sign of severe respiratory distress
Nasal flaring	Flaring of the nostrils. Seen in respiratory distress in infants
Stridor	High-pitched noise on inspiration, indicating laryngeal or tracheal obstruction
Wheeze	Indicates lower airway narrowing. Usually more evident on expiration
Recession	Drawing in of the rib cage on inspiration. Can be intercostal, subcostal, sternal or suprasternal (tracheal tug) and indicates increased work of breathing. Degree of recession (mild, moderate, severe) indicates the severity of respiratory distress
Head bobbing	The head bobs up and down with each breath due to the use of the sternomastoid muscle. Seen in infants and indicates increased work of breathing
Auscultation	The act of using a stethoscope to listen to breath sounds within the chest
Crackles/ crepitations (rales)	Crackling sounds heard on inspiration or expiration. Can be fine or coarse and may indicate the reopening of a small airway, or the presence of fluid, mucus or pus
Rhonchi	Low-pitched noise, sounds similar to snoring and may indicate presence of secretions in the larger airways
Friction (pleural) rub	Harsh grating sound with respiration, which indicates a pleural rub

Auscultation

Auscultation involves using a stethoscope to listen to the chest, so that breath sounds can be heard more clearly. This is a skill that takes practice. Interpretation of breath sounds is not easy (Fergusson, 2008) but it is a useful skill to add to your repertoire as a student. All children have breath sounds that can be heard on auscultation and these can be very loud in young children as their chest wall is thin, and difficult to hear in the crying child. The aim of auscultation is to ascertain if the chest is clear, in which case only normal breath sounds will be heard, or if there are any adventitious sounds, such as crackles, wheezes or rhonchi. Listen first for normal breath sounds, then listen for adventitious sounds. To hear adventitious sounds, go to https://study.sagepub.com/essentialchildnursing

WEBLINK: DIFFERENT BREATH SOUNDS

The deteriorating child

Children, especially young children, can deteriorate very quickly when unwell and their survival depends on prompt recognition of the situation (Miall et al., 2012). Rapid assessment of the acutely ill child should identify 'red flags' that raise a concern and these should be reported to your mentor or a doctor immediately. Using a paediatric early warning system (PEWS) can help to identify the child in need of urgent or emergency medical review, but it is also important that you use your knowledge and skills in alerting appropriate personnel. Prompt recognition and intervention alert nursing and medical staff to impending respiratory failure and can prevent cardiorespiratory arrest.

COMMON RESPIRATORY CONDITIONS

Bronchiolitis

Usually caused by the respiratory syncytial virus (RSV), bronchiolitis is an infectious lower respiratory tract disease seen most commonly in children under one year. Bronchiolitis is seasonal, with the peak incidence occurring between November and March (Knott, 2013). Most children will recover in the community with no specific treatment, but severity can vary and some children will require admission to hospital, with a small percentage needing admission to intensive care. As a nursing student, you will almost certainly care for children with bronchiolitis during at least one hospital-based placement. Premature babies and those under 3 months of age have an increased risk of severe bronchiolitis, as do children with chronic lung disease, congenital heart disease and immunodeficiency (Knott, 2013; NICE, 2015).

Bronchiolitis presents initially as coryza (runny or stuffy nose), followed by cough, low fever, increased respiratory rate and wheeze. The virus results in cell debris that blocks and irritates the bronchioles, causing inflammation and mucus production. Current guidelines recommend taking a pulse oximetry reading in children where bronchiolitis is suspected and any child who presents to the GP with difficulty feeding, clinical dehydration or a respiratory rate above 60 breaths/minute should be referred to hospital for further assessment. Children must be referred to hospital immediately for emergency care and admission if they present with any of the following:

- Severe respiratory distress – for example, grunting, marked chest recession, respiratory rate above 70 breaths/minute
- Observed or reported apnoea
- Difficulty in feeding, taking 50–75 per cent of usual feed volume
- Appearing unwell visually
- Central cyanosis
- Persistent oxygen saturations below 92 per cent in air

(NICE, 2015)

Treatment for bronchiolitis in hospital is supportive and involves oxygen therapy if the oxygen saturations are persistently below 92 per cent in air; upper airway suctioning if the child has respiratory distress, apnoea or difficulty feeding; and enteral feeding if the child is unable to take adequate feeds orally. IV fluid therapy is recommended for children unable to tolerate enteral feeding (NICE, 2015). The use of bronchodilators, antibiotics and saline nose drops are no longer recommended.

Children with mild bronchiolitis can safely be cared for at home, but their caregiver should be advised of 'red flags' that indicate deterioration and how to get help. 'Red flags' include increased work of breathing, decrease in fluid intake, apnoea or cyanosis, and signs of exhaustion such as difficulty in waking. The caregiver should also be aware that smoking in the child's home increases the risk of severe symptoms developing (NICE, 2015).

Asthma

Asthma is the most common chronic condition in children in the UK (Tidy, 2016), affecting approximately 1 in 11 children (Asthma UK, 2016a). The symptoms include cough, wheeze and difficulty in breathing due to mucosal inflammation and narrowing of the bronchi and bronchioles (Miall et al., 2012). In asthma, the airway is more sensitive and an asthma attack can be triggered by a number of factors (see Table 18.4). During an asthma attack, the lining of the bronchioles become swollen in response to a trigger, causing epithelial cells to slough away from the airway walls. The cells then mix with mucous and thick plugs form, resulting in bronchoconstriction which causes wheezing, coughing, shortness of breath and difficulty in breathing (Glasper et al., 2015). Asthma can be life threatening and the UK currently has one of the highest death rates from asthma in Europe (Asthma UK, 2016b). Status asthmaticus occurs when the asthma attack fails to respond to inhaled reliever medication, steroid and oxygen therapy (Dixon, 2012).

VIDEO LINK 18.1:
ASTHMA ATTACK

Table 18.4 Examples of asthma triggers

Cold and flu	Cigarette smoke
House dust mites	Cleaning products
Mould spores	Air fresheners
Animal hair	Deodorants/perfume
Bedding	Paint, glue, varnish
Pollution	Pollen
Stress/anxiety	Cold, damp weather
	Adapted from Asthma UK (2016c)

There is no cure for asthma, so the focus is on treatment and management. All children and their families should be offered education in self-management of their asthma, with a written personalised asthma action plan alongside regular review by a healthcare professional. In managing asthma, the aim is to control the disease with minimal medication side effects, increasing treatment when necessary to achieve control and decreasing when control is good (British Thoracic Society and Scottish Intercollegiate Guidelines Network, 2016).

Most asthma treatments involve the use of inhalers. In the first instance, the child is prescribed a bronchodilator ('reliever') to relax the smooth muscle, making it easier to breathe during an asthma attack (Glasper et al., 2015). Reliever inhalers are intended for use on an 'as needed' basis. However, if this is used three times a week or more, then a preventative inhaler should also be considered (British Thoracic Society and Scottish Intercollegiate Guidelines Network, 2016). Preventative inhalers work by reducing the reactivity of the airway to triggers, and in the UK can be colour-coded brown, orange, red, pink, purple or yellow, whereas reliever inhalers are usually colour-coded blue (Asthma UK, 2016d). In addition, there are other add-on asthma therapies that can be used to improve control of asthma, and once control has been gained, these therapies would be reduced and stopped (British Thoracic Society and Scottish Intercollegiate Guidelines Network, 2016).

VIDEO LINK
18.2: INHALER
TECHNIQUE

Inhaler technique is important in ensuring correct delivery of the asthma drug. Use of a pressurised metered dose inhaler and a spacer device is recommended for children, alongside training in their use. In young children, a facemask is required until the child is old enough to use the spacer device mouthpiece (British Thoracic Society and Scottish Intercollegiate Guidelines Network, 2016). Compliance with preventative inhalers is improved if built into the child's daily routine.

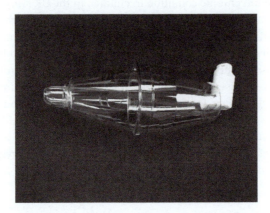

Figure 18.1   Spacer device with pressurised metered dose inhaler (note the inhaler is a placebo for training purposes)

SAFEGUARDING STOP POINT

You are on placement in the children's emergency department when 8-year-old Noah is brought in by ambulance from school. Noah has asthma and this is his third admission to the ED in four weeks. On Noah's last admission, his mum admitted that she hadn't collected his prescription for the 'brown' inhaler as it 'doesn't do anything'. Noah also uses a 'blue' inhaler, but forgot to take it to school today. Noah's teacher says that he often forgets his inhaler and when you check his previous ED admission card, you notice that he had not taken his inhaler to school then either.

- What are the differences between the 'brown' inhaler and the 'blue' inhaler?
- Should Noah be taking a preventative inhaler as well as a reliever?
- Is Noah's current asthma management a potential safeguarding concern?
- What health promotion could be put into place to improve control of Noah's asthma?

SAFEGUARDING
STOP POINT
ANSWER 18.1

Cystic fibrosis

Cystic fibrosis (CF) is a recessive genetic disease, caused by gene mutations found on chromosome 7 (Knott, 2015) and is one of the most common life-limiting conditions you will see as a nursing student. The abnormal gene causes the body to produce higher levels of sodium in sweat and excessively sticky secretions, which causes obstruction to the airways and recurrent chest infections. Although CF predominantly affects the lungs, other organs can be involved, including the liver, gastrointestinal tract, pancreas and the male reproductive system where again, sticky secretions cause obstruction or reduce the organ's ability to work efficiently. For a child to have cystic fibrosis, they must inherit the faulty gene from both parents. Carriers of the faulty gene are unaffected and there is a 1 in 4 chance of a child having CF when both parents are carriers. It is estimated that 1 in 25 people are carriers for CF, with 1 in 2,500 babies born with the condition each year (Knott, 2015).

Since 2007, all babies are screened for CF as part of the Newborn Screening Programme. This involves taking a small amount of blood via a heel prick test at 5 days of age and is usually carried out by a midwife. Newborn screening can be carried out up to a year of age, but if the child is over 8 weeks old when their heel prick test is carried out, the test for CF is excluded, as the results are no longer reliable (Public Health England, 2013). Meconium ileus (bowel obstruction) is a strong indicator for CF and approximately 10–15 per cent of children with CF present in this way within 24 hours of birth (Cystic Fibrosis Trust, 2017a). Other indicators are recurrent chest infections, malabsorption and failure to thrive from infancy. Diagnosis at this stage would normally be confirmed via a sweat test or genetic testing (Miall et al., 2012).

Treatment for CF depends on the severity of the disease and the presence of infection (See Table 18.5). One aim of treatment is to maintain lung health and prevent scarring which can lead to deterioration in lung function. Two bacteria in particular are of concern – *Pseudomonas aeruginosa* and *Burkholderia cepacia*. Colonisation with either can result in chronic respiratory infection and rapid lung function deterioration. For this reason, segregation within hospital and at respiratory clinics is recommended to reduce the risk of cross-infection (Miall et al., 2012).

Table 18.5 Treatment for cystic fibrosis

Treatment	Rationale
Daily oral antibiotic therapy	Prophylactic to prevent infections which result in lung scarring
Daily physiotherapy, which may increase in frequency during infections	Helps to break down secretions and clear the airways
Nebulised DNAse	Helps to break down mucus in the lungs
Bronchodilators	Relaxes the smooth muscle to open the airways
Fat-soluble vitamin supplementation	Pancreatic failure leads to failure to break down fatty foods and may result in malnutrition and vitamin A, D, E and K deficiency
Intravenous antibiotics	Used when symptomatic of infection. Hospitalisation may be required
Creon (enzyme capsules)	Aids digestion of fats and absorption of vitamins and minerals
Salt supplementation	Abnormal sweat gland function leads to the loss of excessive amounts of sodium (salt)
Ursodeoxycholic acid	May help bile flow if the bile ducts become sticky and the bile flow is sluggish
Steroid therapy	Suppresses lung inflammation
High calorie diet	A high calorie diet is required to meet the high metabolic demand created by CF
Enteral feeding overnight	Enteral feeding may be required to maintain a good weight
Glucose monitoring and treatment for CF-related diabetes	Some children develop CF-related diabetes, which requires glucose monitoring and control of blood sugars with either diet or insulin
Oxygen therapy	24-hour oxygen therapy may be needed in severe CF

WHAT'S THE EVIDENCE?

The antibiotic azithromycin is usually taken for three days and is licensed for the treatment of infections such as bronchitis, tonsillitis, ear and skin infections.

Regardless of infection status, where patients are deteriorating on conventional therapy, current guidelines recommend the consideration of a six-month trial of azithromycin, but azithromycin is not licensed to treat cystic fibrosis (Cystic Fibrosis Trust, 2009). To obtain a licence, the manufacturer must be able to demonstrate evidence for the effectiveness and safety of the medicine when used to treat a certain condition or a certain group of patients. Currently, it isn't clear how azithromycin works to treat CF, but it is thought that it might reduce inflammation in the lungs and prevent infection by *Pseudomonas aeruginosa*. When azithromycin is used to treat CF, the prescriber is prescribing it 'off label'. This means that azithromycin has been prescribed differently to the terms set out in its licence as it's being used for a different condition and is prescribed over a longer period of time.

The National Institute for Health and Care Excellence (NICE) reviewed the evidence for azithromycin as a treatment for CF and found that because each study researched azithromycin differently, the results could not be compared with confidence (NICE, 2014). The long-term safety of azithromycin could not be established either, although no serious adverse events had been reported.

- Why is it important to have an evidence base for treatment decisions?
- What are the reasons why a child and their family might agree to a trial of azithromycin?

WHAT'S THE
EVIDENCE?
ANSWER 17.1

SEEALSO
CHAPTER 12

Management of CF requires a high level of commitment from the family and compliance with treatment from the child. Families may find that their lives revolve around the child with CF and the disease can be isolating because segregation is advised. This is done to reduce the risk of cross-infection, but it means that children with CF cannot meet face-to-face and gain support from each other. With the advent of Internet technology, support has become easier using social media. One of the hardest times is during adolescence as the young person begins to develop independence from their parents and adopts responsibility for managing their condition. During this period, young people frequently find compliance to be difficult as they juggle to maintain their treatment regime and a social life with their peers.

ACTIVITY 18.1: CRITICAL THINKING

Using your knowledge of cystic fibrosis and its treatment regime, make a list of the ways in which living with the condition impacts on the child and their family.

ACTIVITY
ANSWER 18.1

There is currently no cure for CF, although with aggressive nutritional and respiratory treatment life expectancy has improved greatly in the last few decades. Currently, over half of children living with CF are expected to reach their 40th birthday and life expectancy continues to increase

(Cystic Fibrosis Trust, 2017b). Lung or heart–lung transplants are offered when CF results in respiratory failure, but due to a scarcity of organs, a third will die whilst waiting on the transplant list (Knott, 2015).

SEE ALSO
CHAPTER 34

SCENARIO 18.1: MIA

You are on placement with a cystic fibrosis nurse specialist. You and your mentor are going to visit Mia, who is 14 years old and has recently been discharged home on IV antibiotics for a chest infection. During the visit, Mia's mother asks to talk to you and your mentor in private. She discloses that Mia has been refusing to comply with her daily physiotherapy routine and she is worried about Mia's long-term health.

- Why is a daily physiotherapy routine important for young people with cystic fibrosis like Mia?
- Why might Mia refuse to comply with treatment?
- What could be the impact on Mia's long-term health?
- What could you do to encourage Mia to comply with treatment?

SCENARIO
ANSWER 18.1

Other respiratory conditions

As a nursing student, you may also care for children with other respiratory disorders. The most common of these are summarised in Table 18.6.

Table 18.6 Other respiratory conditions

Condition	Description
Croup	Mainly affects children from 6 months to 3 years old. The main cause is parainfluenza infection of the upper airway, causing inflammation and potential obstruction. Symptoms include coryza, stridor, wheeze and a barking cough. Most cases self-limit, but severe croup may require hospital admission. Ventilator support is rare, but necessary in severe airway oedema
Acute epiglottitis	Medical emergency, due to life-threatening nature of the illness. Caused by *Haemophilus influenzae*, it presents in children aged 2–5 years, but is now rare since the introduction of the Hib vaccine. Inflammation of the epiglottis creates difficulty in swallowing and drooling. Symptoms include high fever, tachycardia and tachypnoea, with signs of sepsis. Do not lay the child down as this will obstruct the airway
Viral induced wheeze	Caused by viral infection. Symptoms similar to asthma, but only occur when the child has a respiratory infection. A reliever inhaler may be prescribed
Inhaled foreign body	Present with stridor and difficulty in breathing. Sudden onset and signs, such as a wheeze, may be one-sided. Treatment involves identification of object and bronchoscopy to remove
Pneumonia	Bacterial or viral lower respiratory tract infection. Presents with fever, cough and respiratory distress, tachypnoea and intercostal recession. Treatment usually involves antibiotics. Oxygen therapy may also be required
Pertussis (whooping cough)	Coughing spasms during expiration, followed by a sharp intake of breath, causing a 'whoop' sound. Can cause apnoea in infants. Coughing can continue for several months and is known as the 100-day cough. Affects young infants and children who are not fully vaccinated against the disease

VIDEO LINK 18.3:
CROUP

PRACTICE
SCENARIO 18:
SHAYMA

ACTIVITY 18.2: REFLECTIVE PRACTICE

Think back over your placements so far and make a list of the respiratory conditions you have encountered.

- Which conditions did you encounter most frequently?
- What nursing care did these conditions require?
- Which diagnostic tests did you see carried out?

Common diagnostic tests

As a nursing student, you will be involved in assisting healthcare professionals to carry out diagnostic tests and collecting specimens for examination by biomedical scientists in the pathology, biochemistry and haematology departments. See Table 18.7.

Table 18.7 Common diagnostic tests

Diagnostic test	Purpose
Chest X-ray	May show lung changes which can assist in diagnosis
Full blood count (FBC)	Raised neutrophils in bacterial pneumonia Raised lymphocytes in pertussis
Blood cultures	Isolate bacteria, so antibiotic treatment can be targeted
Sputum	Isolate causative organisms so treatment can be targeted
Nasopharyngeal aspirate (NPA)	Diagnose RSV bronchiolitis
Bronchoscopy	Used to perform diagnostic bronchio-alveolar lavage or to remove a foreign body
Per-nasal swab	Isolate *Bordetella pertussis* and diagnose whooping cough
Peak expiratory flow rate (see Figure 18.2)	Measures the ability to breathe out. May be recorded in a peak flow diary to monitor changes over time
Allergy tests	Identify allergy triggers in asthma
Sweat test	Diagnostic test for CF in which the sodium concentration in sweat is high. Measurements made by passing a small electric current across the skin

VIDEO LINK 18.4:
BRONCHOSCOPY

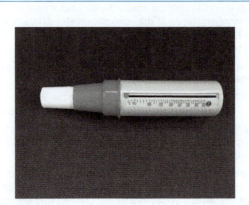

Figure 18.2 Peak expiratory flow meter

NURSING CARE AND MANAGEMENT

Alongside respiratory assessment, the main nursing care you will be involved in is the delivery of respiratory support. This involves oxygen therapy, suctioning and positioning.

Oxygen therapy: Includes head boxes, nasal cannula (see Figure 18.3) and facemasks. Nasal cannula deliver an oxygen flow of less than 2 litres, whereas head boxes and facemasks can be used to deliver higher concentrations of oxygen. A non-rebreathe facemask (see Figure 18.4) is the most effective method of oxygen delivery in the acutely unwell child.

FURTHER INFO
18.1: OXYGEN THERAPY STUDY GUIDE

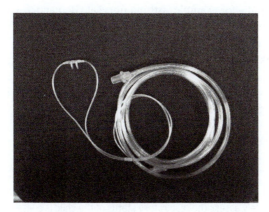

Figure 18.3 Infant size nasal cannula

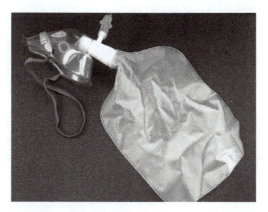

Figure 18.4 Child size non-rebreathe facemask

Suctioning: May be required to help clear secretions from the airway. Suctioning can be traumatic, causing desaturation and should only be used when necessary.

Positioning: Can help open the airways and improve oxygenation and children will sometimes adopt the optimum position themselves. Positions known to be effective include lying prone (face down), sitting upright, leaning forward over the back of a chair, or for infants, lying over someone's shoulder. If snoring is present, readjusting the airway into the 'sniffing' or 'neutral' position can relieve the obstruction.

DISCHARGE PLANNING AND CONTINUING CARE IN THE COMMUNITY

As with all discharge planning, this should start on admission. As a student, you may be involved in helping the child and their family prepare for discharge. If inhalers are to be continued in the community, inhaler technique should be taught and assessed to ensure the child receives maximum benefit.

Other considerations for discharge include:

- Medication management – times, amounts, repeat prescriptions
- Outpatient appointments
- Specialist nursing input – for example, asthma nurse at GP practice, CF nurse specialist
- Contact with support groups
- When to seek medical advice
- Maintenance of peak expiratory flow rate diary

Go to https://study.sagepub.com/essentialchildnursing for tips on preparing for placements and health promotion when working with children with respiratory conditions.

PLACEMENT
ADVICE 18:
RESPIRATORY
PROBLEMS

CHAPTER SUMMARY

- The ability to accurately assess the respiratory status of the child is a vital aspect in children's nursing
- Early recognition of the deteriorating child in relation to respiratory status is essential
- Ensuring an effective transition to community care requires early planning and partnership working with the family

HEALTH
PROMOTION 18:
RESPIRATORY
PROBLEMS

BUILD YOUR BIBLIOGRAPHY

Books

- Fergusson, D. (2008) *Clinical Assessment and Monitoring in Children*. Oxford: Blackwell.

  Very useful book containing two chapters on respiratory assessment and monitoring.

- Dixon, M., Crawford, D., Teesdale, D. and Murphy, J. (2009) *Nursing the Highly Dependent Child or Infant: A Manual of Care*. Chichester: Blackwell.

  Detailed chapter on respiratory nursing of the high dependency child.

- Glasper, A., Coad, J. and Richardson, J. (eds) (2015) *Children and Young People's Nursing at a Glance*. Chichester: Wiley Blackwell.

  Easy to use for quick reference. Contains pages on respiratory conditions, monitoring and assessment.

Journal articles

Go to https://study.sagepub.com/essentialchildnursing for further free online journal articles related to this chapter.

FURTHER
READING:
ONLINE
JOURNAL
ARTICLES

- Ference, E.H., Min, J., Chandra, R.K., Schroeder, J.W., Ciolino, J,D., Yang, A., Holl, J. and Smith, S.S. (2016) 'Antibiotic prescribing by physicians versus nurse practitioners for pediatric upper

respiratory infections'. *Annals of Otology, Rhinology & Laryngology*, 125 (12): 982-91.
This American article explores the prescribing rate differences between doctors and nurse practitioners and is transferable to the UK.

- Lomas, P. (2014) 'Enhancing adherence to inhaled therapies in cystic fibrosis'. *Therapeutic Advances in Respiratory Disease*, 8 (2): 39-47.

  Explores reasons for non-adherence, providing an overview of living with cystic fibrosis. Transferable to the UK.

- Terre, L. (2011) 'Psychosocial factors in pediatric asthma'. *American Journal of Lifestyle Medicine*, 5 (1): 40-43.

  Provides an overview of psychosocial factors which impact on asthma. Transferable to the UK.

Weblinks

Go to https://study.sagepub.com/essentialchildnursing for further weblinks related to this chapter.

FURTHER
READING:
WEBLINKS

- Easy Auscultation, *Easy Auscultation: Lessons, Quizzes & Guides*

  www.easyauscultation.com
  This website contains audio material of different breath sounds to help you learn what to listen for on auscultation.

- NHS Choices, *Ashma: Inhaler Techniques*

  www.nhs.uk/Video/Pages/Childrensasthmainhaler.aspx
  Useful video on inhaler technique in children.

- Spotting the Sick Child

  www.spottingthesickchild.com
  Supported by the Department for Health and Royal College of Paediatrics and Child Health, this website is a training tool for healthcare professionals. You can use this to learn about respiratory assessment and management of the acutely unwell child.

──── ACE YOUR ASSESSMENT ────

Revise what you have learned by visiting https://study.sagepub.com/essentialchildnursing

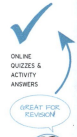

ONLINE
QUIZZES &
ACTIVITY
ANSWERS

GREAT FOR
REVISION

- Test yourself with multiple-choice and short-answer questions
- Do the chapter activities in the book and check your answers online

REFERENCES

Advanced Life Support Group (ALSG) (2016) *Advanced Paediatric Life Support: A Practical Approach to Emergencies,* 6th edn. Chichester: Wiley Blackwell.

Asthma UK (2016a) *What is Asthma?* Available at: www.asthma.org.uk/advice/understanding-asthma/what-is-asthma (accessed 20 February 2017).

Asthma UK (2016b) *Frequently Asked Questions.* Available at: www.asthma.org.uk/advice/understanding-asthma/faqs/#attack (accessed 20 February 2017).

Asthma UK (2016c) *Asthma Triggers*. Available at: www.asthma.org.uk/advice/triggers (accessed 20 February 2017).

Asthma UK (2016d) *Inhalers and Spacers*. Available at: www.asthma.org.uk/advice/inhalers-medicines-treatments/inhalers-and-spacers (accessed 20 February 2017).

British Thoracic Society and Scottish Intercollegiate Guidelines Network (2016) *QRG 153: British Guideline on the Management of Asthma*. Available at: www.brit-thoracic.org.uk/document-library/clinical-information/asthma/btssign-asthma-guideline-quick-reference-guide-2016 (accessed 22 February 2017).

Cystic Fibrosis Trust (2009) *Antibiotic Treatment for Cystic Fibrosis*, 3rd edn. London: Cystic Fibrosis Trust.

Cystic Fibrosis Trust (2017a) *How is Cystic Fibrosis Diagnosed?* Available at: www.cysticfibrosis.org.uk/what-is-cystic-fibrosis/diagnosis# (accessed 24 February 2017).

Cystic Fibrosis Trust (2017b) *CF in Adulthood*. Available at: www.cysticfibrosis.org.uk/life-with-cystic-fibrosis/growing-old (accessed 24 February 2017).

Dixon, M. (2012) 'Care of an infant or child with a respiratory illness and/or the need for respiratory support', in M. Dixon and D. Crawford (eds), *Paediatric Intensive Care Nursing*. Chichester: Wiley Blackwell.

Fergusson, D. (2008) *Clinical Assessment and Monitoring in Children*. Oxford: Blackwell.

Glasper, A., Coad, J. and Richardson, J. (2015) *Children and Young People's Nursing at a Glance*. Chichester: Wiley Blackwell.

Harding, M. (2016) *Common Cold (and other Upper Respiratory Tract Infections*. Available at: http://patient.info/health/common-cold-and-other-upper-respiratory-tract-infections (accessed 19 February 2017).

Knott, L. (2013) *Bronchiolitis*. Available at: http://patient.info/doctor/bronchiolitis-pro (accessed 19 February 2017).

Knott, L. (2015) *Cystic Fibrosis*. Available at: http://patient.info/doctor/cystic-fibrosis-pro (accessed 24 February 2017).

Miall, L., Rudolf, M. and Smith, D. (2012) *Paediatrics at a Glance*, 3rd edn. Chichester: Wiley Blackwell.

NICE (2014) *Cystic Fibrosis: Long-term Azithromycin: Evidence Summary (ESUOM37)*. Available at: www.nice.org.uk/advice/esuom37/chapter/Key-points-from-the-evidence (accessed 24 February 2017).

NICE (2015) *Bronchiolitis in Children: Diagnosis and Management*. Available at: www.nice.org.uk/guidance/ng9 (accessed 19 February 2017).

Public Health England (2013) *Newborn Blood Spot Screening Programme: Programme Overview*. Available at: www.gov.uk/guidance/newborn-blood-spot-screening-programme-overview (accessed 24 February 2017).

Resuscitation Council (UK) (2015) *Paediatric Basic Life Support*. Available at: www.resus.org.uk/resuscitation-guidelines/paediatric-basic-life-support (accessed 27 February 2017).

Tidy, C. (2016) *Asthma*. Available at: https://patient.info/doctor/asthma-pro (accessed 24 February 2017).

CARE OF CHILDREN AND YOUNG PEOPLE WITH CARDIOVASCULAR PROBLEMS

ZOE VEAL AND JO BAILEY

19

THIS CHAPTER COVERS

- Congenital heart disease
- Acquired heart disease
- Arrhythmias
- Nursing considerations

REQUIRED KNOWLEDGE

It would be helpful to have an understanding of the cardiac anatomy and embryology before you start this chapter. Go to the A&P link: 'Cardiac anatomy and embryology' at https://study.sage pub.com/essentialchildnursing

A&P LINK
19.1: CARDIAC
ANATOMY

> " It was very important for my daughter to have a nursing team who were keen to find out about her likes, dislikes, interests and anxieties. We found that she bonded with those who took the time to help her with word searches and scrabble. Time spent chatting is so important. "
>
> **Alison, parent**

Visit https://study.sagepub.com/essentialchildnursing to access a wealth of online resources for this chapter – watch out for the margin icons throughout the chapter.

INTRODUCTION

The heart is not only necessary for life, but is also associated with emotion, love and affection, and we describe ourselves and others as being 'led by the heart', 'wearing our hearts on our sleeves', being 'broken hearted' or 'heartless'. The ancient Egyptians considered the heart to be our soul, the very centre of our being and, alongside the brain, the heart is probably considered to be the most significant of all our organs. In reality of course, the heart is nothing more than a physical organ and the emotional side that we attribute to the heart is really part of our very complex brain and nervous system. In children, heart disease can be either congenital or acquired, the most common being congenital heart disease (CHD), which affects 8.2 children in every 1,000 live births (Gandhi, 2016). Where children are concerned, the heart can malfunction in three areas: its structure (plumbing), its function (mechanics) and its conduction (wiring). Although significant advances in cardiac care have occurred, some cardiac conditions remain life limiting with palliative treatment rather than curative. As a nurse, your role will be to support children and their families through their cardiac journey, enabling them to understand their condition, to manage it, to transition from child to adult services, and to maximise their quality of life through health promotion and psychological support to achieve a sense of normality.

ACTIVITY 19.1: CRITICAL THINKING

Think about how you view the heart and the image that the word 'heart' conjures in your mind. Do you see the heart as physical, emotional or both?

In the opening quote to this chapter, Grace's mum talks about how the nurses developed a therapeutic relationship with her daughter. Think about how family-centred care can be used to address the emotional needs of children and their families and answer the questions below.

- Why is knowledge of the person behind the disease so important?
- What concerns do you think the child and family might have related to the heart?
- How do you think family-centred care could help?

ACTIVITY
ANSWER 19.1

This chapter will consider the main types of cardiovascular problems that children can develop, and will guide you to develop the knowledge needed to care for this group's particular needs.

CONGENITAL HEART DISEASE

Congenital heart disease (CHD) is the largest group of congenital abnormalities, accounting for 30 per cent of all congenital birth defects (Horrox, 2002) and the most common congenital condition diagnosed in neonates (Gandhi, 2016). Although it is associated primarily with children, adults with CHD now outnumber children as survival rates have increased (Ávila et al., 2014), with a need for transitional care as the young person moves into adulthood. Congenital cardiac defects are classified according to their complexity (simple/complex) (Horrox, 2002) or according to their pathological features (cyanotic/acyanotic) (Gandhi, 2016). According to Horrox (2002), 80 per cent fall into the simple category and 20 per cent are classified as complex, indicating that complex congenital cardiac defects are rare. Children can present with a combination of conditions, requiring individualised surgical and nursing plans.

The cause of congenital cardiac defects is thought to be primarily idiopathic, but they are also associated with certain environmental factors, chromosomal defects, syndromes or other congenital

Table 19.1 Examples of congenital cardiac defects

Simple	Complex
Ventricular septal defect (acyanotic)	Interrupted aortic arch (acyanotic)
Atrial septal defect (acyanotic)	Aortic atresia
Patent ductus arteriosus (acyanotic)	Pulmonary atresia with ventricular septal defect (cyanotic)
Pulmonary stenosis (acyanotic)	Pulmonary atresia with intact ventricular septum (cyanotic)
Coarctation of the aorta (acyanotic)	Total anomalous pulmonary venous drainage (cyanotic)
Aortic stenosis (acyanotic)	Hypoplastic left heart syndrome (cyanotic)
Transposition of the great arteries (cyanotic)	Tetralogy of fallot (cyanotic)

birth defects. Approximately 30 per cent of children born with a chromosomal abnormality will have CHD (Horrox, 2002).

The impact of diagnosis is considerable. Not only is there the immediate anxiety of surgical intervention, there are considerable long-term ramifications to come to terms with alongside the shock of diagnosis. Although congenital cardiac defects are present from birth, not all children with CHD will be diagnosed immediately and around a third are discharged home before a diagnosis is made (Wren et al., 2008). These children may present to their GP or local emergency department with faltering weight or in a collapsed state, increasing the distress felt by the family.

Some defects require open-heart surgery, involving a cardiopulmonary bypass. Go to https://study.sagepub.com/essentialchildnursing to find out more about this procedure. Other defects can be corrected using cardiac catheterisation, where a fine tube is inserted into the heart through a vein/artery in the groin/neck. After surgery, most children will need regular check-ups with a cardiologist – some will require additional surgery and many need to adhere to a medication regime. Table 19.2 provides a brief overview of four conditions you may encounter.

WEBLINK: CARDIOPULMONARY BYPASS

Table 19.2 Common congenital heart defects

Ventricular septal defect (VSD)	Brief explanation:	Hole in the wall (septum) separating the two ventricles. Oxygen-rich blood passes from the left to the right ventricle causing increased pressure in the lungs
	Presentation:	Breathlessness, problems feeding and gaining weight
	Treatment:	Open-heart surgery to close the hole with a patch. Sometimes, a band is placed around the pulmonary artery to restrict the amount of blood to the lungs, thereby reducing pressure, until surgical closure is appropriate. You can watch the webcast at https://study.sagepub.com/essentialchildnursing on open-heart surgery
	Prognosis:	Most children will not require further surgery and should be able to live normal, active lives
Coarctation of the aorta	Brief explanation:	A narrowing of the aorta, usually just after the branches which supply the upper part of the body (which then have increased blood pressure) whilst the lower part of the body receives insufficient blood. In addition, the left ventricle needs to work harder to pump blood around the body, which can cause it to become enlarged
	Presentation:	This depends on the severity of the narrowing. It can sometimes be picked up during pregnancy. If severe, neonates can deteriorate quickly

VIDEOLINK 19.1: OPEN HEART SURGERY

(Continued)

Table 19.2 (Continued)

	Treatment:	Either by surgery where the narrowed part of the aorta is removed and the ends sewn back together, or under cardiac catheter using a balloon to stretch the narrow section of the aorta
	Prognosis:	Narrowing may re-develop, or the aorta wall may become weak, requiring additional surgery
Tetralogy of Fallots (TOF) 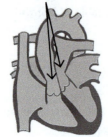	**Brief explanation:**	A large VSD and a narrowing of the pulmonary valve (pulmonary stenosis) that causes the right ventricle to become overworked and thicker (hypertrophied). There is also an overriding aorta: the aorta sits above the VSD resulting in deoxygenated blood getting pumped around the body
	Presentation:	Sometimes identified during pregnancy scans. Babies may appear blue, depending on the severity of the pulmonary stenosis. Some babies have hypercyanotic 'spells' where they become blue very suddenly
	Treatment:	If the child's oxygen levels are very low, an initial 'shunt' operation will be required to increase blood supply to the lungs – this involves placing a shunt (tube) between an artery coming off the aorta to the pulmonary artery, thereby increasing oxygenated blood to the lungs. The child will usually require a full repair under open-heart surgery within a year to correct the VSD and repair the pulmonary stenosis
	Prognosis:	Although children can expect to have a normal quality of life afterwards, their heart should not be considered fully repaired. It is likely that they will have problems with the pulmonary valve leaking (regurgitation). Children may also suffer from arrhythmias in later life
Transposition of the great arteries (TGA)	**Brief explanation:**	The positioning of the pulmonary artery and the aorta are transposed: the pulmonary artery comes out of the left ventricle instead of the right, and the aorta comes out of the right ventricle instead of the left
	Presentation:	Babies are likely to appear blue, particularly when they cry
	Treatment:	Dinoprostone is given to keep the ductus arteriosus open to enable sufficient oxygenated blood to circulate. Babies may also require a balloon septostomy (cardiac catheter procedure) which creates a hole between the two atria of the heart, ensuring sufficient oxygen circulation. Usually within the first three weeks of life the child will require a 'switch procedure' to correct the transposition. Sometimes a switch procedure is not possible and other palliative routes must be considered
	Prognosis:	The pulmonary artery and coronary arteries may narrow and there may be regurgitation from the aortic valve – all of which may require further surgery

You can also watch the video on heart defects at https://study.sagepub.com/essentialchildnursing

WEBLINK:
CARDIAC
CATHETER

VIDEO LINK
19.2: HEART
DEFECTS

SCENARIO 19.1: OLIVER

You are overseeing the admission of Oliver with your mentor. Oliver is a 3-month-old baby with a VSD who has been admitted for surgical repair. Oliver's heart defect was identified following a concern from his health visitor that his weight was faltering. Oliver's mum, Katie, looks very young and appears very anxious.

- During the admission process, what information would you need to gain from Katie?
- What concerns might Katie have?
- What members of the interprofessional team can help support Oliver and Katie?

CHECK YOUR ANSWERS ONLINE!

SCENARIO ANSWER 19.1

SAFEGUARDING STOP POINT

Whilst you are doing Oliver's baseline observations (vital signs), you overhear Katie having a heated conversation on her mobile phone. Katie leaves the ward briefly and, on return, she is visibly upset and appears to be more agitated and anxious than previously. You ask Katie if everything is all right – she smiles and tells you that Oliver's father will be visiting. You notice Katie is shaking.

- What concerns might you have?
- What would you say to Katie?
- Who would you tell?
- Where would you document your concerns?
- How would you promote family-centred care?

SAFEGUARDING STOP POINT ANSWER 19.1

Although cardiac care is carried out in a specialist setting, increased susceptibility to illness leads to frequent admissions to hospital and you could care for a child with CHD in a general ward setting. Similarly, the physical and psychological impact of CHD means that children and their families may have increased contact with health visitors, school nurses and community children's nurses. Community support is an important aspect in supporting the child and family with CHD.

WHAT'S THE EVIDENCE?

Quality of life is an important consideration for children with cardiovascular problems. The World Health Organization defines quality of life (QOL) as 'an individual's perception of their position in life in the context of the culture and value systems in which they live and in relation to their goals, expectations, standards and concerns' (WHOQOL group, 1993. p.153). Within healthcare, QOL measurement is important in understanding the everyday lived experience of people with chronic health conditions, but how or what to measure is contentious (Wray et al., 2009). Generic QOL measures enable comparisons with the general population (e.g. CHD versus non-CHD) whereas disease-specific measures enable discrimination between disease subgroups (e.g. VSD versus TGA) but do not allow for comparison with the general population. In 2009, a systematic review of 33 studies

(Continued)

(Continued)

into QOL and psychological adjustment identified significant risk of psychological maladjustment in children following open-heart surgery and impaired QOL for those with severe CHD (Latal et al., 2009). Further research was recommended, with the impact of parental wellbeing on the child's psychological adjustment being highlighted.

- What aspects of childhood/adolescence do you think would be important when measuring QOL?
- How might the QOL aspects you identified above be affected by a cardiovascular problem?

ACQUIRED HEART DISEASE

Acquired heart disease is normally associated with adults, but a small percentage of children will acquire heart disease in infancy or childhood. Although most children with CHD are at increased risk of developing infective endocarditis (Tidy, 2015), acquired heart disease can affect all children and is a serious diagnosis. The acquired heart diseases you may encounter are explained below.

Table 19.3 Acquired heart diseases

Infective endocarditis	Brief explanation:	Infection of the heart lining, endocardium and valves, which can be bacterial, viral, parasitic or fungal, although 80–90% of cases are bacterial. Bacterial endocarditis occurs in CHD when bacteraemia is present and a high-pressure gradient or turbulent blood flow resulting from a structural defect causes endothelial damage. Platelets and fibrin adhere to the endocardium to create vegetation (thrombosis)
	Presentation:	Fever, lethargy, headache, weight loss, pallor, changed heart murmur. Localised pain, seizure, hemiplegia, blood in urine, chest pain, respiratory distress may indicate embolisation
	Treatment:	Four to six weeks, high dose antimicrobial therapy, tailored to the causative organism, plus pain and fever management, and possible treatment for weight loss and anaemia
	Prognosis:	Despite medical advances, prognosis is poor with an overall mortality of 30% (Cahill and Prendergast, 2015). Children with CHD have an increased risk of infective endocarditis, however, routine antibiotic prophylaxis following dental or surgical procedures is no longer recommended, unless there is infection at the surgical site (NICE, 2016).
Cardiomyopathy picture depicts dilated cardiomyopathy with a large baggy left ventricle	Brief explanation:	Disease of the myocardium affecting overall cardiac function. Several types: dilated, hypertrophic, restrictive or endocardial fibroelastosis. Dilated cardiomyopathy is most common
	Presentation:	Cardiac failure, arrhythmias, respiratory difficulties, fatigue, weakness and reduced exercise tolerance
	Treatment:	Management of cardiac failure and arrhythmias with prevention of thromboembolism and sudden death, using beta-blockers, vasodilators, inotropes, anti-coagulation and diuretic therapy, depending on clinical need. Transplantation may also be required

You can go to https://study.sagepub.com/essentialchildnursing and watch the video on cardiomyopathy

VIDEO LINK 19.3: CARDIOMYOPATHY

Prognosis:	Varies depending on diagnosis. Risk of sudden death is a concern	

Kawasaki Disease

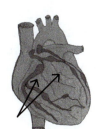

Diagram depicts coronary artery aneurisms

Brief explanation:	Acute, febrile systemic vasculitis, a major complication of which is coronary artery aneurysm formation
Presentation:	Fever lasting ≥ 5 days, irritability, bilateral conjunctivitis, inflamed mucus membranes, rash, peeling skin on hands and feet, enlarged lymph nodes, tachycardia or gallop rhythm. Symptoms often missed or misinterpreted
Treatment:	Management of the inflammatory process with aspirin and intravenous immunoglobulin, to reduce fever and myocardial inflammation with the aim of preventing coronary aneurysm formation
Prognosis:	Discovered in 1967, long-term follow-up results are not yet known (Harding, 2015). Prognosis is dependent on the depth of cardiac impairment, but generally appears to be good if diagnosed early and treated appropriately

Rheumatic heart disease

Diagram depicts aortic valve on left and damaged aortic valve on the right. The valves are open in the top diagrams and closed in the bottom. A leak is visible in the bottom right hand corner

Brief explanation:	Complication of rheumatic fever causing damage to the heart valves. An inflammatory disease, rheumatic fever begins with a strep throat and is most common in children aged 5-15 years. No longer common in the UK, it remains prevalent in developing countries (Knott, 2014)
Presentation:	Symptoms vary and the heart damage is often not readily noticeable. Typical presentation includes fever and feeling unwell one to five weeks after a streptococcal throat infection, painful joints, rash and shortness of breath
Treatment:	Bed rest, management of the infection and inflammatory process with antibiotics and non-steroidal anti-inflammatory drugs (usually aspirin), management of cardiac failure, surgery to repair damaged heart valve(s), prophylactic antibiotics to prevent reoccurrence
Prognosis:	30-45% of patients with rheumatic fever will develop rheumatic heart disease. Long-term follow up of cardiac status required; reoccurrence of rheumatic fever may be seen - usually within first five years (Knott, 2014)

ARRHYTHMIAS

The final type of cardiovascular problem in children is arrhythmia (or dysrhythmia), which means that the heart is beating either irregularly or abnormally fast/slow. Arrhythmias can occur at any life stage, including during fetal life, and can be seen in children with cardiomyopathies, or during the pre- and postoperative period following cardiac surgery, caused either by the structural defect itself, or by the surgical intervention (Dhillon et al., 2009). Cardiac arrhythmias can also be inherited and are most commonly present during adolescence (Dhillon et al., 2009). Arrhythmias can originate anywhere within the heart's conduction system.

A&P LINK

A&P LINK
19.2:
CONDUCTION
SYSTEM

To remind yourself of the relevant anatomy and physiology, please read the A&P link: 'Conduction system' at https://study.sagepub.com/essentialchildnursing

WEBLINK:
RHYTHM
STRIPS

Some arrhythmias (e.g. asystole/ventricular fibrillation) are associated with cardiac arrest and are incompatible with life, but most are not immediately life threatening. A few common arrhythmias seen in children are overviewed here. For examples of rhythm strips, visit the links available at https://study.sagepub.com/essentialchildnursing

Sinus rhythm

This is the 'normal' expected rhythm – deviations from this are known as arrhythmias/dysrhythmias.

The heart rate and rhythm are normal for the age of the patient. The electrical impulse originates in the sinoatrial node and is conducted to the atrioventricular node and through to the bundle of His, bundle branches and Purkinje fibres. It is important to recognise normal before looking at abnormal rhythyms.

Sinus bradycardia

Characteristic of sinus rhythm, but the rate is too slow for the age of the patient, potentially affecting cardiac output and oxygenation. Causes vary, but prolonged bradycardia is normally a pre-terminal sign and should not be ignored. Treatment involves treating the underlying cause.

Sinus tachycardia

Characteristic of sinus rhythm, but the rate is too fast and variable for the age of the patient. In sinus tachycardia, cardiac output may be affected, which can be detrimental in the ill child. Causes include anxiety, fever, hypovolemia, circulatory shock, cardiac failure and myocardial disease. Treatment involves treating the underlying cause.

Supraventricular tachycardia (SVT)

This refers to the three different types of tachycardia (nodal, atrial and AV re-entrant) which originate in the atria to provide a fixed, abnormal rate and rhythm. Heart rate is extremely rapid at over 200 beats/min. and may cause shortness of breath, dizziness/light headedness and a fluttering sensation in the chest. AV re-entrant SVT is associated with Wolff-Parkinson-White syndrome, where an accessory conduction pathway, the bundle of Kent, exists. Treatment consists of an ice pack to the face in infants, or the Valsalva manoeuvre in children. If these fail, then a rapid intravenous injection of adenosine is given to briefly block the AV conduction and sinus node pacemaking activity in the hope of restoring sinus rhythm. Synchronised DC shock may be used if cardiac output becomes compromised. In Wolff-Parkinson-White, the accessory pathway can be ablated to prevent further episodes of SVT.

Long QT syndrome

This is a genetic condition affecting around 1 in 5,000 people, in which the time between depolarisation and repolarisation of the heart (the QT interval) is lengthened. In the normal heart, electrical activity is generated through the flow of sodium, calcium and potassium ions through ion channels in the heart muscle cells. In Long QT syndrome, the faulty gene affects the ion channels and delays the flow of potassium, lengthening the time in which the heart repolarises. Symptoms, if present, range from dizziness to sudden cardiac death and may be triggered by stress, sudden loud noise, strenuous exercise, or sleep.

Heart block

This occurs when there is a disturbance in conduction between the normal sinus impulse and the ventricular response. It is classified according to severity as either first, second or third (complete) degree.

SCENARIO 19.2: MALACHI

Malachi is 14 years old and has Wolff-Parkinson-White syndrome. Malachi enjoys sport and has had several recent episodes of SVT that have required hospital treatment. Malachi has been admitted for catheter ablation of his extra pathway to prevent further episodes of SVT.

- Who should be approached to give consent for Malachi's procedure?
- What care would Malachi require following his catheter procedure?
- What might be the challenges in providing Malachi with privacy and dignity during his admission?
- What are the issues that need to be considered as Malachi transfers between child and adult services?

SCENARIO
ANSWER 19.2

NURSING CONSIDERATIONS

Children with a cardiovascular problem require additional monitoring, depending upon their specific circumstances. Some will be recovering from open-heart surgery; others will have had a cardiac catheter procedure or require medical management for their condition. This section highlights key factors you need to consider, common tests and medications you may encounter, and members of the interprofessional team who help support the recovery of the child.

ACTIVITY 19.2: REFLECTIVE PRACTICE

Reflect on a young person that you (or a colleague/fellow student) have cared for recently.

- How did their heart condition impact on their daily activities and on family life?
- What long-term considerations or worries might they have?
- How could you support them during their stay in hospital?

General nursing considerations

Vital sign observations are a major aspect of cardiac nursing and all patients will have regular observations taken. This will be an opportunity for you to refine and perfect your skills in this area. Following an increase in medication or post-cardiac catheter/surgery, observations need to be completed more frequently.

Table 19.4 Vital signs in cardiac nursing

Vital sign	Rationale
Temperature	As well as indicting infection, temperature can also be indicative of cardiac output and both core and peripheral temperatures should be taken. A high core and a low peripheral temperature may indicate low cardiac output
Pulse	Palpating a pulse will give you information about rate, rhythm (regular/irregular) and pulse volume (weak/thready/bounding). In the neonate/infant an apex pulse is more accurate than a peripheral pulse. (Note – when listening to an apex pulse, a heart murmur may be heard, making it harder to count the pulse until you have become familiar with the sound.) Femoral pulses are checked if coarctation of the aorta is suspected. Pedal pulses are checked post-cardiac catheterisation
Respiration	Visual inspection of respiration for rate, regularity, depth, equal movement and respiratory effort
Blood pressure	For accuracy, use the right arm wherever possible. Blood pressure is not a reliable indicator of cardiac output in children due to their ability to compensate and a low BP may be a pre-terminal sign. Four limb blood pressures may be requested by the cardiologist
Oxygen saturations	Indicates the level of oxygen perfusion in the circulating bloodstream and can be significantly reduced in children with CHD. Check with the child/family or cardiologist the expected oxygen saturation for their condition – this is important to ensure the PEW score is calculated correctly
Capillary refill	Prolonged capillary refill times, especially when mixed with 'mottling' of the skin, indicate poor systemic perfusion
General appearance	Observe for pallor and mottling, which may indicate low cardiac output. Look for cyanosis (in cyanotic CHD, there may also be clubbing of the fingers and toes) – children who are 'spelling' will be very cyanosed. Observe for increased work of breathing, sweating, oedema and clamminess of the skin, which may indicate heart failure

All observations must be carefully recorded so that any deterioration can be quickly identified.

Child safety

Ensure that all bedside safety equipment is present at the start of each shift, is in working order and alarms are set at appropriate levels for the age of the child you are caring for. Make sure also that you have easy access to the bed space. In an emergency, clutter and lack of functioning and appropriately sized equipment can seriously impede medical staff and adversely affect patient outcome. Some children with cardiac conditions must not receive oxygen for reasons of their physiological safety: ensure this and the reasons for it are clearly identified in the bed space and nursing notes.

Positioning

Ensure the child is positioned to ensure optimum breathing, circulatory and neurological function appropriate for their age. Children unable to move themselves should be turned regularly to avoid pressure area deterioration and scrupulous tissues viability recording must be documented and monitored at prescribed intervals.

Mobilisation

Encouraging mobilisation is important in a child's recovery post-surgery. Those recovering from surgery with wounds, drains and intravenous medication may be very apprehensive about mobilising. Pain assessment and management is an essential element of care when expecting children to move freely.

Nutrition and fluid

Prior to surgery/cardiac catheter, required nil by mouth times must be adhered to according to local evidence-based policy. Children are often fluid restricted in the post-operative period, or whilst in cardiac failure to ensure the heart is not placed under increased pressure. Accurate fluid balance is essential and all children with cardiac conditions should be weighed daily to identify possible fluid retention, which may require urgent treatment. Ideally, you should weigh the child at the same time each day, before food is taken and record the results prominently.

Discharge planning and continuing care in the community

Go to https://study.sagepub.com/essentialchildnursing for tips on preparing for placements with children with cardiovascular problems.

PLACEMENT ADVICE 19: CARDIOVASCULAR PROBLEMS

Discharge planning should start on admission. Patient/parental education is an important part of the nursing role and, as a nursing student, you may be involved in assessing parental clinical competence and providing information. The type of information likely to be needed for discharge preparation includes:

- Wound care/pain assessment and symptom relief
- Medication – times, amounts, how long for and how to get repeat prescriptions. Safe storage and administration is also a concern
- Dental treatment/immunisations schedules and surveillance for complications
- Things to look out for, when to worry and who to contact, including out of hours
- Outpatient appointments
- Returning to nursery/school and general day-to-day activity

You should ensure parents receive written instructions regarding their child's care and are given contact numbers for the hospital, should they need at any time to ask a question or seek advice.

Many families find support groups to be a useful source of help and support away from the hospital environment and the ward should hold details of relevant support groups, or you can search for groups on the Internet.

SEE ALSO CHAPTER 30

PRACTICE
SCENARIO 19:
BEN

SEE ALSO
CHAPTER 11

ACTIVITY 19.3: CRITICAL THINKING

Many of the patients you will nurse with cardiovascular problems will be infants. Whilst it is essential they receive the appropriate medical care, it is also important for their cognitive development that you focus on various aspects of appropriate developmental care.

- How could you promote this ethos?
- What good practice have you seen whilst on placement?
- What barriers are there to this?

ACTIVITY
ANSWER 19.3

SEE ALSO
CHAPTERS
3 & 17

Post-surgery care

Following surgery, children may have drains and pacing wires in situ. Drains could be placed in the pleural or mediastinal spaces and will require hourly observations of the entry site and drainage volume. Familiarise yourself with local policy and safety procedures, including infection control matters regarding drain care. Postoperative temporary pacing wires are attached to the atria and ventricles and are visible externally – a specific protocol is followed for their removal. Surgical wounds, particularly thoracotomies, are very painful, and pain assessment and management are fundamental to your nursing care. This will also reduce child and parent anxieties and increase the likelihood of early mobilisation, thus reducing the incidence of complications associated with immobility.

Postoperative wounds require regular visual assessment and recording for signs of infection (pain, redness, swelling, signs of non-healing, abnormal/excessive exudate or bad odour) and wound swabs may need to be taken and treatment commenced if infection is suspected or present.

Common diagnostic tests

Alongside patient history and physical examination, cardiologists will also request diagnostic tests to assess and monitor the child's ongoing cardiac status to assist them in ongoing clinical decision-making.

ACTIVITY 19.4: REFLECTIVE PRACTICE

Using your previous knowledge and learning from placement, reflect on the purpose of each of the following diagnostic tests:

- Chest X-ray
- Echocardiogram (echo)
- ECG (electrocardiogram)
- Cardiac MRI
- CT scan
- Cardiac catheterisation and angiography

What psychological preparation might the child undergoing a diagnostic test require?

ACTIVITY
ANSWER 19.4

Medication

The majority of children with cardiovascular problems will be prescribed medication to help their heart function more efficiently and prevent further damage. Table 19.5 includes some common examples of medications used in the care of cardiac conditions.

Table 19.5   Common medications used in cardiology

Type	Use	Common examples
Diuretics	Treat/prevent fluid retention	Furosemide, Spironolactone
Angiotensin-converting enzyme (ACE) inhibitors	Treat hypertension	Captopril, Enalapril
Beta blockers	Treat hypertension and arrhythmias	Atenolol, Propranolol
Vasodilator antihypertensive drugs	Reduce blood pressure	Hydralazine, Sildenafil
Antibiotics	Treat bacterial infections; 24 hours of antibiotic treatment post-surgery is common	
Anticoagulants	Reduce clotting – often used when children have had a mechanical valve/shunt fitted	Heparin, Warfarin, Aspirin
Inotropes	Affect the contractility of the myocardium	Milrinone, Dopamine, Dobutatime

Interprofessional team

As well as nurses, medical staff and surgeons, a number of other professionals are involved in the care of the child with cardiovascular problems. Below are some examples of other healthcare professionals who have expert input to children's cardiac care.

Dietician: Ensures optimum calorie intake is received for growth and healing and provides a specific feeding regime or supplements. Dieticians also liaise with community teams prior to discharge.

Play specialist: Provides appropriate toys/activities to help promote a sense of normality; provides distraction during painful procedures and can be successfully employed in preparing a child psychologically for procedure or interventions which are required.

Physiotherapist: Provides chest physiotherapy post-surgery and gives advice on positioning and mobilising the child, and suctioning secretions.

Children's cardiac nurse specialist: Provides additional in-house and outreach expertise and support, liaising with children and families pre-admission and as a point of expert contact between hospital visits.

Speech and language therapist: Assists with babies struggling to establish successful oral feeding regimes following a period of tube feeding.

ACTIVITY 19.5: TEAMWORKING

Imagine you are taking verbal handover of a patient from the paediatric cardiac intensive care unit.

- What questions will you need to ask prior to the child arriving on the unit?
- What information will you need to obtain and from whom when the child arrives?
- What non-medical information might you need in order to provide appropriate holistic care to the child and family?

Reflect on handovers that you have observed or participated in. Were they performed in a structured manner to ensure all aspects were covered? Was a tool such as SBAR utilised (Situation, Background, Assessment, Recommendation)? Go to https://study.sagepub.com/essentialchildnursing and access the Institute for Healthcare Improvement website.

WEBLINK: IHI

ACTIVITY ANSWER 19.5

HEALTH PROMOTION 19: CARDIOVASCULAR PROBLEMS

Go to https://study.sagepub.com/essentialchildnursing for tips on health promotion when working with children with cardiovascular problems.

CHAPTER SUMMARY

The ability to support the child and their family safely and effectively through their cardiac journey is vital. This chapter and the corresponding online resources will have provided you with basic knowledge and an understanding of cardiac conditions which affect structure, function and conduction of the heart whilst also introducing you to the role of other healthcare professionals involved in the child and family's care experience. Remember always to listen to the views of the child and the parents as well as heeding the technological and physiological presentations – this is one of the hallmarks of professional excellence in children's nursing practice.

In this chapter we covered:

- Presentation, treatment and prognosis of common CHD, acquired heart disease and arrhythmias
- Nursing considerations and care of the cardiovascular patient
- Common tests and medications involved in the care of the cardiovascular patient

BUILD YOUR BIBLIOGRAPHY

Books

- Chamley, C.A., Carson, P., Randall, D. and Sandwell, M. (2005) *Developmental Anatomy and Physiology of Children: A Practical Approach*. London: Elsevier Churchill Livingstone.

  Contains a very useful chapter on the development of the cardiovascular system.

- Gleason, M.M., Rychik, J. and Shaddy, R.E. (2012) *Pediatric Practice: Cardiology*. New York: McGraw-Hill Medical.

  American textbook which covers foetal development and detailed explanations of heart defects, as well as aspects of care.

- Hampton, J.R. (2013) *The ECG Made Easy*, 8th edn. London: Elsevier Churchill Livingstone. User-friendly guide to understanding ECG and heart rhythms.

Journal articles

Go to https://study.sagepub.com/essentialchildnursing for further free online journal articles related to this chapter.

FURTHER READING: ONLINE JOURNAL ARTICLES

- Etoom, Y. and Ratnapalan, S. (2014) 'Evaluation of children with heart murmurs'. *Clinical Pediatrics*, 53 (2): 111–17.

  Useful article on heart murmurs, a frequent physiological finding in children with CHD.

- Wheeler, D.S., Jeffries, H.E., Zimmerman, J.J., Wong, H.R. and Carcillo, J.A. (2011) 'Sepsis in the pediatric cardiac intensive care unit'. *World Journal for Pediatric and Congenital Heart Surgery*, 2 (3): 393–9.

  This technical article overviews the epidemiology, pathobiology and management of sepsis in paediatric cardiac intensive care.

- Wong, J.J.M., Cheifetz, I.M., Ong, C., Nakao, M. and Lee, J.H. (2015) 'Nutrition support for children undergoing congenital heart surgeries: a narrative review'. *World Journal for Pediatric and Congenital Heart Surgery*, 6 (3): 443–54.

  Useful article on nutrition post-cardiac surgery.

Weblinks

Go to https://study.sagepub.com/essentialchildnursing for further weblinks related to this chapter.

FURTHER READING: WEBLINKS

- Cincinnati Children's, *Heart Institute Encyclopedia*

  www.cincinnatichildrens.org/patients/child/encyclopedia/defects/default
  The Cincinnati Children's Hospital website offers comprehensive information for both health professionals and patients/families.

- The Children's Heart Federation

  www.chfed.org.uk
  The Children's Heart Federation website has annotated diagrams of heart conditions, useful fact sheets which can be printed off and links to other useful sites such as the British Heart Foundation and Great Ormond Street Hospital.

- Congenital Hearts Defects UK, *Types of CHD and Operations*

  www.chd-uk.co.uk/types-of-chd-and-operations
  This is a very useful website. It contains information about anatomy and physiology of CHD, provides details regarding presentation, signs/symptoms and types of treatment/surgery, and includes syndromes linked to cardiac defects.

ACE YOUR ASSESSMENT

ONLINE QUIZZES & ACTIVITY ANSWERS

Revise what you have learned by visiting https://study.sagepub.com/essentialchildnursing

- Test yourself with multiple-choice and short-answer questions
- Do the chapter activities in the book and check your answers online

REFERENCES

Ávila, P., Mercier, LA., Dore, A., Marcotte, F., Mongeon, FP., Ibrahim, R., Asgar, A., Miro, J., Andelfinger, G., Mondésert, B., de Guise, P., Poirier, N. and Khairy, P. (2014) 'Adult congenital heart disease: a growing epidemic'. *Canadian Journal of Cardiology*, 30 (12): S410–19.

Cahill, T.J. and Prendergast, B.D. (2015) 'Infective endocarditis'. *The Lancet*, 387 (100210): 882–93.

Dhillon, R., Sharland, G., Robinson, A., Clay, C. and Bearne, C. (2009) 'Presentation and diagnosis', in K. Cook and H. Langton (eds) *Cardiothoracic Care for Children and Young People: A Multidisciplinary Approach*. Chichester: Wiley-Blackwell.

Gandhi, A. (2016) *Congenital Heart Disease in Children*. Available at: http://patient.info/doctor/congenital-heart-disease-in-children (last accessed 20 May 2017).

Harding, M. (2015) *Kawasaki Disease*. Available at: http://patient.info/doctor/kawasaki-disease-pro (last accessed 20 May 2017).

Horrox, F. (2002) *Manual of Neonatal and Paediatric Heart Disease*. London: Whurr Publishers.

Knott, L. (2014) *Rheumatic Fever*. Available at: http://patient.info/doctor/rheumatic-fever-pro (last accessed 20 May 2017).

Latal, B., Helfricht, S., Fischer, J.E., Bauersfeld, U. and Landolt, M.A. (2009) 'Psychological adjustment and quality of life in children and adolscents following open-heart surgery for congenital heart disease: a systematic review'. *BMC Pediatrics*, 9 (6).

NICE (2016) *Prophylaxis against infective endocarditis: antimicrobial prophylaxis against infective endocarditis in adults and children undergoing interventional procedures*. Clinical guideline [CG64]. Available at: www.nice.org.uk/guidance/cg64 (last accessed 26 June 2017).

Tidy, C. (2015) *Infective Endocarditis*. Available at: http://patient.info/doctor/infective-endocarditis-pro (last accessed 20 May 2017).

WHOQOL Group (1993) 'Study protocol for the World Health Organization project to develop a quality of life assessment instrument'. (WHOQOL). *Quality of Life Research*, 2 (2): 153–9.

Wray, J., Green, C. and Kennedy, F. (2009) 'Impact of heart disease on young people and their families: an introduction', in K. Cook and H. Langton (eds) *Cardiothoracic Care for Children and Young People: A Multidisciplinary Approach*. Chichester: Wiley-Blackwell.

Wren, C., Reinhardt, Z. and Khawaja, K. (2008) 'Twenty-year trends in diagnosis of life-threatening neonatal cardiovascular malformations'. *Archives of Diseases in Childhood: Fetal and Neonatal Edition*, 93 (1): F33–5.

CARE OF CHILDREN AND YOUNG PEOPLE WITH NEUROLOGICAL PROBLEMS

20

STUART HIBBINS

THIS CHAPTER COVERS

- Intracranial physiology in infants and children
- Late signs of raised ICP
- Neurological observations
- Acute and long-term conditions

REQUIRED KNOWLEDGE

It would be helpful to have an understanding of the anatomy and physiology of the nervous system before you start this chapter. Go to the A&P link: 'Nervous system' at https://study.sagepub.com/essentialchildnursing

A&P LINK
20.1:
NERVOUS
SYSTEM

> " I have really enjoyed learning more about the care of children with neurological problems that I can honestly say it has opened my eyes to the complexities of neurosurgical and neurology nursing and also made me realise how much I like my job.
>
> **Fiona, children's nurse** "

INTRODUCTION

The chapter will provide information useful to children's nurses working with patients with a neurological illness. The opening quotation highlights the complex nature of caring for children with neurological problems and their families. Thus, before studying this chapter the reader should gain an awareness of a range of practical knowledge and skills in managing a child with a neurological illness during the acute and long-term phase whether in hospital or a community setting.

INTRACRANIAL PHYSIOLOGY IN INFANTS AND CHILDREN

Many children and young people who present with an acute neurological condition have raised intracranial pressure (RICP), a potentially life threatening situation. An understanding of intracranial physiology and early recognition is a prerequisite for managing patients with raised ICP.

Intracranial Pressure

The intracranial vault (skull) is filled with three components. Brain tissue constitutes approximately eighty per cent of the volume, cerebral blood accounts for approximately ten per cent and CSF makes up the remaining ten per cent. These components coexist within the rigid confines of the skull and exert a pressure known as intracranial pressure (Mestecky, 2011).

Raised intracranial pressure

A good way to understand the concept of raised ICP is by using the Monro-Kellie Doctrine. This states that the volume of the three components of the rigid skull (brain, blood and CSF) remain relatively constant. According to the Monro-Kellie Doctrine there are compensatory mechanisms that allow an increase in one component and a corresponding reduction in one or two of the other components. If this does not occur there will be an increase in ICP.

Compensatory mechanisms

There are several compensatory mechanisms that occur to maintain normal ICP. These include the displacement of cerebral spinal (CSF) and the compression of CSF spaces (arachnoid spaces); the compression of cerebral venous sinuses and large veins and the displacement of venous blood. Anatomical features that allow greater compensation in neonates and young infants include greater pliability of the skull; open fontanelles and patent cranial sutures. This is why the signs of RICP differ through the age groups from infancy through to the ages where the skull sutures are fixed and cannot accommodate a rise in ICP without disastrous results.

The brain is able to withstand small increases in intracranial pressure using the compensatory mechanisms outlined above. However, if the cause of the intracranial volume is not treated (see section on medical management) then the compensatory mechanisms will eventually run out and the brain will be in a decompensated state and extremely vulnerable to further increases in volume. Brain tissue itself is capable of significant distortion to allow increases in volume but will eventually give way to the high intracranial pressure and in extreme cases will herniate through the foramen magnum (the opening at the lower part of the skull). This is referred to as coning and is considered a terminal state.

WHAT'S THE EVIDENCE?

The Monro-Kellie Doctrine is one of the fundamental principles on which the treatment of raised intracranial pressure (ICP) is based. It was first developed and named after two Scottish doctors Alexander Monro (1733-1817) and George Kellie (1770-1829). Learn more about this by reading the article.

Table 20.1   Causes of raised intracranial pressure (ICP)

Cause	Pathology
Head injury, stroke	Intracerebral bleed
Brain swelling (cerebral oedema)	Infection (e.g. meningitis), head injury, hypoxic brain injury, metabolic abnormality (e.g. diabetic ketoacidosis)
Space occupying lesion	Brain tumour
Hydrocephalus (blocked VP shunt)	Congenital or acquired

Early signs and symptoms of raised ICP

Early signs and symptoms of raised ICP can be subtle and include the following: excessive drowsiness; decreased consciousness; confusion; vomiting; headache and visual disturbances. In infants and young children there can be 'sun-setting' eyes where the eyes appear to be in a permanent downward gaze and the sclera is observable between the upper eyelid and the iris.

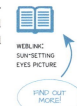

WEBLINK:
SUN-SETTING
EYES PICTURE

FIND OUT
MORE!

LATE SIGNS OF RAISED ICP

Changes to vital signs are generally thought of as late and indicate that the progression of the rising intracranial pressure is at a critical and life threatening stage which needs effective and speedy management in order to preserve life. Cushing's triad is the name given to a situation where there is a 'triad' of signs: raised blood pressure, abnormal breathing patterns and pronounced bradycardia. It is usually preceded by the early signs and symptoms of RICP.

Table 20.2   Signs and symptoms of raised intracranial pressure (adapted from NICE, 2014)

All or some features may be present with the last three signs regarded as very late features:

- Poor feeding and vomiting/nausea
- Tense bulging anterior fontanelle in infants
- High pitched cry (cerebral cry)
- Irritability especially on handling
- Lethargy
- Headaches
- Seizures

(Continued)

Table 20.2 (Continued)

- Changes in the level of consciousness
- Changes in pupil reaction, impaired, upward gaze (sun-setting eyes), new or evolving symptoms or signs such as unequal pupils, asymmetry of limb or facial movement
- Cushing's triad (irregular respiration, bradycardia and hypertension). This is a very late sign and at this stage the child is already extremely unwell
- False localising signs which reflect dysfunction distant or remote from the expected anatomical locus(site) of pathology (disease)

WHAT'S THE EVIDENCE?

Harvey Cushing (1869-1939) was an American surgeon working in Berne, Switzerland who studied the effects of increasing intracranial pressure on vital signs. His paper was published in 1903 and remains one of the fundamental principles on which the management of raised ICP is based. You can learn more by finding and reading the article.

Raised blood pressure

Blood pressure is relatively stable in both infants and children during the early stages of raised ICP. Changes in vital signs are related to the medulla oblongata (lower part of the brainstem) being directly compressed as a result of raised ICP. This causes the capillaries of the medulla to become ischaemic. This initiates a sympathetic response where vasoconstriction occurs and the systemic blood pressure increases to restore the blood supply to the medulla at the same time as overcoming the high ICP. If the raised ICP is not treated and further rises occur and BP cannot match it then brain herniation (often known as 'coning') occurs and the medulla becomes terminally ischaemic and the patient will die (Brunker, 2011).

Abnormal breathing pattern

Changes in respiration usually follow a decrease in conscious levels. When ischaemic changes to the medulla occur breathing becomes slow and irregular. Breathing will cease completely if blood supply to the medulla is not restored. Signs of increased effort of breathing often associated with respiratory distress are not usually evident with raised ICP.

Pronounced bradycardia

Like blood pressure, the heart rate is relatively stable in both infants and children during the early stages of raised ICP. However, in cases where ICP increases to dangerous levels there is a parasympathetic slowing of the heart which is counter-productive as it reduces cardiac output (Brunker, 2011).

Investigations for raised ICP (RICP)

Computed tomography (CT scan) is the preferred choice of investigation (NICE, 2014). It is fast, widely available and generally well tolerated by infants and young children. It is very sensitive and good for detecting the presence of RICP; the cause, size and location of lesions; and for seeing enlarged ventricles in hydrocephalus. However, one of the disadvantages of the CT scan is it that it uses radiation, which is known to be harmful to the developing brain. Repeated use should therefore be avoided (NICE, 2014). Cranial ultrasound is the preferable method of investigation in neonates and infants. Performing a lumbar puncture is contraindicated if RICP is suspected as it can cause a serious pressure gradient (a sudden change from high to low pressure) resulting in an acute brain herniation where the brain stem is forced through the foramen magnum (the opening at the base of the skull). The neural pathways in the brain stem for BP, heart rate and breathing can become irrepairably damaged and can result in death.

VIDEO LINK 20.1: NEURAL TUBE DEFECTS

WATCH A VIDEO ONLINE!

Medical management

Severe or complex cases should be managed in the paediatric intensive care unit (PICU). Treatment may include the use of intravenous (IV) osmotic agents such as hypertonic saline or mannitol. Both of these work by drawing fluid from the cerebral tissues and into the circulatory system. Surgical removal of the cause may be another option (e.g. tumours, lesions, blood clots). If the RICP is due to hydrocephalus, the surgical insertion of a shunting device, an external ventricular drain or a CSF tapping device would be considered.

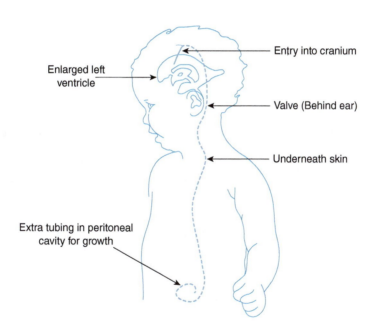

Figure 20.1 A ventriculo peritoneal (VP) shunt device, which is commonly used to treat raised intracranial pressure in hydrocephalus. Cerebral spinal fluid (CSF) drains from the enlarged ventricles into the peritoneal cavity via valve and tube

Nursing management

This will depend on how acutely ill the patient is and on the cause of raised ICP. Initial management would be based on a structured approach to assessment and intervention of airway, breathing and circulation (APLSG, 2016). If RICP is suspected, senior clinical help should be sought immediately. Positioning the patient at 30 degrees with the child's head up and in the midline may help alleviate intracranial pressure by allowing venous drainage from the cranial vault. Temperature should be kept within normal parameters and seizures should be controlled with anti-convulsant drugs.

SEE ALSO
CHAPTER 28

Careful management of IV fluids will be required if the patient is hypertensive. All nurses need to be aware of the hazards of fluid management therapy, in particular risks associated with hypo- and hyper-natraemic states. Scrupulous record-keeping and regular blood levels should be maintained.

ACTIVITY 20.1: REFLECTIVE PRACTICE

Reflect on the care management of a patient you have looked after who had signs of raised intracranial pressure. Discuss with your mentor the expected steps to be taken and why these are necessary.

NEUROLOGICAL OBSERVATIONS

The next section will focus on the use of the Glasgow Coma Scale (GCS) in children (Paediatric Glasgow Coma Scale) and the assessment of pupils and limb power as these are traditionally the areas which cause nursing students most concern regarding accurate measurement, interpretation and reporting.

What is consciousness?

Philosophers and scientists have been discussing the complex nature of consciousness for centuries (Malik, 2000). For nurses carrying out neurological observations the concept of consciousness is about the ability of an individual to be aware of themselves and their surrounding environment. Because of developmental constraints, young children have an incomplete understanding of these concepts. Assessing consciousness in children under five (particularly infants) can therefore be difficult. Nurses need to use their knowledge of child development, play and diversion as well as rely on information from the family. Listening to the parents is very important as they will pick up very quickly on the often subtle changes in ther child's behaviours. This is one of the key skills of a children's nurse, working alongside the parents.

Consciousness relies on the functioning of the reticular formation, which is a network of ascending and descending nerve fibres that extend from primitive areas located in the brain stem to the higher functioning areas of the cerebral cortex (Cole et al., 2005). When a healthy individual is awake and conscious the reticular formation is intact and functional. In the context of brain damage (e.g. RICP) an interruption of the reticular formation occurs and consciousness is affected. This is why assessing consciousness is considered as an assessment of brain function and an important part of neurological observations.

The Glasgow Coma Scale

WEBLINK:
GLASGOW
COMA SCALE

The GCS was originally developed to assess consciousness in adults and has been modified for use with children (Kirkham et al., 2005). It is based on the nurse's observation of the patient's ability to perform three activities: best eye opening, best motor response and best verbal response (see the appendix in the Build Your Bibliography section on pp. 315–6). Each activity is given a score and added together to produce a coma score. Three is the lowest score and indicates the patient is in a deep coma and 15 is the highest score and indicates the patient is fully conscious. For more information on the Glasgow Coma Scale go to https://study.sagepub.com/essentialchildnursing

Modified forms of the Glasgow Coma Scale for use with children

Modified Glasgow Coma Scales are more suitable for use in children aged over 5 years because they assess verbal response and motor response which rely on a child's ability to understand and respond to verbal instructions. For example, an infant will not talk or obey commands; a new born baby demonstrates reflexive movement; the expected best motor response at six months is flexion with spontaneous movement.

Eye opening is the only activity which can be measured in all age groups. There have been various adapted versions of the GCS for use in children (Kirkham et al., 2008). The Adelaide Scale, Pinderfield Scale and James Coma Scale are all examples in use but none is as widely used as the PGCS.

For more information on modified Glasgow Coma Scales, read the article available via https://study.sagepub.com/essentialchildnursing

WEBLINK:
MODIFIED
GLASGOW
COMA SCALES

Which brain structures are being tested?

Eye opening

Eye opening tests a primitive response initiated by the reticular activating system (RAS). This is a network of neural circuitry extending from the brain stem through the thalamus to the cerebral cortex.

Best verbal response

The best way to determine whether someone is orientated is to ask them their name, where they are and what time of day it is. Younger children will respond better to the sound of their mum's voice. This activity tests two areas of the cerebral cortex associated with speech. The first is Wernicke's area in the left temporal lobe which processes what has been said (reception of speech). The other area is Broca's area in the frontal lobe which is linked with the ability to articulate a reply (expression of speech). The nerve pathway called the internal arcuate fasciculus, which connects these two structures, is also being tested.

Best motor response

Asking a child to move his limbs also tests nerve pathways for several higher neurological functions in the brain. For example, neural circuitry for movement is associated with the motor strip in the cerebral cortex as well as the cerebellum and basal ganglia.

Physical stimulus

If a child is not responding to a tactile or verbal stimulus you will need to apply a physical stimulus. Various types of physical stimulus can be used and the specific age of the child will determine which method is used. The National Paediatric Neuroscience Benchmarking Group recommends use of supraorbital pressure to test for localisation, and nail bed pressure to test for flexion (NICE, 2014). While there is generally a consensus on which methods are appropriate, there is no universal agreement as to which method is optimal (Waterhouse, 2009; Teasdale, 2009; Hibbins, 2009). In the context of children this is complicated further by the fact that some methods are suited better for older children than for younger ones. Physical stimulus should be applied forcefully and cause no injury. The general principle of 'do no harm' applies here and the nurse should ensure that he or she applies the least painful method possible to achieve a result. Always listen to what the parents have to say as well as they are best placed to know what is usual for their child and may well pick up sooner on more subtle changes. Local guidance should also be sought in the clinical setting.

Assessment of pupils

Assessment of pupils tests cranial nerves II and III. Cranial nerve II is responsible for vision and cranial nerve III controls pupillary constriction and eye movement. Both may become compressed by increased intracranial pressure and in extreme cases the pupils can become fixed and dilated.

Assessment of limb response

Assessment of limbs or posture identifies any focal neurological deficits caused by damage to specific nerve pathways. Focal signs of neurological problems could include damage to the motor pathways (e.g. hemiplegia, hypertonia and hypotonia).

Assessment of vital signs

See above section on the late signs of RICP (Cushing's triad).

Frequency of observations

NICE (2014) recommend that observations for head injured patients should be performed and recorded half-hourly until the GCS is 15. The frequency of observations after the initial assessment for patients with GCS equal to 15 should be as follows: half-hourly for two hours; then hourly for four hours; two-hourly thereafter. If the patient deteriorates after the initial two-hour period, observations should revert to half-hourly and follow the original frequency schedule (NICE, 2014). If these observations are indicated in a child's care they should be assiduously carried out as ordered and not omitted because, for example, the child is sleeping. The child may not be sleeping. They may in fact have a deteriorating level of consciousness. Always seek senior advice when considering whether CNS sign measurement is to be altered in frequency.

ACUTE AND LONG-TERM CONDITIONS

Hydrocephalus

Hydrocephalus is the most common paediatric neurosurgical disorder. Most cases present in infancy during the first year and in children within the first decade (Hibbins, 2011). It is caused by a number of different disease processes, which can be either congenital or acquired (see Table 20.3). It occurs because of an imbalance between the production of cerebral spinal fluid (CSF) in the cerebral ventricles and its absorption by the arachnoid villi in the subarachnoid space, which creates an over-accumulation of CSF within the CSF pathways. This results in the dilatation and enlargement of the ventricles and can result in RICP.

A&P LINK

To remind yourself of the relevant anatomy and physiology, please read the A&P link: 'The CSF pathways' at https://study.sagepub.co.uk/essentialchildnursing

A&P LINK 20.2:
THE CSF
PATHWAYS

Non-communicating and communicating hydrocephalus

Hydrocephalus is commonly described as having either a non-communicating or a communicating cause. Non-communicating hydrocephalus is caused by an abnormal anatomical obstruction within the CSF pathways. For example, in aqueduct stenosis, infants are born with a narrowing of the cerebral aqueduct which blocks the flow of CSF and results in hydrocephalus. In communicating hydrocephalus there is a functional obstruction to the sites of CSF reabsorption. For example, in meningitis the arachnoid villi are damaged by infection and CSF absorption is impaired resulting in hydrocephalus. It is also thought that in some cases it is possible to have a combination of both types. For example, infants with intraventricular haemorrhage (IVH) have large blood clots that obstruct CSF pathways and blood in the CSF which impairs reabsorption (Hibbins, 2011).

Table 20.3 Congenital and acquired causes of hydrocephalus

Congenital causes	Acquired causes
Spina bifida aperta (e.g. myelomeningocele)	Subarachnoid haemorrhage
Aqueduct stenosis	Intraventricular haemorrhage
Dandy-Walker syndrome	Brain tumours
Chiari malformations	Head injury
	Meningitis

Treatment

CSF shunt devices are the principle method of treating hydrocephalus. These devices shunt CSF from its site of production within the cerebral ventricles past the site of obstruction to an area where the CSF can be reabsorbed. The ventriculo-peritoneal (VP) shunt is the most commonly used system used today.

WEBLINK: VP
SHUNTS

For further reading on the VP shunt, read the article available at https://study.sagepub.com/essentialchildnursing. Another method which avoids the use of shunt devices is third endoscopic ventriculostomy. This has become more popular in recent times because it avoids the complications associated with VP shunts (infection, blockage and displacement).

For further reading on third endoscopic ventriculostomy, read the article available at https://study.sagepub.com/essentialchildnursing

WEBLINK: THIRD
ENDOSCOPIC
VENTRICULOSTOMY

SCENARIO 20.1: SIMON

Simon, aged 9 years, had a three-week history of vomiting and headaches. He had visited the GP four times and was diagnosed with childhood migraines and given pain killers. Mum and Dad were unhappy with his diagnosis and took Simon to his local Emergency Department. He was seen by the on-call paediatrician and sent for a head CT scan. This showed a large posterior fossa lesion (brain tumour) and dilated ventricles (hydrocephalus) with signs of RICP. Simon was transferred to a paediatric neurosurgical unit.

- How would you describe Simon's raised ICP using the Monro-Kellie Doctrine?
- Does Simon have a non-communicating (obstructive) or a communicating type of hydrocephalus?

SCENARIO
ANSWER 20.1

Acquired brain injury

Many children are admitted to hospital with acquired brain injury (ABI) each year, and for some the consequences can be very severe, requiring ongoing care in the community or at a residential rehabilitation centre. 'Acquired' refers to the way the injury occurred – as a result of either an accident or illness that happened after birth.

ABI is classified into two main types:

- Traumatic brain injury (TBI)
- Non-traumatic brain injury

Traumatic brain injury (TBI)

A TBI is caused by an impact to the head and there are three types:

Closed head injury: This refers to a severe head injury where the skull is not fractured. It can result from a deceleration injury (e.g. car accident) where the brain has become severely damaged as a result of movement within the skull. Damage is usually widespread and is referred to a diffuse brain injury (Cartwright and Wallace, 2013). The most common cause of severe head injury in infants under 12 months is non-accidental injury (NAI). It is often referred to as 'shaken baby syndrome', but now known as abusive head trauma (AHT).

WEBLINK:
DANGERS OF
SHAKING BABIES

SAFEGUARDING STOP POINT

To learn more about abusive head trauma (AHT) and non-accidental injury (NAI) read the BBC article on the dangers of shaking babies via https://study.sagepub.com/essentialchildnursing

Shaken Baby Syndrome is an area of ongoing controversy and debate within the scientific community. You can hear the view of a doctor who is openly critical of the science behind shaken baby syndrome.

- Consider the different arguments presented
- What impact does this have for the future role of the expert witness?

VIDEO LINK
20.2: SBS
CRITIQUE

SAFEGUARDING STOP POINT

To learn more about cycle helmets, go to the child safety charity Cycle Smart Foundation via https://study.sagepub.com/essentialchildnursing

WEBLINK:
CYCLE SMART
FOUNDATION

Open or penetrating injury: A head injury where the skull is fractured and the brain exposed. It can be caused by deceleration injury, explosion or gunshot.

Crushing injuries: This is the least common type of brain injury. It can be caused by falling heavy objects such as furniture or a walled-mounted television. Younger children who have more pliable skulls are most at risk.

For further reading on head injuries in children, see Pennington (2009).

Non-traumatic brain injury

A non-traumatic acquired brain injury is caused by an illness rather than an impact to the head. The following are all examples of possible causes: brain tumours, meningitis, encephalitis, hypoxic brain injury, stroke, arteriovenous malformation, cerebral aneurysm (see Table 20.4).

> After he came out of PICU he was moved to a chest unit with a ratio of one nurse to eight patients and they could not cope ... he was waking up from his coma and was confused, agitated and required constant attention and care. We were relieved when he was eventually transferred to the rehabilitation centre ... the doctors and nurses there understood his injuries better there because they'd looked after other head injured children. They didn't take his disinhibited behaviour to heart.
>
> **Sofia, parent**

> One characteristic common to many people after an ABI is lack of self-awareness ... I have no memory of the initial post-injury weeks, and my recollections of the subsequent months and years of recovery are fragmentary.
>
> **Sheena, an adult who recovered from an early ABI, McDonald, 2008**

Long-term outcome

Children with severe ABI are likely to need some form of rehabilitation. This may take place either at the hospital or in a residential rehabilitation centre. Rehabilitation can be a slow and complicated journey for both the affected and their families. Recovery may be ongoing and last for years. The aim is not to cure the individual but to help the child compensate for any changes to their abilities and promote independence through different therapies with help from the multidisciplinary team (MDT) (Woodward and Waterhouse, 2009).

Problems after ABI are complex and result from widespread neurological damage, and no two individuals will present with the same clinical symptoms. Damage to the immature or developing nervous system means that although the initial damage to the brain does not progress, symptoms may appear to worsen as the brain matures and problems become more evident as the child gets older (Scrutton et al., 2004).

Symptoms vary and can include: problems with mobility; disturbances in balance and coordination abilities; difficulty in controlling and maintaining posture; epilepsy and intellectual development. The rehabilitation team includes different therapies and may include the following: physiotherapy, occupational therapy, speech and language therapy (SLT), play therapy, music therapy, social work, clinical psychology, neuropsychology, educational psychology and family therapy. Nurses are in a unique position as they are the most consistent carers and provide continuity of care (May, 2001). This means they play a key role within the rehabilitation programme by coordinating care while providing family support as well as leadership of the MDT.

PRACTICE
SCENARIO 20:
JAMES

ACTIVITY 20.2: REFLECTIVE PRACTICE

Reflect upon a patient with an ABI you have looked after and make a list of the things you found challenging. Try to identify what made this care challenging – was it communication, skills, their unpredictable behaviours?

Epilepsy

Epilepsy is the most common neurological condition found in children. It is often perceived as a single condition but there are many different types of epilepsy and conditions which cause it. Most have their epilepsy controlled with anti-epilepsy drugs (AEDs). However, those whose epilepsy is not controlled with AEDs can have other forms of treatment (e.g. surgery). The management of epilepsy in children is aimed at improving their health and general quality of life as well as minimising the detrimental impact on educational, social and family life. This can be achieved by effective clinical management and enabling the family to manage their child's epilepsy.

Table 20.4 Terminology associated with epilepsy and seizures

Term	Definition
Seizure	A seizure can be a single event that results in an altered state of brain function. Seizures occur because of abnormal neuronal activity in the brain. The appearance of the seizure depends on the site of the abnormal electrical activity. It can occur in a specific area (focal seizure) or it can occur throughout the brain (generalised seizure) (May, 2001)
Epilepsy	An individual can be diagnosed as having epilepsy if repeated and unpredictable seizures occur. Epilepsy can be caused by a variety of disorders (see below)
Seizure disorder	This term is sometimes used as an alternative to 'epilepsy'
Epilepsy syndrome	Epilepsy syndrome is a term that refers to various types of epilepsy which can be grouped together because of shared characteristics (e.g. benign rolandic epilepsy, childhood absence epilepsy and juvenile myoclonic epilepsy)
Febrile convulsion	The most common form of epileptic seizure seen in children under 4 years. It occurs following a fever arising from an infection outside of the central nervous system (e.g. an upper respiratory infection)

Term	Definition
Movement disorder	Movement disorders are neurological conditions, caused by damage to the brain that result in uncontrolled abnormal movement such as excessive or involuntary movements (e.g. ataxia). Movement disorders are not considered to be a form of epilepsy
Status epilepticus	A generalised convulsion lasting 30 minutes or longer or when successive convulsions occur without a period of recovery in between (APLSG, 2016)

ACTIVITY 20.3: CRITICAL THINKING

NICE have produced guidelines for the diagnosis and management of epilepsy in children and adults, which you can access via https://study.sagepub.com/essentialchildnursing. Using these guidelines, answer the following questions:

- How is epilepsy diagnosed?
- Which investigations do the guidelines recommend for those with suspected epilepsy?
- How should those with complex or intractable epilepsy be managed and which alternative treatment other than anti-epilepsy drugs (AEDs) are available?

WEBLINK:
EPILEPSY
GUIDELINES

SCENARIO 20.2: SARAH

Sarah is 15 years old and has a history of runny nose and headache. Her mother reported that she has had a fever for the past three days. While waiting in A&E she had a generalised tonic clonic seizure.

- What action would you initially take?
- How would you manage Sarah's seizure?
- How would you explain to Sarah and her mother what is happening?

✓

SCENARIO
ANSWER 20.2

Table 20.5 Neurological conditions, age of presentation, and signs and symptoms

Condition	Average age of presentation	Signs and symptoms
Seizure and epilepsy	Seizures can occur at any age and most cases of epilepsy are diagnosed under 18 years of age	Focal or generalised seizures
Spinal cord abnormalities Encephaloceles Arachnoid cysts Dandy-Walker syndrome Arnold Chiari malformation Spina Bifida aperta (e.g. myelomeningocele) Spina Bifida occulta (e.g. tethered cord)	Present at birth (origins are congenital)	Hydrocephalus, nerve damage resulting in neurological, orthopaedic and urological dysfunction

(Continued)

Table 20.5 (Continued)

Condition	Average age of presentation	Signs and symptoms
Cerebral palsy (movement disorder)	Diagnosis before 5th birthday	Motor and sensory problems
Neurodegenerative disorders Neurometabolic (e.g. Batten's disease)	Birth and pre-birth, or any stage of childhood	Presenting features are commonly loss of motor and cognitive abilities. Other signs and symptoms include: epilepsy, regression of skills, visual disturbances, spasticity and muscle spasm, hypotonia
Spinocerebellar (e.g. Huntington's disease) Neuromuscular (e.g. Duchenne musculardystrophy) Acquired (e.g. Rasmussen's encephalitis)		gastro-oesophageal reflux, feeding difficulties, aspiration, chest infections, constipation, change in sleep patterns, excessive oral secretions, change in behaviour, irritability
Brain tumours (Most common solid tumour in children, usually confined to the CNS) Types: Astrocytoma Medulloblastoma Ependymoma brain stem tumour Midline tumour (e.g. craniopharyngioma)	Can present during infancy or childhood.	Focal neurological signs (symptoms vary and depend on the location in the brain of the tumour), signs of raised ICP, headache, endocrine disturbances, hemiparesis, seizures, changes in behaviour, seizures, ataxia, hydrocephalus
Cerebral vascular abnormalities Occlusive arteriopathies (e.g. Moya Moya syndrome) Neurovascular abnormalities (e.g. AVM and aneurysms, Vein of Galen malformation) Cerebrovascular (e.g. acute stroke)	Can present during infancy or childhood	Focal neurological signs (symptoms vary and depend on the location in the brain of the bleed), deterioration in consciousness, sudden collapse, severe headache, signs of raised ICP, hemiparesis

Go to https://study.sagepub.com/essentialchildnursing for tips on preparing for placements and health promotion when working with children with neurological problems.

PLACEMENT ADVICE 20: NEUROLOGICAL PROBLEMS

HEALTH PROMOTION 20: NEUROLOGICAL PROBLMS

CHAPTER SUMMARY

A sound understanding of the nervous system – and the impact that disease and injury can have on it – is a prerequisite for nurses caring for children with acute or long-term neurological problems. More importantly, for nurses working in this area, having a basic grasp of the complexities not only enhances performance but also enjoyment of their role. This results in a more rounded, empathetic and fulfilled carer. Having an appreciation of this can only be positive for patients and families. In this chapter you will have:

- Reviewed intracranial physiology in infants and children
- Considered the dynamics of raised intracranial pressure and identified early and late change in children's condition
- Reviewed neurological observations tools and observations and how to record these
- Identified acute and long-term neurological conditions and their associated care (hydrocephalus, acquired brain injury and epilepsy)

───── BUILD YOUR BIBLIOGRAPHY ─────

Books

- Costandi, M. (2013) *50 Ideas You Really Need to Know: The Human Brain*. London: Quercus Publishing.

  An easy-to-read book that includes good introductory sections on A&P as well as chapters explaining many contemporary findings of neuroscience.

- Crossman, A. and Neary, D. (2014) *Neuroanatomy: An Illustrated Colour Text*. Edinburgh: Churchill Livingstone.

  A book dedicated to neuroanatomy for students who want to explore the nervous system in more depth. The introductory chapter provides an excellent overview.

- Smith, J. and Martin, C. (2008) *Paediatric Neurosurgery for Nurses: Evidence-based Care for Children and Their Families*. London: Routledge.

  This text provides accessible and up-to-date information for nurses working in paediatric neurosurgery.

Journal articles

Go to https://study.sagepub.com/essentialchildnursing for further free online journal articles related to this chapter.

FURTHER READING: ONLINE JOURNAL ARTICLES

- Khoo, T.-B. (2012) 'Classification of childhood epilepsies in a tertiary pediatric neurology clinic using a customized classification scheme from the International League against Epilepsy 2010 Report'. *Journal of Child Neurology*, 28 (1): 56-9.

  For further reading on the classification of seizures.

- Bui, A.D., Alexander, A. and Soltesz, I. (2015) 'Seizing control: from current treatments to optogenetic interventions in epilepsy'. *The Neuroscientist*, 23 (1): 68-81.

  For a review of current and future treatments.

- Moseley, B.D., Nickels, K. and Wirrell, E.C. (2011) 'Surgical outcomes for intractable epilepsy in children with epileptic spasms'. *Journal of Child Neurology*, 27 (6): 713-20.
  For more information on epilepsy surgery.

Websites

Go to https://study.sagepub.com/essentialchildnursing for further weblinks related to this chapter.

FURTHER READING: WEBLINKS

- Neuroscience for Kids

  https://faculty.washington.edu/chudler/neurok.html

(Continued)

(Continued)

This site has been created for all students and teachers who would like to learn about the nervous system.

* Young Epilepsy (The National Centre for Young People with Epilepsy)

www.youngepilepsy.org.uk
This site provides information about epilepsy for young people, parents and professionals.

* Headway: the brain injury association

www.headway.org.uk
For information about support services for families with children with acquired brain injury.

Apendix: Glasgow Coma Scale (GCS)

The GCS was originally developed to assess consciousness in adults and has been modified for use with children (Kirkham et al., 2005). It is based on the nurse's observation of the patient's ability to perform three activities: best eye opening, best motor response and best verbal response. Each activity is given a score and added together to produce a coma score. Three is the lowest score and indicates the patient is in a deep coma and 15 the highest score which indicates the patient is fully conscious. For more information on the Glasgow Coma Scale go to their website.

Modified forms of the Glasgow Coma Scale for use with children

There have been various adapted versions of the GCS for use in children; the Adelaide Scale, Pinderfield Scale and James Coma Scale are all examples (Kirkham et al., 2008). Modified Glasgow Coma Scales are more suitable for children who have developed language and motor skills because they rely on a child's ability to understand and respond to verbal instructions. Infants without language skills are not able to talk or obey commands; a new born baby can only demonstrate reflexive movement; the expected best motor response at six months is flexion with spontaneous movement. Eye opening is the only activity which can be measured in all age groups.

ACE YOUR ASSESSMENT

ONLINE
QUIZZES &
ACTIVITY
ANSWERS

Revise what you have learned by visiting https://study.sagepub.com/essentialchildnursing

* Test yourself with multiple-choice and short-answer questions
* Do the chapter activities in the book and check your answers online

REFERENCES

Advanced Paediatric Life Support Group (APLSG) (2016) *The Practical Approach*, 6th edn. Chichester: Wiley-Blackwell.

Brunker, C. (2011) 'Assessment, interpretation and management of altered cardiovascular status in the neurological patient', in S. Woodward and A.-M. Mestecky (eds), *Neuroscience Nursing: Evidence-based Theory and Practice*. Oxford: Wiley-Blackwell.

Cartwright, C. and Wallace, D. (2013) *Nursing Care of the Pediatric Neurosurgery Patient*. New York: Springer.

Cole, M. Levitin, K. and Luria, L. (2005) *The Autobiography of Alexander Luria*. New York: Psychology Press.

Hibbins, S. (2009) 'Painful stimulus in the paediatric setting'. *British Journal of Neuroscience Nursing*, 5 (5): 215.

Hibbins, S. (2011) 'Management of patients with hydrocephalus', in S. Woodward and A.-M. Mestecky (eds), *Neuroscience Nursing: Evidence-based Theory and Practice*. Oxford: Wiley-Blackwell.

Kirkham, F., Newton, C. and Whitehouse, W. (2008) 'Paediatric coma scales'. *Developmental Medicine and Child Neurology*, 50: P267–74.

Malik, K. (2000) *Man, beast and zombie: what science can and cannot tell us about human nature*. London: Weidenfield and Nicolson.

May, L. (2001) *Paediatric Neurosurgery: A Handbook for the Multidisciplinary Team*. London: Whurr Publishers.

McDonald, S. (2008) 'Travels in the land of no self awareness'. *British Journal of Neuroscience Nursing*, 4 (10): 510.

Mestecky, A.-M. (2011) 'Intracranial physiology' in S. Woodward and A.-M. Mestecky (eds), *Neuroscience Nursing: Evidence-based Theory and Practice*. Oxford: Wiley-Blackwell.

NICE (2014) *Head Injury: Assessment and Early Management*. Available at: www.nice.org.uk/guidance/cg176 (last accessed 20 May 2017).

Pennington, N. (2009) 'Head injuries in children'. *Journal of School Nursing*, 26 (1): 26–32.

Scrutton, D., Damiano, D. and Mayston, M. (2004) *Management of the Motor Disorders of Children with Cerebral Palsy*, 2nd edn. London: Mac Keith Press.

Teasdale (2009) 'The use of painful stimulus: simple yet fundamental'. *British Journal of Neuroscience Nursing*, 5 (5): 215.

Waterhouse, C. (2009) 'The use of painful stimulus in relation to Glasgow Coma Scale observations'. *British Journal of Neuroscience Nursing*, 5 (5): 209–14.

Woodward, S. and Waterhouse, C. (eds) (2009) *Oxford Handbook of Neuroscience Nursing*. Oxford University Press.

CARE OF CHILDREN AND YOUNG PEOPLE WITH URINARY AND RENAL PROBLEMS

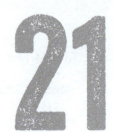

MARY BRADY AND LINDA MOORE

--- **THIS CHAPTER COVERS** ---

- Normal anatomy
- Acquired renal conditions
- Ecalation of concerns to appropriate staff

--- **REQUIRED KNOWLEDGE** ---

It would be helpful to have an understanding of the anatomy and physiology of the renal system before you start this chapter. Go to the A&P link: 'Renal anatomy' at https://study.sagepub.com/essentialchildnursing

A&P LINK
21.1: RENAL
ANATOMY

> " Having a child who suffers from repetitive UTIs caused by an overactive bladder and dysfunctional voiding is challenging. As a parent I find the juggle of her physical and emotional needs challenging. The emotional consequences of her condition at present outweigh the physical side and I often feel under supported in relation to this. The nurse specialists are a very good point of contact for me as a parent when I don't understand what is happening or I need support myself, they are very patient with me as a parent.
>
> **Marsha, parent** "

Visit https://study.sagepub.com/essential childnursing to access a wealth of online resources for this chapte – watch out for the margin icons throughout the chapter.

INTRODUCTION

The kidneys are important organs that maintain homeostasis, control waste elimination and maintain fluid levels within the body. This chapter will guide you with the nursing assessment of a child/young person with a renal condition. Renal conditions can be divided into congenital or acquired disorders. This chapter will explore the aetiology as well as the manifestation of the physical signs of ill health linked to renal pathophysiology such as pyrexia, hypertension, weight gain due to oedema, skin condition, the monitoring of urinary output and urinalysis. Thereafter, aspects of holistic nursing care provision will be discussed covering the early detection of deterioration and cascading that information succinctly and efficiently to other members of the healthcare team. The specific nursing care required for relatively common renal conditions will be discussed, such as in maintaining appropriate fluid and dietary input (in particular fluid volumes, sodium, potassium and protein intake), alongside the observation of fluid output. Medication that is commonly used (antibiotics, steroids and analgesia) will be mentioned but for issues related to the administration of medication you should refer to Chapter 4.

SEE ALSO
CHAPTERS
4 AND 28

The manifestation of renal disorders can have a wide-reaching effect on the child since the disorder can affect body image, school education and family life, as indicated in the opening quotation from a parent. Aspects of caring for a child with an altered body image due to oedema or a chronic renal condition will be discussed as well as the impact of ill health on their school education, alongside the nurse's role in facilitating education. The psychosocial impact of having a child with a renal condition will also be covered as well as any related renal educational provision that is required for the family.

NORMAL ANATOMY

The renal system consists of two bean-shaped kidneys, each connected by a muscular tube called the ureter to the bladder. The kidneys produce a waste product called urine that collects in the bladder and in the continent child passes along the urethra for elimination at a convenient time. Internal and external sphincter muscles at either end of the urethra control when this occurs (Gormley-Fleming, 2015).

SEE ALSO
CHAPTER 28

The renal system develops during the third week of uterine life from the mesoderm and subsequently embryological errors can result in a variety of conditions:

- Total absence of both kidneys (agenesis), which is often incompatible with life although in the absence of other conditions could be treated with dialysis
- Unilateral absence of a kidney
- Fusion of the two kidneys into one horse-shoe-shaped kidney
- Duplex ureters
- Ureteric stenosis
- Malposition of the ureter at the ureteric junction with the bladder or pelvis of the kidney
- The development of valves along the internal urethral walls that prevent the flow of urine
- Bladder extrophy
- Ambiguous genitalia

ACQUIRED RENAL CONDITIONS

With antenatal scanning, some of these defects can be diagnosed and corrected or potential damage to the kidneys minimised with intrauterine surgery (Ruano et al., 2015). After birth, various surgical techniques (described below) may be used to prevent further damage to the kidneys and maximise renal function.

Hydronephrosis

Normally the ureter is a muscular tube that has a funnel-shaped opening which connects with the pelvis of the kidney. In some cases, there is an obstruction due to a kink in the ureter, an aberrant blood vessel or a renal stone. This causes dilation above the obstruction with subsequent scarring and damage to the kidney.

Hypospadias and epispadias

In some male infants, the urinary meatus exits the penis on the ventral (hypospadias) or dorsal side of the penis (epispadias). Surgical repair is usually done when the child is about one year of age.

Bladder extrophy

This is a very rare condition where the abdominal wall has failed to close in utero leaving an exposed bladder (Kumar et al., 2015). It often coexists with epispadias and requires surgery during the neonatal period within a specialist centre.

Ambiguous genitalia

One's sex is a fundamental aspect of existence, so this condition requires sensitive handling and consideration. Genetic information and endocrine tests are required to ascertain the best plan of treatment. During this difficult time for the parents and family, support needs to be collaborative amongst a multidisciplinary team of professional experts.

Urinary tract infections

A urinary tract infection (UTI) is a relatively common childhood condition that requires immediate diagnosis, treatment and investigative management. A small infant may present with a fever or febrile convulsion and a clean urine sample is a routine test. Indeed a UTI is commonly found in about 1:10 girls and 1:30 boys, and if untreated the ensuing renal scarring may lead to hypertension and renal morbidity (Coultard et al., 1997). Diagnosis and treatment are therefore important, so much so that the National Institute for Clinical Excellence (NICE) (2013) has produced guidance and a quality standard to minimise kidney damage, which covers diagnosis, assessment of risk factors for underlying causes, treatment and subsequent management including surgery. Assessment and care should centre round the individual needs of the child and be carried out in partnership with the family. Care, treatment and management can impact the child in the long term as indicated by Melanie's voice below.

I have an overactive bladder and recurrent UTIs which have caused permanent renal damage. I take medicine which stops me from having to go to the toilet as much but my bladder is still naughty and makes me feel desperate every time I need to go. I don't like going into hospital as I don't like blood tests because it hurts and makes me sad. I like the big hospital where I go to see the nurses and doctors, they put jelly on my belly and we look at my insides, it's gross. There is a big slide there and I love it, I go round and round a hundred times but then I have to go and listen to the doctors and that's boring as there aren't many fun things to do in the rooms

> only in the bit where we wait. I like the lady who plays with me best, we do colouring together and I tell her when I'm sad about my bladder and kidneys. I sometimes wish I wasn't poorly as it annoys me when I have to be in hospital and I miss my friends, but it's not too bad as I always make new friends and the nurses are always really nice, they give me jelly and I love that.
>
> **Melanie, child**

SCENARIO 21.1: DANNY

PRACTICE
SCENARIO 21:
ISAAC

Danny is 14 months old. He was admitted again following a second febrile convulsion thought to be induced by a urinary tract infection (UTI). On admission it was noted that although his length is on the 75th centile his weight is on the 50th centile. He was generally irritable, especially when voiding urine.

Urine testing on the ward revealed some proteinuria. He was prescribed a five-day course of antibiotics.

- What care will Danny require for this hospitalisation and why?
- Danny's parents are worried. What short- and long-term consequences might they be worried about?

SCENARIO
ANSWER 21.1

Children who present with urinary tract infections are often assessed for the extent of renal damage using radioactive isotopes such as dimercaptosuccinic acid scan (DMSA) and MCUG (mercapto-acetyltriglycine) scans.

VIDEO LINK
21.1: UTI

ACTIVITY 21.1: CRITICAL THINKING

The consultant arranged for Danny (Scenario 20.1) to have a DMSA scan as a day case and this revealed that he has vesico-ureteric reflux on his left kidney with some renal scarring. The consultant decided that Danny will require surgery to re-implant his left ureter and has referred Danny to a paediatric renal surgeon.

- What can the nurse do to allay parental fears?

ACTIVITY
ANSWER 21.1

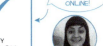

CHECK YOUR
ANSWERS
ONLINE!

Reimplantation of ureters

It is possible to surgically re-implant the ureters either at the pelviureteric junction or the bladder depending on the defect. However, it is important that postoperatively the urinary output is monitored closely and the nurse is vigilant for signs of infection and blood loss and that these are escalated quickly to the surgical team.

Glomerulonephritis

Glomerulonephritis tends to affect more boys than girls and of age range between 6 and 7 years old and is an autoimmune condition where the body reacts to toxins produced following a streptococcal infection elsewhere in the body (e.g. 10–14 days after a β-haemolytic streptococcal throat infection). The antigen–antibody–antigen response results in swelling of endothelial cells in glomeruli that leak blood cells and protein out of the body. The child develops oedema which is peri-orbital in the morning but becomes more generalised around the body as the day progresses, plus, cloudy, smoky brown urine of reduced volume. S/he may also complain of headaches and have slight pyrexia with a slight rise in blood pressure.

Treatment involves intravenous antibiotics and input from a dietician when low potassium, low protein diet and reduced fluids are required. It is important that the nurse also supports the child who will be feeling unwell and bored, and have an altered body image. The family will also be concerned about the long-term outcome since glomerulonephritis may cause permanent damage to the glomeruli with subsequent renal failure. See Table 21.2 for details of further care.

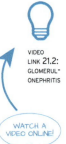

VIDEO LINK 21.2: GLOMERUL-ONEPHRITIS

WATCH A VIDEO ONLINE!

Nephrotic syndrome

This condition, which is also more prevalent in boys, affects 1:50,000 children. The epithelial cells of the glomeruli become swollen, causing protein to leak out into the filtrate, resulting in oedema with a low circulating blood volume and serum albumin. The child may be prone to coagulation issues (thrombosis) and will be susceptible to infection due to a low level of gamma globulin. Blood pressure monitoring may show blood pressure to be normal or reveal slight hypotension due to low serum albumin (see Table 21.1 for differentiation).

Treatment includes steroids, low sodium diet and accurate monitoring of fluid balance and weight measurements. Support is required for the child and family who will be concerned about future renal function, although with nephrotic syndrome the condition may resolve with or without future exacerbations and compromised renal function.

VIDEO LINK 21.3: NEPHROTIC SYNDROME

Haemolytic uraemic syndrome (HUS)

There are three main aspects to this syndrome:

- Haemolytic anaemia caused by the destruction of red blood cells
- Acute kidney failure
- Low platelet count (thrombocytopenia)

Table 21.1 Differentiation between glomerulonephritis and nephrotic syndrome

	Glomerulonephritis	Nephrotic syndrome
Cause	Post β-haemolytic streptococcal infection	Unknown
Urine	Haematuria, proteinuria	Proteinuria
	Cloudy, smoky brown urine	Dark opalescent frothy urine
	Reduced urine output	Reduced urine output
Blood test		High levels of cholesterol, phospholipids and triglycerides
		Low level of albumin
		Hypovolaemia
Blood pressure	Mild to moderate rise	Normal to slightly low
Temperature	Pyrexia	
Oedema	Periorbital-generalised	Periorbital-generalised
Weight	Weight gain	Weight gain
Further infection		Susceptibility to infection due to loss of gamma globulins
Other symptoms	Headaches	General malaise
Prognosis	May lead to permanent damage and chronic renal failure	

HUS usually occurs in children under 5 years old and is the main reason children present with acute kidney failure and often occurs after a gastrointestinal infection with bloody diarrhoea caused by ingesting bacteria such as Escherichia coli, Shigella, or Campylobacter. The toxins these bacteria produce affect the lining of the glomerulus triggering kidney failure. Whilst most children make a full recovery, some will develop chronic kidney failure and require dialysis. There is also a 5–10 per cent mortality rate.

Henoch Schönlein purpura (HSP)

HSP is more common in 3–10-year-old boys and tends to occur in the winter months. Often the child has had a respiratory illness and it is thought that immunoglobulins (IgA and IgG) interact to trigger inflammatory responses. Typically, the child may present with:

- An initially urticarial rash that becomes purpuric
- A rash mainly over the buttocks and extensor surfaces of the legs
- Painful and swollen joints
- Colicky abdominal pain
- Glomerulonephritis with microscopic or macroscopic haematuria

As well as supportive nursing care, the child needs to be monitored for proteinuria, hypertension, oedema and renal deterioration. Those children with renal involvement have to be monitored for a year to detect ongoing and long-term urinary abnormalities.

Wilms tumour

This is an embryonic tumour and is the commonest renal tumour seen in children. It is believed to have a genetic link and usually presents between 5 and 10 years of age when the child develops an

SEE ALSO
CHAPTER 33

abdominal mass with or without other symptoms such as weight gain and poor appetite. After radiological diagnosis treatment usually includes chemotherapy and a nephrectomy.

Table 21.2   General care of the child with an acute renal condition with rationale

Care	Rationale
Skin care: keep skin clean and dry Avoid excessive use of tapes Change positions and use a pressure-relieving mattress	Due to oedema the skin may be fragile and prone to breakdown and sores
Monitor for pyrexia	Hypoalbuminaemia may render the child susceptible to infection due to reduced immunoglobulins
Blood pressure	Hypotension may indicate a low circulating fluid volume
Full blood count, urea and electrolytes	Patients with renal problems may not produce sufficient erythropoietin to stimulate the bone marrow to produce red blood cells Proteinuria results in low serum protein levels such as low albumin which moderates osmotic pressure and will have an ensuing effect on blood pressure Low serum Gamma globulin which will reduce the immune response
Monitor weight	Oedema will cause weight to increase. Ultimately weight gain due to fluid will affect how much of any drug that needs to be given. In children, medication is calculated according to weight so monitoring weight is vital to ensure that therapeutic doses are given
Body image/self-esteem	Excess weight gain and facial oedema will alter how the child views him/herself
Boredom due to inability to move due to tiredness and general malaise	Access to a hospital play specialist and a variety of age-appropriate toys Plan care to enable rest periods
Morbidity and mortality	Depending on the age and maturity of the child, he/she will have a variable understanding of the impact of the condition on their life potential and invincibility. Access to a psychologist may be required

ESCALATION OF CONCERNS TO APPROPRIATE STAFF

WEBLINK:
PEWS CHART

As a nursing student, you will work alongside a registered nurse observing your patients' physiological data. Many hospitals now use age-related paediatric early warning score charts (PEWS) to document observations and facilitate the identification of unwell and deteriorating children. PEWS charts can also be used in conjunction with the Situation, Background, Assessment, Recommendation (SBAR) technique to escalate concerns so that accurate and relevant information can be conveyed succinctly to the senior nurse and medical staff.

WEBLINK:
SBAR

Enuresis: Childhood incontinence in children

SCENARIO 21.3: BECKA

Becka is an 11-year-old girl who has enjoyed being a Brownie but has never been away on a weekend trip. She has recently moved up to be a Girl Guide and would like to be able to join in the Guide weekends and go on sleepovers with her friends. However, on occasions she has wet the bed at home, so her mother has refused to allow her to go until she 'grows out of this habit'.

- What help and support could be made available to enable Becka to participate in more independent activities?

SCENARIO
ANSWER 21.3

Enuresis is a relatively common problem in childhood and early adolescence with about 3 per cent of girls and 2 per cent of boys experiencing daytime incontinence at least once a week (ERIC, 2016). Night time incontinence affects more children (about 8 per cent of 9½-year-olds) and the problem may continue into adulthood. The causes may be multifactorial. Underlying problems such as urinary tract infections and diabetes (mellitus and insipidus) should be excluded. Other causes can be due to defects in the normal renal anatomy or innervation (e.g. with spina bifida), low levels of vasopressin (antidiuretic hormone) and bladder instability. Enuresis is a distressing condition that affects the child's self-esteem and future psychological development; however. there is a variety of help available such as alarms, medication, pelvic floor exercises and self-help groups via the ERIC website.

Renal failure

Renal failure in children falls into two main categories – acute and chronic. In both conditions the kidneys do not filter out the waste or excess fluid from the body, leaving the child with waste and fluid overload and electrolyte imbalance. Treatment varies depending on the severity of kidney failure, ranging from fluid/diet restrictions to dialysis.

Acute renal failure

Also known as acute kidney injury (AKI), this condition lasts for a short time and it is possible that the kidneys will recover and the child's kidney function may return to normal. The need for long-term treatment is therefore variable.

Causes of AKI include:

- Birth trauma
- Sepsis
- Obstructive uropathy
- Glomerulonephritis
- Nephrotic syndrome

Signs and symptoms can develop over hours/days and include:

- Poor/no urine output
- Oedema
- Nausea/vomiting
- Hypertension
- Confusion/seizures

Chronic renal failure

Chronic renal failure (CRF) is an irreversible condition resulting in permanent kidney damage and can be divided into five stages (I-V) depending on the severity of the damage with stage V covering end stage renal failure (ESRF) and these children will need dialysis.

Causes of CRF include:

- Obstructive uropathy
- Hypoplastic/dysplastic kidneys
- Reflux nephropathy

Signs and symptoms:

- Poor appetite
- Stunted growth
- Anaemia
- Low glomerular filtration rate

Dialysis options

Dialysis means 'removal of waste products/fluid' and this is done by filtering out the unwanted material through a semi-permeable membrane. There are two options for dialysis – peritoneal dialysis and haemodialysis.

Peritoneal dialysis

Here the child's semi-permeable peritoneal membrane is used by inserting a peritoneal dialysis catheter into the child's abdominal cavity. The catheter can remain in situ for many months and fluid is passed via this catheter into the child's abdominal cavity. By the processes of diffusion and ultra-filtration, waste is drawn across the peritoneum into the fluid. After three to four hours the fluid is drained out with the waste products/excess fluid, thereby removing waste/fluid from the body. Afterwards another cycle of exchange fluid is introduced into the abdomen and the process repeated with these exchanges running throughout the day. However, they can also be managed by a machine overnight, allowing the child to have a relatively uninterrupted daily routine which minimises the impact on the child's education and social life. There are complications associated with peritoneal dialysis, such as peritonitis and infections at the catheter exit site. For some children who have undergone extensive abdominal surgery or who have adhesions, peritoneal dialysis is contraindicated and haemodialysis is the preferred option.

Haemodialysis

In contrast to peritoneal dialysis, an artificial filter external to the body provides the semi-permeable membrane. The child's blood is drawn out of their body and is transported via tubes to the filter and back to the child in a continuous loop. For this form of dialysis, it is essential to create special vascular access, such as a central line or an arterio-venous fistula. To obtain arterio-venous fistula access, the child undergoes a surgical procedure in which an artery and vein are joined together and the high pressure in the artery causes the vein to dilate which allows easy venepuncture for haemodialysis.

Haemodialysis is performed over three to four hours and needs to occur three or four times a week, depending on the child's individual needs. If a home dialysis machine is available, haemodialysis may be delivered in the child's home; otherwise the child will need to travel to a dialysis centre.

There are complications that can arise associated with haemodialysis and these include hypotension, infection, blood clotting in the circuit and hypothermia. Ultimately these children will require transplantation in order to live independent lives.

VIDEO LINK
21.4: DIALYSIS

WHAT'S THE EVIDENCE?

Swallow et al. (2014) describe caring for children with chronic illness, in this case kidney disease. It is likely that there will be many health professionals involved. Whilst each professional has their own area of expertise it is important to appreciate the value of the contribution others make in the education of the child and family to manage the condition. In this paper, a variety of professionals involved in the care of the child and family are interviewed to explore their experience of multidisciplinary involvement.

Read the paper and consider the different professionals that may be involved in the care of a child with a renal condition.

CHAPTER SUMMARY

- Renal conditions in childhood are wide ranging
- You will be expected to explain the pathophysiology in age-appropriate terminology to children and their families and to refer them to further sources of information
- As a children's nurse you need to be aware of the psychological impact of renal conditions on the child and their family, and to be able to provide the necessary support
- Care of the child with a renal condition is carried out by a range of professionals using an interdisciplinary approach

BUILD YOUR BIBLIOGRAPHY

Books

- Boore, J., Cook, N. and Shepherd, A. (2016) *Essentials of Anatomy and Physiology for Nursing Practice*. London: Sage.

  This book will provide a useful foundation for your knowledge of normal anatomy and physiology so that you can develop your understanding of abnormal anatomy or pathophysiology.

- Collie, M. and Hunter, D.J. (2015) 'Assisting patients with elimination needs', in C. Delves-Yates (ed.), *Essentials of Nursing Practice*. London: Sage.

  Evidence-based guide to a variety of clinical nursing skills.

Journal articles

Go to https://study.sagepub.com/essentialchildnursing for further free online journal articles related to this chapter.

FURTHER
READING:
ONLINE
JOURNAL
ARTICLES

- Flurry, M., Caflisch, U., Ullmann-Bremi, A. and Spichiger, E. (2011) 'Experiences of parents with caring for their child after cancer diagnosis'. *Journal of Pediatric Oncology Nursing*, 28 (3): 143-53.

(Continued)

(Continued)

This paper describes a qualitative study examining the experiences of parents whose child had been recently diagnosed with cancer. The findings revealed the new caring expectations for these parents and how nurses can help proactively to support them.

- Gannoni, A.F. and Shute, R.H. (2009) 'Parental and child perspectives on adaptation to childhood chronic illness: a qualitative study'. *Clinical Child Psychology and Psychiatry*, 15 (1): 39–53.

This paper describes a qualitative study of how children and families adapt to a variety of chronic illnesses, including renal conditions. Data were obtained from both children and their families and revealed the impact of the disease on their lives; many of the themes were similar whilst others related to specific illnesses. Trying to rationalise a meaning for the disease, and process the stress involved in planning for the future are explored with implications for the provision of clinical services.

- Poursanidou, K., Garner, P. and Watson, A. (2008) 'Hospital–school liaison: perspectives of health and education professionals supporting children with renal transplants'. *Journal of Child Health Care*, 12 (4): 253–67.

This paper explores how a multidisciplinary team of health and education staff can work collaboratively to ensure good educational provision for children following renal transplants.

- Roupakias, S., Sinopidis, X., Karatza, A. and Varvarigou, A. (2013) 'Predictive risk factors in childhood urinary tract infection, vesicoureteral reflux, and renal scarring management'. *Clinical Pediatrics*, 53 (12): 1119–33.

Over recent years there has been much debate over how best to manage urinary tract infections to minimise renal scarring. The authors acknowledge that since some renal issues resolve with age and others require surgery, and despite the current availability of scanning, further research is required to identify definitive risk factors.

Weblinks

FURTHER
READING:
WEBLINKS

Go to https://study.sagepub.com/essentialchildnursing for further weblinks related to this chapter.

- NICE, *Urinary Tract Infection in under 16s: Diagnosis and Management*

www.nice.org.uk/guidance/CG54
Evidence-based research regarding best practice regarding urinary tract infection.

- Spotting the Sick Child

www.spottingthesickchild.com/about
A website to help healthcare professionals identify children who have serious illnesses. It incorporates national guidelines with videos and interactive material to increase the learner's knowledge.

- NHS Choices, *Urinary Tract Infections in Children*

www.nhs.uk/conditions/Urinary-tract-infection-children/Pages/Introduction.aspx
The website gives access to information about the treatment and management of urinary tract infections.

- ERIC

www.eric.org.uk/our-story
A website that provides a variety of learning resources for healthcare professionals who care for children with continence issues.

─────── ACE YOUR ASSESSMENT ───────

Revise what you have learned by visiting https://study.sagepub.com/essentialchildnursing

- Test yourself with multiple-choice and short-answer questions
- Do the chapter activities in the book and check your answers online

REFERENCES

Coultard, M.G., Lambert, H.J. and Keir, M.J. (1997) 'Occurrence of renal scars in children after their first referral for urinary tract infection'. *British Medical Journal*, 315 (7113): 918–19.

ERIC (2016) www.eric.org.uk

Gormley-Fleming, E. (2015) 'The renal system', in I. Peate and M. Nair (eds) *Fundamentals of Children's Anatomy and Physiology: A Textbook for Nursing and Healthcare for Students*. Oxford: Wiley-Blackwell.

Kumar, S., Mammen, A. and Varma, K.K. (2015) 'Pathogenesis of bladder exstrophy: a new hypothesis'. *Journal of Pediatric Urology*, 11: 314–18.

Ruano, R., Sananes, N., Sanghi-Haghpeykar, H., Hernandez-Ruano, S., Moog, R., Becmeur, F., Zalosyc, A., Girons, M., Morin, A.M. and Favre, R. (2015) 'Fetal intervention for severe lower tract obstruction: a multicenter case-control study comparing fetal cystoscopy with vesicamniotic shunting'. *Ultrasound Obsteteric Gynacology*, 45: 452–8.

Swallow, V., Smith, T., Webb, N.J.A., Wirz, L., Qizalbash, L., Brennen, E., Birch, A., Sinha, M.D., Krischock, L., van der Voort, J., Kind D., Lambert, H., Milford, D.V., Crowther, L., Saleem, M., Lunn, A. and Williams, J. (2014) 'Distributed expertise: qualitative study of a British network of multidisciplinary teams supporting parents of children with chronic kidney disease'. *Child: Care, Health and Development*, 41 (1): 67–75.

CARE OF CHILDREN AND YOUNG PEOPLE WITH ENDOCRINE PROBLEMS

22

KATE DAVIES

THIS CHAPTER COVERS

- Recognition and nursing management of children with Type 1 Diabetes
- Recognition and nursing management of children with short stature
- Recognition and nursing management of children with congenital hypothyroidism

---

REQUIRED KNOWLEDGE

It would be helpful to have an understanding of the anatomy and physiology of the endocrine system before you start this chapter. Go to the A&P link: 'Endocrine system' at https://study.sagepub.com/essentialchildnursing

A&P LINK
22. 1:
ENDOCRINE
SYSTEM

> " Building a relationship and gaining trust with the patient and family is paramount. There is such satisfaction when you can see the difference in the patients and their families once this has been achieved, and how the care given improves outcomes on so many levels.
>
> **Paediatric endocrine specialist nurse**

Visit https://study.sagepub.com/essentialchildnursing to access a wealth of online resources for this chapter – watch out for the margin icons throughout the chapter.

INTRODUCTION

Endocrinology is the study of hormones, and along with the nervous and immune systems, is one of the most important systems in the body to maintain normal homeostasis (Davis, 2006, 2007). Glands in the body release hormones in response to hormones released from the pituitary gland in the brain. A lot of what is seen in a paediatric endocrine clinic focuses on growth and development, as growth problems are very common, and children with pubertal disorders are also seen. Diabetes also is commonly seen within paediatric endocrinology, with an incidence of around 1 in every 500 children (Raine et al., 2011), and various factors will be highlighted here with signposting to other resources. The importance of neonatal screening will also be discussed with reference to congenital hypothyroidism. Growth, diabetes and congenital hypothyroidism are the most common conditions seen in paediatric endocrinology (Raine et al., 2011). Whilst investigating these conditions, even though there is a medical focus, the children's nurse must not lose sight of the nursing process of Assess, Plan, Implement and Evaluate (Emerson and Northway, 2015): these will be demonstrated within the case studies.

SEE ALSO
CHAPTER 6

When caring for children with endocrine conditions and their families a team approach is paramount. The role of the endocrine specialist nurse within such an approach is key as indicated in the opening quotation. There are many more disorders within this speciality, which can be seen in Table 22.1.

Table 22.1 Conditions seen in paediatric endocrinology

WEBLINK:
BSPED
GUIDELINES

Condition	Average age of presentation	Signs and symptoms	Key guidelines/references
Type 1 diabetes	11–14 years	Blood glucose >11.1mmol/L	Guidelines from the British Society for Paediatric Endocrinology and Diabetes cover the management of Diabetic Keto-Acidosis (DKA) in children for Type 1 and Type 2 diabetes: www.bsped.org.uk/clinical/docs/DKAguideline.pdf British guidelines for the management of diabetes: www.nice.org.uk/guidance/ng18 International guidelines for the management of diabetes: http://web.ispad.org/resource-type/idfispad-2011-global-guideline-diabetes-childhood-and-adolescence
Congenital hyperinsulinism	Within 72 hours of birth	Hypoketotic hypoglycaemia	(Arnoux et al., 2010) www.unicef.org.uk/BabyFriendly/Resources/Guidance-for-Health-Professionals/Writing-policies-and-guidelines/Hypoglycaemia-policy-guidelines
Short stature	Childhood	Height <2 SD below the mean	www.childgrowthfoundation.org/CMS/FILES/01_Growth_and_Disorders.pdf
Turner syndrome	Prenatal, birth, childhood, adolescence	Short stature, some dysmorphia, ovarian dysgenesis	www.tss.org.uk/ UK support group www.bsped.org.uk/patients/docs/Turner_syndrome.pdf UK guidelines on the management of girls with Turner syndrome
Noonan syndrome	Childhood	Short stature, some dysmorphia, cardiac defects	

(Continued)

Table 22.1   (Continued)

Condition	Average age of presentation	Signs and symptoms	Key guidelines/references
Growth hormone insufficiency/ deficiency	Childhood	Short stature	(NICE, 2010) www.nice.org.uk/guidance/ta188
Small for gestational age	Birth	Small for dates	(Lee et al., 2001) Management of short children born short for gestational age *Pediatrics* 111 pp. 1253-1261
Tall stature	Childhood	Height > 2 SD above the mean	www.bsped.org.uk/patients/docs/TALL_ STATURE_2011_v2.pdf
Early puberty	Before 8 years in girls, 9 years in boys	Early pubertal development	www.bsped.org.uk/patients/docs/ PRECOCIOUS_PUBERTY_TR_VERSION.pdf
Delayed puberty	Adolescence	No secondary sexual development in girls by age 13 years, and boys age 14 years	www.bsped.org.uk/patients/docs/DELAYED_ PUBERTY_TR_version.pdf
Congenital hypothyroidism	Birth	Guthrie test	(Leger et al., 2014) (Vanderpump et al., 1996) Consensus statement for good practice and audit measures in the management of hypothyroidism and hyperthyroidism *British Medical Journal* 313 pp. 539-544 www.bsped.org.uk/patients/docs/NN_ CONGENITAL_HYPOTHYROIDISM_June2011.pdf
Graves' disease	Adolescence	Goitre, thyroid storm	www.bsped.org.uk/patients/docs/NN_GRAVES_ DISEASE_(THYROTOXICOSIS)_june2011.pdf
Neonatal thyrotoxicosis	First few days of life	Goitre, tachycardia, arrythmias	
Disorders of sex development	Birth	Genital ambiguity	www.bsped.org.uk/patients/docs/DSD.pdf
Cushing's syndrome	Childhood	Obesity, slow growth, cushingoid habitus	(Savage et al., 2008) Advances in the management of paediatric Cushing's disease *Hormone Research* 69 pp. 327-333
Adrenal insufficiency	Congenital or acquired	Hypoglycaemia, jaundice (newborn), tiredness, lack of energy (older children)	
Congenital adrenal hyperplasia	Congenital	Birth (females), first 2 weeks of life (males) (21-OHD)	(Clayton et al., 2002) www.bsped.org.uk/patients/docs/CAH_21_ HYDROXYLASE_revised.pdf

Condition	Average age of presentation	Signs and symptoms	Key guidelines/references
Diabetes insipidus	Congenital or acquired	Polyuria, polydipsia	www.bsped.org.uk/patients/docs/DIABETES_INSIPIDUS.pdf
Panhypopituitarism	Congenital or acquired	Combination of pituitary hormone deficiency symptoms	www.childgrowthfoundation.org/CMS/FILES/11_Multiple_Pituitary_Hormone_Deficiency.pdf
Rickets	Infancy, puberty	Family history, associated disease e.g. renal failure, malabsorption	(Wagner et al., 2008) Prevention of Rickets and Vitamin D Deficiency in Infants, Children, and Adolescents *Pediatrics* 122, 5 pp.1142-1152
Obesity	Birth, acquired	Increased weight gain	www.nationalobesityforum.org.uk www.bsped.org.uk/patients/docs/Overweight_old.pdf
Endocrine effects of cancer treatment	After treatment for cancer	Post treatment testing for hormone deficiencies	(Skinner, 2005) (Gleeson & Shalet, 2004) The impact of cancer therapy on the endocrine system in survivors of childhood brain tumours *Endocrine Related Cancer* 11 pp. 589-602 www.macmillan.org.uk/Documents/AboutUs/Newsroom/Consequences_of_Treatment_June2013.pdf www.aftercure.org

(Adapted from Raine et al. 2011)

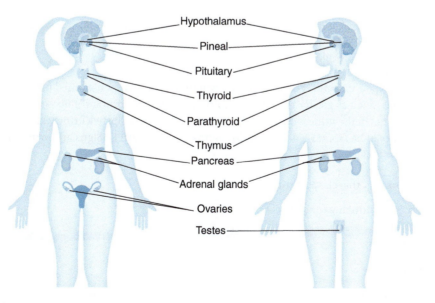

Figure 22.1 Major endocrine organs

RECOGNITION AND NURSING MANAGEMENT OF CHILDREN WITH TYPE 1 DIABETES

Diabetes Mellitus is classified as a group of metabolic disorders, with the overall characteristic of chronic hyperglycaemia, or an increased blood glucose level. There are many types, with Type 1 diabetes being the most commonly seen in childhood (McEvilly, 2003), but Type 2 has seen an increase in recent years (Dmitri, 2012). In 2009, around 25,000 children were living with Type 1 diabetes in the United Kingdom, which equates to approximately 1 in every 4,000–5,000 children. You would probably see one or two children per secondary school with Type 1 diabetes (Dmitri, 2012), so it is likely that you as a children's nurse will come across a child with Type 1 diabetes at some stage in your clinical practice.

In Type 1 diabetes, the pancreas fails to make insulin, due to autoimmune destruction of the beta cells in the Islets of Langherhans (McEvilly, 2003). This lack of insulin means the body fails to utilise the glucose, resulting in hyperglycaemia. The pancreas is about as big as your hand and is situated under the left rib cage towards the back of the abdominal cavity.

This hyperglycaemia leads to what is called an 'osmotic diuresis', which happens when the renal threshold for glucose is exceeded. This leads to polyuria – excessive urination – and polydipsia, which is excessive drinking. This can potentially lead to the child becoming dehydrated, especially if they have been vomiting. The lack of insulin also causes the breakdown of lipids, causing an excess of free fatty acids and ketones, which leads to ketones in the urine. This can cause a metabolic acidosis: acetone is responsible for the sweet-smelling breath, a bit like pear drops. If left untreated, the combination of this dehydration, acidosis and hyperosmolality can cause 'diabetic ketoacidosis', or DKA, and the child may become unconscious, with the potential to lead to a coma and eventually death (Raine et al., 2011).

ACTIVITY 22.1: CRITICAL THINKING

Critically reflect with your mentor on placement on how a child may present with DKA. How would you assess them, and how would you plan their care?

ACTIVITY
ANSWER 22.1

WEBLINK:
DIABETIC
KETOACIDOSIS

Read the article available at https://study.sagepub.com/essentialchildnursing to learn more about diabetic ketoacidosis.

Diagnosis of Type 1 diabetes is confirmed in a symptomatic child with a raised blood glucose level: this would be classified as greater than 11.1mmol/L, alongside glycosuria – glucose in the urine, and ketonuria – ketones in the urine, which can be easily tested for by a dipstick urine test. A normal blood glucose level should be around 3.9–5.8mmol/L (Butler and Kirk, 2011). Signs and symptoms are:

Early

- Most common – the 'classical triad':

    o   Excessive drinking (polydipsia)
    o   Polyuria
    o   Weight loss

- Less common:

    o   Enuresis (secondary)
    o   Skin sepsis
    o   *Candida* and other infections

Late – diabetic ketoacidosis

- Smell of acetone on breath
- Vomiting
- Dehydration
- Abdominal pain
- Hyperventilation due to acidosis (Kussmaul breathing)
- Hypovolaemic shock
- Drowsiness
- Coma and death. (Dmitri, 2012)

As the pancreas is not making any insulin, insulin replacement is needed, and a child is started on a regime of subcutaneous insulin. This is always a big shock for the child and their family, as the therapy will be lifelong, so an intensive, thorough multidisciplinary team educational programme is needed, which can involve the following members:

- Consultant paediatrician with a special interest in diabetes
- Consultant paediatric endocrinologist
- Paediatric diabetes specialist nurse
- Paediatric dietician
- Clinical psychologist
- Social worker
- Adult diabetologist for joint adolescent clinics
- Parent/patient support groups (Dmitri, 2012)

The diabetes team role is to support young people and their families in learning to manage 'their' diabetes in the way that they decide to, whilst optimising care to ensure good health in the present and their futures.

Kirsty Dring, clinical nurse specialist, paediatric diabetes

Now have a look at Scenario 22.1

SCENARIO 22.1: ADAM

A 15-month-old boy, Adam, presents to the local Accident and Emergency Department with a history of polyuria, polydipsia and lethargy. His blood glucose level is 23mmols/l and he is ketotic and acidotic. Type 1 diabetes is diagnosed and he is admitted to the ward. Once Adam has stabilised a discussion is had with his parents about the best insulin regimen for him to go on, and together the diabetes team and family decide that continuous subcutaneous insulin pump therapy is the way they would like to proceed. Adam and his parents meet with the different members of the diabetes team

(Continued)

(Continued)

to learn about the diagnosis. They meet with the dietician and begin to learn about carbohydrate counting and the diabetes specialist nurses to learn about Type 1 diabetes and how to use the insulin pump and test blood glucose levels. Adam often stays at his maternal grandparents' house so they are also invited to the ward to learn about the diagnosis and treatment. Prior to discharge, the parents' knowledge is assessed and they are deemed ready to go home. There is regular telephone contact with the diabetes nurses and Adam comes to weekly multidisciplinary clinic appointments whilst the family get used to managing diabetes at home.

- Who else might need to be educated to help the family manage diabetes?
- What other healthcare professionals might it be useful for the family to meet with at diagnosis?

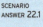

SCENARIO
ANSWER 22.1

VIDEO LINK
22.1: BLOOD
GLUCOSE
MEASURING

Focus here needs to be given on important factors, such as a good understanding of diabetes, how to give the insulin injections, a healthy diet, how to manage hypoglycaemic episodes, or 'hypos', and blood glucose fingerprick testing (Dmitri, 2012).

Watch the video on blood glucose measuring at https://study.sagepub.com/essentialchildnursing

Education needs to be child focused as well as for the family. Watch the video for children at https://study.sagepub.com/essentialchildnursing There are many resources available for children and families, and on how to manage diabetes in schools.

There are various types of insulin available, with differences in the onset and duration of action. These include:

VIDEO LINK
22.2:
DIABETES
CHILDREN'S
GUIDE

- Short-acting insulin, which starts working within 30 to 60 minutes, peaks at two to four hours, and lasts for five to eight hours
- Rapid-acting analogues, which start working within 15 minutes, peak at one to three hours and last for up to five hours
- Intermediate-acting insulin, which starts to work after two to four hours, peaks at 4 to 12 hours, and lasts between 12 and 24 hours

There are also longer-acting insulins and analogues, which can last for 24 hours, and pre-mixed insulins which are a mix of short- and intermediate-acting insulins.

Commonly used regimes for insulin therapy include twice-daily injections three times a day, multiple daily injections, and more recently continuous subcutaneous insulin infusion, commonly known as 'pumps' (Butler and Kirk, 2011).

Table 22.2 Different types of insulin

- Rapid-acting analogues can be injected just before, with or after food and have a peak action at 0–3 hours. They tend to last 2–5 hours and only last long enough for the meal at which they are taken. They are clear in appearance.
- Long-acting analogues tend to be injected once a day to provide background insulin, lasting for approximately 24 hours. They don't need to be taken with food because they don't have a peak action. They are clear in appearance.

- Ultra long-acting analogues are mainly used by people who are unable to inject themselves as they can provide background insulin for up to 42 hours. They should be injected once at any time of the day, preferably at the same time. They don't need to be taken with food because they don't have a peak action. They are clear in appearance.
- Short-acting insulins should be injected 15-30 minutes before a meal to cover the rise in blood glucose levels that occurs after eating. They have a peak action of 2-6 hours and can last for up to eight hours. They are clear in appearance.
- Medium- and long-action insulins are taken once or twice a day to provide background insulin or in combination with short-acting insulins/rapid-acting analogues. Their peak activity is 4-12 hours and can last up to 30 hours. They are cloudy in appearance.
- Mixed insulin – a combination of medium- and short-acting insulin.
- Mixed analogue – a combination of medium-acting insulin and rapid-acting analogue.

Hypoglycaemia or 'hypos'

Hypoglycaemia is classified as a blood glucose level less than 4mmol/L, and hypos can happen occasionally (Hanas, 2015). There are many reasons why a hypo can occur, and there are many symptoms that children may experience:

- Too little to eat, or a delayed meal
- Skipping a meal
- Neglecting to eat, despite symptoms of hypoglycaemia
- Physical exercise, which increases the risk of hypoglycaemia for the rest of the day and the following night
- Too large a dose of insulin
- New site for the injection – for example, from the thigh to the abdomen or to a site free of fatty lumps (lipohypertrophy)
- Recent hypoglycaemia – the glucose stores in the liver may be depleted, or there are fewer warning symptoms of hypoglycaemia (hypoglycaemic unawareness)
- Very low HbA1c (increased risk of hypoglycaemia awareness)
- Drinking alcohol
- Not mixing the cloudy insulin thoroughly enough
- Variable insulin absorption
- Gastroenteritis or tummy upset
- Certain drugs used for the treatment of high blood pressure (Hanas, 2015. Reproduced with kind permission of Class Publishing)

The way to deal with a hypo is to raise the blood glucose level back to within normal limits, which is 4–7mmol/L. This can include giving glucose tablets, orange juice or a fizzy drink, and then some complex carbohydrates, such as a biscuit or bread. If it is more severe, then a sugary gel can be rubbed into the lips or gums, or a glucagon injection may need to be administered. It is essential that children are educated early on the importance of recognising their symptoms and how to manage them.

VIDEO LINK
22.3: HYPOS
AND HYPERS

See the video on a guide to hypos and hypers at https://study.sagepub.com/essentialchildnursing

Long-term management

The aim is for the child and family to live as normal a life as possible, both at home and at school, with good diabetic control. Education on diet is essential, avoiding too many sugary foods and optimum blood glucose measuring. Liaising with the diabetes team is essential, including regular contact in the outpatients' clinic, where discussion will focus on overall wellbeing, growth and development, compliance and assessing HbA1c. This is a small blood test measuring glycosylated haemoglobin, and can give a view of overall control from the previous 6–12 weeks (Dmitri, 2012). Plans need to be in place with school, and diabetes nurse specialists can form and implement care plans, which will need to be evaluated regularly to ensure the child's continuing progress.

As the child enters adolescence, the diabetes can interfere with several elements (see Table 22.3).

Table 22.3 How diabetes interferes with normal adolescence

Normal adolescence	How diabetes interferes with normal adolescence
Physical and sexual maturation	Delayed sexual maturation
	Invasion of privacy with frequent medical examinations
Conformity with peer group	Meals must be eaten on time
	Frequent injections and blood tests
Self-image	Hypoglycaemic attacks show that they are different
Self-esteem	Impaired body image
Independence from parents	Parental over-protection and reluctance to allow their child to be away from home
	Battles over diabetes
Economic independence	Loading of insurance premiums
	Discrimination by employers
	Statutory rules against becoming a pilot or driving heavy goods or public service vehicles

Source: Dmitri (2012)

Again, close liaison with the healthcare professionals involved can help in dealing with these issues in a way that is individualised to the child and increases compliance.

Children with diabetes do need regular assessment and these assessments can help the child grow and develop optimally.

Some key aspects of diabetic assessment in children:

- Any episodes of hyopoglycaemia, diabetic ketoacidosis, hospital admission?
- Is there still awareness of hypoglycaemia?
- Absence from school? School supportive of diabetes care?
- Interference with normal life?
- HbA1c results – 58mmol/mol (7.5%) or less?
- Diary of blood glucose results – if monitoring, are they reacting to results?
- Insulin regimen – appropriate? Correction bolus doses given?
- Lipohypertrophy or lipoatrophy at injection sites?
- Diet – healthy diet, manipulating food intake and insulin to maintain good control?

General overview (periodic):

- Normal growth and pubertal development, avoiding obesity – measure each visit
- Blood pressure – check for hypertension yearly (age-specific centiles)

- Renal disease – screening for microalbuminuria yearly from 12 years
- Eyes – photography for retinopathy or cataracts, yearly from 12 years
- Feet – maintaining good care – yearly
- Screening for coeliac and thyroid disease at diagnosis, thyroid screening yearly, coeliac again after three years or if weight gain is poor
- Annual reminder to have flu vaccination

Knowledge and psychosocial aspects:

- Good understanding of diabetes – would participation/holidays with other diabetic children be beneficial? Member of Diabetes UK?
- Becoming self-reliant, but appropriate supervision at home, school, diabetic team?
- Taking exercise, sport? Diabetes not interfering with it?
- Leading as normal a life as possible?
- Smoking, alcohol?
- Is 'hypo' treatment readily available? Is stepped approach known?
- What are the main issues for the patient? Are there short-term goals to allow engagement with improving control? (Dmitri, 2012)

WHAT'S THE EVIDENCE?

Now that you understand a little bit about diabetes in children, please study the guidelines developed by The British Society of Paediatric Endocrinology and Diabetes (BSPED), www.bsped.org.uk/clinical/clinical_endorsedguidelines.aspx). Here, you will find guidance for medical and nursing staff, as well as families, on DKA, and managing diabetes when a child is ill. See if these guidelines are in place in the clinical environment you are in. If not, what is in place instead and why do you think it is managed differently?

RECOGNITION AND NURSING MANAGEMENT OF CHILDREN WITH SHORT STATURE

To have a full understanding of the diagnosis of short stature, it is important to have an idea of what normal growth in childhood is like. Growth is affected by an interaction of genetic, nutritional and hormonal factors. Adequate nutrition is mostly responsible for growth in infancy, whereas hormones such as growth hormone (GH), insulin-like growth factor (IGF-1) and thyroid hormones play more of a central role throughout childhood (Shetty and Warner, 2012). Genetics are also important – short parents are more likely to have short children, and short stature is also associated with syndromes such as Turner syndrome and Down's syndrome. Growth in childhood can be split into three categories: infancy, childhood and puberty (Raine et al., 2011) (see Table 21.4).

Growth assessment

This area is one of the most important aspects to consider when assessing a child, and it is important that it is done correctly. In the UK, children are measured in Reception class (age 4) and in Year 6 (at the end of primary school).

Table 22.4   Growth in childhood

Infancy

- First two years of life
- Driven by nutrition
- Rapid growth

Grow approximately 25cm in the first year

Childhood

- Dependent on growth hormone
- Period of time when children with growth hormone deficiency present with short stature
- Height velocity is around 4-8 cm/year

Little difference in the growth rate between boys and girls

Puberty

- Height velocity doubles
- Pubertal growth spurt starts two years earlier in girls than boys
- Growth hormone and sex steroids now involved
- Girls grow around 8cm/year at their peak height velocity, and boys 10cm/year

Puberty hormones also end growth, by fusing the growth plates at the ends of the bones

Source: Martin and Collin (2015)

WEBLINK:
MEASURING
IN SCHOOLS

VIDEO LINK
22.4:
GROWTH IN
CHILDREN

VIDEO LINK
22.5:
MEASURING
CHILDREN

WEBLINK:
MEASURING
CYP

WEBLINK:
GROWTH
CHARTS

WHAT'S THE EVIDENCE?

Have a look at the information on https://study.sagepub.com/essentialchildnursing regarding measuring in schools.

What do you think about measuring all children in schools? Do you think it is a good idea? Some parents may refuse for their child to be weighed and measured. Why do you think they might do this? Watch the video on growth in children at https://study.sagepub.com/essentialchildnursing to help you.

Many measurements are taken when assessing a child's growth, including their height (Figure 21.3), their sitting height (most often usually done in paediatric endocrine clinics), length in babies, head circumference in babies (Figure 22.2) and their weight. Watch the clip on https://study.sagepub.com/essentialchildnursing to see how it is done properly. There is additional information here from the website at Great Ormond Street Hospital for Children.

Once the measurements are taken, they need to be properly plotted on an appropriate growth chart (Cole, 2002). Go to https://study.sagepub.com/essentialchildnursing to see the growth charts used in the UK.

Specific centile lines on the charts can show you the percentage of measurements that have higher or lower values than the measurements you have plotted (Martin and Collin, 2015). It is important to take measurements over a period of time to show the child's height velocity – the speed at which they are growing – and whether it is in the normal limits for their age and sex, and in line with their parents' heights (Martin and Collin, 2015). Only now can the diagnosis of short stature be considered. Data can also be collected in the parent-held 'red books' for children under the age of 5.

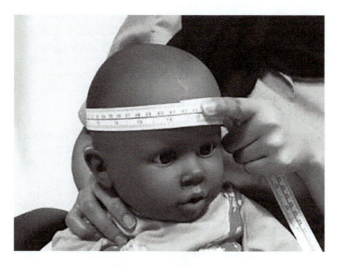

Figure 22.2   Correct measurement of head circumference

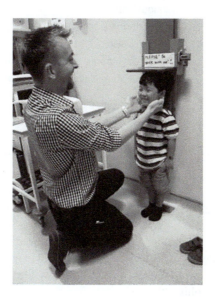

Figure 22.3   Measuring a child

Causes of short stature

Short stature is one of the most common reasons a child is referred to a paediatric endocrine clinic (Martin and Collin, 2015; Raine et al., 2011). There are many causes for a child to be small, as seen in Table 22.5 below:

Table 22.5 Causes of short stature

Non-pathological	Constitutional delay of growth and puberty
	Familial short stature
	Nutritional issues
	Emotional deprivation
	Intrauterine growth retardation
Intrauterine growth retardation/ restriction	Syndromes – including Russell Silver syndrome
	Non-syndromic
Systemic disorders	Cardiovascular disease
	Renal, including chronic renal failure
	Respiratory, including asthma and cystic fibrosis
	Gastrointestinal, including inflammatory bowel disease, Crohn's, coeliac disease
	Neurological
	Psychosocial, including anorexia, child abuse and neglect
Endocrine causes	Growth hormone-related causes
	Growth hormone deficiency, isolated or combined with multiple pituitary hormone deficiency
	Growth hormone resistance
	Hypothyroidism
	Cushing's syndrome
	Exogenous steroid administration and glucocorticoid excess
Chromosomal and genetic causes	Turner syndrome
	Noonan syndrome
	Down's syndrome
	Skeletal dysplasia
	Prader-Willi syndrome

Source: Laing (2014)

From *British Journal of Nursing.* © 2015 MA Healthcare Ltd. Reproduced by permission of MA Healthcare Ltd.

To ascertain the cause of the short stature, other investigations need to be performed, including blood tests. These blood tests can rule out other reasons why the child may be short – for example, anaemia, malabsorption, renal disease, Crohn's disease, or even Turner syndrome (Raine et al., 2011; Cheetham and Davies, 2014; Davies and Collin, 2015).

The most common endocrine reason for a child being short is growth hormone deficiency (Raine et al., 2011). This is seen in around 1 in every 4,000 children (Martin and Collin, 2015). Treatment is given by a once daily injection of growth hormone. To enable children to be prescribed this treatment, they need to be investigated further beyond simple blood tests, by being admitted to a children's ward for day case investigations (Davies and Collin, 2015). This is because a simple one-off blood test to look at growth hormone levels would not work, as the levels in the blood are known as 'pulsatile' – that is, they go up and down throughout the day. The correct diagnosis is then made by examining the results of these tests in order for the child to receive the correct treatment.

SCENARIO 22.2: JOHNNY

Johnny is a 21-month-old boy referred to the paediatric endocrine and growth clinic for poor growth. Johnny was referred by his health visitor who reported his growth was within the lower end of normal range but his parent had 'insisted' on the referral. On assessment at his first clinic appointment Johnny was below the 1st centile on his growth chart, but his projected height in accordance with his parents' heights was on the 31st centile.

Johnny's growth was monitored in clinic over the next year and he continued just below the 1st centile. Johnny's growth hormone production was assessed using a Glucagon stimulation test, showing his highest growth hormone (GH) level to be only 4.4micrograms/L (normal range: >7micrograms/L) which qualified him for GH treatment.

The paediatric endocrine nurse (PEN) then met with Johnny's parents in clinic to demonstrate a range of GH delivery devices. There was discussion about the pros and cons of each device, plus nursing and prescription support offered by each of the homecare delivery companies.

- Good compliance to GH treatment is essential for it to work effectively. What factors do you think contributed to Johnny's good compliance?
- Growth hormone is delivered by subcutaneous injection. What are some nursing considerations regarding subcutaneous injections in children?

SCENARIO
ANSWER 22.2

Children have to remain on growth hormone until they have stopped growing (Clayton et al., 2005; Davies and Ibbotson, 2008), and then sometimes even longer (Brod et al., 2014), especially if they are still growth hormone deficient when final height is achieved. Children and their parents/carers can choose which growth hormone pen device to have: this has been shown to possibly increase compliance (Spoudeas et al., 2014; van Dongen and Kaptein, 2012) as obviously children will not like taking an injection every day.

As there are so many causes for short stature, as a children's nurse you should keep up to date in your clinical practice. Children are weighed and measured as part of best practice not only within the outpatients' department during clinic visits, but also when they are admitted to children's wards. The nursing process is very clear during the assessment of short stature, as accurate growth assessment is vital to aid diagnosis.

> It's a relief to finally reach a point where we will be starting the growth hormone and to see how much difference it will make in Henry's growth … I feel very happy for him that he had this opportunity to have growth hormone
>
> **Karen, parent**

Read more about growth hormone in the article on https://study.sagepub.com/essentialchildnursing

WEBLINK:
GROWTH
HORMONE

RECOGNITION AND NURSING MANAGEMENT OF CHILDREN WITH CONGENITAL HYPOTHYROIDISM

The diagnosis of congenital hypothyroidism is one of the most common conditions seen in a paediatric endocrine clinic, with an incidence of around 1 in every 4,000 births in the UK (Raine et al., 2011). There are many causes, including an error in thyroid synthesis, iodine deficiency, thyroid stimulating hormone (TSH) deficiency, which is linked with multiple pituitary hormone deficiency, but the most common cause is where the thyroid gland has not positioned itself where it should be from foetal development, or 'maldescent of the thyroid' (Dmitri, 2012). Girls are twice as likely to be affected as boys, and there is an increased risk in babies born with Down's syndrome (Butler and Kirk, 2011; Tuysuz and Beker, 2001).

A&P LINK 22.2: THYROID

A&P LINK

To remind yourself of the relevant anatomy and physiology, please read the A&P link: 'Thyroid gland' at https://study.sagepub.com/essentialchildnursing

The hypothalamus in the brain releases thyrotropin releasing hormone (TRH), which in turn stimulates the release of thyroid stimulating hormone (TSH) from the pituitary gland. TSH tells the thyroid gland to make triiodothyronine (T3) and thyroxine (T4) (Bursell and Warner, 2007). The main job of the thyroid gland is to regulate the body's metabolism (Sanders, 2003).

Newborn screening

Testing for congenital hypothyroidism is now done on day five of life in the 'Guthrie test' – a heelprick blood test done by the midwife in hospital or at home (see Figure 22.4).

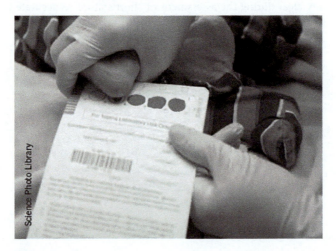

Figure 22.4 The Guthrie test

Source: www.sciencephoto.com

ACTIVITY 22.2: CRITICAL THINKING

- Have a look at the NHS screening programme guide on testing for congenital hypothyroidism via https://study.sagepub.com/essentialchildnursing
- What other conditions are screened for during the newborn screening test?

ACTIVITY
ANSWER 22.2

WEBLINK:
TESTING FOR CH

PRACTICE
SCENARIO 22:
RUBY

You can read more on hypothyroidism in the article at https://study.sagepub.com/essentialchildnursing

Since babies are screened so early on in life, it is unlikely that they will show any symptoms. Early detection, and therefore treatment, is vital as it can prevent neurodevelopmental disability (Leger et al., 2014) and growth failure (Jones et al., 2006). However, if babies are not tested, the symptoms described below may become apparent:

WEBLINK:
HYPOTHYROIDISM

- Failure to thrive
- Feeding problems
- Prolonged jaundice
- Constipation
- Pale, cold, mottled, dry skin
- Coarse facies (for example a large bulging head or prominent scalp veins)
- Large tongue
- Hoarse cry
- Goitre (occasionally)
- Umbilical hernia
- Delayed development
- Wide posterior fontanelle
- Hypothermia
- Peripheral cyanosis
- Oedema (Dmitri, 2012; Raine et al., 2011)

SEE ALSO
CHAPTERS
14 AND 32

Diagnosis is confirmed by a raised TSH level in the blood from the heelprick test. Diagnostic limits vary around the UK, but if the TSH level is ≥ 10mU/L, a second sample is usually requested a week later. If this is still high, the baby's diagnosis is confirmed. A normal level of TSH in the blood is 0.27 – 4.20mU/L (Butler and Kirk, 2011). Radioisotope scanning of the baby's thyroid gland is sometimes performed (Perry et al., 2006; Raine et al., 2011), which may show a kind of transient hypothyroidism, or sometimes an ultrasound scan.

Treatment is with levothyroxine, which comes in liquid or tablet formation, and is lifelong. Clinic visits will be necessary as the child grows for regular blood tests and dose changes.

ACTIVITY 22.3: REFLECTIVE PRACTICE

Think about the role of patient support groups whilst watching the BTF video on https://study.sage pub.com/essentialchildnursing

VIDEO
LINK 22.6:
THYROID
PROBLEMS
IN CHILDREN

> " Having a placement on an endocrinology ward is really exciting and such a valuable experience. As a student you will be able to learn and gain practice in many clinical skills that are very rare on other wards. For example, you will be able to engage in performing blood glucose measurements under supervision, To prepare for this, it is recommended that you look up the acceptable parameter for blood glucose and what the intervention would be if the reading was outside of the parameter, what equipment is needed to measure blood glucose and how to document the blood glucose reading. Another clinical skill that can be undertaken as a student is administering injections under supervision. It is recommended that you look up the main routes of injections, sub-cutaneous and intra-muscular, the angle they need to be administered at for full effectiveness, how to dispose of the sharps and what to do if you obtain a sharps injury. It would also be helpful to read about the endocrine system: what hormones are, where they are specifically secreted from and what their role is within the body.
>
> **Natalie, 3rd-year children's nursing student** "

PLACEMENT ADVICE 22: ENDOCRINE PROBLEMS

Go to https://study.sagepub.com/essentialchildnursing for tips on preparing for placements and health promotion when working with children with endocrine problems.

HEALTH PROMOTION 22: ENDOCRINE PROBLEMS

CHAPTER SUMMARY

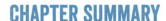

- Diabetes is one of the most common endocrine conditions in children with an incidence of around 1 in every 500 children
- Many of the endocrine conditions affecting children relate to growth and development
- Recognising that endocrine conditions have a wide-ranging impact on the child and family is essential
- Team working is crucial and this should straddle hospital, school and home

BUILD YOUR BIBLIOGRAPHY

Books

- Hanas, R. (2015) *Type 1 Diabetes in Children, Adolescents and Young Adults*. Bridgwater: Class Health.

  This has been described as the 'bible' for everything you need to know about type 1 diabetes in children. It is written in a very easy to understand style, and is a useful resource for the whole multidisciplinary team.

- Raine, J.E., Donaldson, M.D.C., Gregory, J.W. and van Vliet, G. (eds) (2011) *Practical Endocrinology and Diabetes in Children*, 3rd edn. Chichester: Wiley-Blackwell.

  Although this book focuses on diabetes as well, it covers all you need to know on paediatric endocrinology. It is medically focused, and it relates the details in a factual manner, and is a 'must go to' initial resource for anyone interested in paediatric endocrinology. There are separate chapters on growth and thyroid disorders.

Journal articles

Go to https://study.sagepub.com/essentialchildnursing for further free online journal articles related to this chapter.

FURTHER READING: ONLINE JOURNAL ARTICLES

- Mallare, J.T., Cordice, C.C., Ryan, B.A., Carey, D.E., Kreitzer, P.M. and Frank, G.R. (2003) 'Identifying risk factors for the development of diabetic ketoacidosis in new onset type 1 diabetes mellitus'. *Clinical Pediatrics*, 42 (7): 591-7.

  Read the above article to learn more about the DKA risk factors.

- Hardin, D.S., Kemp, S.F. and Allen, D.B. (2007) 'Twenty years of recombinant human growth hormone in children: relevance to pediatric care providers'. *Clinical Pediatrics*, 46 (4): 279-86.

  Read more information on the history of the use of growth hormone in children

- Cameo, T., Gumer, L.B., Williams, K.M., Gomez, J., McMahon, D.J. and Oberfield, S.E. (2013) 'A retrospective review of newborn screening for congenital hypothyroidism and newborn thyroid disease at a major medical center'. *Clinical Pediatrics*, 52 (11): 1054-8.
  Read more on newborn screening here.

Weblinks

Go to https://study.sagepub.com/essentialchildnursing for further weblinks related to this chapter.

FURTHER READING: WEBLINKS

These are the key support groups with excellent resources and societies providing care pathways and guidelines.

- Diabetes UK

  www.diabetes.org.uk
  www.jdrf.org

- Child Growth Foundation

  www.childgrowthfoundation.org

- The Pituitary Foundation

  www.pituitary.org.uk

- Living with CAH

  www.livingwithcah.com

- Verity

  www.verity-pcos.org.uk

- British Thyroid Foundation

  www.btf-thyroid.org

- Turner Syndrome Support Society

  http://tss.org.uk

- DSD Families

  www.dsdfamilies.org

- British Society for Paediatric Endocrinology and Diabetes

  www.bsped.org.uk

- European Society for Paediatric Endocrinology

  www.eurospe.org

- Society for Endocrinology

  www.endocrinology.org

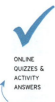

ONLINE
QUIZZES &
ACTIVITY
ANSWERS

GREAT FOR
REVISION!

ACE YOUR ASSESSMENT

Revise what you have learned by visiting https://study.sagepub.com/essentialchildnursing

- Test yourself with multiple-choice and short-answer questions
- Do the chapter activities in the book and check your answers online

REFERENCES

Arnoux, J-B., de Lonlay, P., Ribeiro, M-J., Hussain, K., Blankenstein, O., Mohnike, K., Valayannopoulos, V., Robert, J-J., Rahier, J., Sempoux, C., Bellanné, C., Verkarre, V., Aigrain, Y., Jaubert, F., Brunelle, F. and Nihoul-Fékété, C. (2010) 'Congenital hyperinsulinism'. *Early Human Development,* 86: 287–94.

Brod, M., Hojbjerre, L., Adalsteinsson, J.E. and Rasmussen, M.H. (2014) 'Assessing the impact of growth hormone deficiency and treatment in adults: development of a new disease-specific measure'. *J Clin Endocrinol Metab,* 99: 1204–12.

Bursell, J.D.H. and Warner J.T. (2007) 'Interpretation of thyroid function in children'. *Paediatrics and Child Health,* 17: 361–6.

Butler, G. and Kirk, J. (2011) *Paediatric Endocrinology and Diabetes.* Oxford: OUP Press.

Cheetham, T. and Davies, J.H. (2014) 'Investigation and management of short stature'. *Arch Dis Child.*

Clayton, P.E., Cuneo, R.C., Juul, A., Monson, J.P., Shalet, S.M. and Tauber, M. (2005) 'Consensus statement on the management of the GH treated adolescent in the transition to adult care'. *European Journal of Endocrinology,* 152: 165–70.

Clayton, P.E., Miller, W.L., Oberfield, S.E., Ritzen, E.M., Sippell, W.G. and Speiser, P.W. (2002) 'Consensus statement on 21 Hydroxylase deficiency from the Lawson Wilkins Pediatric Endocrine Society and the European Society of Paediatric Endocrinology'. *The Journal of Clinical Endocrinology & Metabolism,* 87: 4048–53.

Cole, T.J. (2002) 'Assessment of growth'. *Best Pract Res Clin Endocrinol Metab,* 16: 383–98.

Davies, K. and Collin, J. (2015) 'Understanding clinical investigations in children's endocrinology'. *Nursing Children and Young People,* 27: 26–36.

Davies, K. and Ibbotson, V. (2008) *Transition in Growth Hormone Therapy.* London: Haymarket Publishing.

Davis, G. (2006/2007) 'Hormonal control and the endocrine system: achieving homeostasis'. *Nurse Prescribing,* 4: 446–53.

Dmitri, P. (2012) 'Endocrine and metabolic disorders', in *Illustrated Textbook of Paediatrics,* 4th edn (Lissauer, T. and Clayden, G. eds). Edinburgh: Mosby/Elsevier.

Emerson, K. and Northway, R. (2015) 'Patient, service user, family and carer perspectives', in *Essentials of Nursing Practice* (Delves-Yates, C. ed.). London: Sage..

Gleeson, H.K. and Shalet, S.M. (2004) 'The impact of cancer therapy on the endocrine system in survivors of childhood brain tumours'. *Endocrine Related Cancer,* 11: 589–602.

Hanas, R. (2015) *Type 1 Diabetes in Children, Adolescents and Young Adults,* 6th edn. Somerset: Class Health.

Jones, J.H., Mackenzie, J., Croft, G.A., Beaton, S., Young, D. and Donaldson, M.D.C. (2006) 'Improvement in screening performance and diagnosis of congenital hypothyroidsim in Scotland 1979–2003'. *Archives of Diseases in Childhood,* 91: 680–5.

Laing, P. (2014) 'Growth failure and hormone therapy'. *British Journal of Nursing,* 23, S3-9.

Lee, P.A., Chernausek, S.D., Hokken-Koelga, A.C.S. and Czernichow, P. (2001) 'Management of short children born small for gestational age'. *Pediatrics,* 111: 1253–61.

Leger, J., Olivieri, A., Donaldson, M., Torresani, T., Krude, H., van Vliet, G., Polak, M., Butler, G., ESPE-PES-SLEP-JSPE-APEG-APPES-ISPAE and Congenital Hypothyroidism Consensus Conference G (2014) 'European Society for Paediatric Endocrinology consensus guidelines on screening, diagnosis, and management of congenital hypothyroidism'. *J Clin Endocrinol Metab,* 99: 363–84.

Martin, L. and Collin, J. (2015) 'An introduction to growth and atypical growth in childhood and adolescence'. *Nursing Children and Young People,* 27: 29–37.

McEvilly, A. (2003) 'Diabetes Mellitus', in *Paediatrics: A Clinical Guide for Nurse Practitioners* (Barnes, K. ed.). Edinburgh: Butterworth & Heinemann.

NICE (2010) *TA188 Human Growth Hormone (Somatropin) for the Treatment of Growth Failure in Children: Guidance.* London: Department of Health.

Perry, R.J., Maroo, S., Maclennan, A.C., Jones, J.H. and Donaldson, M.D.C. (2006) 'Combined ultrasound and isotope scanning is more informative in the diagnosis of congenital hypothyroidism than single scanning'. *Archives of Diseases in Childhood,* 91: 972–6.

Raine, J.E., Donaldson, M.D.C., Gregory, J.W. and van Vliet, G. (2011) *Practical Endocrinology and Diabetes in Children,* 3rd edn. Chichester: Wiley-Blackwell.

Sanders, S. (2003) *Endocrine and Reproductive Systems,* 2nd edn. London: Mosby.

Savage, M.O., Chan, L.F., Afshar, F., Plowman, P.N., Grossman, A.B. and Storr, H.L. (2008) 'Advances in the management of paediatric Cushing's disease'. *Hormone Research,* 69: 327– 33.

Shetty, A. and Warner, J. (2012) 'An approach to the evaluation and assessment of a short child'. *Welsh Paediatrics Journal,* 37: 6–11.

Skinner, R. (2005) *Therapy Based Long Term Follow Up: Practice Statement.* Pfizer & UKCCSG.

Spoudeas, H.A., Bajaj, P. and Sommerford, N. (2014) 'Maintaining persistence and adherence with subcutaneous growth-hormone therapy in children: comparing jet-delivery and needle-based devices'. *Patient Prefer Adherence,* 8: 1255–63.

Tuysuz, B. and Beker DB (2001) 'Thyroid dysfunction in children with Down's syndrome'. *Acta Paediatrics,* 90: 1389–93.

van Dongen, N. and Kaptein, A.A. (2012) 'Parents' views on growth hormone treatment for their children: psychosocial issues'. *Patient Prefer Adherence,* 6: 547–53.

Vanderpump, M.P.J., Ahlquist, J.A.O., Franklyn, J.A. and Clayton, R.N. (1996) 'Consensus statement for good practice and audit measures in the management of hypothyroidism and hyperthyroidism'. *British Medical Journal,* 313: 539–44.

Wagner, C.L., Greer, F.R., and the Section on Breastfeeding and Committee on Nutrition (2008) 'Prevention of rickets and vitamin D deficiency in infants, children, and adolescents'. *Pediatrics,* 122: 1142–52.

The author would like to thank the following practitioners for their assistance:

Christine Davies, Paediatric Endocrine Specialist Nurse, Children's Hospital for Wales, Cardiff
Kirsty Dring, Clinical Nurse Specialist in Paediatric Diabetes, St. George's Hospital, London
Lee Martin, Clinical Nurse Specialist in Paediatric Endocrinology, The Royal London Hospital, London

CARE OF CHILDREN AND YOUNG PEOPLE WITH IMMUNOLOGICAL PROBLEMS

23

KATIE WARBURTON

THIS CHAPTER COVERS

- Anatomy and physiology
- How do childhood immunisations work?
- Primary immune deficiencies
- HIV

REQUIRED KNOWLEDGE

A&P LINK 23.1:
IMMUNE SYSTEM

It would be helpful to have an understanding of the anatomy and physiology of the immune system before you start this chapter. Go to the A&P link: 'Immune system' at https://study.sagepub.com/essentialchildnursing

> "
> The trembling fear of 'Will I be neglected by the ones I call my friends?' Will I meet the end? Or will I be trapped by the stigma? My strength is only becoming stronger, not weaker. I fight my emotions with a smile on front. When nobody knows the true feelings; how can I be happy when I can't be me? It seems like the only way of being happy is being free. I am a fighter and I've fought this long, soon, very soon, the happiness, it won't be long. It's me against the world. What could possibly go wrong?
>
> **Zoe White, CHIVA Youth Committee, 2015**
> "

Visit https://study.sagepub.com/essentialchildnursing to access a wealth of online resources for this chapter–watchout for the margin icons throughout the chapter.

INTRODUCTION

The immune system must identify foreign agents and stimulate a defence to protect the body. An ineffective response may be caused by a deficiency of the immune system, whereas an inappropriate immune response may result in allergy, transplant rejection or autoimmune diseases. An ineffective immune system leaves the host susceptible to infections including viruses, bacteria, protozoa, fungi, worms and tumours. Common infections seen in children's nursing include those caused by bacteria and viruses. Bacteria are organisms able to reproduce independently. In practice they are seen to cause disease such as Pneumococcal, Meningitis and Pneumonia. However, viruses – including measles, chickenpox and HIV – cannot replicate without the use of cells within the person. Infection is a common reason for hospitalisation and community nursing input. You should be able to assess, plan, implement and evaluate care with the necessary knowledge to underpin decision-making. Children with an immune deficiency may present with minimal symptoms of severe infection.

ANATOMY AND PHYSIOLOGY

It is important that you have a good understanding of the immune system to understand immunological problems. Table 23.1 will help you revise the important components of the immune system. For further help see 'required knowledge' at the start of this chapter.

A&PLINK
23.2: IMMUNE
SYSTEM

Table 23.1 Components of the immune system

Lymphocytes	White blood cells are produced in the bone marrow and travel in the lymphatic and circulatory systems, identifying or responding to foreign agents. B and T lymphocytes have important roles in the acquired immune response. They are found in circulating blood or lymph or at specific lymphatic sites. T lymphocytes travel to the thymus where they mature and later further divide in to cytotoxic, helper or suppressor T cells. Cytotoxic T lymphocytes destroy infected cells and instruct phagocytes to support the destruction of pathogens. B lymphocytes can become plasma cells and produce antibodies to target antigens when instructed to do so by T lymphocytes
Antibodies	Also known as immunoglobulins. They are plasma proteins split in to five main classes: IgM, IgA, IgG, IgE and IgD. Immunoglobulins are Y-shaped molecules that are able to bind to antigens. Antibodies, produced by B lymphocytes, respond to specific antigens. They may individually neutralise and destroy the antigen, be destroyed with the antigen by macrophages or neutrophils, or trigger the complement cascade to destroy the antigen
Major histocompatibility complex (MHC)	MHC is a group of genes; MHC molecules allow T lymphocytes to identify cells containing foreign organisms by expressing peptides on the outside of the invaded cell. MHC plays an important role in tissue typing and tissue rejection
Natural killer cells	Are a type of lymphocyte and capable of destroying virus-infected cells and some tumour cells. They work closely with cytokines as part of the initial response to viruses
Macrophages	Developed from monocytes. They are phagocytic cells, which means they can ingest foreign substances or damaged cells. Some macrophages relate to the specific tissue in which they are found (e.g. Kupffer cells are found in the liver). They are one of the body's first defence mechanisms when a foreign agent is seen
Cytokines	Small proteins initially released following the attempt of macrophages to destroy foreign agents. They have a key signalling role

(Continued)

Table 23.1   (Continued)

Dendritic cells	These cells have the important role of presenting antigens to T lymphocytes. Langerhans Cells are specific dendritic cells found in the skin
Complement	A cascade of proteins that highlight and support the destruction of antigens by following a pathway of triggers. Complement is often activated by antibodies. The complement system plays an important role in phagocytosis
Neutrophils	A type of white blood cell with phagocytic properties. They particularly attack bacteria

Immune system deficiencies may be described as innate or acquired. Primary immune deficiencies predominantly have a genetic cause and are evident from birth. Acquired immune deficiencies include human immunodeficiency virus (HIV), an infection the body is unable to eradicate.

Innate immunity

Innate immune responses are the body's natural defence mechanisms. These defences include the skin, gastric acid, cilia, cytokines, complement cascade and phagocytic cells. The innate immune system has no memory of exposure or response.

If this is not successful, the acquired immune response is stimulated through chemical signalling by cytokines, which work as part of the innate and acquired immune system.

Acquired immunity

Acquired immunity is developed through exposure to infection generated through disease or vaccination. Memory will be developed so further exposure will result in immediate defence. Young children are exposed to infection through socialisation, amongst other things, which also supports the development of the immune system. However, immunisations are a vital part of developing acquired immunity.

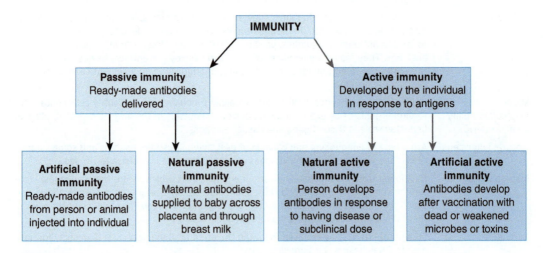

Figure 23.1   Types of immunity

HOW DO CHILDHOOD IMMUNISATIONS WORK?

The World Health Organization (WHO, 2015a) highlighted that 19.2 million children did not receive basic immunisations in 2015 despite recognition that immunisation prevents 2–3 million childhood deaths a year. The purpose of vaccines is to create long-term immunity, similar to that which would follow disease, but without illness. Health practitioners involved in the administration of vaccines must be competent, have the ability to provide current, accurate information to children and families and deliver safe, effective, high standards of care (Health Protection Agency, 2005).

The history of vaccination could be said to commence with the development of the smallpox vaccine in 1798. Although Edward Jenner was not the first to identify the process of inoculation or immunisation, his work is described as instrumental in the eradication of the disease and development of immunology (Riedel, 2005).

Vaccines are produced using live attenuated or killed organisms. Live attenuated vaccines have the ability to replicate within the body and create a response similar to that of infection, whereas killed or inactivated vaccines create a less effective response. The live or killed organism, known as an antigen or an immunogen, creates an immune response. The intention is to create adequate immunity to an infection without causing disease. Vaccines also contain antibiotics, stabilisers, adjuvants and preservatives in differing amounts to improve the stability and effectiveness of the vaccine.

The roll of T lymphocytes in vaccine response is crucial. T helper lymphocytes instruct B lymphocytes to produce antibodies. The initial production of antibody is predominantly IgM antibody, which creates memory of the antigen. IgG production follows and will be the dominating antibody when a second dose of the same vaccine is administered; IgG is a longer-lasting antibody. When B lymphocytes are stimulated or recognise an antigen they will produce specific antibodies to target that antigen; they attach to the antigen through a lock and key technique. Re-exposure to an antigen results in a faster immune response.

Adverse reactions to vaccines are rare and anaphylaxis following vaccination is reported at a risk of one in a million (Public Health England, 2013). Despite the low risk the practitioner must be competent in anaphylaxis management.

Maternal antibodies provide protection for the newborn; however, this is not long lasting (Public Health England, 2013). Vaccines should not be delayed for premature infants. Babies born before 28 weeks' gestation should be given their first dose in hospital followed by respiratory monitoring for 48–72 hours. If there are any concerns when giving the first dose, the second dose should be given under observation (Public Health England, 2013). To review your understanding of how vaccines work, visit https://study.sagepub.com/essentialchildnursing to watch a video.

VIDEO LINK 23.1: HOW VACCINES WORK

Herd immunity

Individuals who cannot receive vaccinations or do not respond to vaccinations rely on 'herd immunity'. The term 'herd immunity' refers to the high number of individuals protected from infection through vaccination. This reduces the risk of infection to unimmunised individuals. Infections can be eliminated from populations through this process, as demonstrated by the elimination of smallpox.

Health promotion

Immunisations remain one of the most successful public health strategies. Every opportunity should be taken to promote the benefit of immunisation, ensure children receive the vaccine schedule and administer missed vaccines. In the case of all established vaccines, risk of adverse events following vaccination versus risk of complications from a vaccine preventable disease make a clear case in support of vaccine. All practitioners must be able to clearly explain risk and benefit. Ensure you access the most up-to-date national schedule. Some parents remain concerned at their perception that vaccinations, particularly the triple combination, are harmful for children. They are reluctant to expose their children to the perceived risk of harm. These parental views should be recognised, listened to attentively and evidence-based information should be provided to assist in allaying their fears. Ignoring their fears or dismissing their concerns is not an ethical or helpful approach in such cases. Working with the parents and towards using the best available scientific evidence is likely to be more effective in assuring parents that they are doing the best thing they can for their children by having them immunised. Always seek informed medical advice in such cases to inform and reassure the parents.

PRIMARY IMMUNE DEFICIENCIES

Primary immune deficiencies (PID) are disorders of the immune system that have a genetic link; the UK PID Registry provides key cohort information (Edgar et al., 2013). A number of signs and symptoms may be linked with an immune deficiency but can often also be assigned to a more common childhood illness, which can inevitably delay diagnosis. Included in this non-exhaustive list are: a family history of PID, frequent or recurrent infections, severe infections, failure to thrive, deep skin or organ abscesses and recurrent fungal infections.

The International Union of Immunological Societies Expert Committee for Primary Immunodeficiency (Al-Herz et al., 2014) classify primary immunodeficiencies in eight categories (see Table 23.2).

Table 23.2 Eight categories of primary immunodeficiencies as classified by the International Union of Immunological Societies Expert Committee for Primary Immunodeficiency

Classification	Example
Combined immunodeficiencies	X-linked severe combined immunodeficiency
Well-defined syndromes with immunodeficiency	DiGeorge syndrome
Predominantly antibody deficiencies	Common variable immune deficiency
Diseases of immune dysregulation	X-linked lymphoproliferative syndrome
Congenital defects of phagocyte number, function, or both	Chronic granulomatous disorder
Defects in innate immunity deficiency	NEMO
Auto-inflammatory disorders	Familial Mediterranean fever
Complement deficiencies	C1 inhibitor deficiency

Treatment is dependent on the diagnosis and may include:

- Prophylactic antibiotics given to prevent infections where there is susceptibility
- Additional vaccinations to improve response and acquired immunity
- Immunoglobulin therapy administered at regular intervals (this is a blood product made from the pooled plasma of donors)

- Gene therapy, which involves introducing a working copy of the faulty gene. Cavazzana-Calvo and Fischer (2007) debate the advantages and limitations
- Bone marrow transplantation is required to cure some immune deficiencies such as severe combined immune deficiency (SCID); infants with this diagnosis are likely to present in the first year of life with severe infections.

Antibody deficiencies are the most common primary immunodeficiency seen in clinical practice (Al-Herz et al., 2014).

Care plan for a child receiving routine IV immunoglobulin therapy on the day unit

Immunoglobulin therapy can be administered intravenously or subcutaneously for a child with an antibody deficiency. The benefits and disadvantages of both methods should be explored with the family. Clinical guidelines for immunoglobulin use (Department of Health, 2011, and subsequest updated information) must be consulted to guide practice as we are in an era of increasing demand and there is concern for supply. The nursing process as outlined in Table 23.3 should be adhered to.

Table 23.3 The nursing process

Assessment	Before therapy, blood tests will be requested by the clinical team. Baseline temperature, blood pressure, heart rate, respiration rate and weight must be recorded. Immunoglobulin therapy must not be administered if the child has a fever or is unwell
Planning	The prescription must be prepared in advance to ensure the product is available. It is essential that nurses are aware of the management of adverse reactions, including anaphylaxis. Ensure a name-band is in situ. IV cannulation should be conducted following local policy, including aseptic non-touch technique and a choice of local anaesthetic cream or spray. Ensure the product is intact and check and record the batch number and expiry date
Implementation	Follow local medicine policy and Nursing and Midwifery Council (2007) guidelines when administering medication. Observe the child closely throughout. Regularly measure vital signs, observe the cannula site and record rates and infusion balance
Evaluation	Evaluation is continuous and includes future investigations to assess the effectiveness of the therapy. Ensure the child and family are kept up to date. The cannula must be removed before discharge home and a follow-up appointment will be necessary for the child

CASE STUDY 23.1: ZARA

Zara is a 3-month-old baby who attended the GP surgery regularly with fever and infection. Zara received the BCG vaccine at birth, administered to the left upper arm. This was appropriate, as her grandparents were born in India, where the incidence of tuberculosis is reported at 167 per 100,000. Zara was taken to A&E by her mother who was becoming increasingly concerned with the large lump under Zara's left arm and her worsening cough. Zara was admitted to the children's ward. A thorough medical history was taken.

(Continued)

(Continued)

Zara was born at 40 weeks' gestation by vaginal delivery. She was the second child of Sumaya and Mohammed who reported no medical complaints. Sumaya was worried as some of her relatives had given birth to children who died in infancy, but as they lived in India there was limited additional information.

Zara appeared to feed well but was not gaining weight and had dropped from the 75th to 25th centile on a growth chart since birth. Blood results indicated that Zara had no B and T lymphocytes.

CASE STUDY
ANSWER 23.1

- What is the likely diagnosis in this scenario?
- How will you nurse Zara on the children's ward before transfer to an immunology centre?

HIV

Human immunodeficiency virus (HIV) is a retrovirus that causes immune deficiency. In 2014, the World Health Organization (WHO, 2015b) estimated that 36.9 million people were living with HIV around the world; 2.6 million of these were children under the age of 15 years. In the United Kingdom, approximately 1,000 children are accessing care for HIV infection at a recognised treatment centre (Collaborative HIV Paediatric Study [CHIPS], 2015).

HIV infection is transmitted through unprotected sexual intercourse, from infected blood to uninfected blood, from mother to baby in utero, during childbirth and through breastfeeding (WHO, 2015c). Nearly all children living with HIV in the UK acquired the virus from their mother and 48 per cent of this cohort were born in the UK (CHIPS, 2015). The average age of the UK cohort is increasing, which is reflective of successful treatment and the prevention of further mother-to-child transmission.

HIV particularly affects T helper lymphocytes that express the CD4 glycoprotein. The protein on the virus allows it to attach to and enter the cell via receptors on the cell wall. An enzyme, reverse transcriptase, allows the viral RNA to change in to DNA and integrates in to the cell nucleus. The virus is able to replicate and release more copies of HIV before it dies. Cytotoxic T lymphocytes expressing the CD8 glycoprotein increase in number as they try to respond to and control HIV.

Over time the CD4 cell count declines as a result of ongoing HIV replication. The CD4 cell count is monitored by a blood test. HIV also infects other cells within the body. The lower the CD4 count the more severe the immune deficiency and consequent risk of infection.

Today, HIV should be discussed as a chronic health condition with life expectancy near normal when effective treatment is available, initiated in a timely manner and taken correctly (May et al., 2014). Today's effective treatment, monitoring and support demonstrates huge medical advances since the first reported cases of acquired immune deficiency syndrome (AIDS) in the 1980s.

The CD4 count and clinical staging are the main indicators for initiating treatment to prevent the risk of severe infections. HIV treatment is often used in combination and described as highly active antiretroviral treatment (HAART). The purpose of treatment is to prevent viral replication and reduce the amount of HIV in the body to an undetectable level. The measurement is referred to as the 'viral load'.

HIV treatment is currently lifelong therapy and adherence is crucial. Children must take the correct drugs at the same time every day. Poor adherence to treatment will result in a rising viral load, falling CD4 count and potentially permanent drug resistance. Challenges today include successful transition to adult care and lifelong treatment (Banford and Lyall, 2015).

ACTIVITY 23.1: CRITICAL THINKING

The importance of adherence to treatment has been highlighted. What would need to be considered before initiating treatment? What reasons may lead to poor adherence in children? How would you support a child and family due to start lifelong treatment?

ACTIVITY
ANSWER 23.1

Stigma

Stigma remains a significant challenge for anyone living with or affected by HIV. This affects the age at which children are informed they are HIV positive. Children should be informed within primary school years by the appropriate healthcare staff and with relevant education and support. Review the CHIVA statement (CHIVA, 2015) on naming HIV to children to understand the challenges and importance. This link can be found at https://study.sagepub.com/essentialchildnursing

WEBLINK:
NAMING HIV

Young people's voice

The chapter opened with a short piece of creative writing by a young person living with HIV and highlights the impact of stigma. Consider the impact of poor understanding of HIV and stigma in education after watching the video at https://study.sagepub.com/essentialchildnursing

The CHIVA Youth Committee has produced a list of important factors for practice to ensure care is appropriate:

VIDEO LINK
23.2: HIV
STIGMA

1. Make sure you know what you're talking about. Misinformation or misunderstanding can affect me. HIV does not stop me from achieving my ambitions
2. Please talk to me and not my parent or guardian
3. If you have a private conversation (which seems to be about me) with a colleague when I'm in the same room, it makes me feel anxious
4. Please take the time to explain my medicine and side effects
5. Please treat me my age. Think about the language you use. Use simple words
6. Don't make assumptions
7. It doesn't matter how/when/why someone got HIV; don't focus on this
8. HIV doesn't define me; I'll always be me first
9. Confidentiality is really important; my health isn't something to gossip about
10. HIV affects my mental health just as much as my physical health; stigma hurts

CASE STUDY 23.2: SUSAN

Susan is 13 years old. She was treated at an HIV specialist family clinic, where her mother also received her treatment and care. They both attended their appointments regularly, their HIV was well controlled with medication and they presented as essentially well.

CASE STUDY:
LAURA

(Continued)

(Continued)

The local children's social care team received a referral from Susan's school due to her poor attendance. A social worker made contact to arrange an assessment.

Mum was very reluctant to allow the social worker to visit. When the social worker visited, their home was found to be in an extremely poor state of hygiene. Medicine was scattered all over the floor and empty take-away food containers were piled high. It was evident that Susan slept in the same bed as her mother as her room was inaccessible due to piles of clothing and belongings. The assessment revealed that mum no longer cooked and they relied on take-away food.

The health information revealed that Susan's physical health had been consistently good. The high level of school absences appeared to be related to mum's need for her daughter to be at home. Susan's mother had become very dependent, and Susan presented little independent identity. It was clear that mum had mental health issues, which were previously unrecognised.

The family's health professionals collaborated in the safeguarding assessment and support plan, which included ongoing community visits to support the family in their home as well as clinic-based care.

The case demonstrates the complex social and psychological impacts HIV can bring to families who struggle to cope, where access to wider support and understanding can be difficult. It reinforces the importance of awareness of how in certain situations the welfare of the child is at risk and needs prompt intervention and support to ensure that the child's welfare is paramount.

(Amanda Ely, social worker and projects manager, CHIVA)

PREP FOR PLACEMENT!

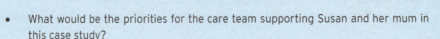

- What would be the priorities for the care team supporting Susan and her mum in this case study?

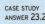

CASE STUDY ANSWER 23.2

PLACEMENT ADVICE 23: IMMUNOLOGICAL PROBLEMS

Go to https://study.sagepub.com/essentialchildnursing for tips on preparing for placements when working with children with immunological problems.

───────────── **CHAPTER SUMMARY** ─────────────

Understanding the immune system will help you to deliver appropriate high-quality evidence-based nursing care to children while also supporting their families. Immunisation remains an essential public health strategy internationally and it is important to note that everyone has a role to play in vaccine promotion. Development and progress are ongoing in the field of immune deficiencies but some understanding can continue to positively influence clinical practice and wellbeing of the child and family.

In this chapter we have looked at the care of a child with immunological problems. We have highlighted:

- Basics of the immune system
- Public health – immunisations
- Caring sensitively for a child with an immune deficiency disorder
- HIV awareness and ongoing education needs
- Safeguarding awareness and considerations for children

BUILD YOUR BIBLIOGRAPHY

Books

- Randall, D. (2005) 'Development of the immune system and immunity', in C. Chamley, P. Carson, D. Randall and M. Sandwell, M. (eds), *Developmental Anatomy and Physiology of Children: A Practical Approach*. London: Elsevier Churchill Livingstone.

  It is important to have some knowledge of normal anatomy and physiology so that illness and changes can be understood.

- Public Health England and and Department of Health (2013) *Immunisation against Infectious Disease*. London: The Stationery Office.

  This book, commonly known as The Green Book, is essential for anybody involved in the care of children requiring immunisation.

- Playfair, J.H.L. and Chain, B.M. (2012) *Immunology at a Glance*, 10th edn. Chichester: Wiley-Blackwell.

  This book will help you develop your understanding of the immune system

Journal articles

Go to https://study.sagepub.com/essentialchildnursing for further free online journal articles related to this chapter.

FURTHER READING: ONLINE JOURNAL ARTICLES

- Banford, A. and Lyall, H. (2014) 'Paediatric HIV grows up: recent advances in perinatally acquired HIV'. *Archives of Disease in Childhood*, 100 (2): 183-8.

  This article highlights the important advances in children's HIV care in the UK since the 1980s.

- Wood, P., Stanworth, S., Burton, J., Jones, A., Peckham, D.G., Green, T., Hyde, C., Chapel, H. and UK Primary Immunodeficiency Network (2007) 'Recognition, clinical diagnosis and management of patients with primary antibody deficiencies: a systematic review'. *Clinical and Experimental Immunology*, 149 (3): 410-23.

  Prompt recognition and diagnosis is important; this article gives some insight to inform practice.

- Cameron, J.C., Allan, G., Johnston, F., Finn, A., Heath, P.T. and Booy, R. (2007) 'Severe complications of chickenpox in hospitalised children in the UK and Ireland'. *Archives of Disease in Childhood*, 92:1062-6.

  Chickenpox is often described as a common childhood illness in the UK. This may lead some to believe that it is not a serious condition. Some countries vaccinate against it, so it is important that the severity of the disease should be appreciated.

Weblinks

Go to https://study.sagepub.com/essentialchildnursing for further weblinks related to this chapter.

FURTHER READING: WEBLINKS

- World Health Organization, *Immunization, Vaccines and Biologicals*

  www.who.int/immunization/en

  Keep up to date with the recommended global immunisation programme.

- PID UK

  www.piduk.org.uk

  Find out more about primary immune deficiencies.

- Children's HIV Association (CHIVA)

  www.chiva.org.uk

  Review children's HIV resources and guidelines in the UK.

- AVERT

  www.avert.org

  Consult the excellent AVERT website for up-to-date global evidence and data on all aspects of HIV and AIDS across the age ranges.

ONLINE
QUIZZES &
ACTIVITY
ANSWERS

ACE YOUR ASSESSMENT

Revise what you have learned by visiting https://study.sagepub.com/essentialchildnursing

- Test yourself with multiple-choice and short-answer questions
- Do the chapter activities in the book and check your answers online

REFERENCES

Al-Herz, W., Bousfiha, A., Casanova, J-L., Chatila, T., Conley, M.E., Cunningham-Rundles, C., et al. (2014) 'Primary immunodeficiency diseases: an update on the classification from the International Union of Immunological Societies Expert Committee for Primary Immunodeficiency'. *Frontiers in Immunology*, 5 (162): 1–33.

Banford, A. and Lyall, H. (2014) 'Paediatric HIV grows up: recent advances in perinatally acquired HIV'. *Archives of Disease in Childhood*. 100(2): 183–8.

Boore, J., Cook, N. and Shepherd, A. (2016) *Essentials of Anatomy and Physiology for Nursing Practice*. London: Sage.

Cavazzana-Calvo, M. and Fischer, A. (2007) 'Gene therapy for severe combined immunodeficiency: are we there yet?' *The Journal of Clinical Investigation*, 117 (6): 1457–65.

Children's HIV Association (CHIVA) (2015) *CHIVA Statement on children's knowledge about their HIV*. Available at: www.chiva.org.uk/professionals/support/chiva-position-statement/ (last accessed 7 June 2017).

Children's HIV Association (CHIVA) *Taking Medication*. Available at www.chiva.org.uk/parent/child-hiv/medication-support (last accessed 22 May 2017).

Collaborative HIV Paediatric Study (2015) *Summary Data*. London: CHIPS. Available at: www.chipscohort.ac.uk/summary_data.asp (last accessed 22 May 2017).

Department of Health (2011) *Clinical Guidelines for Immunoglobulin Use*, 2nd edn. London: Department of Health.

Edgar, J.D.M., Buckland, M., Guzman, D., Conlon, N.P., Knerr, V., Bangs, C., et al. (2013) 'The UK Primary Immune Deficiency (UK-PID) Registry: a report of the first 4 years' activity 2008–2012'. *Clinical and Experimental Immunology*, 175: 68–78.

Health Protection Agency (2005) *National Minimum Standards for Immunisation Training*. London: Health Protection Agency.

May, M.T., Gompels, M., Delpech, V., Porter, K., Orkin, C., Kegg, S., et al. (2014) 'Impact on life expectancy of HIV-1 positive individuals of CD+ cell count and viral load response to antiretroviral therapy'. *AIDS*, 28 (8): 1193–202.

Nursing and Midwifery Council (2007) *Standards for Medicine Management*. London: NMC.

Public Health England (2013) *Immunisation Against Infectious Disease*. London: HMSO.

Riedel, S. (2005) 'Edward Jenner and the history of smallpox and vaccination'. *BUMC Proceedings*, 18: 21–5.

World Health Organization (WHO) (2015a) *Immunizations*. Available at: www.who.int/topics/immunization/en/ (last accessed 7 June 2017).

World Health Organization (WHO) (2015b) *HIV/AIDS Data and Statistics*. New York: WHO. Available at: www.who.int/hiv/data/en (last accessed 22 May 2017).

World Health Organization (WHO) (2015c) *Guideline on When to Start Antiretroviral Therapy and on Pre-exposure Prophylaxis for HIV*. Available at: www.who.int/hiv/pub/guidelines/earlyrelease-arv/en (last accessed 22 May 2017).

CARE OF CHILDREN AND YOUNG PEOPLE WITH MUSCULOSKELETAL PROBLEMS

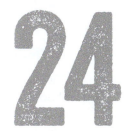

JULIA JUDD

THIS CHAPTER COVERS

- Assessment of the child with a musculoskeletal problem
- Bone health
- Common children's orthopaedic conditions
- Development dysplasia of the hip
- Legg–Calvé–Perthes disease
- Congenital talipes equinovarus or club foot
- Amplified musculoskeletal pain syndrome (AMPS)
- Limb lengthening
- Fracture in the child or young person

REQUIRED KNOWLEDGE

It would be helpful to have an understanding of the anatomy and physiology of the musculo-skeletal system before you start this chapter. Go to the A&P link: 'Skeletal and muscle anatomy' at https://study.sagepub.com/essentialchildnursing

A&P LINK 24.1:
SKELETON &
MUSCLES

Step into my shoes and walk the life I'm living and if you get as far as I am, just maybe you will see how strong I really am.

Unknown, www.wisdomquotesandstories.com/step-into-my-shoes-walk-my-life

Visit   https://study.sagepub.com/essentialchildnursing to access a wealth of online resources for this chapter – watch out for the margin icons throughout the chapter.

INTRODUCTION

The children's orthopaedic specialism covers a wide range of disorders affecting the child's growing skeleton, and includes trauma, infection, syndromic and neoplastic conditions, known collectively as musculoskeletal (MSK) conditions. The challenge in nursing the orthopaedic child is to apply specific knowledge of children's orthopaedic conditions and encompass generic medical and surgical knowledge and skills. As a children's nurse working in this area, you will need a true understanding of the differences of a child's anatomy and be able to adapt the basic principles of orthopaedic management to meet their needs. Throughout this chapter you will see how this knowledge crosses the boundaries of specialisms. The chapter focuses on some common musculoskeletal problems, although you will need to read more widely to gain a fuller understanding of these conditions (see the 'Build your bibliography' section at the end of the chapter and further online resources at https://study.sagepub.com/essential-childnursing). The chapter will begin by looking at the first step for any nurse working with a child presenting with an MSK condition, which is a thorough assessment.

ASSESSMENT OF THE CHILD WITH A MUSCULOSKELETAL PROBLEM

There are key aspects to any assessment of a child who presents with an MSK problem, which are summarised in Table 24.1.

Table 24.1   The nurses' role in assessment of a child with an MSK problem

Listen to the history given by the child and family. Formulate in your mind a potential diagnosis Sometimes this is not obvious, hip pain is frequently manifested as knee pain (i.e. the pain is 'referred' pain)	• Focus on the child. Build a rapport with them. • Assess the family and child's understanding. Is English their first language? • Is there a past or family history relevant to this assessment? • In your mind, consider what is normal for the child. What are the normal milestones for a young child? • If the child has an underlying diagnosis, for example cerebral palsy, their mobility and range of movement will be affected • Document the history
Look at the child	• Start looking as soon as possible - i.e. even before the formal assessment has begun. Children are often self-conscious, which can alter the true representation of the problem • Look at how they stand, sit down, stand up • Look at their leg alignment. Watch them walk (ideally when they walk into the clinic room or ward) • Look at their range of movement in their joints • Look and assess the colour of the limb • Look for swelling and compare with the contralateral side • Document your findings. E.g. grade a pressure ulcer - so comparison can be made in follow up assessment

WEBLINK:
PRESSURE ULCER

Feel the affected area	• Feel for swelling, warmth. Feel for pain. Is there pain at a specific point/area? • Document your findings
Move the affected area	• Assess movement of the presenting problem and move the child's joints above and below the problem area (unless impossible due to immobilisation with a cast or traction). Does this induce pain? • Document your findings
Neurovascular assessment Investigations	• Depending on the reason for the assessment, the nurse performs a formal neurovascular assessment, to ensure normality and exclude acute limb compartment syndrome • Document your findings

WEBLINK:
NEUROVASCULAR
ASSESSMENT

You can use the above table as a quick reference guide when working with a variety of MSK conditions. The chapter will explore a selection of these conditions in more detail, but first will look at key aspects of bone health that are essential to children's health and that you should be aware of.

SEE ALSO
CHAPTER 15

BONE HEALTH

Strong bones are essential for long-term health and well-being.

Children need to build strong bones ... by doing plenty of weight-bearing exercise and eating a well-balanced, calcium-rich diet. (National Osteoporosis Society, www.nos.org.uk)

Vitamin D is essential to ensure the body's absorption of calcium. Inadequate serum levels of vitamin D have resulted in a prevalence of musculoskeletal symptoms, deformity, fractures and noticeably a rebirth of rickets (Davies et al., 2011; Clarke and Page, 2012). Table 24.2 shows the normal levels of vitamin D.

Table 24.2 Vitamin D values

Serum25-hydroxy vitamin D Nmols/L (Nanomoles per Litre)		
Serum 25OHD	< 30 nmol/L	Deficient level
Serum 25OHD	30–50 nmol/L	Insufficient level
Serum 25OHD	> 50 nmols/L	Sufficient level

National Osteoporosis Society, 2013

Typical presentations of vitamin D deficiency in children are those which describe a history of musculoskeletal pain, which in essence is non-specific and termed as 'growing pains'. Normal variants such as physiological genu varum (bow legs) or valgum (knock knees) are commonly associated with vitamin D deficiency. Supplementation is usually beneficial in treating MSK symptoms and is recommended to facilitate resolution of bony deformity.

WHAT'S THE EVIDENCE?

There is growing evidence of the links between vitamin D deficiency and a variety of health problems. In children particularly, bony deformity, fractures and muscle pain are a feature.

You can find this evidence in a number of publications, including:

- NICE public health guidelines: www.nice.org.uk/guidance/ph56
- NHS Choices: www.nhs.uk/conditions/rickets
- Judd, 2013
- Clarke and Page, 2012
- Davies et al., 2011

Read through one of the above articles and consider what this might mean for health promotion opportunities.

Rickets

Rickets is prevalent again today and whilst sometimes thought to be exclusive to children from ethnic minorities due to skin colour, this is not the case. Children's nurses and other healthcare professionals are responsible for identifying the problem early, initiating appropriate management and directing parents and carers to resource information regarding healthy dietary intake and recommendations for oral supplementation.

PROMOTING HEALTH

WEBLINK:
INCREASE
VITAMIN D

NICE have published an interactive flowchart on how to increase vitamin D supplement use among at-risk groups (Nice Guideline [PH56] 2014: Recommendation 8), which you can access from https:// study.sagepub.com/essentialchildnursing The key messages for you as a nurse to bear in mind when working with children and their families are:

Ensure health professionals recommend and record vitamin D supplement use, among at-risk groups (and other family members, as appropriate) whenever possible. This could take place during registration appointments with new patients in general practice, flu, other vaccine and screening appointments. It could also take place during routine appointments and health checks including, for example:

- NHS Health Check
- diabetes check-ups
- falls appointments and check-ups
- health assessments for looked-after children
- the first contact with someone who is pregnant
- antenatal and postnatal appointments
- medicine use and prescription reviews
- health visitor appointments
- developmental checks for infants and children.

These are not specific to children, but take into account the importance of the role of the nurse in caring for the whole family.

Developers of standardised electronic and handheld maternity notes and developers of personal child health records (the 'red book') should add specific questions about the use of vitamin D supplements.

The classical picture of rickets is bony deformity, specifically noted at the wrists and lower limbs. Normalising the child's serum levels of 25 hydroxyvitamin D may rectify the deformity. However, in some cases, surgery is required to correct leg alignment. During this stressful time, the parents need vital support and reassurance from nurses.

ACTIVITY 24.1: EVIDENCE-BASED PRACTICE

Using your research skills to find appropriate evidence, list the factors that may be contributing to the growing problem of vitamin D deficiency in the UK.

CHECK YOUR ANSWERS ONLINE!

ACTIVITY ANSWER 24.1

COMMON CHILDREN'S ORTHOPAEDIC CONDITIONS

Caring for children with an orthopaedic problem requires medical and surgical nursing skills. Children may present with complex problems and often with comorbidities to manage. The common disorders affecting children require a variety of treatment interventions dependent on the child's age at presentation. Table 24.3 summarises these disorders, symptoms and the main guidelines that you should read and refer to when working with children and their families affected by these conditions. The chapter will then consider a selection of these in more detail.

Table 24.3 Common orthopaedic disorders affecting infants and children

WEBLINK: COMMON ORTHOPAEDIC DISORDERS

Musculoskeletal disorder	Body part	Common age range	Signs/ Symptoms	Investigations	Key guidelines/references
Developmental dysplasia of the hip - abnormal hip growth ranging from instability of the hip to a fixed dislocation	Hip	0-6 months Can be identified older - i.e. late presentation	Reduced hip abduction Leg length inequality	Ultrasound hip scan (under 8 months) Anteroposterior view (AP) hips and pelvis X-ray (over 8 months)	The website for the International Hip Dysplasia Institute contains lots of information and real patient stories: www.hipdysplasia.org

(Continued)

Table 24.3   (Continued)

Musculoskeletal disorder	Body part	Common age range	Signs/ Symptoms	Investigations	Key guidelines/references
					Newborn and infant physical examination: clinical guidance: www.evidence.nhs.uk Clarke NM, Taylor C, Judd J. 2016. Diagnosis and management of developmental hip dysplasia. 2015. Paediatrics and Child Health.
Legg-Calvé-Perthes disease (or Perthes) - a disruption of the blood supply to the head of the femur, causing it to collapse and deform	Hip	5-7 years	Persistent limp and pain Reduced hip abduction	AP and frog leglateral views hips and pelvis X-ray MRI (if diagnosis equivocal)	The Perthes Association is a charitable organisation offering families help and advice: www.perthes.org.uk For the management of Perthes disease, see: www.ncbi.nlm.nih.gov/pmc/articles/PMC4292319
Slipped capital femoral epiphysis - the femoral head slips off the neck of the femur, at the top, through the growth plate	Hip	Adolescence	Limp/unable to bear weight Pain Leg lies in external rotation	AP and frog leg lateral views hips and pelvis X-ray	For an overview of slipped capital femoral epiphysis, see: http://emedicine.medscape.com/article/91596-overview#a6 and Judd (2014)
Genu varum/ valgum (bow legs/ knock knees)	Knees/ Tibia	6 months-6 years	Angular deformity (bowed legs - inward or outward)	Whole lower limb X-ray (i.e. both legs)	Medscape give a complete over-view of bow legs and knock knee: http://emedicine.medscape.com/article/1355974-overview#a2 http://emedicine.medscape.com/article/1259772-overview
Bone deformity e.g. Infantile Blounts/rickets	Knees/ Any bone	Newborn-adolescence	Angular leg deformity Rickets: affects any bone	X-ray	Medscape gives an overview of Blount disease: http://emedicine.medscape.com/article/1250420-overview
Congenital talipes equinovarus ('club foot')	Feet	Newborn	Feet are turned inward, supinated and the heel is high	Clinical assessment	This website provides a wealth of information for health professionals and families: www.ponseti.info
Amplified pain (increased pain sensitivity)	Any	Adolescence	Abnormal pain sensitivity		Dr Sherry in Philadelphia has published extensively on amplified musculoskeletal pain. These two websites will give the reader a real insight into the condition: www.chop.edu/conditions-diseases/amplified-musculoskeletal-pain-syndrome-amps/about#.V3P6WLgrKW8 www.clinexprheumatol.org/article.asp?a=1186

Musculoskeletal disorder	Body part	Common age range	Signs/ Symptoms	Investigations	Key guidelines/references
Trauma – a physical injury to bones, joints, or soft tissues, e.g. muscles, tendons, ligaments	Any	Any	Pain, deformity, neurovascular compromise	X-ray CT	Take a look at this website to better understand how children are different from adults: www.rch.org.au/paed_trauma/manual/11_How_are_children_different/ See also Clarke and Liggett (2014)

DEVELOPMENTAL DYSPLASIA OF THE HIP

Developmental dysplasia of the hip (DDH) is a descriptive term used to cover the spectrum of disorders affecting the infant hip. The UK incidence is 1–2 per 1,000 live births, varying elsewhere to 4–20 per 1,000 (Clarke et al., 2016). Presentation is either a dysplastic (abnormal development), subluxing (partial dislocation) or unstable hip (ligaments are loose, so the hip is not stable within the joint), or a frank (complete) dislocation. The cause is unknown, although there are a number of identified risk factors. The primary risk factors include:

- Family medical history of DDH
- Breech presentation (baby is born bottom first)
- Twin delivery
- Reduced abduction (frog-leg position)

Other associated risk factors include:

- Oligohydramnios (reduced amniotic fluid in the uterus)
- Firstborn child
- Large baby for gestational age
- Packaging disorders (minimal room in the uterus) – for example, torticollis, positional/structural club foot
- Caesarean section delivery
- Cerebral palsy (Public Health England, 2016)

DDH is usually detected in the infant presenting at birth, or to their health visitor or GP with a hip click or reduced abduction. However, diagnosis may be dependent on clinical expertise. Whilst hip clicks are often innocent in nature, clinical examination by a trained practitioner will test for hip dislocation and stability (the Ortolani and Barlow manoeuvres) (Davis, 2009; Public Health England, 2016).

Criteria for referral by a trained health professional include a positive clinical examination and those with a true risk factor. Ultrasound is the gold standard to diagnose hip dysplasia/dislocation in the cartilaginous hip joint (Eastwood and de Gheldere, 2010).

Treatment

Treatment is started when there is an abnormal clinical and ultrasound examination (Clarke and Castenada, 2012). In the infant, treatment is non-surgical, using a Pavlik harness (Figure 24.3), with a

VIDEO LINK 24.1: OSCAR'S STORY

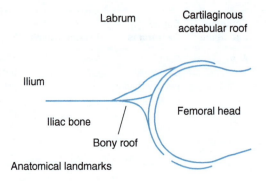

Figure 24.1 **Hip ultrasound showing normal hip position**

http://bonepit.com/Reference/Neonatal%20hip%20Ultrasound.htm

success rate of 95 per cent. A later diagnosis for an older child requires a closed or open hip reduction and possibility of subsequent reconstructive surgery (Bolland et al., 2010). Parents will seek information, so it is important that you have an understanding of the management options of DDH for the different age groups, as outlined in Table 24.4.

ACTIVITY 24.2: REFLECTIVE PRACTICE

Sometimes one of the hardest things to deal with emotionally is the fact that you assume you should handle this easily and well, because hip dysplasia is treatable. (www.hipdysplasia.org)

- Look at the advice for parents and carers given by the International Hip Dysplasia Institute (www.hipdysplasia.org) and reflect on the support and reassurance you can give parents at this difficult time.

ACTIVITY
ANSWER 24.2

Table 24.4   **Treatment for developmental dysplasia of the hip**

WEBLINK:
TRACTION

Newborn to 4 months	Pavlik harness (minimum six weeks, 24 hours/day and a further six weeks part-time wear until stable)
Months Failed Pavlik harness or late diagnosis	Closed or open hip reduction +/− preoperative gallows traction (using skin traction the baby's legs are suspended so that the buttocks are just clear of the bed)
	Postoperative management:
	Hip spica 6 to 12 weeks +/− sequential broomstick and night splint casting (subsequent casts after the hip spica gradually enable more hip movement)
>18 months	Open hip reduction + femoral shortening Hip spica +/− sequential broomstick and night splint casting

WEBLINK:
HAMISH'S
JOURNEY

(Clarke et al., 2016)

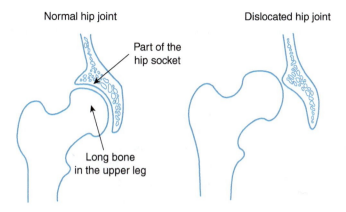

Normal hip joint

Part of the
hip socket

Long bone
in the upper leg

Dislocated hip joint

Figure 24.2 A normal and a dislocated hip

Pavlik harness

The Pavlik harness is a soft brace that places the baby's legs in an optimal position to facilitate normal hip development. The fabric straps secure the harness around the baby's chest and legs, allowing movement of the hip joint to encourage deepening of the hip joint socket. The legs straps are positioned to hold the hips in 90 degrees of flexion and 60 degrees of abduction. The role of the nurse is to support parents during this stressful time and ensure they have confidence in caring for their baby in the harness. Written information on hygiene, nappy care, clothing, handling, feeding and

VIDEO LINK 24.2:
PAVLIK HARNESS
OF CARE

WEBLINK:
PARENTS' GUIDE

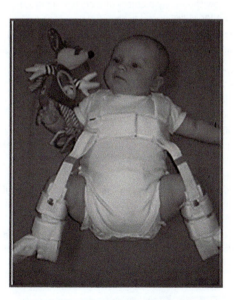

Figure 24.3 Pavlik harness

90 degrees hip flexion/60 degrees hip abduction

Reproduced with permission from Clarke and Santy-Tomlinson, *Orthopaedic and Trauma Nursing: An Evidence-based Approach to Musculoskeletal Care*, 2014, Wiley

transporting should be provided. Further information can be found on the Steps website (www.steps-charity.org.uk), which has some great resources to read and share with families caring for infants in Pavlik harnesses.

Further surgical procedures and hip spica care

WEBLINK:
SPICA LIFE

The success of DDH treatment is dependent on age at diagnosis. Between 2 and 17 per cent of children who are diagnosed will require subsequent surgical procedures to treat residual hip dysplasia (Cashman et al., 2002). This may be due to failure of the Pavlik harness or a late diagnosis of dysplasia (the harness is only effective before 4 months of age). A late diagnosis of hip dysplasia is the commonest reported risk factor for total hip replacement under the age of 40 years (Engesæter et al., 2011). Surgery for hip dysplasia varies depending on the severity of the condition and age of the child. Either a closed (manipulation) or an open procedure is performed to reduce the hip into the socket (acetabulum), with or without pelvic surgery to augment the shape of the socket. Postoperatively the child is managed in a hip spica cast for up to three months, with sequential cast changes to allow for growth and assessment of the hip. As a nurse, an important part of your role is to explain and support the family in postoperative care when the child is in a hip spica cast. Table 24.5 outlines some important considerations.

Table 24.5   The role of the nurse in caring for the child in a hip spica

Care aspect	Nursing support considerations
Support and information resources for the family	Provide written information on how to care for the child in a spica - for example, hygiene, sponge bathing, nappy care, toileting, seating and positioning, keeping the cast dry, preventing soiling and pressure sores
	It is helpful to show the family pictures of a child in a hip spica before the surgery, so they have an idea of what it looks like
	If possible introduce the parents to another family whose child has been in a spica
	Direct the family to appropriate websites - for example, IHDI (www.hipdysplasia.org) and STEPS (www.steps-charity.org.uk).
	Liaise with the occupational therapy and physiotherapy teams to contact and meet with the family to give advice and reassurance regarding car seat (only certain models are suitable for children in spicas), manual handling, buggies and toileting
Child support	Make recommendations to the family regarding appropriate play for their child whilst in a spica. Consider the use of a hip spica table for the child to sit at (discuss with the occupational therapist and with the STEPS charity regarding a loan)
Pain relief and comfort	Ensure the child is comfortable and pain free. An epidural is commonly used for 48 hours after an open hip reduction. Once at home paracetamol is usually sufficient. Try alternative ways to console the child. They may be fretful because they are too hot or cold in the spica, need their positon changed or are bored
Clothing	Suggest suitable clothing for a child in a spica. Some clothes can be adapted. More information is on the STEPS and IHDI websites, plus online companies accessible via https://study.sagepub.com/essentialchildnursing

(Judd, 2014, Clarke and McKay, 2006)

WEBLINK:
HIP-POSE

LEGG-CALVÉ-PERTHES DISEASE

Legg–Calvé–Perthes disease (LCPD), named after the three orthopaedic surgeons who first described it in 1910, is a condition of unknown aetiology affecting the child's hip. The vascular supply to the femoral head (ball) of the hip joint is interrupted, causing bony necrosis (death of bone) and loss of hip joint congruency (ability to fit or work together). This results in a painful limp and reduced hip movement, and may also affect leg length, due to flattening of the head of the femur. During this time, the aim is to maintain movement within the hip joint, reduce pain and spasm, and with either non-surgical or surgical management, protect the deforming femoral head (Daly et al., 1999).

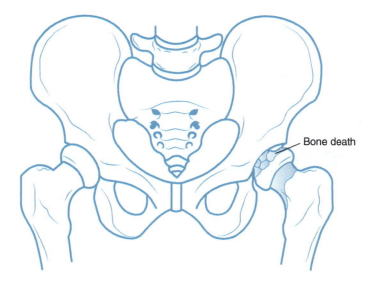

Figure 24.4 Perthes disease left hip

Perthes disease can last between two and four years, going through four distinct phases which are visible on the child's X-ray. This information gives guidance with regard to treatment and can inform parents of their child's progression through the disease process.

The stages of Perthes are:

- *Stage 1*: Necrosis (bone death)
- *Stage 2*: Fragmentation (the dead bone is replaced with softer, weak bone which breaks into pieces)
- *Stage 3*: Reossification (the blood supply returns to the head of the femur and new bone forms)
- *Stage 4*: Remodelling (the new bone heals; the shape of the head of the femur is dependent on the severity of the condition and the age of the child)

As a nurse, your support at diagnosis and throughout the duration of the disease process is vital for the parents and child. You should give guidance on avoiding activities which provoke pain and suggest or consider alternative activities to help reduce the child's symptoms. The condition is more prevalent in boys and helping them to understand the connection between impact activities (such as football) and their symptoms can be challenging.

VIDEO LINK 24.3: PERTHES PATIENT

ACTIVITY 24.3: CRITICAL THINKING

- What suggestions can you make to enable parents to help their child who has LCPD?

Think, for example, about switching activities, offloading the hip during painful episodes (crutches, bed rest).

ACTIVITY
ANSWER 24.3

Treatment

VIDEO LINK
24.4:
PERTHES
DISEASE – A
PATIENT CASE
STUDY

LCPD is one of many children's orthopaedic conditions in which the cause and the best treatment option continue to be debated by orthopaedic surgeons. However, the principles of management are agreed: to prevent further deformity of the head of the femur and to contain it within the socket of the hip joint. This will facilitate the best long-term outcome of a joint that has good movement and minimal symptoms (Bowen et al., 2011).

Table 24.6 outlines the surgical options.

WHAT'S THE EVIDENCE?

Look at historical management of the condition and review how treatment has advanced by reading Wenger and Pandya, 2011.

The two main surgical procedures are listed below.

Both aim to protect the deforming femoral head to achieve good remodelling at the final stage of the disease. Note that the roundness of the femoral head is dependent on it being located in the acetabulum (socket).

As the disease worsens and the femoral head flattens, there is potential for it to extrude out of the acetabulum.

Table 24.6 Surgery for Perthes

Operation	Average age	Further reading
Shelf acetabuloplasty Aims: Bone graft provides additional cover for the extruding femoral head Femoral head remodels in the new hip socket	< 8 years (dependent on the stage of LCPD)	Van der Geest et al., 2001 Carsi et al., 2015 (These two papers describe the surgery and discuss patient outcomes)
Varus derotation femoral osteotomy Aims: Realigns the proximal femur Redirects the force through the hip when weight bearing Achieves improved containment and facilitates femoral remodelling ability	Age not specific	Tripathy et al., 2010 Gives a complete overview of Perthes and treatment options

CONGENITAL TALIPES EQUINOVARUS OR CLUB FOOT

Congenital talipes equinovarus (CTEV), or club foot, is a deformity of the foot and ankle that can be present from birth. A club foot is diagnosed by the following features:

- Forefoot is turned inward (adducted)
- Sole is turned upward (supinated)
- Arch is high (cavus)
- Heel is high (equinus)

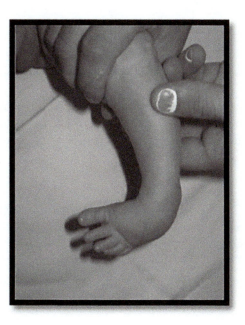

Figure 24.5 Left club foot

Reproduced with permission from Clarke and Santy-Tomlinson, *Orthopaedic and Trauma Nursing: An Evidence-based Approach to Musculoskeletal Care*, 2014, Wiley

Treatment

The gold standard for club foot treatment is the Ponseti method: gentle manipulation and serial casting to gradually correct the foot position, subsequently maintained with boots on an abduction bar until age 4 (see Table 24.7). Compliance with these is key to the success of the treatment and parent support is imperative. The Internet has provided access to advanced knowledge with regard to club foot treatment, with parents driving the demand for the Ponseti method. The nurse's role in supporting parents at diagnosis, whether antenatally or at birth, is very important. Many parents are given the wrong impression by untrained and uniformed health practitioners – for example, that their child will have problems walking and not have normal function.

VIDEO LINK
24.5:
PARENT'S
GUIDE TO CLUB
FOOT

ACTIVITY 24.4: EVIDENCE-BASED PRACTICE

Browse the Internet to explore the information available to parents about club foot.

- How would you as a nurse direct them to the appropriate information?
- Consider your opinion of social media information. For example, are Facebook groups helpful or otherwise?

(Continued)

WEBLINK:
GLOBAL CLUB
FOOT

(Continued)

Now explore the Global Clubfoot Initiative website (www.globalclubfoot.com).

This takes you straight to the home page with links on blogs from India, Pakistan, Solomon Islands, etc.

- Look at how some of the third world countries have advanced their ability to treat club foot through training. What can we learn from this?

Access to the Ponseti method is dependent on availability of competent practitioners within the family's locality. Some parents source practitioners via the Internet and travel long distances for their baby's treatment (Judd, 2004). Alternative management involves surgical correction of the foot deformity, resulting in a stiffer, less flexible foot with scars.

WEBLINK: CLUB
FOOT PATIENT

> When we were told he had fixed talipes we didn't know what that meant, but his left foot was completely turned in. We were concerned about him not being able to walk … and not being able to run or play football and other sports was at the back of my mind.
>
> **James, parent, www.uhs.nhs.uk**

VIDEO LINK
24.6: THE
PONSETI
METHOD

Table 24.7 Ponseti method pathway

Club foot determined on ultrasound at 20 weeks
↓
Parents meet health professional to discuss treatment pathway
↓
Information pointers given to parents
↓
Baby seen by 2 weeks of age
↓
Deformity assessed (Pirani +/– Dimeglio score)
↓
Gradual correction with gentle manipulation and weekly serial casting (average five weeks)
↓
+/– Achilles tenotomy (70-85%)
↓
Final cast for three weeks in maximum ankle dorsiflexion
↓
Boots and bar full time (23 hours per day) for three months
↓
Boots and bar naps and night time up to 4 years of age

Note: Approximately 25% of children require tibialis anterior tendon transfer at approximate age 3

AMPLIFIED MUSCULOSKELETAL PAIN SYNDROME (AMPS)

Pain is:

> An unpleasant sensory and emotional experience normally associated with tissue damage or described in terms of such damage (International Association for the Study of Pain, www.iasp-pain.org)

Amplified pain is a descriptive term for the problem. It is challenging to diagnose and treat, requiring the expertise of a multidisciplinary team to facilitate resolution.

Associated factors frequently identified with the initiation of AMPS are minor trauma, an episode of psychological stress and personal or family illness. The pain fails to settle within the expected time frame and dysfunction results due to muscle disuse. AMP is prevalent in female adolescents, who are frequently high achievers. The lower limbs are the most commonly affected and intrusive symptoms result in school non-attendance. The child may present with some of the following symptoms:

- Hyperalgesia – disproportionate extreme sensitivity to pain
- Allodynia – pain from light touch
- Swelling – may occur over the painful region
- Skin temperature changes
- Skin colour changes (Miller, 2003)

SEE ALSO CHAPTER 5

The cause is unknown although associations between personality type and contributing factors have been made. Early recognition and prompt initiation of a therapy plan is vital to avoid functional deterioration.

Diagnosis requires exclusion of pathology with normal radiological and laboratory investigations. The child and the family need a clear explanation of the problem supported with evidence in a patient-information leaflet. This encourages their full commitment to the rehabilitation programme, provided by the whole MDT, which will address all the influencing factors to lead to the child's improvement and ultimate cure (Judd, 2014).

WEBLINK: MDT APPROACH

ACTIVITY 24.5: CRITICAL THINKING

Think about how different people express or interpret pain.

- What does pain mean to you?
- How can we as nurses assess pain? What tools are available?
- What are the options for managing the child's AMP so they can participate in their physical therapy to regain normal function?

ACTIVITY ANSWER 24.5

PRACTICE SCENARIO 24.1: LILY

LIMB LENGTHENING

CASE STUDY 24.1: JOHN (1)

John is a 17-year-old male who had spent much of his childhood having numerous surgical procedures to correct deformity and lengthen bones. He had a residual 5 centimetre leg length

(Continued)

VIDEO LINK 24.7: LIMB LENGTHENING

(Continued)

discrepancy and he decided to undergo one final procedure before moving onto higher education and leading a 'normal' university life. As he was skeletally mature he was offered lengthening using the Precice nail, a relatively new magnetically driven internal rod.

John's preoperative X-ray (Figure 24.6) shows his previous pelvic support osteotomy and right leg length discrepancy.

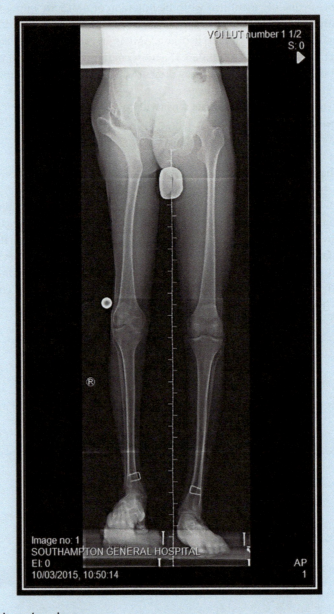

Figure 24.6   Long leg views

Table 24.8 Comparison of external lengthening device versus internal device

External fixator	Internal lengthening
Joint stiffness	Less joint stiffness
Muscle contracture	Less pain
Pin infection	No pin site infections
Malalignment	Improved activity level whilst lengthening
Re-fracture	Faster rehabilitation

Table 24.8 outlines the main advantages to the patient in using the new internal Precice nail rather than an external lengthening circular frame, or monolateral rail.

As a lengthening device, the Precice nail has been shown to be patients' preferred option (Herzenberg et al., 2013), mainly due to the non-requirement for pin site cleaning and the ease of returning to mobility without the encumbrance of an external frame. The Precice nail is an intramedullary locked nail (a nail placed down through the middle (medulla) of the bone), which is lengthened by placing a magnet over osteotomised bone (bone that has been cut). Below are radiographs and pictures illustrated with John's words showing the stages of lengthening and recovery.

CASE STUDY 24.1: JOHN (2)

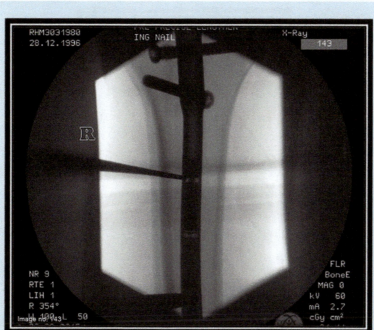

Figure 24.7 Osteotomised tibia with Precice nail in situ

(Continued)

(Continued)

Met with the anaesthetist – decided a nerve block at the front and back of my right leg would be sufficient to help deal with pain. Lasted 24 hours... My leg felt numb and insensitive. Had trouble urinating, but not serious enough to have a catheter. The medication I had post-op was morphine and paracetamol.

Sleeping that night was okay because my leg was still numb, although a nurse called Belle kept tapping my foot at various times throughout the night.

WEBLINK:
RCN
CONSENSUS

- Consider why the nurse kept tapping John's foot?
- Look up the research for neurovascular compromise and peripheral neurovascular limb observations. For example, *Peripheral Neurovascular Observations for Acute Limb Compartment Syndrome: RCN Consensus Guidance* (2014), available via https://study.sagepub.com/essentialchildnursing

Once at home, John started the lengthening process by placing the magnet over the marked site on his leg (where the bone was cut). He did this three times a day.

CASE STUDY 24.1: JOHN (3)

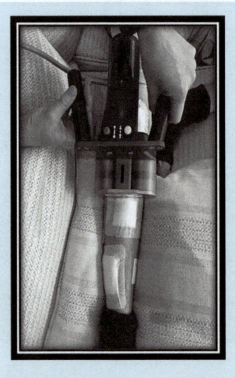

Figure 24.8 Magnet placed over the marked site on the patient's shin to achieve lengthening

The lengthening process begins after 7 days with 3 x 0.25 mm turns each day, hoping to achieve 4 cm after 5/6 months. The magnetic device is very heavy so caused discomfort to my knee.

Day 3: I decided to shower this morning ... I had a waste bag wrapped around my right leg and tied up (to keep dry). I sat on a shower seat and my Mum showered me as I could not possibly shower myself alone.

Over the next few weeks, X-rays showed the distraction of the bone ends (cut bone ends moving apart to make a gap) and clinically John's leg was longer.

Figure 24.9 shows the distracted tibia with evidence of early callus formation. The nail is usually removed at approximately 12–18 months after this.

CASE STUDY 24.1: JOHN (4)

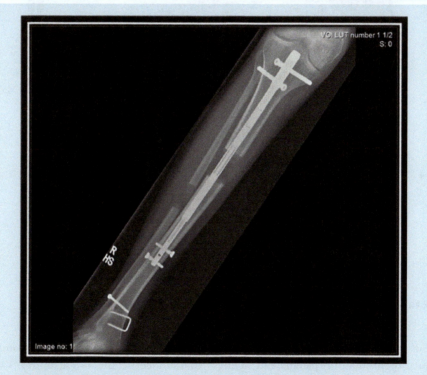

PRACTICE SCENARIO 24.2: SOPHIE

Figure 24.9 Distracted tibia with evidence of early callus formation

Day 20-14th: Tibia lengthening but quality of the new bone is poor. This means I will have to increase my Vitamin D intake and recline on a sun-lounger!

Day 27: a set back. Not enough new bone. Magnet reprogrammed to compress the bone and use ultrasound machine for 3 weeks to stimulate growth.

Delay or failure of bone formation can delay weight bearing and increase the period of disability and recovery. The advantage of the Precice over other intramedullary nails is that it can be stopped or reversed. Nine months after nail insertion, on Day 55, the tibia is still not united (see Figure 24.10). Although this is longer than usual, John is very happy with the outcome and is currently leading a relatively normal life continuing his university studies.

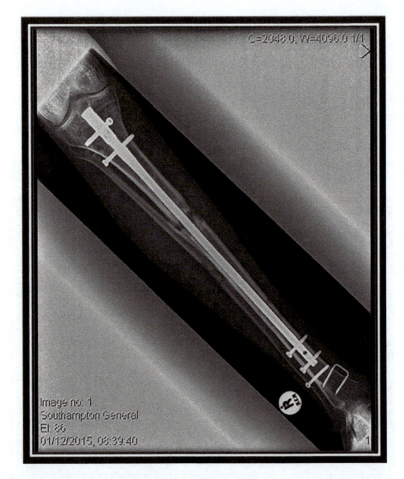

Figure 24.10   Evidence of bone healing

The role of the MDT in John's treatment was encompassing and cohesive, but his successful outcome was secured by his, and his parents and siblings', commitment to the long haul of his treatment. Throughout John's management it was imperative he, his family and the MDT worked closely together with agreed aims for a successful outcome. Lengthening procedures are often prolonged and can be fraught with complications. For some children and families, psychology input is useful.

FRACTURE IN THE CHILD OR YOUNG PERSON

Children's fractures are different from those of adults ... The causes for bone injuries in children are usually simple ... The fact most fractures in children heal fairly well with indifferent treatment has led the unwary to neglect the fact that other fractures terminate disastrously unless expertly handled. (Blount, 1955, p 1)

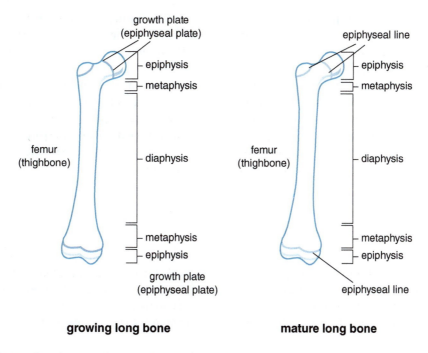

growing long bone   **mature long bone**

Figure 24.11 Growing long bone and mature long bone

http://kidshealth.org/en/parents/growth-plate-injuries.html

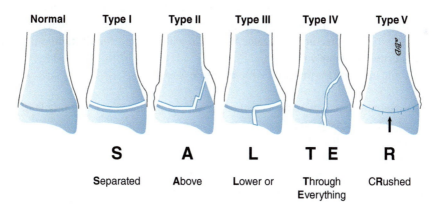

Figure 24.12 Salter Harris classification

This quotation is still relevant today: treating a child's fracture can be simple or necessitate significant expertise, depending on the nature of the fracture. Similarly, the nursing care of the child with a
fracture requires knowledge and competence to detect signs of compartment syndrome, and manage
pain, swelling and immobility.

The child's long bone is made up of the diaphysis, metaphysis, physis and epiphysis (Figure 24.11).

A fracture through the physis (growth plate) will injure the growing cells of the bone. The severity of the injury is assessed using the Salter Harris (SH) classification (Figure 24.12). An SH 1 fracture is least likely to cause any long-term problems, whilst an SH 5 fracture will affect the growth of the bone and require follow-up.

Diagnosing a fracture in a child is not always straightforward. An X-ray of the injured limb may be ambiguous due to the cartilaginous components of the bone (dependent on the age of the child). It therefore requires a clear history and a thorough clinical examination, looking for reduced range of movement, deformity and pain. It is important to note whether the history fits the pattern of the fracture, and any discrepancies in the description of the injury should alert the practitioner. Any fracture sustained in the non-ambulant child requires careful investigation.

SAFEGUARDING STOP POINT

WEBLINK:
SAFEGUARDING
DISABLED
CHILDREN

Every NHS Trust has a local child protection policy and lead consultant. As nurses it is our duty of care to appreciate the vulnerability of all children to potential abuse, in particular those with disability. A child who presents with an unexplained fracture requires investigation, but it is also important to recognise that disabled children are at greater risk of abuse than non-disabled children, and it is essential that safeguarding strategies are in place to protect them from harm and ensure their needs are met.

Treatment of the fracture is to realign the bone ends, and whilst a degree of angulation can be accepted (depending on the bone involved and the age of the child), rotational deformities require correction. Immobilisation of a fracture may be achieved by a plaster cast, traction or internal fixation with metal work. Generally, the child will recover quickly following treatment for a fracture. Once out of immobilisation, when the fracture has healed, the child will self-limit their activities until confident. Physiotherapy is therefore rarely required.

The nurse's role in caring for the child with a fracture is to:

- Assess for peripheral neurovascular deficit (signs and symptoms of vascular problems to the limb) and report any concerns promptly
- Elevate the limb to reduce swelling
- Ensure the child receives optimal pain relief
- Reassure and explain the reason for immobilisation
- Educate the child and family in the care of the cast/splint

Go to https://study.sagepub.com/essentialchildnursing for tips on preparing for placements when working with children with musculoskeletal problems.

PLACEMENT
ADVICE 24:
MUSCULOSKELETAL
PROBLEMS

CHAPTER SUMMARY

- The delivery of expert care for the child with a musculoskeletal disorder requires the nurse to be knowledgeable about the differences in a child's anatomy and have the skills to adapt orthopaedic interventions to meet the needs of the child

- Specialist paediatric orthopaedic nursing is becoming centralised into the larger 'hub' hospitals. However, whether a fracture or a child presenting for the first time with undiagnosed hip pain, the nurse is at the forefront in ensuring the child receives appropriate evidenced-based care

BUILD YOUR BIBLIOGRAPHY

Books

- Clarke, S. and Santy-Tomlinson, J. (eds) (2014) *Orthopaedic and Trauma Nursing. An Evidence-based Approach to Musculoskeletal Care*. Oxford: Wiley Blackwell.

  This book provides practitioners with up-to-date evidence and knowledge which underpins safe and effective nursing practice. It includes a specific section on the management of children.

- Judd, J. (2008) 'Application and care of traction', in J. Kelsey and G. McEwing (eds), *Clinical Skills in Child Health Practice*. London: Churchill Livingstone.

  This chapter gives a complete pictorial overview of the application of Thomas splint traction. It can be read in conjunction with the Traction benchmark in the RCN guidance *Benchmarks for Children's Orthopaedic Nursing Care*. Available at: www2.rcn.org.uk/__data/assets/pdf_file/0007/115486/RCN_CYP_ortho_WEB.pdf (last accessed 23 May 2017).

- Staheli, L.T. (2016) *Fundamentals of Pediatric Orthopaedics*, 5th edn. Seattle, WA: Lippincott Williams & Wilkins.

  This book is an excellent resource covering children's orthopaedic conditions in a question and answer format.

Journal articles

Go to https://study.sagepub.com/essentialchildnursing for further free online journal articles related to this chapter.

FURTHER READING: ONLINE JOURNAL ARTICLES

- Hainsworth, K.R., Miller, L.A., Stolzman, S.C., Fidlin, B.M., Hobart Davies, W., Weisman, S.J. and Skelton, J.A. (2012) 'Pain as a comorbidity of pediatric obesity'. *ICAN: Infant, Child, & Adolescent Nutrition*, 4 (5): 315-20.

  Read this article and reflect on the increasing problem of obesity in children and how it impacts on their growing skeleton. Obesity is also linked to slipped capital femoral epiphysis and vitamin D deficiency.

- Griffin, A. and Christie, D. 'Taking the psycho out of psychosomatic: using systemic approaches in a paediatric setting for the treatment of adolescents with unexplained physical symptoms'. *Clin Child Psychol Psychiatry*, 13 (4): 531-42.

  Although not related to an orthopaedic problem, this article describes a multidisciplinary psychological approach to treating the adolescent with amplified pain syndrome.

- Sims-Gould, J., Race, J., Hamilton, L., MacDonald, H., Mulpuri, K. and Mckay, H. (2016) '"I fell off and landed badly": Children's experiences of forearm fracture and injury prevention'. *J Child Health Care*, 20 (1): 98-108.

  Using a research method called Photovoice this article presents children's views on their injury experience and reviews fracture prevention.

(Continued)

(Continued)

Weblinks

FURTHER
READING:
WEBLINKS

Go to https://study.sagepub.com/essentialchildnursing for further weblinks related to this chapter.

- RCN, *Benchmarks for Children's Orthopaedic Nursing Care*

  www2.rcn.org.uk/__data/assets/pdf_file/0007/115486/RCN_CYP_ortho_WEB.pdf

- International Hip Dysplasia Institute

  www.hipdysplasia.org
  A wealth of evidence-based literature for the practitioner and essential information and advice for parents.

- RCN, *Guidance on Pin Site Care*

  www2.rcn.org.uk/__data/assets/pdf_file/0009/413982/004137.pdf
  Report and recommendations from the 2010 Consensus Project on pin site care.

ONLINE
QUIZZES &
ACTIVITY
ANSWERS

GREAT FOR
REVISION!

——— ACE YOUR ASSESSMENT ———

Revise what you have learned by visiting https://study.sagepub.com/essentialchildnursing

- Test yourself with multiple-choice and short-answer questions
- Do the chapter activities in the book and check your answers online

REFERENCES

Blount, W.T. (1955) *Fractures in Children*. Baltimore, MD: Williams & Wilkins.

Bolland, B.J., Wahed, A., Al-Hallao, S., Culliford, D.J. and Clarke, N.M.P. (2010) 'Late reduction in congenital dislocation of the hip and the need for secondary surgery: radiologic predictors and confounding variables'. *J PediatrOrthop*, 30 (7): 676–82.

Bowen, J.R., Guille, J.T., Jeong, C., Worananarat, P., Oh, C-W., Rodriquez, A., Holmes, L. and Rogers, K.J. (2011) 'Labral support shelf arthroplasty for containment in early stages of Legg-Calve-Perthes disease'. *J PediatrOrthop*, 31 (2) Supplement: S206–11.

Carsi, B., Judd, J. and Clarke, N.M.P. (2015) 'Shelf acetabuloplasty for containment in the early stages of Legg-Calve-Perthes disease'. *J PediatrOrthop*, 35 (2): 151–6.

Cashman, J.P., Round, J., Taylor, G. and Clarke, N.M.P. (2002) 'The natural history of developmental dysplasia of the hip after early supervised treatment in the Pavlik harness'. *J Bone Joint Surg*, 84 (3): 418–25.

Clarke, N.M.P. and Castanada, P. (2012) 'Strategies to improve non-operative childhood management'. *Orthopaedic Clinics of North America*, 43: 281–9.

Clarke, N.M.P. and Page, J.E. (2012) 'Vitamin D deficiency: a paediatric orthopaedic perspective'. *CurrOpin Pediatr*, 24: 46–9.

Clarke, N.M.P., Taylor, C.C. and Judd, J. (2016) 'Diagnosis and management of developmental dysplasia of the hip'. *Paediatrics and Child Health*, 26 (6), 252–6.

Clarke, S. and Liggett, L. (2014) 'Key issues in caring for the child and young person with an orthopaedic or musculoskeletal trauma condition', in S. Clarke and J. Santy-Tomlinson (eds), *Orthopaedic and Trauma Nursing: An Evidenced-based Approach to Musculoskeletal Care*. Oxford: Wiley Blackwell.

Clarke, S. and McKay, M. (2006) 'An audit of spica cast guidelines for parents and professionals caring for children with developmental dysplasia of the hip'. *Journal of Orthopaedic Nursing*, 10 (3): 128–37.

Clarke, S. and Santy-Tomlinson, J. (eds) (2014) *Orthopaedic and Trauma Nursing: An Evidenced-based Approach to Musculoskeletal Care*. Oxford: Wiley Blackwell.

Daly, K., Bruce, C. and Catterall, A. (1999) 'Lateral shelf acetabuloplasty in Perthes' disease. A review at the end of growth'. *Journal of Bone & Joint Surgery*, 81: 380–4.

Davies, J.H., Reed, J.M., Blake, E., Priesemann, M., Jackson, A.A. and Clarke, N.M.P. (2011) 'Epidemiology of vitamin D deficiency in children presenting to a pediatric orthopaedic service in the UK'. *J PediatrOrthop*, 31: 798–802.

Davis, A. (2009) 'Developmental dysplasia of the hip. Screening for developmental dysplasia of the hip'. *BMJ*, 339: b4454.

Eastwood, D.M. and de Gheldere, A. (2010) 'Clinical examination for developmental dysplasia of the hip in neonates: how to stay out of trouble'. *BMJ*, 340: c1965.

Engesæter, I.Ø., Lehmann, T., Laborie, L.B., Lie, S.A., Rosendahl, K. and Engesæter, L.B. (2011) 'Total hip replacement in young adults with hip dysplasia. Age at diagnosis, previous treatment, quality of life, and validation of diagnoses reported to the Norwegian Arthroplasty Register between 1987 and 2007'. *ActaOrthopaedica*, 82 (2): 149–54.

Herzenberg, J.H., Standard, S.C. and Specht, S.C. (2013) 'Limb lengthening in children with a new, controllable internal device'. Poster. *European Paediatric Orthopaedic Society (EPOS)*, April 17–20, 2013; Athens, Greece.

Judd, J. (2004) 'Congenital talipes equino varus – evidence for using the Ponseti method of treatment'. *Journal of Orthopaedic Nursing*, 8 (3):160–3.

Judd, J. (2013) 'Rickets in the 21st century: a review of the consequences of low vitamin D and its management'. *International Journal of Orthopaedic and Trauma Nursing*, 17 (4): 199–208.

Judd. J. (2014) 'Common childhood orthopaedic conditions, their care and management', in S. Clarke and J. Santy-Tomlinson (eds), *Orthopaedic and Trauma Nursing: An Evidenced-based Approach to Musculoskeletal Care*. Oxford: Wiley Blackwell.

Miller, R.L.S. (2003) 'Reflex sympathetic dystrophy'. *Orthopaedic Nursing*, 22 (2): 91–9.

Public Health England (2016) *Newborn and Infant Physical Examination Screening Programme Standards 2016/17*. Available at: www.gov.uk/government/uploads/system/uploads/attachment_data/file/524424/NIPE_Programme_Standards_2016_to_2017.pdf (accessed 14 September 2017)

Tripathy, S., Sen, R., Dhatt, S. and Goyal, T. (2010) 'Legg-Calve-Perthes disease: current concepts'. *WebmedCentral Orthopaedics*, 1 (11). Available at: www.webmedcentral.com/article_view/1173 (last accessed 23 May 2017).

Van Der Geest, I.C.M., Kooijman, M.A.P., Spruit, M., Anderson, P.G. and De Smet, P.M.A. (2001) 'Shelf acetabuloplasty for Perthes disease: 12 year follow up'. *ActaOrthopædicaBelgica*, 67 (2): 126–31.

Wenger, D.R. and Pandya, N.K. (2011) 'A brief history of Legg-Calvé-Perthes disease'. *J PediatrOrthop*, 31 (2 Suppl): S130–6.

CARE OF CHILDREN AND YOUNG PEOPLE WITH HAEMATOLOGICAL PROBLEMS

25

LOUISE HOLLIDAY AND CARLA KIERULFF

THIS CHAPTER COVERS

- What is blood?
- Blood cell disorders
- Bleeding disorders
- Blood groups
- Care during a blood transfusion

REQUIRED KNOWLEDGE

A&P LINK 25.1:
HAEMATOLOGICAL
SYSTEM

It would be helpful to have an understanding of the haematological system before you start this chapter. Go to the A&P link: 'Haematological system' at https://study.sagepub.com/essential childnursing

> **"** Blood disorders can restrict children and young people when participating in physical activity, which can exclude them from lots of health and wellbeing benefits.
>
> **Alison Bain, senior physiotherapist** **"**

Visit https://study.sagepub.com/essentialchildnursing to access a wealth of online resources for this chapter – watch out for the margin icons throughout the chapter.

INTRODUCTION

The quotation that opens this chapter highlights how blood disorders can significantly affect quality of life. Some are life-limiting. If any child is seriously injured, obvious haemorrhage is the immediate priority, even before moving on to a structured 'ABCDE' assessment (Advanced Life Support Group, 2016). Beliefs about blood are so powerful in human culture that they may determine what people will eat, if they will accept a blood transfusion, their understanding about family and the expression of emotions.

This chapter will include an overview of the composition of blood. Some of the blood disorders you may encounter in practice will be highlighted and three will be explored in more depth: aplastic anaemia, sickle cell disease and haemophilia A. Management of blood disorders may require transfusions, so blood groups and care during transfusions will also be discussed.

WHAT IS BLOOD?

Blood is composed of 45 per cent cells and 55 per cent plasma (see Table 25.1). Blood is vital in carrying oxygen and other chemicals around the body, fighting infection and repairing damaged tissue.

Table 25.1 The composition of blood

Constituent		Action
Hematopoietic stem cells		These cells in the bone marrow are pluripotent so can develop into all types of blood cells
Lymphoid progenitor cells	B cells	These white blood cells respond to specific microbes based on previous encounters (adaptive response). NK cells are also involved in the innate immune response (see below)
	T cells	
	Natural killer (NK) cells	
Myeloid progenitor cells	Neutrophils	These white blood cells are all responsible for the inborn (innate) immune response. They secrete substances to kill invading microorganisms and/or attract other blood cells to come and help. Some ingest the microorganisms
	Eosinophils	
	Basophils	
	Mast cells	
	Monocytes	
	Dendritic cells	Guide the immune response by providing a vital link between innate and adaptive responses
	Erythrocytes (red blood cells)	Contain haemoglobin which carries oxygen around the body
	Thrombocytes (platelets)	Gather together to stop bleeding by plugging the gap in the endothelium
Plasma (about 55% of blood)	A liquid which carries the blood cells and contains a complex mixture of proteins and other vital substances. It helps maintain blood pressure and body temperature	
	Albumin	The most abundant plasma protein. Prevents fluid from leaking out of blood vessels. Carries other vital substances
	Clotting factors	Proteins which work together in a series of chemical reactions to stop bleeding
	Immunoglobulins	Protective proteins produced by the immune system in response to the presence of a foreign substance

ACTIVITY 25.1: CRITICAL THINKING

Before reading more of this chapter, consider how a lack of one or more of the constituents listed in Table 25.1 could affect health and wellbeing.

ACTIVITY
ANSWER 25.1

BLOOD CELL DISORDERS

Lack of stem cells leads to lack of all blood cells (pancytopenia; see Case study 24.1 about aplastic anaemia). Lack of mature white blood cells, including neutrophils (neutropenia), makes the child at risk of sepsis. Lack of red blood cells (anaemia) causes fatigue, paleness, tachypnoea, headaches, dizziness, tachycardia and cold extremities. Long-term anaemia impairs growth, motor and cognitive development, reduces school achievement and increases morbidity and mortality (World Health Organization, 2017). Signs of low platelets (thrombocytopenia) include easy and excessive bruising, petechiae (pinprick red/purple spots), purpura (larger, flat purple patches), bleeding nose, bleeding gums, bloody urine or faeces, and heavier periods in older girls.

PRACTICE
SCENARIO 25:
BRYAN

CASE STUDY 25.1: LUCY

Lucy was a 7-year-old girl diagnosed with aplastic anaemia following a history of a petechial rash and pallor. Clinicians initially adopted a 'watch and wait' approach to see if she would make a spontaneous recovery. When this did not occur, Lucy was admitted into hospital for insertion of a Hickman line and commencement of immunosuppressive therapy of anti-thymocyte globulin (ATG) horse and cyclosporin. The therapy was generally well tolerated, but Lucy needed many platelet and red blood cell transfusions and intravenous antibiotics to treat infections. This required Lucy to stay in hospital for prolonged periods, as she lived a two-hour drive from the hospital in a rural home she shared with her parents and younger brother.

Initially there was not a clear response to treatment, and a bone marrow transplant was considered. Gradually an increase in haemoglobin and platelets demonstrated a slow but satisfactory response to treatment. Weekly blood counts, reviews and platelet transfusions still meant regular trips to the hospital.

Cyclosporin doses were slowly reduced. Lucy was able to attend clinic every two weeks. To allow Lucy to stay at home, oncology nurses from the hospital taught local district nurses to manage her central line.

- What support would help Lucy and her family cope with her hospitalisation?
- How might the disease have an impact on her family?
- What advice was required to help Lucy's family promote her health while she was pancytopenic?

CASE STUDY
ANSWER 25.1

WATCH A
VIDEO ONLINE!

VIDEO
LINK 25.1:
APLASTIC
ANAEMIA

Go to https://study.sagepub.com/essentialchildnursing and watch the video which shows what happens to the blood cells in aplastic anaemia.

Iron deficiency is the most common cause of anaemia (World Health Organization, 2017). This may be prevented through a diet which includes iron-rich food and is high in vitamin C, which enhances iron absorption. Tea and coffee should be avoided. In some cases, iron supplements may be required. Side effects of daily oral iron supplements include nausea, constipation and stained teeth. Benefits can be obtained with fewer side effects by taking iron supplementation once, twice or three times a week, on non-consecutive days (De-Regil et al., 2011).

Haemaglobinopathies are disorders caused by mutations of the genes which control haemoglobin manufacture. These include sickle cell disease (see Scenario 25.1) and alpha and beta thalassemia. Mutation of the gene that controls red blood cell membrane proteins causes hereditary spherocytosis.

Another gene mutation results in pyruvate kinase deficiency, pyruvate kinase being an enzyme required in red blood cells. These conditions all cause haemolytic anaemia, as the abnormal red blood cells are fragile and are broken down more quickly than usual. This causes jaundice and an enlarged liver and spleen, as well as all the signs and symptoms of anaemia described earlier. Damage to the spleen reduces the body's ability to fight infection. Mutation of the gene which makes the enzyme glucose-6-phosphate dehydrogenase (G6PD), causes G6PD deficiency. This only causes a haemolytic crisis on exposure to certain foods and some medicines (G6PD Deficiency Association, 2017).

SCENARIO 25.1: HOLLY

Holly is a 15-year-old with sickle cell disease. She takes regular penicillin to prevent infection, and folic acid to promote the production of red blood cells. She tries to drink plenty of fluids, and stay warm and free from stress. However, recently, with school exams approaching, she has had a couple of painful crises. This has meant time off school and in hospital, where she required opioid analgesia, oxygen, intravenous antibiotics and fluids. Holly is worried that she might not do as well as expected in her exams. She is also aware that the severe pain she experienced was due to blockage of her blood vessels by the sickle-shaped red blood cells. She knows such blockages could cause permanent damage to her organs and bones. She is scared she might have a stroke and die. This happened to a relative. Holly does not feel able to discuss her fears with her family.

CHECK YOUR
ANSWERS
ONLINE!

- Who do you think could provide support for Holly?

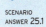

SCENARIO
ANSWER 25.1

Immune (idiopathic) thrombocytopenia (ITP) is a blood disorder in which the immune system attacks the platelets, often following a viral infection or vaccination (Grainger, 2017). About three quarters of children with ITP will recover spontaneously within six months. Tranexamic acid may be given to promote clotting. A short course of steroids, intravenous immunoglobulin or anti-D may be given to try to reduce platelet destruction.

VIDEO LINK
25.2:
SICKLE CELL
INHERITANCE

Go to https://study.sagepub.com/essentialchildnursing and watch the film exploring how sickle cell inheritance can affect a family.

SAFEGUARDING STOP POINT

Multiple bruises on an infant should raise concerns about whether the child is being cared for in an unsafe environment or has been harmed. However, large amounts of bruising can also be a sign of low platelets (thrombocytopenia, see above) caused by rare conditions such as Glanzmann's thrombasthenia.

SEE ALSO
CHAPTER 33

- How would you respond to the parents of an infant who claim they have no knowledge of how such bruising has occurred?
- What blood tests do you think would be required?

SAFEGUARDING
STOP POINT
ANSWER 25.1

BLEEDING DISORDERS

Clotting factor deficiencies are often inherited. Haemophilia A is caused by a deficiency of factor VIII and haemophilia B is caused by a deficiency of factor IX: both of these are X-linked disorders, usually inherited from the mother (see Figure 25.1).

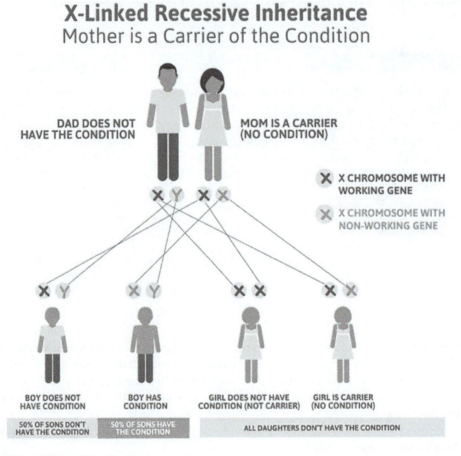

Figure 25.1   X-linked inheritance

www.geneticsupport.org/genetics-101/inheritance-patterns/x-linked

The more severe the condition, the earlier the age of presentation (Haemophilia Society, 2017). There will be a tendency to bruise easily, excessive and prolonged bleeding from cuts, and a tendency to bleed into joints and muscles causing pain, swelling, limitation of movement and long-term damage. Haemophilia is managed by replacing the missing clotting factor through an intravenous infusion of clotting factor concentrate. Research suggests it is beneficial for children with haemophilia to be treated prophylactically with the missing clotting factor, as young as possible, before joint damage has occurred (Lambert et al., 2014). Any bleeding episodes must be treated promptly, preferably within two hours. Physiotherapy, to maintain muscle strength and functional ability, is an important part of management.

SCENARIO 25.2: KYLE

Kyle is a two-year-old with haemophilia A. His mother Catherine is a carrier. Kyle has been on prophylactic factor VIII therapy for a year. A decision was made to insert an implanted port and both his parents agreed to be trained in its use. His father Bruce is not as confident as Catherine at accessing the port, but Catherine needs his help to hold Kyle still. Catherine is frustrated that Bruce often arrives home late from work, which delays the time Kyle can be given his prophylaxis and settled to sleep. This causes frequent rows between Catherine and Bruce.

- As a nurse how could you support Kyle, Catherine and Bruce?

SCENARIO
ANSWER 25.2

Von Willebrand disease (vW), the most common inherited bleeding disorder, is caused by a deficiency of von Willebrand factor (vWf). Type 1 or 2 usually occurs when one parent has passed on a faulty gene. Type 3, the most severe, occurs if both parents pass on a faulty gene. Both men and women are affected by vW, though women experience more problems because of menstruation, pregnancy and childbirth. The disorder causes little or no disruption to the lives of most people with vW. In severe cases, internal bleeding to muscles and joints can occur in a similar way to haemophilia. Management will depend on the person's specific condition. Options include tranexamic acid, desmopressin and vWf replacement therapy.

Disseminated intravascular coagulation (DIC) is an acute crisis in which there is a sudden systemic activation of coagulation, involving the whole body (Levi et al., 2009). It is usually caused by sepsis, malignancy, trauma or liver disease. Widespread fibrin deposition leads to microvascular thrombosis, causing tissue necrosis and organ failure. As platelets and coagulation factors are used up in the clotting process, thrombocytopenia and coagulation factor deficiency may also result, causing bleeding.

Either thrombosis or bleeding may predominate at any given time, and this may change as a situation evolves. Where thrombosis predominates, heparin may be given. If the child is bleeding, or if an invasive procedure is required that entails a risk of bleeding, then platelet transfusion and/or fresh frozen plasma (FFP) (and, in some severe cases, fibrinogen concentrate or cryoprecipitate) will be required. If thrombosis predominates, but the child is also bleeding, tranexamic acid may be given.

BLOOD GROUPS

There are over 300 human blood groups, but the two most important for clinical practice are the ABO and RhD systems (Norfolk, 2013).

ABO

A person is identified as A, B, AB or O based on the combination or absence of A or B antigens on their red blood cells (see Figure 25.2 below).

In the first few months of life, you normally develop antibodies to the A or B antigens that are not present on your own red cells. People with blood group O are sometimes known as 'universal donors' as their red cells have no A or B antigens. However, if a group O donor's plasma contains high levels of anti-A and anti-B their platelets may only be suitable for recipients with group O blood and group O fresh frozen plasma must only be given to people with group O blood.

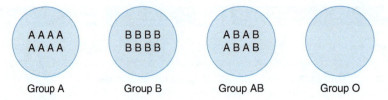

Figure 25.2   ABO blood group antigens on red blood cells

Rh

There are several Rh antigens on red cells for which individuals can be positive or negative. RhD negative individuals only develop antibodies to RhD ('anti-D') in two specific circumstances: if an RhD negative male or female is transfused with RhD positive red blood cells, and if an RhD negative women becomes pregnant with an RhD positive baby.

If an RhD negative person who has developed anti-D antibodies in either of these circumstances is subsequently exposed to RhD positive blood, their anti-D antibodies will attack it. It is therefore important to avoid exposing RhD negative individuals of both sexes to RhD positive red blood cell transfusions, except in extreme emergencies. This is particularly important with females of child-bearing potential, in order to avoid haemolytic disease of the foetus or newborn.

CARE DURING A BLOOD TRANSFUSION

WEBLINK:
LEARNBLOOD
TRANSFUSION

Transfusion of blood components may be required due to acute or chronic conditions or following intensive treatments such as immunosuppressive therapy. Nurses must ensure they are fully informed and appropriately educated to be competent to assist or carry out transfusions. The e-learning resource *LearnBloodTransfusion* (http://betterblood.org.uk) is recommended by blood transfusion services in the British Isles.

Local policies must be followed.

Compatibility

When a blood transfusion is required it is essential that blood from a compatible blood type is given. Giving incompatible blood can be fatal. It is vital that staff check a patient's identity both verbally (with patient, their parent or carer) and with name band, when obtaining blood samples for cross matching, as well as when starting a transfusion. Staff must equally ensure blood tubes are labelled accurately. Transfusion of even a small amount of incompatible blood can trigger a major immune response, and children can die from circulatory collapse or renal failure. Ideally people should receive their own precise blood type. If this is not possible, a different but compatible blood type must be given.

Potential change in blood group

In finding a suitable match for bone marrow transplant or peripheral blood stem cell transplant, it is human leukocyte antigen (HLA) rather than red blood cell antigen compatibility which is most vital (Helming et al., 2007; Worel and Kalhs, 2008). A patient's blood group will change to the donor's blood type. It is therefore vital that nurses are vigilant in checking that components from the correct blood group are administered during and after engraftment of cells.

Red blood cell transfusion

Red blood cells may be required when a child is severely anaemic. They must be stored within a designated blood fridge and the infusion started within 30 minutes of the pack leaving this fridge. The whole unit of red blood cells (or the amount required, calculated on the child's weight and haemoglobin) must be infused within four hours of being removed from the cold storage system. Blood must be transfused using a dedicated blood-giving set with filter and not be mixed with other medication or fluids. Normal saline must be used to check patency of the intravenous (IV) access device.

Platelet transfusion

Signs of low platelets (thrombocytopenia) have already been discussed. Platelet transfusions are given in a unit bag. It is a straw-coloured liquid, which is usually administered over 30 minutes. Platelets are stored at room temperature on a platelet agitator to prevent clumping. Platelet infusions require a blood transfusion set with filter, and nurses must ensure infusion pumps are suitable and will not crush the platelets during infusion.

Consent

Other than in an emergency, consent must be obtained prior to transfusion. The type of transfusion needed, the reason transfusion is required and the risks and benefits of the transfusion must be explained and documented when seeking such consent. Literature about transfusion is available from the national blood transfusion service for children (NHS Blood and Transplant, 2012) and parents (NHS Blood and Transplant, 2014). If consent is not given for blood transfusion, which the treating clinician considers is life-saving or essential for the wellbeing of the child, a court order can be obtained (Norfolk, 2013).

Observations

A prior assessment must be made to determine if the child is fit for a planned blood transfusion. This must include a baseline set of observations of blood pressure, pulse, temperature and respiratory rate. Any changes in condition must be reported to medical staff prior to transfusion. After the transfusion is commenced, observation and monitoring will be required as per hospital policy, which will usually involve a minimum of recording observations 15 minutes into transfusion, then hourly throughout transfusion, and at the end.

Haemolytic reactions

Haemolytic reactions can occur if there is an ABO, RhD or other incompatibility between the donated blood unit and patient's blood. Such reactions usually appear within 5 to 15 minutes after commencement of transfusion, although they may develop later, either during or even some days after the infusion.

Signs and symptoms of an acute haemolytic reaction include hypotension, fever, rigors, chills, lower back and chest pain, anxiety, nausea, vomiting, bloody urine, dizziness, and DIC (see above). If any of these signs appear, the transfusion must be stopped immediately and experienced help summoned. Management will include: maintaining the airway, breathing and circulation; observation of vital signs; administration of high flow oxygen; and hydration and diuretics. Blood samples will be required from the recipient to confirm this was a haemolytic reaction.

Hypersensitivity reactions

Signs and symptoms of an allergic reaction include urticaria (hives), facial swelling, wheezing, respiratory distress, nausea, abdominal cramps, vomiting, diarrhoea, fever, hypotension, shock and loss of consciousness. Reactions may initially be mild, often with an itchy rash. At this point the transfusion must be discontinued, while maintaining intravenous access, and then an anaphylaxis algorithm must be followed.

Immunoglobulins can be given intravenously to help individuals fight infection. Although there are five types of immunoglobulins found in plasma, it is usually IgG that is transfused. It can be administered for a variety of conditions as well as low immunity. It is sometimes given to treat autoimmune neurological disease such as Guillain-Barré syndrome. A cross match is not required but the patient should be monitored for hypersensitivity reactions.

Albumin may be used to restore and maintain circulating blood volume, although its use is now controversial (Norfolk, 2013). Different concentrations are available, usually ranging between 5 and 25 per cent. A cross match is not required, but nurses should monitor for fluid overload and hypersensitivity reactions.

Irradiated blood products have been treated with radiation to prevent transfusion associated graft versus host disease. These are required for all patients with Hodgkin's disease, unborn babies who require an exchange transfusion, patients who are undergoing a stem cell transplant or those who are receiving certain medication (NHS Blood and Transplant, 2016).

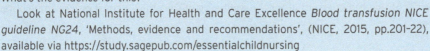

WHAT'S THE EVIDENCE?

Different centres have different cut-off levels for transfusing platelets for invasive nursing interventions, such as intramuscular injection and passing nasogastric tubes. What's the evidence for this?

Look at National Institute for Health and Care Excellence *Blood transfusion NICE guideline NG24*, 'Methods, evidence and recommendations', (NICE, 2015, pp.201–22), available via https://study.sagepub.com/essentialchildnursing

WEBLINK:
BLOOD
TRANSFUSION

WHAT'S THE
EVIDENCE?
ANSWER 25.1

Go to https://study.sagepub.com/essentialchildnursing for tips on preparing for placements when working with children with haematological problems.

PLACEMENT
ADVICE 25:
HAEMATOLOGICAL
PROBLEMS

CHAPTER SUMMARY

- Blood is vital in carrying oxygen around the body, fighting infection and repairing damaged tissue
- Blood disorders in children are wide ranging and can greatly impact quality of life for the child and family
- Children having a blood transfusion need specific care and monitoring

BUILD YOUR BIBLIOGRAPHY

Journal articles

Go to https://study.sagepub.com/essentialchildnursing for further free online journal articles related to this chapter.

FURTHER
READING:
ONLINE
JOURNAL
ARTICLES

- Erskine, R. (2011) 'Adolescent boys with sickle cell disease: a qualitative study'. *Clinical Child Psychology and Psychiatry*, 17 (1): 17–31.

  This article gives an insight into the experience of young people with sickle cell disease.

Weblinks

Go to https://study.sagepub.com/essentialchildnursing for further weblinks related to this chapter.

- The British Psychological Society, *Good Practice Guidelines: Evidence-based Guidelines for the Management of Invasive and/or Distressing Procedures with Children* (Gaskell, 2010)

  www.bps.org.uk/system/files/Public%20files/cat-606.pdf

  Diagnosis and monitoring of blood disorders involves venepuncture. Read more about ways of reducing the distress for children.

- SHOT (Serious Hazards of Transfusion)

  www.shotuk.org

  Since 1996, Serious Hazards of Blood Transfusion (SHOT) has collected and analysed anonymised information on adverse events and reactions in blood transfusion from all healthcare organisations that are involved in the transfusion of blood and blood components in the UK. Where risks and problems are identified, SHOT produces recommendations to improve patient safety. The recommendations are put into its annual report which is then circulated to all the relevant organisations including the four UK Blood Services, the Departments of Health in England, Wales, Scotland and Northern Ireland and all the relevant professional bodies as well as to all the reporting hospitals. As haemovigilance is an ongoing exercise, SHOT can also monitor the effect of the implementation of its recommendations:

- JPAC (Joint United Kingdom (UK) Blood Transfusion and Tissue Transplantation Services Professional Advisory Committee), *Blood Products*

  www.transfusionguidelines.org.uk/transfusion-handbook/3-providing-safe-blood/3-3-blood-products

  For further information and guidance, JPAC provide best practice guidance on various blood products mentioned in this chapter, which can be required in caring for children with blood disorders.

- GOV.UK, *Clinical Guidelines for Immunoglobulin Use* (Department of Health, 2011)

  www.gov.uk/government/publications/clinical-guidelines-for-immunoglobulin-use-second-edition-update

  For further information about use of immunoglobulin.

FURTHER READING: WEBLINKS

ACE YOUR ASSESSMENT

Revise what you have learned by visiting https://study.sagepub.com/essentialchildnursing

- Test yourself with multiple-choice and short-answer questions
- Do the chapter activities in the book and check your answers online

ONLINE QUIZZES & ACTIVITY ANSWERS

REFERENCES

Advanced Life Support Group (2016) *Advanced Paediatric Life Support: A Practical Approach to Emergencies (APLS)*, 6th edn. London: BMJ Books Wiley-Blackwell.

De-Regil, L.M., Jefferds, M.E., Sylvetsky, A.C. and Dowswell, T. (2011) 'Intermittent iron supplementation for improving nutrition and development in children under 12 years of age'. *Cochrane Database of Systematic Reviews*. Available at: www.ncbi.nlm.nih.gov/pubmed/22161444 (last accessed 23 May 2017).

G6PD Deficiency Association (2017) *What Is G6PD Deficiency?* Available at: www.g6pd.org/en/G6PDDeficiency.aspx (last accessed 23 May 2017).

Grainger, J. (2017) *What Is Childhood ITP?* Available at: www.itpsupport.org.uk/index.php/en/information/itp-in-children (last accessed 23 May 2017).

Haemophilia Society (2017) *Bleeding Disorders*. Available at: http://haemophilia.org.uk/bleeding-disorders (last accessed 23 May 2017).

Helming, A.M., Brand, A., Wolterbeek, R., van Tol, M.J., Egeler, R.M. and Ball, L.M. (2007) 'ABO incompatible stem cell transplantation in children does not influence outcome'. *Pediatric Blood & Cancer*, 49 (3): 313–17.

Lambert, T., Auerswald, G., Benson, G., Hedner, G., Jiménez-Yuste, V., Liung, R., Morfini, M., Remor, E., Santagostino, E. and Zupančić Šalek, S. (2014) 'Joint disease, the hallmark of haemophilia: what issues and challenges remain despite the development of effective therapies?' *Thrombosis Research*, 133: 967–71.

Levi, M., Toh, C.H., Thachil, J. and Watson, H.G. (2009) 'Guidelines for the diagnosis and management of disseminated intravascular coagulation. British Committee for Standards in Haematology'. *British Journal of Haematology*, 145 (1): 24–33.

National Institute for Health and Care Excellence (2015) *Blood Transfusion NICE Guideline NG24*. London: NICE. Available at: www.nice.org.uk/guidance/ng24/evidence (last accessed 23 May 2017).

NHS Blood and Transplant (2012) *Amazing You and Voyages on the Microsub Discovery*. Oxford: NHSBT. Available at: http://hospital.blood.co.uk/patient-services/patient-blood-management/patient-information-leaflets (last accessed 23 May 2017).

NHS Blood and Transplant (2014) *Will Your Child Need a Blood Transfusion?* Oxford: NHSBT. Available at: http://hospital.blood.co.uk/patient-services/patient-blood-management/patient-information-leaflets (last accessed 23 May 2017).

NHS Blood and Transplant (2016) *Information for Patients Needing Irradiated Blood*. Oxford: NHSBT. Available at: http://hospital.blood.co.uk/patient-services/patient-blood-management/patient-information-leaflets (last accessed 23 May 2017).

Norfolk, D. (2013) *Handbook of Transfusion Medicine United Kingdom Blood Services*, 5th edn. London: The Stationery Office. Available at: www.transfusionguidelines.org/transfusion-handbook (last accessed 23 May 2017).

Worel, N. and Kalhs, P. (2008) 'ABO-incompatible allogeneic hematopoietic stem cell transplantation'. *Heamatologica*, 93, 1605–7.

World Health Organization (2017) *Anaemia*. Available at: www.who.int/topics/anaemia/en (last accessed 23 May 2017).

CARE OF CHILDREN AND YOUNG PEOPLE WITH DERMATOLOGICAL PROBLEMS

26

JOAN MYERS AND DOLORES D'SOUZA

THIS CHAPTER COVERS

- Physiology of the skin
- Atopic eczema
- Discoid eczema
- Seborrhoeic eczema
- Eczema herpeticum
- Acne
- History taking and skin assessment

REQUIRED KNOWLEDGE

It would be helpful to have an understanding of the anatomy and physiology of the skin system before you start this chapter. Go to the A&P link: 'Skin system' at https://study.sagepub.com/essentialchildnursing

A&P LINK 26.1: SKIN

> 66
> Eczema is a hard thing to deal with and a hard thing to clear. Knowing that I can't do things like other people is hard, like playing with play dough.
>
> **Kai, child**
> 99

Visit https://study.sagepub.com/essentialchildnursing to access a wealth of online resources for this chapter – watch out for the margin icons throughout the chapter.

INTRODUCTION

Mason reveals how his eczema impacts on his ability to play. As children's nurses it's important to understand how common dermatological conditions affect children and their quality of life. This will be covered in the chapter along with a brief overview of the anatomy and physiology of the skin. We will also examine how to recognise common dermatological conditions in childhood and how to take a history and carry out a skin assessment. By the end of the chapter you should be able to write a care plan and evaluate treatment given.

CASE
STUDY 26.1:
TAAIBAH

This chapter explores common features of atopic eczema, seborrhoeic eczema, discoid eczema, eczema herpeticum, acne and fungal infections of the skin. Management of these dermatological conditions will be discussed, including common treatments used, such as emollients and topical corticosteroids. The opening quotation gives an indication of the impact eczema has on the child, and the case studies in the chapter will explore the impact of other dermatological conditions on quality of life. By the end of this chapter you will be able to understand and recognise the principles of skin assessment, and will gain an understanding of how to manage and treat the dermatological conditions identified.

PHYSIOLOGY OF THE SKIN

The skin is the largest organ of the body as it provides a continuous covering for the whole surface of the body. The skin, also known as stratified squamous epithelium, is composed of three layers: the epidermis, the dermis, and subcutaneous tissue (see Figure 26.1). Each layer has a distinct role in the overall function of the skin. The skin has many functions, including protection against external physical, chemical and biologic attack. It also prevents excessive water loss from the body and has a role in thermoregulation and synthesis of vitamin D.

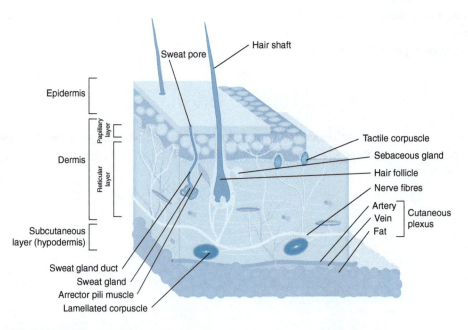

WEBLINK: SKIN
STRUCTURE
AND
FUNCTIONS

Figure 26.1 Accessory structures of the skin

Boore et al. (2016) *Essentials of Anatomy and Physiology for Nursing Practice*. London: Sage.

The outer layer of the skin, the epidermis, is affected by several factors including: age, diet, disease, ethnicity, the environment, internal and external stresses, and soaps and cleansers.

ACTIVITY 26.1: CRITICAL THINKING

In what ways might age, diet, disease, ethnicity, the environment, internal and external stresses, and soaps and cleansers affect the function of the skin in a child with eczema?

ACTIVITY
ANSWER 26.1

ATOPIC ECZEMA

Changes in the skin's appearance are often referred to as a rash. Most rashes are caused by simple skin irritations, but there are others that are formed as a result of a dermatological condition. 'Dermatitis' is a general term for skin that is inflamed. Atopic eczema is the most common type of skin inflammation, causing an irritating pruritic (itchy) rash in the epidermal layers of the skin. It usually manifests at 3 months of age, but can occur at any age, and is considered to be a chronic recurring condition which has exacerbations or flares followed by remissions.

Atopic eczema is a genetically determined disorder arising out of the interaction of environmental factors and an abnormal immune system. Cork et al. (2009) discuss three groups of genes which cause a defective epidermal barrier and predispose an individual to the development of eczema. The most important of these is the FLG gene, which encodes the structural protein filaggrin. Filaggrin is an important gene in the maintenance of a healthy stratum corneum, which is the outer layer of the skin. When healthy, this layer keeps pathogens and allergens out and maintains moisture by preventing water loss by evaporation (please refer to Case study 26.1 and photographs). You can watch the NHS video on 'Eczema in babies and young children' accessible via https://study.sagepub.com/essentialchildnursing

VIDEO LINK
26.1: ECZEMA
IN CHILDREN

ACTIVITY 26.2: CRITICAL THINKING

List some irritants and inhaled allergens that could trigger eczema to worsen.

ACTIVITY
ANSWER 26.2

CASE
STUDY 26.2:
TARA

Diagnosing atopic eczema

There is no specific laboratory diagnostic test for atopic eczema. A diagnosis of atopic eczema is therefore usually made on clinical evidence. NICE guidance provides diagnostic criteria for disgnosis of eczema (NICE, 2007).

To be diagnosed with atopic eczema the child must have an itchy condition (or reported scratching or rubbing), plus three or more of the following:

1. A history of itchiness in skin creases, such as folds of the elbows, behind the knees, front of ankles or around the neck (or the cheeks in children under 4 years)
2. A history of asthma or hay fever (or a history of atopic disease in a first-degree relative in children under 4 years)
3. General dry skin in the past year
4. Visible flexural eczema (or eczema affecting the cheeks or forehead and outer aspects of limbs in children under 4 years). Darkly pigmented skin is more likely to have eczema in the extensor surfaces of limbs
5. Onset in the first two years of life (not always diagnostic in children under 4 years)

It is important to be aware that in Asian, black Caribbean and black African children atopic eczema may appear discoid (circular) or follicular (around hair follicles).

Treating atopic eczema

Emollients are the first-line treatment for atopic eczema. They are available as ointments, creams, lotions, gels, sprays and paste. Emollients increase the amount of water held in the stratum corneum. They work in two specific ways depending on their ingredients: greasy emollients such as petroleum trap moisture in the skin; emollients containing humectants work by penetrating the epidermis and drawing water in from the dermis to the stratum corneum of the epidermis (BDNG, 2012).

There is a wide variety of emollients available for use. It is therefore essential to allow parents and children to sample different types of emollients to find one they prefer. Patient preference is more important than professional choice when considering an emollient, as parents and children are more likely to use what they like and this is an important factor in compliance with treatment.

CASE STUDY 26.1: SALEH

Saleh was diagnosed with eczema when he was 2 months old. At the age of four his eczema was poorly controlled and he found it very itchy and annoying, particularly at night when he would scratch until his skin bled. At the age of 5 Saleh started seeing a dermatology nurse, who provided creams and educated the family in the application. The nurse reviewed Saleh's skin regularly. After some time his skin began to improve, and now, at the age of 6, his body is clear and most of the eczema is gone.

- Why was Saleh's skin so itchy?
- What can be done to ease the itch?
- What is the itch–scratch cycle?

CASE STUDY
ANSWER 26.1

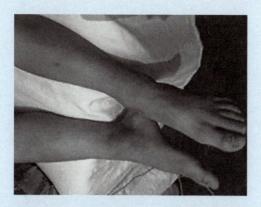

Figure 26.2 Saleh's skin before regular emollients and steroids

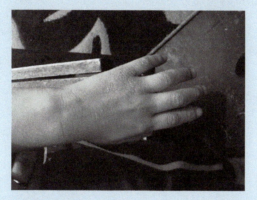

Figure 26.3 Saleh's skin after regular emollients and steroids

Once the skin is moisturised there is less risk of irritants affecting it and causing it to feel itchy. Emollients protect the skin by forming a barrier against allergens while moisturising the skin, so there is less risk of the skin becoming infected. Emollients are effective rehydrating agents and are one of the most important tools in controlling and managing dry skin conditions. It is therefore important that a complete emollient therapy of soap substitute, emollient bath oil and emollient cream or ointment is used so that the child's skin can be kept adequately hydrated.

CASE STUDY 26.2: BEN

Five-year-old Ben was referred to the primary care nursing clinic by his GP to have his eczema reviewed. Ben has had eczema since he was 2 months old. His GP has been managing his eczema by prescribing various creams. He has also been referred to the dermatology clinic twice, but the appointments were not attended. In children's nursing there is a recent drive to say the child 'was

(Continued)

(Continued)

not brought' to the appointment rather than say the child 'did not attend'. This recognises the fact that attending clinics is beyond the ability of the individual child and the responsibility for this lies with the parent or family members. It is another example of respecting the rights of the child.

Ben's arms, legs, hands and feet were covered in severe active eczema with areas of thickened skin. He also had small scabs on his wrists and hands from previous scratching that caused bleeding. After assessing Ben's skin, taking a full history and making a new eczema care plan, it was decided that it would be more appropriate to visit Ben and his mother at home, where adequate time could be spent educating and supporting.

There was no initial improvement in Ben's skin. However, after demonstrating how to use the cream, Ben's skin quickly showed signs of improvement.

The assessment and treatment of eczema often require more than a ten-minute consultation. Many families are unable to comply with the specialist's instructions as they do not know how to apply creams. Spending time with Ben and his mother in their home was an essential aspect of care and education, and highlighted their needs. With support and encouragement, they are were empowered in their understanding and treatment of Ben's eczema. As a result, Ben's skin improved and he now lives a much happier life.

- Name five skin symptoms of atopic eczema
- What is an emollient?
- How often is emollient used?
- How do topical corticosteroids work?

CASE STUDY
ANSWER 26.2

My recent practice placement with the community children's nursing service has brought new light on the physical and mental difficulties children face with chronic skin conditions. Equally, the challenges that parents and families experience with managing skin conditions. One case of childhood atopic eczema stands out in my mind whilst working alongside my mentor in the nurse-led eczema clinic. A 9-year-old girl was brought to clinic by her father as her mother was at work. The child's skin was infected as a result of continuous scratching and poor management. During the assessment and observation it was gathered that dad lacked the knowledge of how to manage his daughter's condition and as a result the child was left to cope on her own.

The child was prescribed emollients and topical corticosteroids and given a care plan. Time was also spent educating the child and her dad verbally alongside practice demonstration. Written instructions were given along with literature about the condition and the importance of adhering to treatment. The identification and management of triggers were also covered. It became clear to me now that in some cases all parents need is more education, support and guidance to relieve the worry that comes with dealing with childhood eczema.

Camesha, 2nd-year children's nursing student

DISCOID ECZEMA

This is another form of eczema, which presents in the form of disc shapes. It is sometimes called num-mular eczema, which means coin shaped. This type of eczema presents with lesions that are highly inflamed and very itchy. It affects the limbs more than the body and can involve the face, although rare, or the scalp. Each area can begin with a small group of red spots and tiny bumps which become bigger and develop into a round patch. The round patches become dry and scaly.

Treatment is by potent steroids used once or twice daily in either cream or ointment form. Steroids should be applied on a step-down approach, weaning off to prevent undesirable rebound effects. Treatment must be initiated at the first sign of recurrence. Emollients in the form of creams and oint-ments should be used routinely and as prescribed.

Topical corticosteroids

Topical steroids are creams, gels or ointments containing corticosteroids. Corticosteroids are hor-mones that assist the body in the reduction of inflammation and, in this instance, they are applied directly on the skin to reduce skin inflammation and irritation. Topical steroids are effective for the management of acute flare-ups of eczema, as they can relieve symptoms of itching and treat inflammation. In practice, parents are often reluctant to use topical steroids as prescribed. They voice perceived risks of skin thinning or effects on growth and development of their children. It is extremely important to provide education and information regarding the use of topical steroids to alleviate anxiety, as this will reduce the risk of non-compliance with treatment. In practice, a care plan is issued to the parent detailing the fingertip unit of steroid application in the different age ranges. Steroids are prescribed in a potency and format suitable to treat the specific skin erythema (redness) and specific location. Different steroid strengths are required for the axilla, femoral, facial, trunk and limb areas.

Topical steroids are classified in four categories: mild, moderate, potent and very potent. This is determined by the amount of vasoconstriction the topical corticosteroid produces and the degree to which it inhibits inflammation. According to the British National Formulary for Children (BNFC, 2016) there are minimal side effects, such as skin thinning and systemic effects, associated with mild and moderately potent topical corticosteroids when used appropriately as prescribed. However, caution should be taken if applying them to large areas of the child or if used under 'wet wraps' or bandages, as this may increase systemic absorption. Watch the video at https://study.sagepub.com/essentialchildnursing on how to apply wet wraps. Effective monitor-ing of topical corticosteroid use is important to reduce the risk of adverse effects. Potent and very potent topical corticosteroids should be used in the management of eczema in line with the NICE (2007) and SIGN (2011) guidelines. The approach is a stepped-up or stepped-down regime – the stepped-down approach is more commonly used.

VIDEO LINK 26.2: WET WRAPS

If children are not responsive to the appropriate treatment with steroids, treatment with calcinuerin inhibitors, such as tacrolimus and primeolimus, known as non-steroidal or immune modulators, may be considered. Calcineurin inhibitors are licensed to be used in children over 2 years old. Calcineurin inhibitors are usually initiated by a specialist dermatologist (SIGN, 2011). These drugs can initially cause flushing and stinging of the skin. SIGN (2011) suggests that this product be used where there is risk from continued steroid use, particularly skin atrophy.

WEBLINK: BNF

FIND OUT MORE!

ACTIVITY 26.3: EVIDENCE-BASED PRACTICE

Using the current British National Formulary (BNF) publication for children, give an example of a topical steroid for each potency level.

ACTIVITY ANSWER 26.3

SEBORRHOEIC ECZEMA

Infantile seborrhoeic eczema, also known as cradle cap, mainly affects the scalp and face. It is a diffuse, greasy scaling of the scalp, which is often not itchy. The rash may also be found in the axilla and nappy area. Seborrhoeic eczema can sometimes cause hypo-pigmentation in darkly pigmented skin. Consequently, the area around the hairline and face of a child from black Caribbean, black African or Asian background may appear very pale. The parents are often distressed by the discolouration. It is therefore very important to reassure them that cases of hypo-pigmentation will resolve spontaneously once the condition improves (Myers, 2015).

Seborrhoeic dermatitis is diagnosed by its clinical appearance and behaviour and can be treated by medicated shampoos. Sometimes steroid scalp applications and emollients to moisturise the scalp and reduce inflammation and itchiness are also used.

ECZEMA HERPETICUM

Eczema herpeticum is a widespread, highly contagious, potentially serious dermatological condition caused by herpes simplex virus HV1, the virus that causes cold sores. The child with this condition may have a herpes simplex or have been in contact with someone who has. If this is suspected then immediate medical attention is required. It presents as a cluster of itchy blisters, which are also sometimes very painful. It can occur anywhere, but it most often appears on the face and neck. It can spread within a week to ten days if left untreated, to cover large areas of the skin, including the eczematous areas. Eczema herpeticum causes itchy sore skin eruptions and is often coupled with pyrexia and swollen glands. The child may therefore feel very unwell. Treatment includes intravenous anti-viral therapy. The child may also need antibiotics if a bacterial infection is present.

WEBLINK: TAAIBAH'S STORY

You can read the 'Hi I'm Taaibah I'm 9 years old and I have eczema, here is something I wrote about it' story at https://study.sagepub.com/essentialchildnursing

ACNE

Acne is common and predominantly affects teenagers. As with other skin conditions, it cannot be hidden and has a profound psychological effect on the young person. Children's nurses should therefore be knowledgeable and sensitive about the appropriate symptoms and treatments.

Acne is a common skin condition affecting the pilosebaceous unit. Sebaceous glands are found all over the body but most frequently on the face, scalp, chest and back. Acne usually presents in adolescence, but can occur in neonates and is thought to be due to the effects of hormones on the production of sebum. Increased sebum production leads to blockage of the sebaceous follicle by keratin and sebum, leading to colonisation of the follicle which results in inflammation.

The patient usually presents with comodenes, commonly known as blackheads and whiteheads. Open comodenes are known as blackheads and closed comodenes are known as whiteheads.

Blackheads are follicles that have a wider opening and contain plugs of sebum and sloughed-off cells, which appear black in colour from the oxidised melanin (Lewis-Jones, 2010). Closed comedones arise when the follicles are obstructed by cells and sebum, but the opening is smaller. Blackheads and whiteheads are the non-inflammatory stage of acne. The blockage of the hair follicle allows a build-up of sebum, which creates a natural breeding ground for bacteria. The bacterium associated with acne is called Propionibacterium acnes (Lewis-Jones, 2010). The presence of this bacteria results in local inflammation.

It is important to ask the young person about their experience and success with past and current treatments, including over-the-counter products. The skin needs to be examined in good light, and the severity of the acne should be graded and any scarring carefully documented. The face, back and chest need to be examined for classical acne lesions, open and closed comedones, papules, pustules and nodules. Advise the patient to wash skin twice daily using a mild cleanser or antiseptic wash and avoid irritants, oil and non-comedonegenic cosmetics. For treatment options please see the Primary Care Dermatology Society, accessible via https://study.sagepub.com/essentialchildnursing

WEBLINK: PCDS

Research the Leeds Acne Grading system (O'Brien et al., 1998) for acne severity. This is a visual aid to scoring and one can see photos of young people with varying degrees of acne severity with a corresponding grade.

Tinea is the fungal infection of keratinised tissues such as the skin, scalp and nails. These are superficial fungal skin infections caused by dermatophytes. Dermatophytes cause scalp ring worm known as tinea capitis, body ring worm known as tinea corporis, and feet infections called tinea pedis. Ring worm present as circular lesions with a darker ring on the outer edge.

Fungal skin infections are contagious and spread by direct contact with an infected person, animal, soil (although rarely) or by indirect contact with a contaminated object. Investigations to confirm diagnosis include skin scrapings and nail examination. Treatment can be given topically for infections of feet and skin. Infections of the scalp may require enteral antifungal agents as they may become resistant skin infections. Parents must be advised to adhere to therapies post-disappearance of lesions as prescribed. Families may need advice on how to prevent spread of infection, such as regular skin hygiene, proper drying and regular washing of clothes and linen.

HISTORY TAKING AND SKIN ASSESSMENT

It is vital to complete a thorough skin assessment of the child who presents with a skin condition. A skin assessment captures the patient's general physical condition, based on careful inspection and palpation of the skin and documentation of findings (Jarvis, 2015). It is important to explain to the child and family what you are going to do and the reason why, and to gain their permission and cooperation.

First, it is important to take a full history of the presenting problem as well as listen and observe for signs of pain or discomfort; this will help to make a diagnosis. In young children the history should include birth weight and current weight and any relevant past medical history (Hess, 2010). Plotting the weight will highlight to the nurse any problems in relation to achieving adequate growth, which is an indicator of good health.

Observing or inspecting the skin will provide visual clues, especially if the child cannot communicate verbally. The nurse should be able to see if there are any areas of broken skin, excoriation or any visible lesions. The nurse's sense of smell may be able to detect poor hygiene, incontinence, or fungal and bacterial infection which could present with a bad odour. The nurse should inspect the skin, taking into consideration colour, uniform appearance, symmetry and hygiene, presence of lesions, tears, bruises, oedema, rashes and flakiness.

SAFEGUARDING STOP POINT

---

1. When undertaking a history and skin assessment, what findings would cause you concern and how would you address this? Reflect on your safeguarding training and how the nurse can protect children
2. Explain what steps you would take to safeguard a child in this situation.

SAFEGUARDING
STOP POINT
ANSWER 26.1

WEBLINK:
VICTORIA
CLIMBIÉ

Read the BBC article which you can access via https://study.sagepub.com/essentialchildnursing about Victoria Climbié whose abuse was overlooked as the first impression was that she had scabies. Look up signs and symptoms of scabies.

Second, the nurse will need to touch or palpate the skin. By touching the skin the nurse will feel the texture, if there is moisture or the skin is hot to touch. By palpating the skin the nurse may be able to detect different lumps and bumps. When assessing a child with atopic eczema it is important to find out what irritants may be exacerbating the eczema. This may include soaps, shampoos, bubble baths and shower gels. The soap powder and softeners used to wash clothes may also irritate the skin, especially if there are fragrances, perfumes or additives in them. Parents should be encouraged to use non-biological soap powder to wash clothes and to avoid fabric softeners. Woollen and manmade fibres, including feathers in pillows and duvets may irritate the skin, so it is best to use cotton clothes next to the skin to reduce the risk of these irritants affecting the child's skin. In some cases pets, such as dogs and cats, may be the allergens that trigger the eczema.

Food allergy

Consultations with families often reveal the main concern is whether the child has an allergy. Often they feel that if a food allergy is detected and the allergen is then removed, the eczema will be cleared. A detailed history should be taken, including birth, weight, feeding, growth, age of onset of eczema, any problems with gastro-oesophageal reflux or 'mucousy' stools, whether breast or formula fed, and when formula was introduced to the diet. If the child has reacted to any foods, record how this presented and what actions were required. If a practitioner feels that an infant has reacted adversely to formula milk then referral to a dietician is needed to support the mother in considering a milk occlusion diet with a lipid formula (NICE, 2011). This can be instituted for a trial of six weeks and a referral to an allergy clinic for skin prick testing to identify the main allergens.

ACTIVITY 26.4: CRITICAL THINKING

Name some foods that infants might be allergic to that may also affect their eczema.

ACTIVITY
ANSWER 26.4

CHAPTER SUMMARY

In this chapter we have looked at the assessment and care of the child with dermatological problems. This chapter has:

- Provided the opportunity for you to review your current understanding of the anatomy and physiology of the skin
- Demonstrated how dermatological conditions can alter the appearance of the skin and adversely affect how the child feels about their appearance
- Presented a brief overview of some of the most common dermatological conditions and their assessment and management
- Introduced a framework for taking a history of the skin and performing a skin assessment
- Provided you with additional knowledge and skills to start to assess, plan, implement and evaluate and re-evaluate care plans for for these more common skin presentations

BUILD YOUR BIBLIOGRAPHY

Journal articles

Go to https://study.sagepub.com/essentialchildnursing for further free online journal articles related to this chapter.

- Carbonell, A., Siu, A. and Patel, R. (2010) 'Pediatric atopic dermatitis: a review of the medical management'. *Annals of Pharmacotherapy*, 44 (9): 1448-58.

  This is a review of the pertinent literature synthesising the medical management of eczema from 2005-2010.

- Bell, M.C., Stoval, I S.H., Scurlock, A.M., Perry, T.T., Jones, S.M. and Harik, N.S. (2012) 'Addressing antimicrobial resistance to treat children with atopic dermatitis in a tertiary pediatric allergy clinic'. *Clinical Pediatrics*, 51 (11): 1025-9.

  This is a research study into skin infection in children with atopic eczema and evaluates antimicrobial resistance and frequent skin infections.

FURTHER READING: ONLINE JOURNAL ARTICLES

Weblinks

Go to https://study.sagepub.com/essentialchildnursing for further weblinks related to this chapter.

- PCDS (Primary Care Dermatology Society), *Acne - Primary Care Treatment Pathway*

  www.pcds.org.uk/ee/images/uploads/general/Acne_Treatment_2015-web.pdf
  Information about acne treatment options.

- BBC, Climbié doctor diagnosed scabies

  http://news.bbc.co.uk/1/hi/uk/1595866.stm
  Victoria Climbié died from abuse in 2000. Her death prompted a major inquiry and changes to the child protection policies in the UK. Her abuse was first overlooked because it was thought she had scabies. This highlights the importance of a thorough assessment.

FURTHER READING: WEBLINKS

ACE YOUR ASSESSMENT

ONLINE
QUIZZES &
ACTIVITY
ANSWERS

Revise what you have learned by visiting https://study.sagepub.com/essentialchildnursing

- Test yourself with multiple-choice and short-answer questions
- Do the chapter activities in the book and check your answers online

REFERENCES

Boore, J., Cook, N. and Shepherd, A. (2016) *Essentials of Anatomy and Physiology for Nursing Practice*. London: Sage.

British Dermatological Nursing Group (BDNG) (2012) 'Best practice in emollient therapy: a statement for healthcare professionals'. *Dermatological Nursing*, 11 (4): 60–79.

British National Formulary for Children (BNFC) www.bnfc.org (last accessed 15 December 2016).

Cork, M.J., Danby, S.G., Vasilopoulos, Y., Hadgraft, J., Lane, M.E., Moustafa, M., Guy, R.H., Macgowan, A.L., Tazi-Ahnini, R. and Ward, S.J. (2009) 'Epidermal barrier dysfunction in atopic dermatitis'. *Journal of Investigative Dermatology*, 129 (8): 1892–908.

Hess, C.T. (2010) 'Performing a skin assessment'. *Nursing*, 40 (7): 66.

Jarvis, C. (2015) *Physical Examination and Health Assessment*, 7th edn. St Louis, MO: Elsevier.

Lewis-Jones, S. (2010) *Paediatric Dermatology: Oxford Specialist Handbooks in Paediatrics*. Oxford: Oxford University Press.

Myers, J. (2015) 'The challenges of identifying eczema in darkly-pigmented skin'. *Nursing Children and Young People*, 27 (6): 24–8.

National Institute for Health and Clinical Excellence (NICE) (2007) *Atopic Eczema in Under 12s: Diagnosis and Management*. NICE Clinical Guideline 57. London: NICE. Available at: www.nice.org.uk/guidance/CG57/chapter/1-Guidance#treatment (last accessed 27 June 2017).

National Institute for Health and Clinical Excellence (NICE) (2011) *Food Allergy in Children and Young People*. Nice Clinical Guideline 116. London: NICE.

O'Brien, S.C., Lewis, J.B. and Cunliffe, W.J. (1998) 'The Leeds Revised Acne Grading System'. *Journal of Dermatological Treatment*, 9: 215–20.

Scottish Intercollegiate Guidelines Network (SIGN) (2011) *Management of Atopic Eczema in Primary Care. A National Clinical Guideline*. Edinburgh: SIGN.

CARE OF CHILDREN AND YOUNG PEOPLE WITH A THERMAL INJURY

27

SHIRIN POMEROY

THIS CHAPTER COVERS

- What is a thermal injury?
- Describing a thermal injury in terms of size and depth
- Treatment options and considerations
- Pain management strategies for the child after thermal injury
- The complexities of caring for children with extensive thermal injuries

---

REQUIRED KNOWLEDGE

It would be helpful to have an understanding of the structure and functions of the skin before you start this chapter. Go to the A&P link: 'Skin' at https://study.sagepub.com/essentialchildnursing A thorough understanding of this will help provide the rationale for why certain treatment modalities are undertaken, as discussed later in the chapter.

A&P LINK
27.1: SKIN
ANATOMY

> ❝ The team approach is imperative to understanding the rehabilitation and emotional, psychological and physiological recovery of burns patients.
>
> **Herndon, 2012, p. 13** ❞

Visit https://study.sagepub.com/essentialchildnursing to access a wealth of online resources for this chapter – watch out for the margin icons throughout the chapter.

INTRODUCTION

Caring for children after thermal injury is both challenging and rewarding. Most people can relate to having had a small burn injury at some point in their life (e.g. from cooking or sunbathing) and afterwards think nothing of it because it heals without any problems. However, a more significant thermal injury can and will impact physically, emotionally and psychologically on the child and the whole family. For some this will have long-term implications.

In recent years, burn care in the UK has acquired a much improved status as a speciality in its own right. The Burn Care Review (NBCR Group, 2001) paved the way for this, enabling burns to be recognised as a specialised field of healthcare within NHS England. Consequently, the organisation and delivery of burn care across the country is more closely monitored, supported and generally better resourced.

There is international recognition that most thermal injuries in children are preventable (WHO, 2008). The majority result from accidents that occur in the home, with the exploring toddler (aged 12 months to 2 years of age) being the most vulnerable age group. Verey et al. (2014) note that they represent half of all burns admissions in England and Wales. Public awareness of the causes and consequences of burn injury for children and their families is generally poor, hence the ongoing need for injury prevention programmes.

This chapter provides clarity on the definition of a thermal injury, and how treatment is determined after assessment. It is intended that greater knowledge and understanding will be gained of how thermal injury affects child development and all activities of daily living.

WHAT IS A THERMAL INJURY?

A thermal injury is defined as damage to the skin or internal organs caused by the transfer of heat from a direct heat source. There are five generally accepted categories of heat transferring sources: wet heat, dry heat, chemical, electrical and radiation (see Table 27.1) (Bosworth-Bousfield, 2002).

Table 27.1 Different categories of thermal injury with examples

Category	Description	Examples
Wet heat	Liquid-based heat sources (excluding chemicals)	Hot drinks, water, soups, sauces, stews
Dry heat	Non-liquid-based heat sources	Fire, ash, hot objects such as an iron, hob/oven, radiator or hair straighteners
Chemicals	Acids or alkalis	Most household cleaning products are alkaline, including bleach
Electrical	High voltage (>2000v) Low voltage/domestic electricity (240v)	Most electrical burns in children occur from touching or biting exposed cables
Radiation	Radiant heat	Ultraviolet light (sunlight) Hair dryers, fan heaters, radiotherapy burns

Not included in this list are burns caused by exposure to cold. These include frostbite, but also encompass deliberate injuries from aerosol sprays or other cold/chemical sources. These injuries are worthy of mention and are part of the burn care team remit. Usually attributed to risk-taking adolescent behaviour or peer pressure, aerosol spray injuries (a combination of cold and chemical injury) can, if deep, leave permanent scars. Another self-injuring activity currently popular in some schools and amongst adolescent children is the 'ice/salt challenge'. Williams et al. (2013) illustrate a case report of such an injury in a young adult, although local unpublished data within the International Burn Injury Database (iBID, 2010) also shows this in younger teenagers. It is important to identify whether there is a history of bullying or self-harming behaviour associated with these self-inflicted injuries. Any child displaying mental health concerns must be directed to appropriately qualified healthcare professionals so that the right assessment and support can be attained.

WEBLINK: IBID

The Royal Society for the Prevention of Accidents (RoSPA) (2015) confirms that scalds (wet heat sources) are the most frequent cause of thermal injury in children internationally. Contact burns or flame burns follow thereafter but this depends on how the data is collected and whether or not out-patient or emergency department figures are included. As a children's nurse it is useful to be aware of what is common, so that safeguarding and health protection questions can be asked when a patient presents with a less common thermal injury.

SAFEGUARDING STOP POINT

The importance of obtaining a detailed history and clinical examination of a child after thermal injury should not be underestimated in the context of safeguarding. While this may not be within the scope of practice for the children's nurse, the recognition of a 'cause for concern' is the responsibility of all members of the burn care team. Since the systematic review article by Maguire et al. (2008), research is evolving in this field wherein the development of a burns and scalds specific triage tool determining the likelihood of intentional versus unintentional injury is soon to be realised. Some additional information about this can be found in the 'Build your bibliography' section at the end of the chapter.

DESCRIBING A THERMAL INJURY IN TERMS OF SIZE AND DEPTH

The extent of a thermal injury is assessed in two ways: the size of the burn in terms of the percentage body surface area affected (the spread of injury), and the depth of injury (how deep through the layers of the skin the damage has occurred) (Chan et al., 2012). It is a combination of both these two assessments and location of injury that determines its significance. A common misconception is that only big burns have a significant impact on the child and family.

Assessing the size of burn injury

The size of injury is described as a percentage of the total body surface area (%TBSA). There are a variety of tools that can be employed to help in this assessment (see Table 27.2).

Table 27.2 Assessment tools to measure size of burn in children

Tool	Description
Adapted rule of nines (for children) (American College of Surgeons, 1997)	An adult's head and each arm equate to 9% TBSA. An adult's front torso, back torso and each leg are 18% TBSA. A child's head and legs differ, being 18% and 14% (each leg) respectively. As the child grows, the head size lessens and the legs increase as a percentage of TBSA

(Continued)

Table 27.2 (Continued)

Tool	Description
Rule of palms or 1% rule (Kyle and Wallace, 1951; Rossiter et al., 1996; Berry et al., 2001)	The size of the patient's hand (palmar surface including fingers) equates to 1% TBSA
Lund and Browder chart (Lund and Browder, 1944)	The burn area is drawn on a body map with predetermined size estimations for each body part. Some sizes change with the age of the patient (in years) and are determined from a table on the chart
Serial halving (Allison and Porter, 2004)	Divides the body into a number of halves - front/back, top/bottom, left/right - it is possible to determine whether the injury is ≥50%, ≥25%, ≥12.5% and so on
Mersey burns application (Barnes et al., 2015)	The burn area is drawn directly into a 'smart phone application' (app) body map. The application determines burn size once the age of the patient is entered

ACTIVITY 27.1: REFLECTIVE PRACTICE

Use the Lund and Browder chart to calculate the estimated burn area drawn. Include all coloured areas in your calculation. Consider what the size of burn would be for a child aged under 1 year with one in a child aged 10 years.

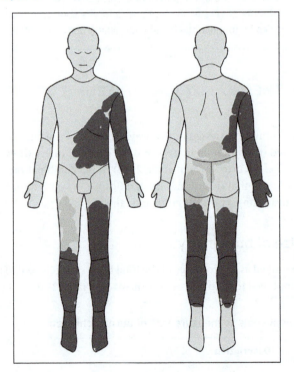

Figure 27.1

Image created from: St Helens and Knowsley Teaching Hospitals NHS Trust (2010-13) *Mersey Burns*. Available at: http://merseyburns.com (accessed 10 November 2015)

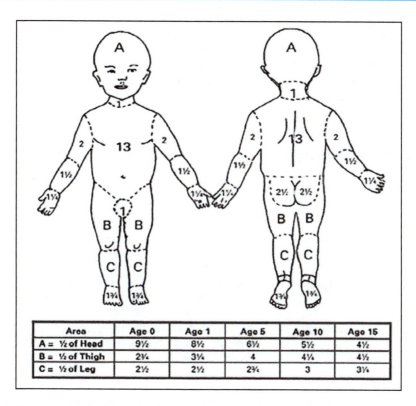

Area	Age 0	Age 1	Age 5	Age 10	Age 15
A = ½ of Head	9½	8½	6½	5½	4½
B = ½ of Thigh	2¾	3¼	4	4¼	4½
C = ½ of Leg	2½	2½	2¾	3	3¼

Figure 27.2 Lund and Browder Chart

From: Harwood-Nuss, A., Wolfson, A. and Linden, C. *The Clinical Practice of Emergency Medicine*. Philadelphia. Wolters Kluwer, 2015, with permissions.

Critical observation of these assessment tools will firstly highlight that they were originally devised for adults and have been modified to fit to children. The literature on burn assessment tools is somewhat mixed, with frequent claims that one tool is more accurate than another. All tools available should be regarded as a helpful aid but with limitations due to inter-rater concordance on their use and interpretation. Giretzlehner et al. (2013) investigated this with a group of just over a hundred clinical staff. Significant discrepancies were found between staff assessments of the same patients. They also found that computer-generated programmes mapping photographic images to 3D-scoring systems were more accurate at burn size calculation. These inaccuracies were also emphasised by Chan et al. (2012) who expressed particular concern for children with increased risk of fluid resuscitation errors if the burn size estimation is correct. The future of burn size estimation may lie in technologically based tools (apps), but an innovative study by Malic et al. (2007) considered the potential for a 'credit card' tool. This has international appeal as all credit cards and most identification badges the world over are made to a standard size of 8.5cm by 5.3cm and equate to 45cm². More accurate burn size estimations can potentially be made by mapping the credit card size to the burn area distribution and then calculating this as a proportion of the total body surface area (BSA) of the patient (BSA is calculated using a formula requiring patient weight and height).

Assessing the depth of thermal injury

Assessing the depth of a thermal injury is a complex clinical skill that improves with experience, but still remains a highly subjective task (Serrano et al., 2015). Most clinicians report that the extremes of depth (either very superficial or very deep) are easier to assess and it is the intermediate or mixed depth injuries that are more difficult. Burn depth classification terminology widely taught and used in the UK, Europe and Australasia differs from that used in the USA, but is more precise (see Table 27.3).

Table 27.3 Burn depth descriptor comparisons between the UK and the USA

Burn depth category	US comparison	Description
Epidermal	1st degree	Epidermis only is affected. Also termed 'superficial burn'. The skin is not broken. The skin looks red
Dermal	2nd degree	Epidermis is denuded or blistered. Also termed 'superficial partial thickness'. The papillary dermis layer is affected. The wound is wet and painful when exposed or touched
	3rd degree	'Deep partial thickness'. The reticular layer of the dermis is affected. The wound looks drier and more leathery. The wound is not as painful due to nerve damage
Full thickness	4th degree	Both layers of skin are destroyed. Subcutaneous tissue and other underlying structures such as muscle, ligaments, or bone may be exposed or charred

Burn depth assessment is generally directed by clinical observation of the wound at the bedside, followed by wound reviews every one to seven days until it is fully healed. The frequency of this review is determined by a number of factors including: the stage of healing, the clinical condition of the patient and the type of dressing used. Deitch et al. (1983) found that if sufficient re-epithelialisation (healing) is observed over a two-week period, then the risk of developing hypertrophic scarring and other longer-term complications is deemed minimal. This risk of scarring increases the longer the wound takes to heal. A more recent interpretation by Cubison et al. (2006) claims that if a burn wound looks like it will heal within two to three weeks, then the need for surgical intervention (skin grafting) is less likely, or would be much smaller in area. This tradition continues today and, although highly subjective, is often employed out of choice due to a lack of other more objective and reliable methods of burn depth assessment.

The National Institute of Clinical Excellence (NICE, 2011) recommends the use of laser doppler imaging to determine the need or avoidance of surgical intervention for intermediate depth wounds. The laser doppler image detects blood flow to the burn injured skin and associated software predicts whether the wound will heal within 14 days, 14–21 days or more than 21 days. At face value the laser doppler seems invaluable to burn care services when used as part of routine burn assessment. Yet the costs of this equipment (initial capital spend, annual servicing and staff training costs) are not insignificant. Other considerations affecting the reliability of the equipment include: taking the image too early or too late, patient movement during the procedure (especially with young children) and interpretation errors of the images obtained. Despite these limitations, Khatib et al. (2014) acknowledge that laser doppler imaging provides a useful contribution to burn depth assessment as an adjunct to clinical observation.

ACTIVITY 27.2: CRITICAL THINKING

The tools illustrated to measure the size of a burn were devised by clinical staff based on the size of patients at the time and all show validation limitations. List what you think the implications are if the burn size is either over- or under-estimated?

ACTIVITY
ANSWER 27.2

PRACTICE
SCENARIO 27:
RUBY

SEE ALSO
CHAPTER 28

WEBLINK: FLUID
RESUSCITATION

Knowledge of the size and depth of injury is necessary for directing initial treatment options of early surgery and fluid management. Fluid management strategies have been subject to much debate in recent years and in children they are a difficult area to research. Go to the 'Build your bibliography' section and read the article which introduces you to this vast topic.

WHAT'S THE EVIDENCE?

Often described as dynamic wounds because they can change over time (Jackson, 1953), the size and depth of a thermal injury is influenced by a number of factors, including:

- The promptness and effectiveness of first aid (cooling)
- Judicious fluid management
- Adequacy of pain control
- Sufficient infection control practices to reduce the risk of infection

Deficiencies in any of these can cause the injury to both deepen as well as widen. The Jackson model as described in Yarrow et al. (2009) offers a simple explanation of what is happening at the wound site and within the microcirculation influencing how the injury might evolve over time.

TREATMENT OPTIONS AND CONSIDERATIONS

Irrespective of the size, depth or type of burn injury, a key priority for the burn care team is to achieve wound closure (healing) as promptly as possible with minimal complication. Healing occurs either by secondary intention (on its own with the support of dressings) or with surgery (debridement alone or with skin grafting). On the surface this can seem straightforward, but becomes more complex depending on where the burns are on the body, how long they take to heal and how much they impact on normal activities of daily living. Burns can be described as 'extraordinarily painful' (Stoddard et al., 2002) and this is corroborated by Meyer et al. (2012) who state that all burns will be painful to a greater or lesser extent. The fear and anxiety of pain and painful procedures can be debilitating irrespective of the age of the patient. At times it can be for this reason alone that the child cannot function as normal. It seems pertinent to utilise the activities of daily living as described by Roper et al. (2000) as a guiding principle in the care of burns patients, even for infants and young children who are largely dependent on carers.

SEE ALSO
CHAPTER 3

ACTIVITY 27.3: REFLECTIVE PRACTICE

Use the 12 activities of daily living (ADL) to highlight the potential problems for a child aged 18 months, 5 years and 12 years for the following burn injuries:

- Burns to the face, including eyes, ears, nose and mouth
- Burns to the hands and feet
- Burns to the neck, axilla, elbows, knees and ankles
- Burns to the perineum
- Smoke inhalational injuries

List how you would care for the child and family in light of the above, considering both the physical and psychological needs of both the child and the parents.

ACTIVITY
ANSWER 27.3

SEE ALSO
CHAPTERS 3,
5 AND 14

Central to burn care is the burn care team. This multidisciplinary team is vitally important in coordinating and delivering treatment/care to children and their families after burn injury, and should not be underestimated. Alongside surgeons and nursing staff, the team might also include general paediatricians, intensivists, anaesthetics/acute pain services, physiotherapy, occupational therapy, play specialists, clinical psychology, dietetics and microbiology, depending on the severity of injury and the needs of the child and family. Effective interdisciplinary working is crucial to the decision-making process in all 'phases' after burn injury, in conjunction with the child (if able) and family (see Table 27.4).

Table 27.4   Thermal injury recovery phases

Phase	Identified priorities
Emergency (first 1-6 hours)	• Airway, breathing, circulation • Fluid resuscitation • Pain control
Acute (first 5 days)	• Fluid management • Eating/drinking • Wound care/management • Pain and anxiety management • Function and mobility
Rehabilitation (from day 1 until healed)	Needs assessed using a range of assessment tools, including ADL
Long term (from healed date to potentially years later)	As per ADL assessment, and including: • Scar management • School/nursery integration

The role of the children's nurse in burn care is to assess and deliver specific interventions such as wound care, and coordinate holistic treatment/care to support children and their families during initial and intermediate phases of care and after discharge from hospital. It may also be necessary for the nurse to act as the child and family advocate, so that painful procedures are not a source of secondary psychological trauma.

Contemporary burn care espouses two main principles: early debridement and skin grafting of notably deep burns, and 'moist' wound healing. Both practices have shown to improve survival rates, reduce length of hospital stay, and produce better outcomes in terms of reduced scarring and infection rates (D'Cruz et al., 2013). The term 'debridement' is often used to describe anything from simple wound cleansing to surgically cutting away necrotic tissue, and all else in between these extremes. The aim of this process is to remove dead particles from the wound, reduce inflammation and potential sources of infection. For children (in conjunction with good pain/anxiety/symptom control), superficial wound cleansing/debridement is achieved in the bath/shower using gauze swabs to rub/wipe debris away from the wounds. Although there is little evidence to support this, it encourages good hygiene practices through washing the whole body as well as the wound and is common practice nationally (Langschmidt et al., 2014). Particular care is needed to ensure the psychological safety of the child is not overlooked in relation to managing the pain experience, both anticipated and actual pain.

Wound care and dressings and associated psychological preparation and care are essential nursing skills in burns inpatient, outpatient and community settings. These are complex interventions, often involving advanced interpersonal skills and engagement in working collaboratively with parents/carers and children.

To learn more about different types of dressings used in burn care, the Cochrane review 'Dressings for superficial and partial thickness burns' (Wasiak et al., 2013) is a useful starting point.

WEBLINK: BURN DRESSINGS

PAIN MANAGEMENT STRATEGIES FOR CHILDREN AFTER THERMAL INJURY

> Whilst on placement I participated in the bathing of burns patients. The primary aim of bathing is to reduce infection through removing the necrotic skin. During bathing/wound cleansing some bleeding can occur. The child can also become vocally distressed, hence they are assessed for pain and given analgesia beforehand. Play specialists are usually involved with the procedure providing valuable therapeutic distraction. Parents/carers understandably may become distressed witnessing their child so upset. Procedural preparation is crucial in burn care.
>
> **Matthew, 1st-year children's nursing student**

Effective pain management for the child after thermal injury cannot be over-emphasised. The student's experience above reflects a common example within burns services whereby staff undertake a range of clinical procedures such as wound care, turns/limb positioning, physiotherapy exercises and stretches, all with the potential to exacerbate pain and distress for the child and family. Two key principles in the assessment and management of pain for these patients are that the pain experience evolves over time post-injury and that regular, dynamic assessment is essential to ensure the effectiveness of the pain assessment and management strategies employed. Hospital acute pain services, anaesthetists, hospital play and clinical psychology are key players in helping the children's nurse implement individualised pain management strategies, which also includes post-burn itching.

Pain management strategies after thermal injury must address all types of pain experienced: background, procedural and breakthrough. Better control is achieved with a combination of both pharmacological and non-pharmacological approaches. Useful summaries of this within burn care can be found in Retrouvey and Shahrokhi (2015) and a more child-centred review by Pardesi and Fuzaylov (2016). Distraction techniques and other forms of non-pharmacological pain management strategies are considered essential armoury within a children's burn care setting, particularly for wound care and dressing changes: television, background music, toys, puppetry, iPad/tablet activities or more sophisticated technological devices such as virtual reality can be employed according to the child's age and stage of development (Miller et al., 2010). The play specialist can be a skilled and welcome ally for the child especially in the initial and intermediate stages of care management.

WHAT'S THE EVIDENCE?

Recognition that a burn injury can be a stressful and painful experience for the child and family is the first step in supporting physical and psychological recovery. Research in this area is limited and often difficult to individualise because each child and family's experience after a burns/thermal injury is very different. The review article by Bakker et al. (2013) in the 'Build your bibliography' reading section at the end of this chapter provides a useful summary of what is known on this subject.

THE COMPLEXITIES OF CARING FOR CHILDREN WITH EXTENSIVE THERMAL INJURIES

In its simplest form, a comprehensive understanding of this is best achieved in the context of a patient example (see Scenario 26.1).

SCENARIO 27.1: RUPERT

Rupert is 4 years old. He was helping his dad build a bonfire to burn rubbish. Something in the bonfire exploded and a fireball occurred. Rupert's clothes caught fire. His dad experienced hand burns as he put the flames out. Rupert has 55 per cent mixed-depth flame burns to his face, torso, arms and hands. Luckily no eye damage or smoke inhalation injury occurred, so his airway and breathing were not of concern after the initial transfer.

- List what supportive measures might help Rupert and family on their journey of recovery after a severe thermal injury
- Consider what package of care Rupert may require in the community after discharge from hospital

Employing the 12 activities of daily living (ADLs), the following table maps out the needs, potential risks and likely care plan for this patient from initial injury, through rehabilitation and into the long term (see Table 27.5). This may help guide your thoughts and responses to the above questions.

Table 27.5 Case example, illustrating the complexities of caring for children with extensive thermal injuries

Activity	Potential problems/needs	Acute stage	Rehabilitation/long term	Interdisciplinary working
Maintaining a safe environment	• Intravenous/arterial lines, urinary catheter • Risk of falls • Risk of infection from wounds/lines • Pain and medication safety • Psychological safety	Single cubicle for protective isolation Nurse in an appropriate cot/bed Observe and monitor for signs of infection	Proactive line removal when no longer required Support child and family in maintaining physical and psychological safety	Anaesthetists/intensivists Infection prevention and control team Play therapists Clinical psychology services
Communication	• Swelling of face, eyes • Limited vision • Disorientation • Difficulty in speaking • Ability to accurately communicate pain and fear	Nurse upright to reduce swelling Provide reassurance Consider communication aids Developmentally appropriate communication strategies	Support family to encourage the child to communicate own needs Child-centred interventions	Ophthalmologist Hospital play Speech and language therapist Clinical psychology
Breathing	• Poor chest expansion from pain of wounds/bed rest/sedative medications • Risk of fluid retention – wet lungs • Risk of chest infection	Nurse upright for better lung expansion Encourage deep breathing/breathing exercises Observe for signs of chest problems (e.g. breathing changes, increasing oxygen requirement)	Support family to encourage active mobilisation and cardio-vascular exercise to prevent long-term chest problems Utilise play and recreation to facilitate normal functions	Physiotherapy Hospital play
Eating and drinking	• Reduced appetite • Increased metabolic demands • Hand injury so unable to self-feed • Risk of reduced gut motility • Fluid losses externally from wounds • Oedema formation due to injury and internal capillary leak	Prescribed supplementary feeding regime via naso-gastric or naso-jejunal tube Continue to offer oral food/drink Prescribed fluid management regime Maintain a strict fluid balance Observe for signs of fluid overload or dehydration Record-keeping	Support family to normalise and encourage oral diet Enable independent feeding	Intensivists/medical staff Dietician Occupational therapy Hospital play – for example, food play

(Continued)

Table 27.5 (Continued)

Activity	Potential problems/needs	Acute stage	Rehabilitation/long term	Interdisciplinary working
Elimination	• Reduced independence in toileting • Catheterised to enable strict fluid monitoring • Risk of constipation due to immobility and opiate medication • Risk of loose stools from liquid-based feeds • Risk of soiling on wounds	Catheter care Consider aperients to aid bowel motions May require incontinence pads	Support family in enabling independent toileting	Physiotherapy Occupational therapy Hospital play
Washing and dressing	• Significant painful wounds covered in dressings • Unable to wash or wear clothes • High risk of infection	Multiple theatre trips to facilitate wound cleansing Pre- and post-op care Observe for 'strike through' on dressings and soiled dressings Support family in following universal infection control procedures	Support family with bathing/showering Support family with wound care and dressings Support family with scar management treatments and reducing contracture formation	Burns surgeons Hospital play Clinical psychology Physiotherapy Occupational therapy Pharmacist
Controlling temperature	• Inflammatory response after injury causes body temperature to rise • Hyper-metabolic state causes body temperature to rise	Nurse in a thermo-neutral environment to maintain body temperature between 37°C-38°C Observe for signs of infection/sepsis Record keeping	Support CYP and family in managing own body temperature	
Mobilisation	• Significant pain on moving and turning • Risk of muscle de-conditioning from prolonged bed rest • Risk of abnormal posturing due to skin tightness	Ensure adequacy of pain assessment using appropriate validated tools Regular appropriate analgesia and non-pharmacological approaches to symptom control Encourage moving and turning on a regular basis Support appropriate positioning when in bed or sitting Follow prescribed splint regime	Support CYP/family in encouraging active stretching and mobilisation	Physiotherapy Occupational therapy Hospital play

Activity	Potential problems/needs	Acute stage	Rehabilitation/long term	Interdisciplinary working
Working and playing	• Reduced concentration ability • Increased fatigue • Risk of developmental/schooling regression • Social deprivation from hospitalisation	Offer play/activities when awake Extra encouragement may be required if low in mood and motivation Ensure adequate rest periods after key stress times (dressing, baths, etc.)	Initiate a daily routine to include play/school activities Support CYP in returning to school	Hospital play Hospital school Clinical psychology
Expressing sexuality	• Fear of scarring and looking different from other boys/girls • For boys: risk of penis deformities • For girls: risk of problems with breast development	Provide realistic expectations for child and family to voice and come to terms with their fears	Support the child and family through puberty	Clinical psychology
Sleeping	• Risk of poor sleep from hospitalisation/pain • Sleep difficulties when weaning off sedative drugs • Risk of flashbacks and nightmares about the injury • Post-traumatic stress disorder potential	Observe and address sleep disturbances as soon as possible May require night time sedation	Encourage the child and family to re-establish a bedtime routine	Hospital play Clinical psychology
Death and dying	• Risk of mortality increases with significant injuries • Post-traumatic stress symptoms at time or later	Support the child and family in voicing their fears of death and dying		Clinical psychology

Traditional burn care practices are gradually being supported, disputed or improved by a greater evidence base and technological advances (particularly within wound assessment and tissue viability). Recovery after thermal injury can be a complex, morbidly painful process with long-term physical and psychological implications even if carefully managed. By employing regular 'activities of daily living', assessments and a team approach, most aspects of burn care can be highlighted and addressed. We should be thankful that children display immense resilience, and with supportive and enabling care from their family alongside healthcare professionals, they can grow to lead able-bodied and meaningful adult lives.

PLACEMENT ADVICE 27: THERMAL INJURY

Go to https://study.sagepub.com/essentialchildnursing for tips on preparing for placements when working with children with thermal injuries.

HEALTH PROMOTION 27: THERMAL INJURY

CHAPTER SUMMARY

This chapter has explored:

- Definitions and explanations of thermal injuries and how such injuries may be effectively assessed and managed
- How thermal injuries can affect all activities of daily living across all developmental stages
- Skilled assessment of pain and other symptoms associated with burn care/thermal injury
- The importance of the whole multidisciplinary team in supporting the child and family so that the child can begin to recover after a thermal injury
- The importance of working in partnership with the child and parents/carers in enabling the child to achieve their full potential after a thermal injury

BUILD YOUR BIBLIOGRAPHY

Books

- Herndon, D. (ed.) (2012) *Total Burn Care*, 4th edn. New York: Elsevier.

  This book, with additional online content, is the internationally recognised authority for the burn care community. Although US centric, it covers every aspect of burn care, is extensively referenced throughout and includes adequate illustrations and images.

- Barret-Nerin, J. and Herndon, D. (2004) *Principles and Practice of Burn Surgery*. New York: Taylor and Francis.

  This book provides a less dense, easier read than *Total Burn Care* although it covers similar subject matter. Focusing on education and training for burn care staff, the various options for the surgical treatment of burns are illustrated.

Journal articles

FURTHER READING: ONLINE JOURNAL ARTICLES

Go to https://study.sagepub.com/essentialchildnursing for further free online journal articles related to this chapter.

- Fodor, L., Fodor, A., Ramon, Y., Shoshani, O., Rissin, Y. and Ullmann, Y. (2006) 'Controversies in fluid resuscitation for burn management: Literature review and our experience'. *Injury*, 37: 374-9.

This article will introduce you to the complex area of fluid management for burn management in children.

- Bakker, A., Maertens, K., Van Son, M. and Van Loey, N. (2013) 'Psychological consequences of pediatric burns from a child and family perspective: a review of the empirical literature'. *Clinical Psychology Review*, 33, 3: 361–71.

  This article highlights the potential psychological consequences of burns for children and their families.

- Wasiak, J., Cleland, H., Campbell, F. and Spinks, A. (2013) 'Dressings for superficial and partial thickness burns'. *Cochrane Database of Systematic Reviews.* DOI: 10.1002/14651858.CD002106.pub4

  This article covers different types of dressings used in burns and is a useful starting point.

Weblinks

Go to https://study.sagepub.com/essentialchildnursing for further weblinks related to this chapter.

- The Scar Free Foundation Centre for Children's Burns Research

  www.bristol.ac.uk/social-community-medicine/childrens-burns/about
  This is a UK-based consortium paving the way in creating a body of new research specific to burns in children. It follows three themes of work: clinical, prevention and psychosocial adjustment and support. Many of the projects are collaborative, multicentre studies involving a number of burn services from all over the UK.

- Core Info, *Scalds Triage Tool*

  www.core-info.cardiff.ac.uk/reviews/burns/scalds-key-messages/triage-tool
  You can explore the work to date on the development of a burns and scalds triage tool that can be used to determine the likelihood of intentional versus unintentional injury.

- Children's Burns Trust

  www.cbtrust.org.uk/burn-prevention
  This is an exemplary resource for children, families and healthcare professionals. A key area of their work is in burn injury prevention – they provide a range of online educational resources and deliver specific awareness campaigns. There is also an opportunity to get involved and support their work.

FURTHER READING: WEBLINKS

GREAT FOR REVISION

ACE YOUR ASSESSMENT

Revise what you have learned by visiting https://study.sagepub.com/essentialchildnursing

- Test yourself with multiple-choice and short-answer questions
- Do the chapter activities in the book and check your answers online

ONLINE QUIZZES & ACTIVITY ANSWERS

REFERENCES

Allison, K. and Porter, K. (2004) 'Consensus on the pre-hospital approach to burns patient management'. *Emergency Medicine Journal*, 21 (1): 112–14.

American College of Surgeons (1997) *Advanced Trauma Life Support*, 6th edn. Chicago: American College of Surgeons.

Bakker, A., Maertens, K., Van Son, M. and Van Loey, N. (2013) 'Psychological consequences of pediatric burns from a child and family perspective: a review of the empirical literature'. *Clinical Psychology Review*, 33 (3): 361–71.

Barnes, J., Duffy, A., Hamnett, N., McPhail, J., Seaton, C., Shokrollahi, K., James, M., McArthur, P. and Pritchard Jones, R. (2015) 'The Mersey Burns app: evolving a model of validation'. *Emergency Medicine Journal*, 32: 637–41.

Berry, M., Evison, D. and Roberts, A. (2001) 'The influence of body mass index on burn surface estimated from the area of the hand'. *Burns*, 27: 591–4.

Bosworth-Bousfield, C. (2002) *Burn Trauma: Management and Nursing Care*, 2nd edn. London: Whurr.

Chan, Q., Barzi, F., Cheney, L., Harvey, J. and Holland, A. (2012) 'Burn size estimation in children: still a problem'. *Emergency Medicine Australasia*, 24: 181–6.

Cubison, T., Pape, S. and Parkhouse, N. (2006) 'Evidence for the link between healing time and the development of hypertrophic scars (HTS) in paediatric burns due to scald injury'. *Burns*. 32: 992–9.

D'Cruz, R., Martin, H. and Holland, A. (2013) 'Medical management of paediatric burn injuries: best practice part 2'. *Journal of Paediatrics and Child Health*, 49: 397–404.

Deitch, E., Wheelahan, T., Rose, M., Clothier, J. and Cotter, J. (1983) 'Hypertrophic burn scars: analysis of variables'. *The Journal of Trauma*, 23 (10): 895–8.

Giretzlehner, M., Dirnberger, J., Owen, R., Haller, H., Lumenta, D. and Kamolz, L. (2013) 'The determination of total burn surface area: how much difference?' *Burns*, 39: 1107–13.

Herndon, D. (ed.) (2012) *Total Burn Care*, 4th edn. New York: Elsevier.

International Burn Injury Database (iBID) (2010) *iBID Introduction*. Available at: www.ibidb.org/ibid (last accessed 24 May 2017).

Jackson, D. (1953) 'The diagnosis of the depth of burning'. *British Journal of Surgery*, 40 (164): 588–96.

Khatib, M., Jabir, S., O'Connor, E.F. and Philp, B. (2014) 'A systematic review of the evolution of laser doppler techniques in burn depth assessment'. *Plastic Surgery International*, 214. Available at: www.hindawi.com/journals/psi/2014/621792 (last accessed 24 May 2017).

Kyle, J. and Wallace, A. (1951) 'Fluid replacement in burnt children'. *British Journal of Plastic Surgery*, 3:194–204.

Langschmidt, J., Caine, P., Wearn, C., Bamford, A., Wilson, Y. and Moiemen, N. (2014) 'Hydrotherapy in burn care: a survey of hydrotherapy practices in the UK and Ireland and literature review'. *Burns*, 40: 860–4.

Lund, C. and Browder, N. (1944) 'The estimation of areas of burns'. *Surgery, Gynecology and Obstetrics*, 79: 352–8.

Maguire, S., Moynihan, S., Mann, M., Potokar, T. and Kemp, A. (2008) 'A systematic review of the features that indicate intentional scalds in children'. *Burns*, 34: 1072–81.

Malic, C., Karoo, R., Austin, O. and Phipps, A. (2007) 'Resuscitation burn card – a useful tool for burn injury assessment'. *Burns*, 33: 195–9.

Meyer, W., Wiechman, S., Woodson, L., Jaco, M. and Thomas, C. (2012) 'Management of pain and other discomforts in burned patients', in D. Herndon (ed.) *Total Burn Care*, 4th edn. New York: Elesvier.

Miller, K., Rodger, S., Bucolo, S., Greer, R. and Kimble, R. (2010) 'Multi-modal distraction: using technology to combat pain in young children with burn injuries'. *Burns*, 36: 647–58.

National Institute for Clinical Excellence (NICE) (2011) *MoorLDI2-BI: A Laser Doppler Blood Flow Imager for Burn Wound Assessment*. Medical Technologies Guidance MTG2. Available at: www.nice.org.uk/guidance/mtg2 (last accessed 24 May 2017).

National Network for Burn Care Review (NBCR) Group (2001) *Committee Report: Standards and Strategy for Burn Care*. Available at: www.britishburnassociation.org/downloads/NBCR2001.pdf (last accessed 24 May 2017).

Pardesi, D. and Fuzaylov, G. (2016) 'Pain management in pediatric burn patients: review of recent literature and future direction'. *Journal of Burn Care and Research*, DOI 10.1097/BCR.0000000000000470.

Retrouvey, H. and Shahrokhi, S. (2015) 'Pain and the thermally injured patient – a review of current therapies'. *Journal of Burn Care and Research*, 36: 315–23.

Roper, N., Logan, W. and Tierney, A. (2000) *The Roper-Logan-Tierney Model of Nursing: Based on Activities of Living*. Edinburgh: Elsevier Health Sciences.

Rossiter, N., Chapman, P. and Haywood, I. (1996) 'How big is a hand?' *Burns*, 22: 230–1.

Royal Society for the Prevention of Accidents (RoSPA) (2015) *Accidents to Children: Scalds and Burns*. Available at: www.rospa.com/home-safety/advice/child-safety/accidents-to-children/#scalds (last accessed 24 May 2017).

Serrano, C., Boloix-Tortosa, R., Gómez-Cía, T, and Acha, B. (2015) 'Features identification for automatic Burn classification'. *Burns*, 41: 1883–90.

Stoddard, F., Sheridan, R., Saxe, G., King, B.S., King, B.H., Chedekel, D., Schnitzer, J. and Martyn, J. (2002) 'Treatment of pain in acutely burned children'. *Journal of Burn Care and Rehabilitation*, 23: 135–56.

Verey, F., Lyttle, M., Lawson, Z., Greenwood, R. and Young, A. (2014) 'When do children get burnt?' *Burns*, 40: 1322–8.

Wasiak, J., Cleland, H., Campbell, F. and Spinks, A. (2013) 'Dressings for superficial and partial thickness burns'. *Cochrane Database of Systematic Reviews*. DOI: 10.1002/14651858.CD002106.pub4

Williams, J., Cubbitt, J. and Dickson, W. (2013) 'The challenge of salt and ice'. *Burns*, 39: 1029.

World Health Organization (WHO) (2008) *World Report on Child Injury Prevention*. Available at: http://apps.who.int/iris/bitstream/10665/43851/1/9789241563574_eng.pdf (last accessed 24 May 2017).

Yarrow, J., Moiemen, N. and Gulhane, S. (2009) 'Early management of burns in children'. *Paediatrics and Child Health*, 19 (11): 509–16.

CARE OF CHILDREN AND YOUNG PEOPLE WITH FLUID AND ELECTROLYTE IMBALANCE

28

ZOE VEAL AND COLIN VEAL

THIS CHAPTER COVERS

- Homeostasis
- Dehydration
- Gastroenteritis
- Sodium imbalance (hyponatraemia and hypernatraemia)
- Potassium imbalance (hypokalaemia and hyperkalaemia)

REQUIRED KNOWLEDGE

A&P LINK 28.1: RENAL SYSTEM

It would be helpful to have an understanding of the anatomy and physiology of the renal system before you start this chapter. Go to the A&P link: 'Renal system' at https://study.sagepub.com/essentialchildnursing

> I don't think it can be emphasised enough that clinical assessment of dehydration can be challenging. The most useful measurement is the degree of weight loss during the illness. I insist that children are reweighed when they re-present to the emergency department with gastroenteritis, as this is by far and away the most accurate way of assessing fluid loss. It is vital to get an actual weight to base fluid calculations on, at the earliest possible opportunity. You don't want to overestimate the weight of a child in diabetic ketoacidosis and prescribe too much fluid, as this puts them at risk of cerebral oedema, etc.
>
> **Nicholas Sargeant, consultant in paediatric emergency medicine**

Visit https://study.sagepub.com/essentialchildnursing to access a wealth of online resources for this chapter – watch out for the margin icons throughout the chapter.

INTRODUCTION

This chapter explores fluid and electrolyte imbalance in children, starting with homeostasis and its role in maintaining the body's fluid balance. All children have a daily fluid requirement that can be affected by illness and disease. There are many reasons for fluid and electrolyte imbalance. However, this chapter focuses on the common causes of fluid imbalance and standard treatment as indicated by current guidelines. As a nursing student, you will be involved in caring for children with fluid and electrolyte imbalance and will be tasked with monitoring and recording their fluid input and output.

HOMEOSTASIS

Homeostasis describes the relatively constant internal state of the body within a narrow range of variables, despite constant changes to the internal or external environment (Patton and Thibodeau, 2013). Maintenance of fluid and electrolyte balance is an important aspect of homeostasis and, at its very basic level, means that the body's 'input' of fluid and electrolytes should be roughly equal to the body's 'output'. If the body takes in too much fluid and electrolytes to maintain its homeostatic balance, the excess will need to be eliminated. If too little is taken in, or an excess loss of fluid and electrolytes occurs – for example, through diarrhoea and vomiting – then those fluids and electrolytes will need to be replaced. Maintaining fluid balance and homeostasis is important for all human life, but it is particularly important in infants and young children as their mechanisms for maintaining homeostatic fluid balance are less well developed (Fergusson, 2008; Macqueen et al., 2012).

Fluid balance

On a daily basis, fluid mainly enters the body via the digestive tract in drink and food, but a small amount of fluid also enters the body through cell catabolism (Patton and Thibodeau, 2013). Likewise, fluid is routinely lost through the kidneys (urine), the gastrointestinal tract (faeces), the skin (sweat and diffusion) and the lungs (water vapour). The body maintains homeostasis by regulating the mechanisms through which fluid is routinely lost and this is one reason why humans sweat more and urinate less in hot weather compared to cold. Go to https://study.sagepub.com/essentialchildnursing to watch a video about what the kidneys do.

VIDEO LINK
28.1: WHAT
THE KIDNEYS
DO

Normal fluid requirements

The normal volume of fluid required by children on a daily basis is shown in Table 28.1. These are general guidelines and some children may require more or less depending on their disease process, renal function, hormone response and level of consciousness. As a nursing student, you will be actively involved in the recording of fluid input and output and in calculating daily fluid requirements. Daily and hourly fluid requirements are calculated using the formula outlined in Table 28.1.

Table 28.1 Daily and hourly fluid requirement calculation

Daily fluid requirement	Hourly fluid requirement
100ml per kg for the first 10kg	4ml per kg for the first 10kg
50ml per kg for the second 10kg	2ml per kg for the second 10kg
20ml per kg for subsequent kg	1ml per kg for subsequent kg

(Continued)

Table 28.1   (Continued)

Daily fluid requirement	Hourly fluid requirement
Example – George is 10 years old and weighs 32 kg. His daily and hourly fluid requirements are calculated as follows	
First 10kg × 100 = 1000ml	First 10kg × 4 = 40ml
Second 10kg × 50 = 500ml	Second 10kg × 2 = 20ml
Subsequent 12kg × 20 = 240ml	Subsequent 12kg × 1 = 12ml
Total daily requirement = 1740 ml	**Total hourly requirement = 72 ml**

PRACTICE
SCENARIO 28:
KAYLEIGH

ACTIVITY 28:1 CRITICAL THINKING

You are working with your mentor and sharing the care of five patients. Your mentor asks you to calculate the daily and hourly fluid requirements for these patients:

- Arthur is 2 years old and weighs 12 kg
- Daisy is 8 years old and weighs 31 kg
- Mohammad is 7 months old and weighs 7.5 kg
- Isabelle is 14 years old and weighs 49 kg
- Elyshia is 5 years old and weighs 18 kg

Daisy and Elyshia are fluid restricted to an 80 per cent daily fluid allowance. Based on their daily fluid requirements, calculate what 80 per cent would be.

ACTIVITY
ANSWER 28.1

Electrolytes

Electrolytes are salts and minerals that conduct electrical impulses around the body to maintain acid-base balance within homeostasis. Found in the blood, they include chemical elements such as sodium and potassium, ions such as chloride and buffers such as bicarbonate. As a nursing student, you will care for children with electrolyte imbalance, as it is frequently seen in conditions such as pyloric stenosis, diabetic ketoacidosis and gastroenteritis.

Normal electrolyte values

Local guidelines mean there is a slight variation in normal values between laboratories. The values given in Table 28.2 are only a guide, so always check the normal value range with the laboratory processing the blood serum level.

Treatment for electrolyte imbalance will depend on which electrolyte is out of balance and by how much. For example, in pyloric stenosis, repeated vomiting and subsequent loss of stomach acid causes low chloride, potassium and sodium concentrations, resulting in the body's acid base becoming too alkaline. By comparison, diabetic ketoacidosis causes a low bicarbonate, with high potassium, urea and creatinine and a very high glucose concentration, which results in the body's acid base becoming too acidic. In diabetic ketoacidosis, the lack of insulin prevents glucose absorption, which in turn results in fatty acid metabolism and ketone production to provide cellular energy. The kidneys become

Table 28.2 Normal electrolyte values

Electrolyte	Lower value	Upper value
Sodium (Na+)	136 mmol/l	145 mmol/l
Potassium (K+)	3.5mmol/l	4.5 mmol/l
Chloride (Cl-)	96 mmol/l	106 mmol/l
Calcium (Ca2+)	2.2 mmol/l	2.6 mmol/l
Magnesium (Mg2+)	0.75 mmol/l	1.0 mmol/l
Phosphate (PO43-)	1 mmol/l	1.8 mmol/l
Bicarbonate (HCO3-)	24 mmol/l	30 mmol/l
Urea	3 mmol/l	7 mmol/l
Creatinine	18 micromol/l	70 micromol/l
Glucose	3.9 mmol/l	6.9 mmol/l

overloaded by both glucose and ketones and will attempt to excrete them both, causing dehydration and a reduction in bicarbonate, which in turn increases the acidic levels in the body.

SEE ALSO CHAPTERS 4 AND 21

ACTIVITY 28.2: CRITICAL THINKING

Return to the earlier section on electrolytes. Make a list of the electrolytes you have come across on placement/in theory. Are you aware of what electrolytes do and why they are so important?

A&P LINK

Drawing on your current knowledge of physiology, spend some time revising the importance of electrolytes in controlling the movement of fluid around the body. To remind yourself of the relevant anatomy and physiology, please read the A&P link: 'Electrolytes' and watch the video at https://study.sagepub.com/essentialchildnursing

A&P LINK 28.2: ELECTROLITES

DEHYDRATION

In children over a year, around 60 per cent of body weight is made up of water, but in infants, body weight is around 80 per cent water. Clinical dehydration occurs when there is a loss of more than 5 per cent of this water (Miall et al., 2012). Feeling unwell can occur before clinical dehydration is reached. Within the body, fluid is held in two main compartments, intracellular and extracellular, and can be lost from either. Table 28.3 indicates how to assess dehydration in children under the age of 5.

One of the most common causes of dehydration in infants and children is diarrhoea and vomiting, most commonly due to gastroenteritis (Miall et al., 2012).

Left untreated, dehydration can lead to shock and death, especially in infants (Tasker et al., 2013), so accurate diagnosis and early assessment is very important. As Nick, Consultant in Children's

SEE ALSO CHAPTERS 15 AND 31

VIDEO LINK 28.2: DEHYDRATION

Table 28.3 Assessing dehydration in children under five years

Increasing severity of dehydration

		No clinically detectable dehydration	Clinical dehydration	Clinical shock
Symptoms (remote and face-to-face assessments)		Appears well	⚑Appears to be unwell or deteriorating	-
		Alert and responsive	⚑ Altered responsiveness (for example, irritable, lethargic)	Decreased level of consciousness
		Normal urine output	Decreased urine output	-
		Skin colour unchanged	Skin colour unchanged	Pale or mottled skin
		Warm extremities	Warm extremities	Cold extremities
Signs (face-to-face assessments)		Alert and responsive	⚑ Altered responsiveness (for example, irritable, lethargic)	Decreased level of consciousness
		Skin colour unchanged	Skin colour unchanged	Pale or mottled skin
		Warm extremities	Warm extremities	Cold extremities
		Eyes not sunken	⚑ Sunken eyes	-
		Moist mucous membranes (except after a drink)	Dry mucous membranes (except for 'mouth breather')	-
		Normal heart rate	⚑ Tachycardia	Tachycardia
		Normal breathing pattern	⚑ Tachypnoea	Tachypnoea
		Normal peripheral pulses	Normal peripheral pulses	Weak peripheral pulses
		Normal capillary refill time	Normal capillary refill time	Prolonged capillary refill time
		Normal skin turgor	⚑ Reduced skin turgor	-
		Normal blood pressure	Normal blood pressure	Hypotension (decompensated shock)

National Institute for Health and Clinical Excellence (2009) *CG84 Diarrhoea and Vomiting Caused by Gastroenteritis in Under 5s: diagnosis and management.* London: NICE. Available at: www.nice.org.uk/guidance/cg84. Reproduced with permission.

Emergency Medicine, stated at the start of this chapter, the clinical assessment of dehydration can be challenging and the most useful measurement is the degree of weight loss during the illness (Lissauer and Clayden, 2012).

GASTROENTERITIS

Gastroenteritis is characterised by the sudden onset of diarrhoea and may or may not include vomiting (NICE, 2009). Gastroenteritis is very common and can range from a minor illness to a life-threatening one, as it affects absorption in the gastrointestinal tract, which in turn can lead to dehydration due to fluid loss. The causes of gastroenteritis can be bacterial, viral or parasitic infection (Glasper et al., 2016) and the majority of children are cared for in the community. However, as a nursing student, you will almost certainly care for young children admitted to hospital with dehydration as a result of gastroenteritis.

SEE ALSO
CHAPTER 29

Treatment and management of gastroenteritis

Initially, infection control measures need to be instigated to prevent cross-contamination. If there is mild to moderate dehydration, then oral rehydration salt (ORS) solutions should be suitable, but if the dehydration is severe, then intravenous fluids will be required. Once rehydration is completed then normal feeding/drinking patterns are recommenced. The use of medications such as antidiarrhoeals, antiemetics or antibiotics are not normally recommended.

Some infections causing gastroenteritis are classed as notifiable diseases under the Public Health (Control of Disease) Act 1984 and Health Protection (Notification) Regulations 2010. This normally only applies to gastroenteritis caused by food poisoning, rather than the more common viral causes such as rotavirus or norovirus. Where the cause is notifiable, a notification form needs to be completed (GOV.UK, 2010).

Where there are no signs of clinical dehydration, current guidelines (see Table 28.4) recommend continuing with breast or formula feeding, encouragement of fluid intake (but not fruit juices or carbonated drinks) and offering ORS solution as supplemental fluid to those whose risk of developing dehydration is high (NICE, 2009).

Table 28.4   Treatment of clinical dehydration and clinical shock based on NICE guidelines

Use of oral rehydration salt (ORS) solution to treat clinical dehydration	Use of intravenous therapy to treat clinical shock
• Use ORS solution to rehydrate children unless intravenous therapy is indicated • Give 50 ml/kg for fluid deficit replacement over four hours on top of maintenance fluid • Give small amounts of ORS solution frequently • Consider supplementing with usual fluids, including breast/formula milk or water if sufficient amounts of ORS solution are refused • Consider using nasogastric tube if vomiting or an inadequate volume of ORS solution is taken • Use regular clinical assessment to monitor response to therapy	• Use intravenous therapy if shock is suspected or confirmed • Treat with rapid infusion of 20 ml/kg of 0.9% saline • Repeat infusion if required and consider consulting paediatric intensive care specialist • If an initial fluid rapid infusion was required for suspected or confirmed shock, then 100ml/kg is recommended on top of the maintenance fluid requirement • Consider other causes of shock rather than dehydration • Monitoring of blood biochemistry should happen from the outset and then be monitored regularly. The composition of the fluid should be altered and infusion rate changed if required

Source: National Institute for Health and Clinical Excellence (2009) *CG84 Diarrhoea and Vomiting Caused by Gastroenteritis in Under 5s: diagnosis and management.* London: NICE. Available from: www.nice.org.uk/guidance/cg84.

Intravenous therapy

As a nursing student, you are not allowed to commence or stop an intravenous infusion as this is an extended role for which the registered nurse requires additional training in intravenous therapy. However, you may be involved in caring for a patient with an intravenous infusion and keeping a record of the amount infused. It is also important that you are familiar with fluid prescription charts and the standard protocol for rehydration through intravenous therapy. NICE (2015) recommends fluid prescription charts be signed, dated, timed and written clearly with fluids prescribed in millilitres (mls) per hour. All input and output should be recorded on an hourly basis and a running total kept, with 12-hourly fluid balance subtotals and reassessment of the fluid prescription and hydration status (NICE, 2015). A 24-hour fluid balance should also be calculated, alongside 12-hourly assessment of whether oral fluids can be re-started (NICE, 2015).

After rehydration, the advice is the same as that for preventing dehydration. Breast/formula feeding should be reintroduced and in older children, fluid intake should be encouraged, avoiding fruit juice or carbonated drinks. In children who continue to be at risk of dehydration, due to the continuation of diarrhoea and/or vomiting, ORS solution should also be considered (NICE, 2009).

WHAT'S THE EVIDENCE?

Modern nursing care is rooted in an evidence base and, as a nursing student, you should be aware of where to find clinical evidence to provide a rationale for your practice and the care you deliver. Publications produced by The National Institute for Health and Care Excellence (NICE) are one example of evidence-based guidance with a reputation for rigour, independence and objectivity.

Go now to *Diarrhoea and Vomiting Caused by Gastroenteritis in Under 5s: Diagnosis and Management* (NICE, 2009) and download the full guideline – you can access it via https://study.sagepub.com/essentialchildnursing

WEBLINK:
GASTROENTERITIS
IN UNDER 5s

- How many articles were reviewed in Chapter 5 'Fluid management', before the recommendations on treating dehydration were made?
- Are you surprised by the detail in this guideline?

WHAT'S THE
EVIDENCE?
ANSWER 28.1

To help consolidate your learning so far, look at a hypothetical scenario based on a common presentation seen in emergency departments. Work your way through the findings presented and answer the questions that follow.

SCENARIO 28.1: ALBERT

Albert is 18 months old and is brought to the emergency department by his parents, following a three-day history of diarrhoea and vomiting. Albert's parents noticed his symptoms had become worse in the last 24 hours. In response to your questions, they inform you that mum and Albert's 3-year-old sibling have both had an 'upset stomach' recently. Examinations indicate:

A – Self-ventilating in air with saturations >95 per cent

B – Respiratory rate: 45 breaths per minute

C – Heart rate: 140 beats per minute; blood pressure 90/45; capillary refill time 2 secs

D – Albert is irritable

E – Temperature: 37.1°C

F – Reduced skin turgor, dry mucous membranes and his eyes appear sunken

When asked, Albert's mum tells you he hasn't had a wet nappy since yesterday evening.

- Using the assessment of dehydration tool in Table 28.3, how dehydrated is Albert?
- What are your key nursing care priorities for Albert?

SCENARIO
ANSWER 28.1

SODIUM IMBALANCE (HYPONATRAEMIA AND HYPERNATRAEMIA)

A sodium imbalance almost always indicates a change in the hydration level of the body (Miall et al., 2012). A sodium level of below 136 mmol/l is known as hyponatraemia and can be caused either through sodium loss resulting from diarrhoea, excessive sweating or renal failure, or by an excess of water that causes the body's sodium concentration to become diluted. Hyponatraemia is a serious condition requiring urgent treatment, as a low sodium level can lead to convulsions, caused by the movement of water from the extracellular compartment to the intracellular compartment, increasing brain volume. Treatment is normally through intravenous infusion of an isotonic solution such as 0.9% saline, or 0.9% saline with 5% glucose. Where shock is suspected or confirmed, rapid intravenous infusion is recommended (NICE, 2009).

Hypernatraemia is the medical term for a high sodium level, which is defined as being above 145 mmol/l. A high sodium level could be caused by dehydration resulting from fluid deprivation or diarrhoea, or through excessive salt intake. Incorrect formula feed preparation or adding salt to solids whilst weaning can cause excessive salt intake, as can deliberate salt poisoning, although this is rare. Hypernatraemic dehydration is very dangerous (Lissauer and Clayden, 2012). The shift in water from the intracellular compartment to the extracellular compartment means that some of the red flag signs of dehydration, such as sunken eyes and reduced skin turgor, are harder to spot. As water is drawn out of the brain, jittery movements, increased muscle tone, altered consciousness, seizures and cerebral haemorrhage may occur. Treatment involves rehydration using either 0.9% saline, or 0.9% saline with 5% glucose via slow intravenous infusion, typically over 48 hours and reverting to oral rehydration therapy as soon as it is tolerated (NICE, 2009).

In both hyponatraemia and hypernatraemia, sodium levels should be monitored, so you should expect your patient to have their blood taken on a regular basis. The NICE guidelines *Intravenous Fluid Therapy in Children and Young People in Hospital* (2015) recommend all children undergoing intravenous therapy have blood taken at least every 24 hours to check electrolyte concentrations, with more frequent measurement of electrolyte levels if an imbalance exists.

POTASSIUM IMBALANCE (HYPOKALAEMIA AND HYPERKALAEMIA)

Potassium imbalance occurs when there is too little (hypokalaemia) or too much (hyperkalaemia) potassium in the bloodstream. It is less common than sodium imbalance, but more serious. Hyperkalaemia (above 5.5 mmol/l) is caused by either ineffective elimination of potassium through the renal system or through excessive release of potassium from the cells. Causes of ineffective elimination include renal failure or a sudden reduced urine volume (oliguria) and congenital adrenal hyperplasia. Some medications such as potassium-sparing diuretics, non-steroidal anti-inflammatory drugs (NSAID) and ACE inhibitors can also interfere with urinary excretion and may result in raised potassium levels. Excessive release of potassium from cells may occur from tissue necrosis, burn injury or massive haemolysis, during which red blood cells are rapidly broken down and their contents released into the surrounding blood plasma. A high potassium blood result can also be a false positive. This is common in very young children for whom there has been difficulty in obtaining a blood sample. Known as pseudohyperkalaemia, this is the result of laboratory artefact rather than actual potassium imbalance, so where this is suspected, the blood test should be repeated.

Hyperkalaemia is potentially very dangerous as it can cause serious, even fatal, cardiac arrhythmias (Miall et al., 2012). Treatment for hyperkalaemia includes salbutamol infusion, insulin and dextrose infusion to encourage potassium into the cells. Calcium may also be given to protect the myocardium (heart) (Tasker et al., 2013).

Hypokalaemia (below 3 mmol/l) is usually less serious, but still requires treatment as it can lead to muscle weakness, lethargy, gastric ileus and in severe hypokalaemia (below 2.5 mmol/l) cardiac arrhythmias. Causes of low potassium include diarrhoea and vomiting, diuretic therapy and an inadequate potassium intake through starvation. As a nursing student, you may care for a young person with anorexia nervosa who has been admitted to hospital with a low potassium level. Depending on the severity of the hypokalaemia, treatment is either via oral potassium supplements or an intravenous infusion of potassium, given over an hour. Where there are ECG changes, correction of the imbalance is considered to be urgent, requiring intravenous potassium infusion (Tasker et al., 2013).

Because potassium can cause cardiac arrhythmias, children with a potassium imbalance should be nursed under ECG monitoring to observe for any changes to the ECG. As with a sodium imbalance, you should also expect your patient to have their blood taken frequently to monitor the potassium level.

A summary of sodium and potassium imbalances is presented in Table 28.5.

Table 28.5 Summary of sodium and potassium imbalance

		Caused by	Signs and symptoms
Sodium (Na+)	Hyponatraemia (<136 mmol/l)	Diarrhoea Excess sweating Renal failure Excess water = dilute sodium concentration	Convulsions
	Hypernatraemia (>145 mmol/l)	Diarrhoea Fluid deprivation Excess salt intake	Jittery movements Increased muscle tone Altered consciousness Cerebral haemorrhage
Potassium (K+)	Hypokalaemia (<3 mmol/l)	Diarrhoea and vomiting Diuretic therapy Intake potassium intake through starvation	Muscle weakness Lethargy Gastric ileus In severe hypokalaemia, cardiac arrhythmias
	Hyperkalaemia (>5.5 mmol/l)	Excessive release of potassium from the cells through: • Tissue necrosis • Burn injury • Haemolysis Renal failure Congenital adrenal hyperplasia Medications such as: • Potassium-sparing diuretics • Non-steriodal anti-infammatory drugs • ACE inhibitors	Nausea and vomiting Dizziness Muscle cramps ECG changes Cardiac arrhythmias which can lead to cardiac arrest

SCENARIO 28.2: CHELSEA

Chelsea is 9 months old and has been brought to the emergency department by her mother and grandmother. She has jittery movements, decreased consciousness, no history of diarrhoea or vomiting, but her urea and electrolytes show a high sodium level. Chelsea is formula fed and was weaned three months ago. Chelsea's grandmother tells you that she makes all of Chelsea's food as 'babies should be encouraged to eat the same food as the rest of the family'.

- What do you think might be the cause of Chelsea's hypernatremia?
- What health promotion may be needed for this family?

SCENARIO
ANSWER 28.2

SAFEGUARDING STOP POINT

Consider Chelsea's scenario. Do you identify any cause for concern in the scenario? The grandmother's phrase 'babies should be encouraged to eat the same food as the rest of the family' may indicate the use of food meant for adult consumption and this may place Chelsea at harm.

Using the weblinks provided at https://study.sagepub.com/essentialchildnursing, explore the case of Leroy Elders who died in 1999 from salt poisoning. What were the factors that contributed to Leroy's death? What weaning advice would you give to parents?

SAFEGUARDING
STOP POINT
ANSWER 28.1

WEBLINK:
LEROY ELDERS

ACTIVITY 28.3: CRITICAL THINKING

Write a plan of care for a child with diarrhoea and vomiting, taking into consideration fluid management and infection control needs. Annotate your care plan with available evidence and discuss this with your mentor. Your care plan could be used as evidence towards achieving your learning competencies while in placement.

ACTIVITY
ANSWER 28.3

PLACEMENT
ADVICE 28: FLUID
& ELECTROLYTE
IMBALANCE

The ability to manage a child's fluid and electrolyte balance is an important skill in children's nursing, as is the knowledge which underpins the process of homeostasis and acid-base balance in maintaining the body's equilibrium. Children, especially very young children, are at particular risk of dehydration and can become clinically dehydrated very quickly. Caring for a child who is dehydrated is a common occurrence and you will almost certainly come across this during placement. This chapter and its online resources will have provided you with the basic knowledge needed to enable you to provide care to the child with a fluid and electrolyte imbalance.

HEALTH
PROMOTION
28: FLUID &
ELECTROLYTE
IMBALANCE

Go to https://study.sagepub.com/essentialchildnursing for tips on preparing for placements and health promotion when working with children with fluid and electrolyte imbalance.

CHAPTER SUMMARY

In this chapter, you have explored:

- Normal fluid requirements and electrolyte levels for children and young people
- Dehydration and electrolyte imbalance, with a focus on gastroenteritis and how it is treated
- Sodium imbalance (hyponatraemia and hypernatraemia)
- Potassium imbalance (hypokalaemia and hyperkalaemia)

In addition, you have enhanced your learning through the application of knowledge and understanding using case studies on dehydration and hypernatraemia.

BUILD YOUR BIBLIOGRAPHY

Books

- Glasper, A. and Richardson, J. (2010) *A Textbook of Children's and Young People's Nursing*, 2nd edn. London: Churchill Livingstone Elsevier.

  This widely accessible textbook contains an in-depth chapter on fluid and electrolyte imbalance.

- Miall, L., Rudolf, M. and Smith, D. (2016) *Paediatrics at a Glance*, 4th edn. Chichester: Wiley Blackwell.

  Intended as a quick reference, this textbook gives a brief, but thorough, overview of paediatric care, including diarrhoea management, dehydration and electrolyte balance.

Journal articles

Go to https://study.sagepub.com/essentialchildnursing for further free online journal articles related to this chapter.

FURTHER
READING:
ONLINE
JOURNAL
ARTICLES

FIND OUT
MORE!

- Falszewska, A., Dziechciarz, P. and Szajewska, H. (2014) 'The diagnostic accuracy of Clinical Dehydration Scale in identifying dehydration in children with acute gastroenteritis: a systematic review'. *Clinical Pediatrics*, 53 (12): 1181–8.

  This systematic review explores the data available on the accuracy of the clinical dehydration scale. It's a useful article to test your skills in research analysis.

- Mathieson, L. (2015) 'Vomiting and diarrhoea in children'. *InnovAiT*, 8 (10): 592–8.

  This easy-to-read article provides an overview of vomiting and diarrhoea in children, including common viral causes, clinical assessment, fluid management and complications.

- Parkin, P.C., Macarthur, C., Khambalia, A., Goldman, R.D. and Friedman, J.N. (2010) 'Clinical and laboratory assessment of dehydration severity in children with acute gastroenteritis'. *Clinical Pediatrics*, 49 (3): 235–9.

  On research carried out in Canada, this article assessing the effectiveness of a clinical dehydration scale and laboratory tests in clinical decision-making, provides a comparison to UK-based care.

Weblinks

FURTHER
READING:
WEBLINKS

Go to https://study.sagepub.com/essentialchildnursing for further weblinks related to this chapter.

- GOV.UK, *Notifiable Diseases and Causative Organisms: How to Report*

  www.gov.uk/guidance/notifiable-diseases-and-causative-organisms-how-to-report

Reporting certain notifiable infectious diseases aims to help prevent their spread and reduce the risk of epidemic. A list of notifiable diseases requiring report is available on this weblink.

- NICE, *Diarrhoea and Vomiting Caused by Gastroenteritis in Under 5s: Diagnosis and Management*
www.nice.org.uk/guidance/cg84
This evidence-based guideline underpins clinical decision-making and care delivery for children under 5 who present with diarrhoea and vomiting.

- Spotting the Sick Child
http://edition3.spottingthesickchild.com
The Royal College of Paediatrics and Child Health and the Department of Health, as well as others, support this educational resource. It contains a section on dehydration.

ACE YOUR ASSESSMENT

Revise what you have learned by visiting https://study.sagepub.com/essentialchildnursing

ONLINE
QUIZZES &
ACTIVITY
ANSWERS

- Test yourself with multiple-choice and short-answer questions
- Do the chapter activities in the book and check your answers online

REFERENCES

Fergusson, D. (2008) *Clinical Assessment and Monitoring in Children.* Oxford: Blackwell Publishing.

Glasper, E.A., McEwing, G. and Richardson, J. (2016) *Oxford Handbook of Children's and Young People's Nursing*, 2nd edn. Oxford: Oxford University Press.

GOV.UK (2010) *Notifiable Diseases and Causative Organisms: How to Report.* Available at: www.gov.uk/guidance/notifiable-diseases-and-causative-organisms-how-to-report (last accessed 24 May 2017).

Lissauer, T. and Clayden, G. (2012) *Illustrated Textbook of Paediatrics*, 4th edn. London: Mosby Elsevier.

Macqueen, S., Bruce, E.A. and Gibson, F. (2012) *The Great Ormond Street Hospital Manual of Children's Nursing Practices.* Oxford: Wiley Blackwell.

Miall, L. Rudolf, M. and Smith, D. (2012) *Paediatrics at a Glance.* Chichester: John Wiley and Sons.

National Institute for Health and Clinical Excellence (NICE) (2009) *Diarrhoea and Vomiting Caused by Gastroenteritis in Under 5s: Diagnosis and Management.* Available at: www.nice.org.uk/guidance/cg84 (last accessed: 24 May 2017).

National Institute for Health and Care Excellence (NICE) (2015) *Intravenous Fluid Therapy in Children and Young People in Hospital.* Available at: www.nice.org.uk/guidance/ng29 (last accessed 24 May 2017).

Patton, K.T. and Thibodeau, G.A. (2013) *Anthony's Textbook of Anatomy and Physiology*, 20th edn. St. Louis, MO: Mosby Elsevier.

Tasker, R.C., McClure, R.J. and Acerini, C.L. (2013) *Oxford Handbook of Paediatrics*, 2nd edn. Oxford: Oxford University Press.

CARE OF CHILDREN AND YOUNG PEOPLE WITH GASTROINTESTINAL PROBLEMS

29

ZOE VEAL, ORLA McALINDEN AND DOREEN CRAWFORD

THIS CHAPTER COVERS

- Common gastrointestinal conditions
- Nursing management of gastrointestinal problems
- Nutrition
- Stoma (Ostomy) management
- Discharge planning and continuing care in the community

REQUIRED KNOWLEDGE

A&P LINK 29.1: GASTROINTESTINAL SYSTEM AND EMBRYOLOGY

It would be helpful to have an understanding of the anatomy and physiology of the gastrointestinal system before you start this chapter. Go to the A&P Link 29.1: Gastrointestinal system and embryology at https://study.sagepub.com/essentialchildnursing

> " You worry that he's getting enough to grow, and that you will be able to manage the tube feeds, then you worry that he won't look like other children of his age because the nasogastric tube is really obvious.
>
> **Ramesh, parent** "

Visit https://study.sagepub.com/essentialchildnursing to access a wealth of online resources for this chapter – watch out for the margin icons throughout the chapter.

INTRODUCTION

The opening quotation illustrates how a parent can feel when their child requires enteral feeding, for whatever reason. They may feel concern that their child cannot feed 'normally' to grow and develop into a 'healthy' child/adult. They may also be worried their child will be treated differently from other children. As a student, you will care for children with a range of gastrointestinal conditions and needs. Some may have acute and short-term conditions that quickly resolve on treatment whereas others may have chronic, lifelong difficulties with eating and digestion, requiring long-term treatment and intervention which impacts on the whole family. A family-focused approach is always essential when delivering child-centred care, and children's nurses are best placed to ensure this happens.

The gastrointestinal system is extensive and complex, consisting primarily of the oesophagus, stomach and small and large intestines, alongside accessory digestive organs: the pancreas, liver and gallbladder. Consequently, there are a number of conditions which can arise, either from a fault during embryological development or via disease process. As a children's nursing student, you may be involved in both the medical and surgical management of gastrointestinal problems, both in hospital and in the community.

COMMON GASTROINTESTINAL CONDITIONS

There are a number of common gastrointestinal conditions that you may come across during your placements. Some, especially those that are congenital/present at birth, require specialist intervention and care from a tertiary children's hospital and are seen less commonly outside of these settings. Others, such as gastroenteritis, are seen more frequently within the community, with children only being admitted to hospital when they become clinically dehydrated.

SEE ALSO
CHAPTER 15

Abdomimal pain

Abdominal pain is very common in children and the pain may be local or generalised. Young children may not be able to locate the exact area of pain within their abdomen and may have their own special words to describe the pain. Older children with localised pain should be able to point to the source. Older children may hold their tummy; infants may draw up their legs to indicate they have abdominal pain. Abdominal pain can have a surgical, medical or psychological cause.

Causes of abdominal pain

Constipation

Constipation is frequently seen in children and has a number of causes/risk factors:

- A diet low in fibre and not drinking enough fluids
- Unwillingness to use a school or public toilet – 'stool holding'
- Distraction or unwillingness to interrupt activity to use the toilet
- Lack of exercise/impaired mobility
- Fear of pain – previous anal fissure or passing a painful, hard stool in the past can lead to toilet delay/avoidance in the future
- Hirschsprung's disease

WEBLINK:
CONSTIPATION
DIAGNOSIS
MANAGEMENT

Around a third of 4–7-year-olds experience constipation, and many children experience constipation during potty training (Miall et al., 2012). In 2010, NICE published guidelines on the diagnosis and management of constipation in children. For more information on this guideline, go to the 'Build your bibliography' section at the end of the chapter.

Functional/idiopathic constipation is the most common seen in children and has no known anatomical or physiological cause. When there have been no bowel movements for several days, the faeces becomes hard and compacted in the rectum, making it more difficult and painful to pass. If the bowel becomes very impacted, then soiling can occur as faecal liquid leaks around the faecal mass. This can be mistaken for diarrhoea and can sometimes cause delay in accepting a constipation diagnosis. Treatment for functional constipation is based on a three-pronged approach – disimpaction of the bowel through the use of laxatives, parent and child education and maintenance therapy consisting of improved diet, exercise and regular toileting, and medication (Glasper et al., 2015).

PRACTICE
SCENARIO 29:
JACK

SCENARIO 29.1: ZAC

You are on placement with the health visitor and you visit Zac, a 4-year-old boy, who according to mum is a 'picky eater'. Zac has a history of constipation and soiling and is due to start school shortly. His mum has asked for advice.

- What advice would you give Zac's mum to help manage his constipation?
- What advice would you give to mum regarding school?

SCENARIO
ANSWER 29.1

Appendicitis/peritonitis

Appendicitis is an infection of the appendix. Perforation of the appendix causes peritonitis, which can lead to septicaemia. Sudden relief of pain can indicate that perforation has occurred. Treatment is usually surgical removal of the appendix and nursing care will follow the routine pre- and postoperative care directed by local policy and surgical instruction. Conservative treatment with antibiotics is sometimes used, but its effectiveness as an alternative to surgery is still uncertain.

SEE ALSO
CHAPTERS 15,
17 AND 28

Gastroenteritis

This is an extremely common condition in children, which causes diarrhoea and vomiting, often with sudden onset. Common viral causes include norovirus and rotavirus which are highly infectious. Bacterial causes include shigella, E. Coli, salmonella and campylobacter. Most cases can be managed successfully at home in the community, but the child may require hospitalisation if symptoms are prolonged and dehydration indicated.

WHAT'S THE EVIDENCE?

Giving medication to stop vomiting or diarrhoea in gastroenteritis is not normally advised. However, ondansetron – an antiemetic licensed for prescription in children for chemotherapy-induced or postoperative nausea and vomiting – has been shown to be of some benefit in treating gastroenteritis. In studies undertaken outside the UK, more children stopped vomiting when given ondansetron compared to children given a placebo and fewer children needed intravenous therapy or hospitalisation to treat dehydration (NICE, 2014).

- Why might some prescribers be reluctant to prescribe ondansetron to treat gastro-enteritis?
- Antiemetic and antidiarrhoeal medication is not normally advised – what might be the reason for this?

WHAT'S THE EVIDENCE? ANSWER 29.1

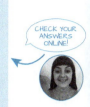

CHECK YOUR ANSWERS ONLINE!

Intussusception

Intussusception is the most common form of bowel obstruction in children under the age of 3 years, accounting for 25 per cent of abdominal emergencies in children under 5 years (Rull, 2016). One part of the bowel telescopes into another part, causing colicky abdominal pain, bile-stained vomiting, pallor, lethargy, irritability, and possible dehydration and shock. A defining feature is the passage of blood and mucus in a 'redcurrant jelly' stool. Depending on the child's clinical condition, treatment is with either an air enema or surgical repair. Untreated intussusception is fatal.

Gastritis/peptic ulcer

Now recognised to be an important cause of abdominal pain in children (Miall et al., 2012). Causes include infection with Helicobacter pylori, use of non-steroidal anti-inflammatory medication, stress and an autoimmune response. Treatment involves symptom management and lifestyle changes (Tidy, 2015a).

Other causes of abdominal pain

Abdominal pain can also be caused by mesenteric adenitis, urinary tract infection, Henoch-Schönlein purpura, pyelonephritis, diabetic ketoacidosis and in adolescent girls, gynaecological causes such as ovarian cysts or ectopic pregnancy. Recurrent abdominal pain can also be caused by irritable bowel syndrome, anxiety and problems at home/school causing psychosomatic presentation of pain.

ACTIVITY 29.1: CRITICAL THINKING

A gynaecological cause may be the source of abdominal pain and in addition, the pregnancy status of females should be known before surgery. NICE states that all women of childbearing potential should be asked sensitively about the possibility of pregnancy and a pregnancy test carried out with consent, if there is doubt (NICE, 2016a). This is because there are associated risks with anaesthesia during pregnancy. However, this NICE guideline does not apply to young people under 16 years of age.

(Continued)

(Continued)

Consider the following:

- Should pregnancy checking be routinely carried out on all adolescent females?
- If you do discuss the possibility of pregnancy with your patient, should you document this?
- Should a pregnancy test be carried out without consent?
- What elements of privacy and dignity do you need to consider?
- Does your placement area have a protocol for pregnancy checking in adolescent female patients? Discuss this with your mentor.

Now read the Royal College of Paediatrics and Child Health (RCPCH, 2012) document *Pre-procedure Pregnancy Checking in Under 16s: Guidance for Clinicians* available via https://study.sagepub.com/essentialchildnursing

WEBLINK: PREGNANCY CHECK

ACTIVITY ANSWER 29.1

Congenital abnormalities of the gastrointestinal system

Gastroschisis/exomphalos (omphalocele)

VIDEO LINK 29.1: ABDOMINAL WALL DEFECTS

Often considered to be similar, these are very different in presentation. In gastroschisis, the intestines are exposed and consequently there is a risk of peritonitis and thickening of the bowel wall. Treatment is via surgical restoration of the bowel to the abdominal cavity and may be carried out as a staged repair if the lesion is extensive. The infant will require intravenous feeding until the bowel can fulfil normal function. Prognosis is usually good. Watch the video explaining abdominal wall defects, such as gastroschisis and exomphalos (omphalocele) at https://study.sagepub.com/essentialchildnursing

Exomphalos (omphalocele) is intestinal herniation into the umbilicus. Defect size may vary, but can involve the liver, spleen or bladder as well as the intestines. Surgical repair is possible, but the condition is associated with chromosomal abnormalities and other midline defects, so prognosis may be uncertain.

Oesophageal atresia/tracheo-oesophageal fistula

Tracheo-oesphageal fistula (TOF) is a passage between the trachea and the oesophagus, whereas oesophageal atresia (OA) means the oesophagus does not connect to the stomach, but ends in a blind pouch. OA can occur in isolation, but this is rare and both defects are usually seen together. Incidence is 1 in 3,000 births (Tidy, 2015b).

SEE ALSO CHAPTER 17

TOF/OA may be suspected antenatally if there is excessive amniotic fluid (polyhydraminos) seen on ultrasound scan, but it is difficult to diagnose before birth. At birth, the infant will present as having 'bubbly' breathing, unable to feed or clear mucus and may have respiratory distress (Tidy, 2015b). Emergency steps are needed to secure the airway and a Repogle tube on low continuous suction is passed into the oesophagus to clear secretions which collect there. This is flushed regularly to maintain patency. Surgical repair is possible, but if the oesophageal gap is large, there may be a period of delay to allow the oesophagus to grow a little. Intravenous nutrition is seldom required, as feeds are usually tolerated through a gastrostomy.

Postoperative complications include stricture (scar tissue) and gastro-oesophageal reflux. TOF/OA is associated with other congenital and chromosomal abnormalities, including VACTERL syndrome, CHARGE association, Trisomy 13, 18 and 21 (Tidy, 2015b). Watch the video on colon interposition at https://study.sagepub.com/essentialchildnursing to find out more on ways to treat severe oesophageal atresia.

VIDEO LINK
29.2: COLON
INTERPOSITION

Malrotation/volvulus

Malrotation, the failure of the midgut to rotate during gestation, occurs in 1 in 500 live births, with 90 per cent presenting during the first year of life, and 80 per cent of these within the first four weeks (Tidy, 2015c). Volvulus is an associated condition, which results from failure of the small intestine to fix correctly into the abdominal cavity, allowing for twisting and occlusion of the blood supply. For both conditions, bilious vomiting is a key presenting sign, indicating partial or complete bowel obstruction. The presentation of a sick child with a paralytic ileus and possibly an abdominal mass of twisted intestines is a surgical emergency. Repair is surgical (Ladd's procedure).

VIDEO LINK
29.3: PRIMITIVE
GUT

Anorectal anomaly

Also known as imperforate anus, this is the term given to a range of anal malformations, from anal stenosis where the anal opening is too tight to allow for the passage of stool, to the complete absence of an anal opening and a rectum that ends as a fistula in the vagina (females) or urethra (males). Failure to pass meconium, or the presence of meconium in the urine are presenting signs. Incidence ranges from 1 in 500 births for minor defects to 1 in 5,000 births for the more severe form (Gandhi, 2014).

Obstructive disorders

Intussusception, malrotation/volvulus and anorectal anomaly could also be classified as obstructive disorders.

Hirschsprung's disease

The absence of ganglion cells in the colon leads to weak/absent peristalsis, so faeces cannot pass through normally. The extent of abnormal bowel can vary and symptoms can range from chronic constipation to bowel obstruction, depending on severity. Failure to pass meconium within 48 hours is an important sign (Gandhi, 2014). Repair is surgical to remove or bypass the portion of affected bowel. Occasionally, temporary or permanent colostomy is required.

Adhesions

Adhesions are fibrous bands that occur as a side effect of abdominal surgery, causing twisting and pulling, resulting in abdominal pain and bowel obstruction. Adhesions are a surgical emergency.

Problems with the gastric sphincters

Pyloric stenosis

An idiopathic overgrowth of the pyloric sphincter causing an obstruction to gastric emptying. Peak incidence is at six weeks old, is more common in first-born male infants and tends to run in families. The infant presents with projectile vomiting after taking a feed, weight loss and dehydration. Treatment is correction of dehydration and surgical incision/dilation (Ramstedt's pyloromyotomy) of the hypertrophied muscle.

SEE ALSO
CHAPTER 28

Gastro-oesophageal reflux disease (GORD)

This is the passage of gastric contents back into the oesophagus, causing pain and discomfort. Common in babies, especially premature infants and those who have had surgery for TOF. GORD is also seen in older children with cerebral palsy or Down's syndrome (Miall et al., 2012).

NICE guidelines currently recommend the following:

- Maintain sleeping position on the back
- Breastfeeding assessment in breastfed infants with marked distress
- Offer smaller, more frequent feeds (maintaining daily amount) in formula fed infants
- Trial of feed thickener or alginate therapy if the above has been unsuccessful
- Trial of proton pump inhibitors or H2 receptor antagonists and review effectiveness
- Jejunal feeding for infants only if at risk of aspiration pneumonia
- Surgery only if medical management has demonstrably failed or the reflux is of long-standing duration (NICE, 2015a)

The routine use of feeding tubes is no longer advised. For more information, read the NICE guideline.

Autoimmune disorders

Crohn's disease and ulcerative colitis

Collectively known as inflammatory bowel disease (IBD), Crohn's disease and ulcerative colitis are autoimmune conditions. Crohn's disease can affect any part of the child's gastrointestinal tract from mouth to anus; ulcerative colitis affects the rectum and colon only. The exact cause is unknown but is most likely a combination of genetic, environmental and immunological factors (Crohn's and Colitis UK, 2013). Presentation includes abdominal pain, diarrhoea, rectal bleeding, weight loss and fatigue. Treatment and management depends on severity, but usually involves nutritional support and hydration, corticosteroid and immunosuppressant medication. Wherever possible, surgery is avoided but a resection and anastomosis surgical technique may be required or a resection and formation of a stoma, which may or may not be permanent (Glasper et al., 2016).

There is separate NICE guidance for both Crohn's disease and ulcerative colitis, alongside a NICE quality standard which can be found in the 'Build your bibliography' section.

Coeliac disease

This is a lifelong autoimmune disorder in which the body reacts to gluten, a protein found in wheat, barley and rye. Although a genetically linked condition, the genetic risks are low (Coeliac UK, 2016). Symptoms appear after weaning and can range from mild to severe, with faltering growth in extreme cases. Other symptoms include diarrhoea, poor appetite, abdominal distension and lethargy. Diagnosis is via antibody testing and depending on these results, possible intestinal biopsy. Coeliac disease, once confirmed, is managed by a gluten-free diet for life and, if necessary, supplements to treat deficiencies in iron, vitamin B12 or folic acid. There is NICE guidance (NICE 2015b) to support healthcare decision-making.

Other gastrointestinal problems

Necrotising enterocolitis (NEC)

NEC is primarily seen in premature infants where sections of the intestine become necrotic, resulting in potential perforation and peritonitis. The exact cause is unknown. Presentation usually occurs while the infant is still in the neonatal unit and signs may be subtle at first – lethargy, reduced feeding, 'not themselves' and not tolerating handling as well as usual. This may progress to more worrying signs such as apnoea, bradycardia, poor thermoregulation, abdominal distention, vomiting and the appearance of blood in the stools.

SEE ALSO
CHAPTER 32

Treatment can be either by medical or surgical approaches. The conservative approach of nil by mouth, naso/orogastric tube to empty stomach of contents, intravenous fluids, total parenteral nutrition (TPN) and triple antibiotics is usually tried first. If the infant's bowel should perforate, surgery is required to resect the diseased bowel and rejoin (anastomose) the healthy ends. The repair is usually protected by the formation of a temporary stoma.

Lactose intolerance and cow's milk protein allergy

Cow's milk protein allergy (CMPA) is an abnormal reaction by the immune system to proteins found in cow's milk. It affects around 7 per cent of formula-fed and 0.5 per cent exclusively breast-fed infants, which suggests that exclusive breast-feeding may protect infants from developing CMPA. It is a common allergy, frequently affecting children in the first year of life (Sambrook, 2017). Symptoms include vomiting, abdominal pain, bloody stools and diarrhoea, hives, eczema, and also wheeze (GI Kids, 2013). Treatment is the elimination of cow's milk from the diet. CMPA is more likely if close family members have asthma, eczema or hayfever. However, prognosis is good with a 90 per cent remission rate by 3 years of age (Sambrook, 2017).

Lactose intolerance is the inability to digest lactose due to deficiency in the lactase enzyme (Harding, 2016). Lactose is a type of sugar found in milk and dairy products. Symptoms include flatulence, bloating, abdominal discomfort and diarrhoea, usually occurring within hours of consuming food/drink containing lactose. Infants with lactose intolerance cannot be breastfed – they must have lactose-free formula instead (Harding, 2016). The symptoms are similar to other gastrointestinal disorders and may be confused with CMPA. However, it should be noted that lactose intolerance is *not* the same as a milk or dairy allergy.

Parasite/worm infection

The most common parasite infection is Giardia lamblia, which causes diarrhoea, weight loss and abdominal pain. Transmission is via faecal contamination in food/drink or hand-to-mouth contact. Excretion of Giardia is intermittent, so collection of three stool samples from different days is advised. Treatment is with antibiotics, usually metronidazole (antimicrobial) (Miall et al., 2012; Henderson, 2016).

Threadworms are common in children. The eggs are laid around the anus, causing itching and are then transferred to fingers when the child scratches. Transmission is via hand-to-mouth contact and because children are very social beings, transmission is particularly easy. Management is via improved hygiene and a single dose of mebendazole. The whole family should be treated at the same time to ensure eradiciation and avoid reinfection (Henderson, 2014).

Roundworm and tapeworms are uncommon in the UK but more serious, and may be seen following a visit overseas. Infection is by the ingestion of contaminated food/water, or from contaminated soil (roundworms) or raw/undercooked meat (tapeworms). Both require medical treatment.

Problems with accessory digestive organs – liver

Neonatal jaundice is very common and usually resolves as the liver enzymes mature during the first week of life. Congenital defects of the liver, such as biliary atresia and choledochal cysts are rare, but result in obstruction of bile flow. Symptoms include jaundice, dark urine, pale stools, abdominal mass, abdominal pain and faltering growth. Early detection of biliary atresia is vital, so infants who remain jaundiced a fortnight after birth should be further investigated, with referral to a specialist centre if biliary atresia is suspected. This is important and has particular implications for the healthcare professional who carries out baby checks during the first few weeks after birth (Children's Liver Disease Foundation, 2011). Surgical treatment to reconstruct or bypass the bile duct is not curative and liver transplantation is usually required by early adulthood.

NURSING MANAGEMENT OF GASTROINTESTINAL PROBLEMS

To a certain extent, the nursing requirement will be dependent on the gastrointestinal problem and whether management is following a medical or surgical route, or being delivered in hospital or at home. However, the type of nursing care you will be expected to deliver is likely to consist of some or all of the following:

SEE ALSO CHAPTERS 3, 15 & 28

- Pain assessment and management
- Assessment of the acutely ill child
- Vital signs observations – temperature, pulse, respiration, blood pressure, oxygen saturations and PEW score
- Management of fluid and electrolyte balance – oral, gastrostomy and intravenous fluid intake and urine and gastric output (faeces/vomit/stoma losses), assessment of and treatment for dehydration
- Infection control – management of diarrhoea and vomiting, wound/stoma care
- Nutritional assessment and support via oral, enteral and parenteral routes
- Stool assessment using the Bristol Stool Chart
- Pre- and postoperative care
- High dependency nursing care
- Medication administration
- Parent/child/young person education

SEE ALSO CHAPTERS 4, 17 & 31

As a nursing student, you will be involved in assisting healthcare professionals to carry out diagnostic tests and collecting specimens for examination by biomedical scientists in the pathology, biochemistry and haematology departments. See Table 29.1 for details.

Table 29.1 Common diagnostic tests

Diagnostic test	Purpose
Urinalysis	Rule out urinary tract infection as cause of abdominal pain. Assess dehydration status
Stool culture	Identify causative bacteria/micro-organisms in gastroenteritis/food poisoning
Full blood count (FBC)	Raised white blood cells in appendicitis and urinary tract infection. Anaemia may indicate blood loss, malabsorption, poor iron intake
Urea and electrolytes (U&E)	Assess for electrolyte imbalance and dehydration
C-reactive protein (CRP)	A raised CRP may be seen with infection/inflammatory bowel disease
Blood gas	Identify any acid-base imbalance in the acutely ill child
Abdominal X-ray	Look for dilated bowel loops (intestinal obstruction), abnormal gas pattern (intussusception) or faecal loading (constipation)

Diagnostic test	Purpose
Abdominal ultrasound scan	May diagnose appendicitis/intussception
Barium enema	Used to see the outline of the large intestine
pH study	Diagnosis and severity of GORD
Upper GI contrast study	May be used in GORD, or following bile-stained vomiting to rule out malrotation of gut
Coeliac antibodies	Test for coeliac disease
Biopsy	A small sample of tissue is taken for examination under a microscope
Endoscopy	Camera investigation of the gastrointestinal tract. Can be either upper GI via the mouth and oesophagus, or lower GI via the rectum

NUTRITION

As a nursing student, an understanding of nutrition and nutritional assessment is important because good nutrition in childhood is vital in maximising growth, development and wellbeing, whereas poor nutrition can cause or complicate childhood ill health. For more information on nutrition go the health promotion section at https://study.sagepub.com/essentialchildnursing

HEALTH
PROMOTION 29:
GASTROINTESTINAL
PROBLEMS

SAFEGUARDING STOP POINT

Malnutrition is defined as a lack of proper nutrition and can refer to either undernutrition, when a child does not get sufficient nutrients, leading to poor growth and development, or overnutrition, when a child receives more nutrients than are needed, leading to obesity.

There are multiple reasons why a child may be underweight for their age. However, as children's nurses, it's important to recognise that one cause could be the deliberate withholding of nutrition by the child's parent/carer.

- What signs might indicate that a child is being deliberately starved?
- When a teacher or a healthcare professional is concerned about a child, it is common for them to speak to the child's parent/carer, but who else should they speak to?
- If you think a child is at risk of harm, who should you report your concerns to?

Now read the Daniel Pelka serious case review *Lessons to Be Learned Briefing No. 16* available at https://study.sagepub.com/essentialchildnursing

WEBLINK: DANIEL
PELKA CASE
REVIEW

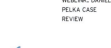

SAFEGUARDING
STOP POINT
ANSWER 29.1

Enteral and parenteral methods of feeding

Sometimes, the child may be unable to eat and drink normally – they may have had surgery, be unable to swallow properly, or it may be unsafe for them to feed orally. Some conditions dictate that the gastrointestinal tract cannot be used, as there may be mechanical dysfunction, the gut may require 'resting', or the stomach is required to be empty.

The nasogastric tube was fairly easy to manage but when it turned out he needed a naso-jejunal tube it all got a bit trickier. It's different, we can't insert it ourselves like the NG tube, neither can the CCNs. It goes into the jejunum and takes much longer to put in … it's very precious, and if it comes out that means a long wait in A&E and then X-rays to check it's where it should be.

You are always keeping a careful eye on it to make sure it doesn't accidentally dislodge, and then if it does his feeds are interrupted! We are waiting for a PEJ … but there's a long waiting list to put one of those in, and although you can't see that under his clothes, it's not straightforward either, you need to care for the site and keep an eye on his skin.

Alice, parent

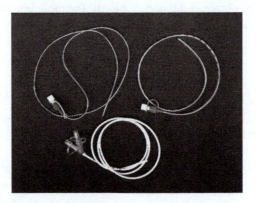

Figure 29.1 Nasogastric tubes

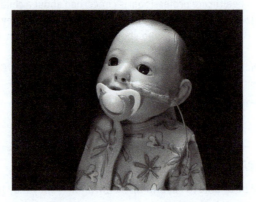

Figure 29.2 Nasogastric tube in position

The decision to move to enteral or parenteral feeding is not taken lightly as the quotation above illustrates. The route chosen will depend on the specific needs of each individual child. Knowledge, care and skill are required by the team around the child to ensure safe and effective nutritional support. Enteral feeds may be delivered by bolus or pump-controlled continuous feeding methods, dependent on the route used. For enteral-fed infants, breast milk is the feed of choice, but where breast milk is not available, an infant feeding formula can be used. Children require dietician input and specialist formula feeds to ensure their nutritional needs are fully met. Infants receiving enteral feeding may benefit from non-nutritive sucking of their thumb, fingers or a soother. This reduces length of hospital stay and the transition time from enteral to oral feeding (Foster et al., 2016).

Table 29.2 Types of enteral feeding

Enteral route	How it works
Nasogastric/orogastric tube	A tube inserted into either the nose or mouth, which is then passed into the oesophagus and stomach. Used to aspirate stomach contents or deliver feeds and medication. Tube position must be checked before every use
Nasojejunal tube	Method of feeding directly into the small bowel, the tube is passed into the nose and through the oesophagus and stomach into the jejunum. Useful in delayed gastric emptying, persistent vomiting or high aspiration risk. Tube position must be checked before every use. Compatibility of medication with the small intestine should be considered, to ensure proper absorption
Gastrostomy/jejunostomy Percutaneous endoscopic gastrostomy/jejunostomy (PEG/PEJ)	Tube inserted through the stomach wall directly into the stomach/jejunem via surgical procedure. Used when long-term feeding is required. Gastrostomy/jejunstomy feeding reduces distress for the child who may not tolerate regular nasogastric/nasojejunal tube insertions. They are also less visible, an important cosmetic and psychological consideration

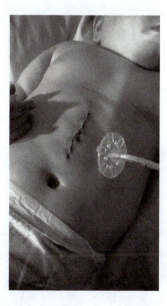

Figure 29.3 Position of gastrostomy

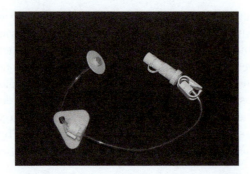

Figure 29.4   Percutaneous endoscopic gastrostomy with internal retention disk and external fixation plate

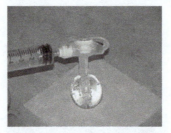

Figure 29.5   Low profile balloon gastrostomy (button) with extension set

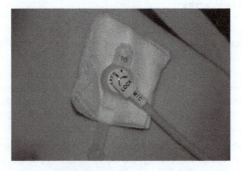

Figure 29.6   Low profile balloon gastrostomy (button) showing inflated balloon

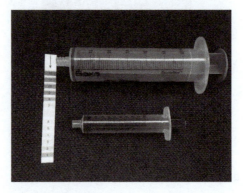

Figure 29.7   Enteral syringes and pH paper

SCENARIO 29.2: MATTHIS

You are looking after Matthis who is 3 weeks old and was born with gastroschisis. Matthis has a nasogastric tube in place and feeds are slowly being introduced. A feed is due now – when you test the tube for its correct position, you cannot draw back any aspirate.

- What should you do now?

Read the policy on nasogastric feeding for your placement area.

- What does the policy advise?
- How practical is this advice for children in the community who have nasogastric feeds?

Discuss and document your thoughts with your mentor.

SCENARIO
ANSWER 29.2

SEE ALSO
CHAPTER 39

Parenteral nutrition (PN) is the administration of specialised pre-prepared nutrients directly into the bloodstream in children with intestinal failure. It is invasive, requiring intravenous access usually through a central venous access device (CVAD) and carries high risks, so should only be used when there is no alternative method of feeding available. As a nursing student, you may care for children receiving PN, but its administration is regarded as an advanced nursing skill requiring registered nurse involvement and strict adherence to aseptic technique and biochemical monitoring.

Because the risk of sepsis is particularly high in invasive procedures like PN, it is important that you become aware of the early signs of sepsis and know how to act accordingly (NICE, 2016b). The UK Sepsis Trust (http://sepsistrust.org) has produced tools to aid early detection and management in various settings and across various age ranges.

WEBLINK:
SEPSIS
TRUST

STOMA (OSTOMY) MANAGEMENT

When a child is unable to use the normal route of faecal elimination, an ostomy or stoma (opening) may be surgically created through the abdominal wall (see Table 29.3). A stoma may be either temporary or permanent.

Table 29.3 Types of stoma

Type	Location
Colostomy – stoma made from portion of colon	Usually left iliac fossa
Ileostomy – stoma made from portion of ileum	Usually right iliac fossa

Where stoma formation is pre-planned, specific multidisciplinary care is required to ensure that the child and family are adequately prepared. Ideally, this involves physical and psychological preparation, familiarisation with the site, appearance, care of the stoma and equipment used such as stoma bags and securing methods. The stoma nurse specialist should be involved as early as possible and the psychological impact of having a stoma should not be ignored.

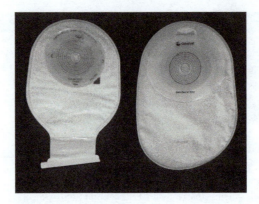

Figure 29.8 Stoma bags – drainable system and closed system

VIDEO LINK
29.4:
STOMA CARE

Stoma loss volume and consistency are dependent on the type and location of the stoma, but in general, the higher the intestinal location of the stoma, the greater the volume of losses. Children with a colostomy will have formed or semi-formed losses, whereas children with an ileostomy will have liquid losses and are at risk of sodium depletion due to the volume of losses they experience.

DISCHARGE PLANNING AND CONTINUING CARE IN THE COMMUNITY

Discharge planning should begin on admission to hospital and will be dependent on the reason for admission. The child and family are likely to require information about the condition itself and ongoing care in the community. Some children may have been hospitalised for a long period of time and if this is the first time the family have been able to take their child home, they also need to adjust to being a family, as well as coping with any additional needs their child may have. If the family have received care from a specialist tertiary centre far from home, they may feel anxious about taking their child to their local hospital for continuing care. Brief admission to their local hospital before full discharge home may help to alleviate this and enable the family to build a therapeutic relationship with staff that will continue their child's nursing care.

It is important to ensure parents/carers are trained and competent in all ongoing care needs their child may have. This is important in maintaining the health and safety of the child, both physically and psychologically. As a nursing student, you may be involved in the education and assessment of families, although overall accountability for this lies with the registered nurse. Care in the community for children with long- term conditions is likely to include:

- Wound care (surgical patients)
- Outpatients appointments
- Medication management and administration
- Nutrition management – healthy eating, enteral feeding, parenteral nutrition
- Specialist nursing input – for example, stoma nurse, children's community nurse, enteral feeding nurse
- Open access arrangements to the local children's ward
- Stoma care and prescriptions for stoma equipment
- Feeding tube care and prescriptions for feeds and equipment

- Bloods and other routine monitoring – particularly important for children on parenteral nutrition
- Listening to the concerns of parents and providing emotional as well as practical support

Go to https://study.sagepub.com/essentialchildnursing for tips on preparing for placements and health promotion when working with children with gastrointestinal problems.

PLACEMENT
ADVICE 29:
GASTROINTESTINAL
PROBLEMS

CHAPTER SUMMARY

The ability to understand the gastrointestinal tract and its altered anatomy and functions is an important aspect of children's nursing care. This chapter and the corresponding on resources will have provided you with information about:

HEALTH
PROMOTION 29:
GASTROINTESTINAL
PROBLEMS

- Nursing assessment and management of children with gastrointestinal conditions in hospital and community settings
- Nutritional awareness and the importance of promoting growth and development
- Ostomy/stoma management, education and support
- Proactive discharge planning and care in the community
- The art of listening to and meeting the needs of children and families with gastrointestinal conditions

BUILD YOUR BIBLIOGRAPHY

Books

- Dixon, M. and Crawford, D. (eds) (2012) *Paediatric Intensive Care Nursing*. Chichester: Wiley-Blackwell.

  Chapter 8 on gastrointestinal and endocrine function and Chapter 12 on nutrition and fluid management explore the care needs when gastrointestinal disturbance moves from 'standard' to higher dependency levels of care.

- Macqueen, S., Bruce, E.A. and Gibson, F. (eds) (2012) *The Great Ormond Street Hospital Manual of Children's Nursing Practices*. Chichester: Wiley-Blackwell.

  This skills-based textbook contains an excellent chapter on nutrition and feeding, including step-by-step guides to enteral and parenteral feeding, as well as a section on stoma care.

- Peate, I. and Gormley-Fleming, E. (2015) *Fundamentals of Children's Anatomy and Physiology: A Textbook for Nursing and Healthcare Students*. Chichester: Wiley-Blackwell.

  This A&P textbook contains a useful chapter on the digestive system and nutrition, along with clinical application sections and other activities.

Journal articles

Go to https://study.sagepub.com/essentialchildnursing for further free online journal articles related to this chapter.

- Ismail, N., Ratchford, I., Proudfoot, C. and Gibbs, J. (2011) 'Impact of a nurse-led clinic for chronic constipation in children'. *Journal of Child Health Care*, 15 (3): 221-9.

FURTHER
READING:
ONLINE
JOURNAL
ARTICLES

(Continued)

(Continued)

The article on UK-based research demonstrates how a nurse-led clinic was more successful at treating chronic constipation than a general paediatric clinic.

- Egnell, C., Eksborg, S. and Grahnquist, L. (2014) 'Jejunostomy enteral feeding in children: outcome and safety'. *Journal of Parenteral and Enteral Nutrition*, 38 (5): 631–6.

This Swedish-based retrospective study explores the safety and effectiveness of jejunal feeding via jejunostomy in children with neurological impairment.

- El-Matary, W. (2011) 'Percutaneous endoscopic gastrojejunostomy tube feeding in children'. *Nutrition in Clinical Practice*, 26 (1): 78–83.

This UK-based article explores the use of gastrosjejunostomy tube feeding in children for whom PEG feeding is not an option.

Weblinks

FURTHER READING: WEBLINKS

Go to https://study.sagepub.com/essentialchildnursing for further weblinks related to this chapter.

- NICE, *Constipation in Children and Young People: Diagnosis and Management*, Clinical guideline CG99

www.nice.org.uk/guidance/cg99
This guideline, published in 2010, outlines the diagnostic criteria and recommended management for constipation in children.

- NICE, *Gastro-oesophageal Reflux Disease in Children and Young People: Diagnosis and Management*, NICE guideline [NG1]

www.nice.org.uk/guidance/ng1
This guideline, published in 2015, outlines the diagnostic criteria and management of children with gastro-oesophageal reflux disease (GORD).

- NICE, Inflammatory Bowel Disease, Quality standard [QS81]

www.nice.org.uk/guidance/qs81
This quality standard describes the high-priority areas for quality improvement in IBD, detailing diagnosis and management of the condition in adults, children and young people.

ACE YOUR ASSESSMENT

Revise what you have learned by visiting https://study.sagepub.com/essentialchildnursing

ONLINE QUIZZES & ACTIVITY ANSWERS

- Test yourself with multiple-choice and short-answer questions
- Do the chapter activities in the book and check your answers online

REFERENCES

Children's Liver Disease Foundation (2011) *Yellow Alert*. Available at: www.yellowalert.org (last accessed 25 June 2017).

Coeliac UK (2016) *Coeliac Disease*. Available at: www.coeliac.org.uk/coeliac-disease (last accessed 26 May 2017).

Crohn's and Colitis UK (2013) *About Inflammatory Bowel Disease*. Available at: www.crohnsandcolitis. org.uk/about-inflammatory-bowel-disease (last accessed 26 May 2017).

Foster, J.P., Psaila, K. and Patterson, T. (2016) 'Non-nutritive sucking for increasing physiologic stability and nutrition in preterm infants'. *Cochrane Database of Systematic Reviews*, 10. DOI: 10.1002/14651858.CD001071.pub3.

Gandhi, A. (2014) *Congenital Gastrointestinal Malformations*. Available at: http://patient.info/doctor/ congenital-gastrointestinal-malformations (last accessed 26 May 2017).

GI Kids (2013) *Cow's Milk Protein Intolerance*. Available at: www.gikids.org/content/103/en/cows-milk-protein-intolerance (last accessed 26 May 2017).

Glasper, A., Coad, J. and Richardson, J. (2015) *Children and Young People's Nursing at a Glance*. Chichester: Wiley Blackwell.

Glasper, E.A., McEwing, G. and Richardson, J. (2016) *Oxford Handbook of Children's and Young People's Nursing*, 2nd edn. Oxford: Oxford University Press.

Harding, M. (2016) *Lactose Intolerance*. Available at: http://patient.info/doctor/lactose-intolerance-pro (last accessed 26 May 2017).

Henderson, R. (2014) *Threadworms*. Available at: http://patient.info/health/threadworms-leaflet (last accessed 26 May 2017).

Henderson, R. (2016) *Giardia*. Available at: http://patient.info/health/giardia (last accessed 26 May 2017).

Miall, L., Rudolf, M. and Smith, D. (2012) *Paediatrics at a Glance*, 3rd edn. Chichester: Wiley Blackwell.

NICE (2014) *Management of Vomiting in Children and Young People with Gastroenteritis: Ondansetron*, Evidence summary [ESUOM34]. Available at: www.nice.org.uk/advice/esuom34/chapter/ Key-points-from-the-evidence (last accessed 26 May 2017).

NICE (2015a) *Guideline on Gastro-oesophageal Reflux Disease in Children and Young People: Diagnosis and Management*, NICE guideline [NG1]. Available at: www.nice.org.uk/guidance/ng1 (last accessed 26 May 2017).

NICE (2015b) *Coeliac Disease: Recognition, Assessment and Management*, NICE guideline [NG20]. Available at: www.nice.org.uk/guidance/ng20 (last accessed 26 May 2017).

NICE (2016a) *Routine Preoperative Tests for Elective Surgery*, NICE guideline [NG45]. Available at: www. nice.org.uk/guidance/ng45 (last accessed 26 May 2017).

NICE (2016b) *Sepsis: Recognition, Diagnosis and Early Management*, NICE guideline [NG51]. Available at: www.nice.org.uk/guidance/ng51 (last accessed 26 May 2017).

Royal College of Paediatrics and Child Health (RCPCH) (2012) *Pre-procedure Pregnancy Checking in Under 16s: Guidance for Clinicians*. London: RCPCH.

Rull, G. (2016) *Intussusception in Children*. Available at: http://patient.info/doctor/intussusception-in-children (last accessed 26 May 2017).

Sambrook, J. (2017) *Cow's Milk Protein Allergy*. Available at: http://patient.info/doctor/cows-milk-protein-allergy-pro (last accessed 26 May 2017).

Tidy, C. (2015a) *Gastritis*. Available at: http://patient.info/health/gastritis (last accessed 26 May 2017).

Tidy, C. (2015b) *Oesophageal Atresia*. Available at: http://patient.info/doctor/oesophageal-atresia (last accessed 26 May 2017).

Tidy, C. (2015c) *Volvulus and Midgut Malrotations*. Available at: http://patient.info/doctor/volvulus-and-midgut-malrotations (last accessed 26 May 2017).

DISCHARGE PLANNING AND TRANSFER FOR CHILDREN AND YOUNG PEOPLE

30

ELIZABETH GILLESPIE AND SUE DUNLOP

THIS CHAPTER COVERS

- Fundamental principles of discharge planning for children
- Simple discharge
- Complex discharge
- Transfers
- Processes and systems

> "
>
> Then I get the news I'm waiting for: if she does well tonight we get home tomorrow. She does well. In the morning we wait, and wait, for rounds. After lunch, we get to speak to a doctor. It now transpires that we can't go home because she's still on oxygen. If the healthcare team had spoken to me about how we manage our daughter at home, they would have known that she is on oxygen at night at home.
>
> **Nandini, parent**
>
> "

Visit https://study.sagepub.com/essentialchildnursing to access a wealth of online resources for this chapter – watch out for the margin icons throughout the chapter.

INTRODUCTION

Since the Platt Report (Ministry of Health, 1959), it has been accepted that children should only be hospitalised when absolutely necessary, and for the briefest time possible to minimise family disruption and decrease stress for all concerned (Lewis and Noyes, 2007). If children are admitted to hospital, they will require discharge home or transfer to another inpatient setting. Although both discharge and transfer are an everyday occurrence, and can appear routine to staff, these processes can be complex and challenging, causing many opportunities for care to become fragmented and for children to 'fall between the gaps' in the various care environments, as will become evident throughout this chapter.

The opening quote is a classic example of miscommunication, which led to a prolonged stay, sub-optimal patient flow ('blocking the bed'), and increased parental anxiety (Häggström and Bäckström, 2014). Throughout this chapter we will explore principles to 'get it right' when you are discharging and transferring children. Discharge planning will be discussed first, followed by transfers, safeguarding practices, health promotion, and a brief consideration of processes and systems.

FUNDAMENTAL PRINCIPLES OF DISCHARGE PLANNING FOR CHILDREN

Discharge planning aims to improve the coordination of service and care when the child and family are discharged from hospital to home (Peters et al., 2011) or elsewhere. As illustrated in the quotation above, the nurses and doctors had not coordinated the child's care needs, so the discharge was delayed. Discharge planning also includes the process of identifying the needs of the child and family to ensure seamless care between hospital and home as well as between primary and secondary care (Domanski et al., 2003). In order to coordinate and identify needs, basic principles need to be adhered to.

Assessment

Effective discharge planning begins with a holistic, thorough and accurate assessment of the child and family's needs to identify any support they may require at home (Hewitt-Taylor, 2012). This will include the family's wishes and consideration of their strengths and resources; the capability of parents/carers to undertake the care of the child (Noyes et al., 2013), any equipment and ongoing supplies required, and potential modifications of the family home (Edwards, 2004). This assessment will identify the potential need for ongoing support from community children's nurses (CCNs), general practitioners (GPs), therapists, and respite services, or increasingly, bespoke package of care (Welsh Government, 2012). Once a robust assessment has been carried out a discharge plan can be formulated, making sure to keep the child and family at the centre of planning.

Communication and knowledge sharing

Communication and knowledge sharing is essential between the child, family and multidisciplinary team to ensure a safe and effective discharge (Limbrick, 2003). Good communication involves speaking a common language, and understanding everyone's roles and responsibilities to avoid misunderstandings (Smith and Coleman, 2009).

Noyes et al. (2013) introduce an aspect of communication which is overlooked in the discharge process: the interface between hospital and community. They suggest using closed-loop communication to

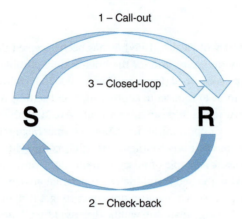

Figure 30.1   Description of closed-loop communication (CLC)

Reproduced from *Emergency Medicine*, Härgestam, M. et al. Volume 3, Issue 10, page 2, 2013 with permission from BMJ Publishing Group Ltd.

ensure sharing of timely information between all concerned. Closed-loop communication is depicted in Figure 30.1 and described by Härgestam et al. (2013) as:

1. The sender (S) transmits the message or call-out (CO)
2. The receiver (R) acknowledges the message by check-back
3. The sender verifies that the message is interpreted correctly: CLC is obtained

In addition, knowledge sharing is a crucial component of the discharge process as parents play a major role in caring for their child at home. Ingram et al. (2016) reported that a child and family-centred approach to education for discharge was most advantageous for parents of premature babies. Previously, Weiss et al. (2008) reported that planned, effective teaching and education plans are integral to ensure parents and carers are confident to carry out care. Bernstein et al. (2007) remind us that education and training should be tailored to each family's abilities and willingness to undertake the prescribed care. We as children's nurses must ensure the family understand the child's condition and disease trajectory, have time to practise any clinical procedures until they are confident and competent (Lerrett, 2009), and know how to recognise any potential changes to the child's health status which may require nursing or medical reassessment (Stephens, 2005). Professionals need to share knowledge through a variety of media and formats that are appropriate to the child development level, family literacy level and chosen language (Department of Health, 2004).

SEE ALSO
CHAPTERS 5
AND 6

ACTIVITY 30.1: REFLECTIVE PRACTICE

Critically reflect on one nurse's experiences of patient education for discharge.

> I explained to the father of a 5-year-old girl with epilepsy the dosage changes of the medication. I also gave him written instructions. After a week, they came back, and it was evident that he had not understood the dosage correctly. (Children's nurse, in Kelo et al., 2015)

- Consider how we can improve knowledge sharing. Discuss the story above with your mentor or peers and ask, 'If this was me what would I have done differently?'

Processes to aid communication and knowledge sharing

The use of discharge policies, procedures and pathways can help with communication and knowledge sharing (Waring et al., 2014). Integral to this is excellence in record-keeping and documentation. Wong et al. (2011) suggest that a single case record shared by all professionals can facilitate safe effective discharge. SIGN (2012) devised such a document for patients discharged back to the care of a GP. However, because of variations in policies and procedures across the UK, local knowledge of documentation and processes is also essential. Remember that when we structure discharge planning, we can reduce readmission and improve family satisfaction (Hesselink et al., 2013). This is an important quality outcome for children and familes.

ACTIVITY 30.2: CRITICAL THINKING

Refer to *The Code: Professional Standards and Behaviour for Nurses and Midwives* for guidance on documentation and record keeping (NMC, 2015). A link is available at https://study.sagepub.com/essentialchildnursing

Consider how keeping clear and accurate records is crucial to good discharge planning. Review the paperwork you have seen within clinical practice and evaluate the extent to which the paperwork meets NMC requirements for documentation and record-keeping.

Consider the principles of good communication as they apply to nursing care and discharge planning for children.

WEBLINK:
NMC CODE

SEE ALSO
CHAPTER 2

Family-centred care and partnership working

Family-centred care and partnership working are essential in the provision of high-quality care and a crucial element of good discharge planning (Coyne et al., 2011). To enable families to care safely and consistently at home, staff must work with families as partners, sharing accessible, current information to aid informed decision-making (Samwell, 2012). Ask yourself, 'Do we really always listen to the child's wishes?'

As you can see in the list below, for some families a multitude of professionals and agencies may need to be involved to ensure consistent care at home.

- Child and family at the centre of the process
- Consultant paediatrician
- Dietician
- Discharge nurse
- CCN
- Health visitor
- Specialist nurse
- School nurse
- Physiotherapists
- Speech and language therapists
- Occupational therapists
- Pharmacy hospital/community
- Social worker
- Education staff
- Voluntary services

PREPARE FOR
PRACTICE 30.1:
PAEDIATRIC
COMMUNITY
PHYSIOTHERAPIST

SEE ALSO
CHAPTERS
8, 9 AND 11

In these cases, effective partnership working and collaboration between all concerned is paramount. The use of shared protocols and documentation can facilitate consistency and continuity in these situations (Penthybridge, 2004), although such 'shared documentation' may not always be apparent within your clinical area.

Go to https://study.sagepub.com/essentialchildnursing to find out more about the role of the paediatric community physiotherapist.

Discharge planning needs to be viewed as a process, and not as a single clinical event when the child and family leave hospital. Planning therefore begins on admission, or in elective cases, before admission and continues as a set of care processes throughout the inpatient period (Lees, 2012).

Effective and timely discharge is crucial for best quality care and continuity. In contrast, poorly planned discharge is a risk to children's safety, inhibits recovery, increases unplanned readmission and increases costs (Waring et al., 2014). This makes for care which is unethical, and does not respect the duty of care and candour owed by professionals to the children concerned.

SIMPLE DISCHARGE

Simple discharges account for approximately 80 per cent of all hospital discharges (NHS London Health Programmes, 2013). A simple discharge is where a child is discharged home with simple ongoing care needs, which do not need complex planning and delivery (Lees, 2012). Children are discharged back to primary care, and are only referred to children's community nursing services for time-limited interventions (RCN, 2014). However, in a study with district nurses they reported the varying ways they are informed of patient discharges (sometimes by the family rather than the ward staff), and that secondary care staff do not understand the roles and demands of community nurses (Pellett, 2016). These findings could apply equally to referral to children's community services.

Read the following experiences of a mother and her child being discharged following a day surgery procedure.

My child was admitted for day surgery for a minor procedure. On admission he was very nervous. I felt helpless while he was in surgery and was not expecting him to be as sore when he woke up. After some stronger pain relief and a bit more observation time, we were ready to go home. Although you feel desperate to get your child home, there is an element of anxiety about being able to cope at home alone after a surgical procedure. At discharge, we were taken into a room by one of the nursing staff. This was really good as it gave privacy to discuss what to expect but it was a nurse that we had not met before. I think it would have been nicer if we had a named nurse who already knew my child. This would have offered him more continuity of his care. The nurse discussed pain management with me and reassured my child that his pain would be well catered for and that he must let me know when he was sore. Some brief details of topical pain relief were given; thankfully I had used this before as the information may not have been specific enough otherwise. My child became upset with the conversation around pain and the discharge nurse was very sensitive towards him and provided a lot of reassurance. Most of the information given to us at discharge was verbal. However, I was concentrating so much on my son, who was upset, I could have forgotten important advice that was given to us. Lastly, we were given written contact details for support should we have any problems at home and advised to return through Accident and Emergency if we had serious concerns. It wasn't until we got home that I realised just how sore he would be once the local anaesthetic had worn off. I felt that I had not been fully prepared for this. I feel that some honest conversation prior to discharge without my son being present could have helped prepare me for what he would experience and, in turn, support him better.

Pamela, parent

My operation had finished and it was time to go home. My mum and I went into a room with one of the nurses. The nurse was smiling at me and was telling us about different medicines that can help ease the pain and what times to take them at. She was kind and made sure everything was OK. Talking about it definitely made me feel a lot better. She also told me to take baths regularly. She said that they might hurt at first, but then I would get used to it. There was a lot to remember because we didn't write any instructions down and we never got a handout. I was given my medicine and it was time to go home. I was happy to be going back home because I knew that I had everything that I needed to help me and also my mum to look after me. I was a wee bit worried because it was sore to move around and go different places. Before leaving, we were told if I got very sore or any had difficulties, I should come back to the A&E department. I was a bit upset and worried about it when I was told that, but my mum gave me a hug and said that everything would be OK. The nurse said she was sad to see me upset but told me that my mum would take very good care of me.

Ross, child

As we can see after reading these family stories, central to effective discharge is the provision of timely and accurate written and verbal communication and/or instructions. The mother pointed out that even though she had been through the process before and knew what to expect it would have been useful to have had written information.

The child commented that as there was a lot to remember a handout would have been useful.

The provision of both written and verbal discharge information for parents is more effective in improving knowledge and satisfaction than providing verbal information alone. The benefits of providing written discharge information include improving confidence, decreasing recovery time, improving satisfaction, reducing readmissions and improving adherence to recommended care.

WHAT'S THE EVIDENCE?

Consider how the communication needs of the child and mother in the scenario could have been met more effectively.

- List three things that mum and child found positive about the discharge
- Could anything have been done differently to ensure the discharge was more effective?

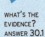

WHAT'S THE
EVIDENCE?
ANSWER 30.1

COMPLEX DISCHARGE

Increasing numbers of children are discharged home with chronic illness, complex or exceptional care needs, or technology dependence, to parents/carers who are providing 24-hour care (Noyes et al., 2013; Carter et al., 2016). Both the child's needs and the process are complex. Complexity can arise from the need to provide individually tailored family support, effective multiagency agreements, robust clinical governance, accessible accommodation and well-functioning acute/community relationships, as well as meeting the needs of the child as an individual at the centre of care (Brenner et al., 2015).

Pivotal to complex discharge is the role of the discharge liaison nurse, key worker or specialist nurse who provides the crucial link between the child, family and other services (Peters et al., 2011).

ACTIVITY 30.3: CRITICAL THINKING

Brenner et al. (2015) interviewed parents who had to become the primary care giver when their child was discharged home. They expressed frustration at the time it took to get everything ready for discharge, they were fearful of the levels of competence in community services and worried about how they were going to cope in the future. While all of the parents interviewed spoke of the value of the staged process to going home, they collectively identified themselves as overwhelmed when they were eventually discharged from hospital. Parents stated that they were often 'petrified' or 'terrified' in their initial days at home despite their perceived clinical readiness and sense of empowerment while in the hospital.

Parents also spoke about 'stepping stones', whereby they had a phased discharge home, with the parent taking increased responsibility of care as the process rolled out.

- Why might the parents have valued a stepping stones approach?

ACTIVITY
ANSWER 30.3

Read the following scenario about a mother who wants to go home.

SCENARIO 30.1: CAROLINE

I can't wait to get home. This is a recurrent theme in my head from the moment we are en route to hospital, never mind the weeks that my daughter is an inpatient.

She's doing great so we are stepping down from PICU [the paediatric intensive care unit] to a ward. She's doing great, but we can't get a transfer back to our local hospital because she is still on oxygen. She will require a drizzle of oxygen for about a month after this infection. It's how she rolls. The healthcare staff would have known that if they had spoken to me. We have oxygen at home and portable oxygen for car journeys. There appears to be a disconnect between the opinions of the staff on the ward and the consultant, whom I have never met.

Then I get the news I'm waiting for: if she does well tonight we get home tomorrow. She does well. In the morning we wait, and wait, for rounds. After lunch, we get to speak to a doctor. It now transpires that we can't go home because she's still on oxygen. After a long discussion we get to go back to our local district general hospital. We stay overnight and they have a much smoother final discharge for us. Yes, we are going home on a drizzle of oxygen. Yes, we have supplies of medicines which we require for home. Yes, I'm confident that we are making the correct and safe choice for my daughter.

How could discharge have been smoother? Mum's view:

- *Anticipate discharge*: you know that you will need supplies of regular medication for discharge so order them up at least 24 hours in advance so that they are ready for discharge
- *Manage my expectations*: give me a clear and concise plan of what is going to happen and when
- *Ask me questions*: if you had spoken to me at all about how we manage my daughter at home you would have known that she is on oxygen at night, but that she habitually requires a 'drizzle' of oxygen (low-flow oxygen) in the daytime for weeks after a bad respiratory virus
- *I know my daughter*: please listen to what I have to say about her day-to-day care
- *Continuity is important*: make sure each health professional has the same opinion before speaking with parents/child
- *A multidisciplinary (MDT) meeting is important*: it would have been easier to assess my daughter's health progress if she wasn't admitted as an unknown entity; don't discharge her like one either
- *It is important to be honest and open with parent/child*: after a long period of having my daughter as an inpatient I am getting less sleep, feeling more exhausted, more worried and less tolerant. Do me the courtesy of paying attention to the little things
- *Update relevant professionals of changes to care needs*: one recurrent problem that we have is that my daughter's medicines change by weight or by condition. If you are discharging a patient with complex care needs it would help to give the patient/parent an updated medicine/dosage list detailing changes to hand in to their GP on discharge. Often when we order new supplies from our GP the latest dosage has not been communicated. I can medicate as per the updated dosage at home. I know it is not 1.8ml but 2ml, as instructed by the doctor during the admission. The problem comes when we have home nursing, or when we have a hospice stay or are admitted again

- After reading this mother's account, what should/could the staff have done to better facilitate her daughter's discharge?
- How can we ensure that the multidisciplinary teams work in partnership with the mother on the detail of the discharge plan?
- What aspects of the discharge process could have been anticipated and arranged prior to the day of discharge?

SCENARIO
ANSWER 30.1

VIDEO LINK
30.1: GOING
HOME

You can watch a video from Great Ormond Hospital on going home and on appendectomy surgery discharge at https://study.sagepub.com/essentialchildnursing

TRANSFERS

The transfer described in Caroline's scenario is known as an inter-hospital transfer (IHT), which may be required when the child requires diagnostic or therapeutic facilities that are not available at a given ward, unit or hospital. IHT may take place from an emergency department, ward or paediatric intensive care unit (PICU) of one hospital to that of another. Due to the need to provide tertiary services regionally – such as for trauma, burns, cardiac or neurology – there is an increase in IHT (Wagner et al., 2013). Occasionally, a child may require an IHT if a bed is not available locally. IHT of children is an integral process and essential component of healthcare systems (Sethi and Subramanian, 2014).

VIDEO LINK
30.2:
DISCHARGE
INSTRUCTIONS

Children frequently require transferring to and from theatres. Utilising evidence-based risk assessment tools, such as the one detailed in *Transferring Children to and from Theatre* guidance (RCN, 2011), will enable you to work safely and competently when you accompany children to and from theatres.

Read this case study about an intra-hospital transfer.

WATCH A
VIDEO ONLINE!

PRACTICE
SCENARIO:
JOHN

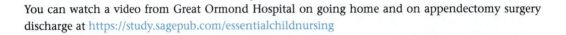

CASE STUDY 30.1: SARAH

Sarah was antenatally diagnosed with a complex heart condition: tetralogy of Fallot. Following delivery, she was admitted to the neonatal unit for observation. She was clinically well and, following a review by the cardiology team, it was decided that she could be cared for on the transitional care unit. This unit provides care for neonates who are essentially well but have additional care needs met by a team of nursery nurses and require ongoing monitoring by neonatal medical staff. Sarah required daily blood pressures and intermittent oxygen saturation monitoring due to her heart condition. She also needed to establish breast feeding. She was transferred to the unit by a neonatal nurse who gave a verbal handover. Written discharge letters were also given to these members of staff. The medical discharge letter did not contain a clear plan for the baby as it was assumed that the following day a member of the medical team would review Sarah. During the following shift, the nursery nurses caring for Sarah expressed concern about the appropriateness of her transfer. They were anxious about her heart condition and doubted their ability to manage her care in a safe manner. Sarah was readmitted to the neonatal unit for ongoing care.

- What assumptions were made about the transfer and how did they contribute to the nursery nurses' anxiety?
- How could this have been avoided?
- What impact do you think readmission to the neonatal unit had on the family?

CASE STUDY
ANSWER 30.1

Transfer from children's services to adult services

Another area of transfer can occur when a child needs to be transferred to adult healthcare. This is usually referred to as transition. Please consider the statement below.

> As a clinical nurse specialist in paediatric diabetes, it is clear to me that the movement of care from children's to adult services is a challenging time for the young person and their family. During the teenage years, many young people experience a worsening of their diabetes control and they represent a particularly vulnerable group, whose care can get lost in the process of transferring between children's and adult services (Allen and Gregory, 2009). In an unpublished audit undertaken in 2002 at the unit where I work, patients' experience of their transition process was investigated. Teenagers reported feeling unprepared, scared and unhappy that their new team didn't know them. They stated that there was no choice to be had regarding the decision to move to a new team. Furthermore, following transition, many felt that the provision of support was reduced, particularly as an out-of-hours emergency contact number is not offered by the adult service. Despite these negative comments, many teenagers described feeling fed up with the environment of the paediatric clinic and wanted to 'move on' and be more independent. This move towards independence was in line with other aspects of their emerging adult status. The same audit sought parents' views of their experiences. Many indicated that there was little preparation for transition and that they felt 'kicked out' of the paediatric service. Moving up to adult care is considered a milestone on the diabetes journey and parents, like the teenagers, typically conveyed the feeling that there was no choice over transition.
>
> **Corinna, children's nurse**

ACTIVITY 30.4: CRITICAL THINKING

- Consider why children need to transition from children's to adult services
- Reflect on the positive aspects of transfer to adult services, and the challenges which transition may present both to the child and family and the practitioners involved in the transition process
- Reflect on the reported experiences of teenagers moving into adult-focused services
- Think about what children's services do to improve transfer and subsequent experiences for teenagers

Transfer to another hospital (in another country)

The narrative below articulates the views of a young person who needed to be transferred to another country to receive specialist proton therapy:

> I personally found the change from healthcare in England to healthcare in America was very easy. All of the nurses in the UK prepared me for the differences in America, such as how the drugs I needed might have different names, so I wasn't worried when I was suddenly prescribed something that sounded completely different! When I was actually in hospital, the

(Continued)

nurses were very understanding and were happy to answer any questions I had. The atmosphere was very relaxed, which helped my family and me to feel more comfortable with the whole situation, and I never felt unsure or scared. The communication between the UK and America was outstanding, meaning I always had everything I needed. I was understandably stressed about my feeding tube, which was put in place in the UK, but when I was in America they managed to sort everything so that my worries were quickly worked through. Despite the UK using different endings on the tube, the Americans dealt with the issue well and I was soon sorted out. As our accommodation and transport were arranged before our arrival, I was always on time to appointments, meaning the stress usually associated with hospital was eradicated. Overall, the whole experience was a whole lot easier than I thought it would be which meant my stress as a patient was minimal.

Eve, child

Consider how good preparation of the young person for the transfer by the nursing staff, excellent communication between healthcare providers, and prior planning and preparation reduced anxiety and stress in this instance.

The key to successful transfers is excellent communication and planning. The aim is to provide a safe experience where there is accuracy and continuity when information is exchanged about the child. The key aspects are those of transfer of responsibility and accountability (CMPA, 2016).

SAFEGUARDING STOP POINT

All organisations involved in caring for children have safeguarding policies to ensure children are protected from harm (NSPCC, 2016). Where there are concerns about possible child protection issues, there must be a multiagency action plan agreed and recorded before the child is transferred or discharged, and the safety of the transfer or discharge must be agreed between children's social care and the child's consultant. All professionals involved with the child need to consider what future support may be required and who else needs to be informed of the situation. Consideration always needs to be given to the sharing of information and confidentiality (Parkin, 2016).

SEE ALSO
CHAPTER 9

PROCESSES AND SYSTEMS

Health services are large complex systems, and within these systems children and families depend on care to be organised to meet their many needs (WHO, 2012). When discussing the discharge of older people, a health ombudsman (Mellor, 2016) recognised that there are structural and systematic barriers to effective discharge planning, which have massive human costs. We as children's nurses need to ensure that we work within existing polices and processes, but also that we look at different ways of working. These may include: 'criteria-led discharge' (Lees, 2012, p.5), which can be used for diseases or conditions where the parameters for discharge are similar (such as acute asthma); care-pathway-led discharge (such as in oncology); and nurse-led discharge. At all times the voice of the child and family should be central to care.

Go to https://study.sagepub.com/essentialchildnursing for tips on preparing for placements and health promotion in discharge planning and transfer.

PLACEMENT
ADVICE 30:
DISCHARGE
PLANNING

HEALTH
PROMOTION
30: DISCHARGE
PLANNING

CHAPTER SUMMARY

- Effective discharge planning improves quality of care for the child, enables continuity of care, improved compliance and ensures good patient outcomes, often preventing readmission
- Discharge planning is is a dynamic ongoing process which should begin as early as possible before or during admission to hospital
- Planning, preparation and communication are vital when transferring and discharging children Effective team working and communication are vital to the success of discharge planning and transfer
- The child and family must be actively engaged and welcomed as partners in the discharge process, goal planning and decision-making

BUILD YOUR BIBLIOGRAPHY

Books

- Lees, L. (2012) *Timely Discharge from Hospital.* Keswick: M&K Publishing.

  A book designed to explore multidisciplinary and multiagency perspectives of discharge planning.

- National Leadership and Innovation Agency for Healthcare (2008) *Passing the Baton: A Practical Guide to Effective Discharge Planning.* Cardiff: NLIAH.

  This book is aimed at practitioners working in acute, community, intermediate and ambulatory care settings; all areas of practice are featured. Each section is arranged in themes but written to stand alone, allowing the reader to dip in and out. The book is further enhanced by a comprehensive selection of case studies.

- Thurston, C. (2013) 'Transferring to adult services for young people with long-term conditions', in C. Thurston (ed.) *Essential Care for Children and Young People: Theory, Policy and Practice.* New York: Routledge.

  This chapter explores the transition from young person to adult and examines the development approach to encouraging independence. It highlights relevant theories and examines the implication for policy and practice. The chapter discusses the changing context of young people's lives and the services they may require, advising that this means that health professionals should develop their capacity to undertake assessments and interpretation in a wide variety of settings. The chapter will also assist practitioners in understanding their role in the context of their statutory duties, agency requirements and the needs and wishes of the young person.

(Continued)

(Continued)

Journal articles

FURTHER READING: ONLINE JOURNAL ARTICLES

Go to https://study.sagepub.com/essentialchildnursing for further free online journal articles related to this chapter.

- Hawthorn, J. and Killen, M. (2006) 'Transferring babies between units: issues for parents'. *Infant*, 2 (2): 44-6.

  This article is based on material from a research study 'Foretelling futures: Dilemmas in neonatal neurology'. It is a social science research project in four neonatal intensive care units (NICUs) exploring how practitioners and parents share information and care of the babies. The researchers found that one of the issues arising from the study concerned parents' emotional experiences when their baby was transferred to another NICU or special care unit, which was the case for 31 per cent of babies in the sample. They found that parents in neonatal units are distressed when their baby is transferred to another hospital or when their baby is moved within the unit or the hospital.

- Ingram, J.C., Powell, J.E., Blair, P.S., Pontin, D., Redshaw, M., Manns, S., Beasant, L., Burden, H., Johnson, D., Rose, C. and Fleming, P.J. (2016) 'Does family-centred neonatal discharge planning reduce healthcare usage? A before and after study in South West England'. *BMJ Open*. 6: e010752.

  This study measures the impact of a neonatal family-centred care intervention on parental self-efficacy on use of emergency department (ED) post-discharge for moderately preterm infants. Using health economic data collection the study found that lack of time for implementing the Train-to-Home intervention meant that some staff were not confident in using the family-centred approach to discharge planning.

- Lees, L. (2013) 'The key principles of effective discharge planning'. *Nursing Times*, 109 (3). Available at www.nursingtimes.net/Journals/2013/01/17/x/l/m/130122-Effective-discharge-planning.pdf (last accessed 26 May 2017).

  This article highlights the complexity of discharge planning and suggests that effective discharge planning is crucial to ensure timely discharge and continuity of care. It discusses in detail ten steps of discharge planning, highlighting the need to plan before or on admission. There is a clear message about the importance of identifying whether the patient has simple or complex needs, and the need for a discharge management plan.

Websites

FURTHER READING: WEBLINKS

Go to https://study.sagepub.com/essentialchildnursing for further weblinks related to this chapter.

- What? Why? Children in Hospital, *Preparing for Hospital*

  www.whatwhychildreninhospital.org.uk
  What? Why? Children in Hospital prepares children, parents and carers for a positive hospital experience by sharing age-appropriate videos and information.

- Children with Exceptional Healthcare Needs Network

  www.cen.scot.nhs.uk
  The National Managed Clinical Network for Children with Exceptional Healthcare Needs (CEN) started in March 2009, with the aim of strengthening specialist services for children with complex and exceptional healthcare needs in Scotland. Parents/carers, voluntary sector organisations and professionals are invited to join the network and attend working group meetings and events. The website provides a good source of information for professionals and carers.

- Great Ormond Street Hospital for Children

  www.gosh.nhs.uk

  Great Ormond Street Hospital is the UK's largest children's hospital. This website has a number of good discharge planning information leaflets for parents and carers.

ACE YOUR ASSESSMENT

Revise what you have learned by visiting https://study.sagepub.com/essentialchildnursing

- Test yourself with multiple-choice and short-answer questions
- Do the chapter activities in the book and check your answers online

ONLINE QUIZZES & ACTIVITY ANSWERS

REFERENCES

Allen, D. and Gregory, J. (2009) 'The transition from children's to adult diabetes services: understanding the "problem"'. *Diabetic Medicine*, 26: 162–6.

Bernstein, H.H., Spino, C., Finch, S., Wasserman, R., Slora, E. and Lalama, C., Touloukian, C.L., Lilienfeld, H. and McCormick, M.C. (2007) 'Decision-making for postpartum discharges of 4300 mothers and their healthy infants: the life around newborn discharge study'. *Pediatrics*, 120 (2): 391–400.

Brenner, M., Larkin, P.J., Hilliard, C., Cawley, D., Howlin, F. and Connolly, M. (2015) 'Parents' perspectives of the transition to home when a child has complex technological health care needs'. *International Journal of Integrated Care*, 15, e035.

Canadian Medical Protective Association (CMPA) (2016) *Improving Patient Handovers*. Available at: www.cmpa-acpm.ca/en/advice-publications/browse-articles/2016/improving-patient-handovers (last accessed 26 May 2017).

Carter, B., Bray, L., Sanders, C., van Miert, C., Hunt, A. and Moore, A. (2016) 'Knowing the places of care: how nurses facilitate transition of children with complex health care needs from hospital to home'. *Comprehensive Child and Adolescent Nursing*, 39 (2).

Coyne, L., O'Neil, C., Murphy, M., Costello, T. and O'Shea, R. (2011) 'What does family-centred care mean to nurses and how do they think it could be enhanced in practice'. *Journal of Advanced Nursing*, 67 (12): 2561–73.

Department of Health (DH) (2004) *Achieving Timely and Simple Discharge from Hospital: A Toolkit for the Multidisciplinary Team*. London: DH.

Domanski, M.D., Jackson, A.C., Miller, J. and Jeffery, C. (2003) 'Towards the development of a paediatric discharge screening tool'. *Journal of Child Health*, 7 (3): 163–83.

Edwards, E.A. (2004) 'Sending children home on tracheostomy dependent ventilation: pitfalls and outcomes'. *Archives of Disease in Childhood*, 89 (3): 251–5.

Häggström, M. and Bäckström, B. (2014) 'Organizing safe transitions from intensive care'. *Nursing Research and Practice*. DOI: 10.1155/2014/175314

Härgestam, M., Lindvist, M., Brulin, C., Jacobsson, M. and Hultin, M. (2013) 'Communication in interdisciplinary teams: exploring closed-loop communication during in situ trauma team training'. *Emergency Medicine BMJ Open*, 3, 10.

Hesselink, G., Schoonhoven, L., Plas, M., Wollersheim, H. and Veernooij-Dassen, M. (2013) 'Quality and safety of hospital discharge: a study on experiences and perceptions of patients' relatives and care providers'. *International Journal of Quality Care*, 25: 66–74.

Hewitt-Taylor, J. (2012) 'Planning the transition of children with complex needs from hospital to home'. *Nursing Children and Young People*, 24 (10): 20–3.

Ingram, J.C., Powell, J.E., Blair, P.S., Pontin, D., Redshaw, M., Manns, S., Beasant, L., Burden, H., Johnson, D., Rose, C. and Fleming, P.G. (2016) 'Does family-centred neonatal discharge planning reduce healthcare usage? A before and after study in South West England'. *BMJ Open*, 6 (3): e010752.

Kelo, M., Martikainen, M. and Eriksson, E. (2015) 'Patient education of children and their families: nurses' experiences'. *Paediatric Nursing*, 39 (2): 71: 9.

Lees, L. (2012) 'What is best practice for timely discharge?' in L. Lees (ed.), *Timely Discharge from Hospital*. London: M&K Publishing.

Lerrett, S.M. (2009) 'Discharge readiness: an integrative review focusing on discharge following pediatric hospitalization'. *Journal for Specialists in Pediatric Nursing*, 14 (4): 245–55.

Lewis, M. and Noyes, J. (2007) 'Discharge management of children with complex health needs'. *Paediatric Nursing*, 19 (4): 26–30.

Limbrick, P. (2003) *An Integrated Pathway for Assessment and Support for Children with Complex Needs and Their Families*. Worcester: Interconnections.

Mellor, J. (2016) *A Report of Investigation into Unsafe Discharge from Hospital*. Parliamentary and Health Service Ombudsman. Available at: www.ombudsman.org.uk/sites/default/files/page/A%20 report%20of%20investigations%20into%20unsafe%20discharge%20from%20hospital.pdf (last accessed 26 May 2017).

Ministry of Health (1959) *The Welfare of Children in Hospital, Platt Report*. London: Her Majesty's Stationery Office.

NHS London Health Programmes (2013) *Quality and Safety Programme: Inter-hospital Transfers – Paediatrics*. London: NHS. Available at: www.londonhp.nhs.uk/wp-content/uploads/2014/12/ FINAL-Paediatric-IHT-standards_updated.pdf (last accessed 26 May 2017).

Noyes, J., Brenner, M., Fox, P. and Guerin, A. (2013) 'Reconceptualising children's complex discharge with health systems theory: novel integrative review with embedded expert consultation and theory development'. *Journal of Advanced Nursing*, 70 (5): 975–96.

NSPCC (2016) *Child Protection in the UK*. Available at: www.nspcc.org.uk/preventing-abuse/child-protection-system (last accessed 26 May 2017).

Nursing and Midwifery Council (NMC) (2015) *The Code: Professional Standards for Nursing and Midwifery*. London: NMC.

Parkin, E. (2016) *Patient Health Records and Confidentiality*. House of Commons Library. Briefing paper 07103. 25 April.

Pellett, C. (2016) 'Discharge planning: best practice in transitions of care'. *British Journal of Community Nursing*, 21 (11). DOI: http://dx.doi.org/10.12968/bjcn.2016.21.11.542

Penthybridge, J. (2004) 'How team working influences discharge planning from hospital: a study of four multi-disciplinary teams in an acute hospital in England'. *Journal of Interprofessional Care*, 18 (1): 29–41.

Peters, S., Chaney, G., Zappla, T., van Veldhusine, C., Pereira, S. and Santamaria, N. (2011) 'Care coordination for children with complex care needs significantly reduces hospital utilization'. *Journal for Specialists in Paediatric Nursing*, 16: 305–12.

Royal College of Nursing (RCN) (2011) *Transferring Children to and from Theatre*. Available at: www2. rcn.org.uk/__data/assets/pdf_file/0003/395760/004127.pdf (last accessed 26 May 2017).

Royal College of Nursing (RCN) (2014) *The Future of Community Children's Nursing*. London: RCN.

Samwell, B. (2012) 'From hospital to home: journey of a child with complex care needs'. *Nursing Children and Young People*, 24 (2): 14–19.

Scottish Intercollegiate Guidance Network (SIGN) (2012) *The SIGN Discharge Document*. Available at: www.sign.ac.uk/pdf/sign128.pdf (last accessed 26 May 2017).

Sethi, D. and Subramanian, S. (2014) 'When place and time matter: how to conduct safe inter-hospital transfer of patients'. *Saudi Journal Anaesthesia*, 8 (1): 104–13.

Smith, L. and Coleman, V. (2009) *Child and Family-centred Care. Concept Theory and Practice*, 2nd edn. London: Palgrave Macmillan.

Stephens, N. (2005) 'Complex care packages: supporting seamless discharge for children and families'. *Paediatric Nursing*, 17 (7): 30–2.

Wagner, J., Iwashyna, T.J. and Kahn, J.M. (2013) 'Reasons underlying interhospital transfers to an academic medical intensive care unit'. *Journal of Critical Care*, 28: 202–8.

Waring, J., Marshall, F., Bishop, S., Sahota, O., Walker, M., Currie, G., Fisher, R. and Avery, T. (2014) 'An ethnographic study of knowledge sharing across the boundaries between care processes services and organisations: the contribution to safe hospital discharge'. *Health and Services Delivery Research*, 2 (29): 1–160.

Weiss, M., Johnson, N.L., Malin, S., Jerofke, T., Lang, C. and Sherburn, E. (2008) 'Readiness for discharge in parents of hospitalized children'. *Journal of Paediatric Nursing*, 23 (4): 282–95.

Welsh Government (2102) *Children and Young People's Continuing Care Guidance*. Available at: http://gov.wales/docs/phhs/publications/121127careen.pdf (last accessed 26 May 2017).

Wong, E., Yam, C. Leung, M., Chan, F., Wong, F. and Yeoh, E. (2011) 'Barriers to effective discharge planning: a qualitative study investigating the perspective of frontline health professionals'. *BMC Health Services Research*, 11 (1): 242.

World Health Organization (2012) *The WHO Strategy on Research for Health*. Available at: www.who.int/phi/WHO_Strategy_on_research_for_health.pdf (last accessed 26 May 2017).

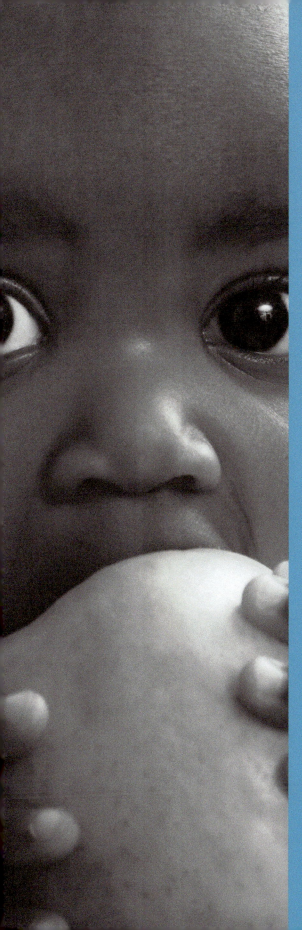

PART 4 CARING FOR CHILDREN AND YOUNG PEOPLE WITH COMPLEX AND HIGH DEPENDENCY NEEDS

31 Care of highly dependent and critically
    ill children and young people   475

32 Care of the neonate   493

33 Care of children and young people
    with a malignant condition   512

34 Care of children and young people
    with life-limiting illness   529

35 Care of children and young people
    at the end of life   539

36 Care of children and young people
    with learning disabilities   556

37 Care of children and young people
    with mental health issues   576

CARE OF HIGHLY DEPENDENT AND CRITICALLY ILL CHILDREN AND YOUNG PEOPLE

31

USHA CHANDRAN AND FIONA LYNCH

THIS CHAPTER COVERS

- An introduction to the paediatric critical care unit (PCCU)
- Assessing and caring for PCC children
- Holistic and child/family-centred care
- PCC outcomes

> 'As a parent my world was tipped upside down completely, unexpectedly and suddenly, with the life of the most precious thing in the world to me hanging in the balance. I was helpless, scared, and shell-shocked. The nurses were our advocates, support, voice of reason, teachers, interpreters, substitute parents, in addition to providing expert medical care to our child. They made us laugh, listened when we were worried, looked after us when we cried. The people we relied on 24 hours a day, who I still think of so incredibly fondly.'
>
> **Leah, parent of 18-month-old girl with multi-organ failure**

> 'I initially dreaded coming to the PCCU. I imagined myself irrelevant and unable to do anything. On the contrary, the staff are always so well organised and prepared. The nurses have taught me so many things and I'm so happy. I now feel ready to take on life as a qualified nurse. I've learnt skills here and gained knowledge at three times the rate I have elsewhere. Consider yourself lucky if you're placed in the PCCU. There are many learning opportunities that await you.'
>
> **Zakinah, 3rd-year children's nursing student**

Visit https://study.sagepub.com/essentialchildnursing to access a wealth of online resources for this chapter – watch out for the margin icons throughout the chapter.

INTRODUCTION

In this chapter we will cover the structure and function of PCCUs in the UK and describe two models for the assessment and management of critically ill children. A range of critical care interventions, common PCC complications and PCC outcomes are highlighted. The principles for delivering safe and high-quality critical care, team work and holistic and child/FCC are emphasised.

First you should revise the anatomy and physiology of the major organ systems of children. A good resource for revising these concepts is *Fundamentals of Children's Anatomy and Physiology: A Textbook for Nursing and Healthcare Students* (Peate and Gormley-Fleming, 2015).

AN INTRODUCTION TO THE PAEDIATRIC CRITICAL CARE UNIT (PCCU)

The Paediatric Intensive Care Society (PICS, 2015) defines the PCCU as 'a discrete area within a ward or hospital where paediatric critical care is delivered' (p.14). The Royal College of Paediatrics and Child Health (RCPCH, 2014), which sets standards for PCC outside of the paediatric intensive care unit (PICU) defines PCC as levels 1, 2 and 3 depending on patient complexity. Levels 1 and 2 PCC can be delivered in dedicated high dependency areas (HDU) whereas level 3 PCC requires an ICU environment.

Table 31.1 Essential bedside equipment

System	Equipment	Comments
Airway	Wall suction	Must be accessible and functional in an emergency or arrest. Portable suction is required for transfers
	Wide-bore rigid suction catheter (Yankauer)	Essential for clearing the airway and for all intubation/ extubation and transfers
	Guedel airways	Maintains a patent airway
	Soft suction catheters	For clearing nasopharyngeal and artificial airways. For artificial airways, suction catheters are twice the size of the endotracheal (ETT) or tracheostomy tube. For example, for size 4 ETT, you will need size 8 FG suction catheters
Breathing	Self-inflating Ambu bag and face mask	Not dependent on gas flow. Mandatory on all transfers
	Ayers T-piece, Mapleson circuit or similar hand-ventilation circuit and face-mask	Requires gas flow to inflate. Most preferred mode of hand/manual ventilation. Essential for intubation/ extubation procedures
	¾ or full oxygen cylinder	In case piped oxygen fails
	Pulse oximetry (SpO_2)	Monitors oxygenation
	End-tidal CO_2 sensor	Monitors carbon dioxide (CO_2) clearance
	Stethoscope	Auscultate breath sounds (BS)
Circulation	ECG monitoring	Monitors heart rate (HR) and rhythm. If patient is paced, pacing spikes must be visible on monitor
	Invasive or non-invasive blood pressure (BP)	Invasive BP must show a reliable waveform on monitor
Disability	Drugs/infusions	Must be checked and verified as correct
Exposure	Health and safety	Adheres to policies and procedures
		Clean and clutter-free environment

Nursing practice

This begins with a clear and comprehensive handover of the child and includes patient demographics, past medical and presenting history, family structures, treatment to date and safeguarding issues. A structured approach (e.g. ABCDE – airway, breathing, circulation, disability and exposure) is used to communicate clinical data, patient problems, needs and treatment goals. Following this, the patient's bedspace is checked to ensure it is safe and appropriate for the child. These tasks are only superseded if an unexpected event occurs that places the child at immediate risk, for example the desaturating child, cardiorespiratory arrest or the patient at risk of harming him/herself. These safety principles also apply to transfers.

SCENARIO 31.1: BILLY

Billy is a 2-year-old little boy with toxic shock secondary to chicken pox. He has been very unwell in his local hospital and a referral has been made to the PCC transport service for ongoing advice and transfer to a level 3 PCCU. He has been intubated and ventilated, volume (fluid) resuscitated and commenced on vasoactive drugs to support his BP.

- What do you think Billy, his family and the transport team will require on arrival to the PCCU?

SCENARIO ANSWER 31.1

Go to https://study.sagepub.com/essentialchildnursing and look up your local PCC transport service. These websites have very useful information on PCC transport principles and process, clinical management of different conditions and information on parental advice.

WEBLINK:
PCC
TRANSPORT
SERVICE

FIND OUT MORE!

PCC monitoring

All PCC children will have basic essential monitoring that includes ECG monitoring, BP, RR, temperature, SpO_2 and pulse rate (PR). However, you must never rely solely on any type of monitoring without first checking your patient. For instance, in pulseless electrical activity – a type of cardiac arrest with normal electrical activity but no cardiac output (CO) or perfusion – the ECG trace can show a normal cardiac rhythm and HR yet the patient is in cardiac arrest and requires cardiopulmonary resuscitation.

Intubated patients will have end-tidal CO_2 ($EtCO_2$) monitoring. $EtCO_2$ provides information on how effectively the child is ventilating and is also a safety device for intubated patients. The device is a non-invasive sensor applied to the CYP's ventilator circuit to detect exhaled CO_2. The loss of the $EtCO_2$ trace on the monitor is a reliable indicator of a dislodged or misplaced airway tube. This is because for $EtCO_2$ to be detected the artificial airway (ETT or tracheostomy) must be positioned correctly in the airway. Basic monitoring may also include capillary or venous blood gas analysis.

A&P LINK

To remind yourself of the relevant anatomy and physiology, read the A&P link: 'Blood gases' at
https://study.sagepub.com/essentialchildnursing

A&P LINK 31.1:
BLOOD GASES

ACTIVITY 31.1: CRITICAL THINKING

When you look after a child with ECG monitoring, you must recognise the normal ECG pattern and what it means. To support this learning, look up the normal PQRST ECG pattern and explain its link to cardiac contraction (systole) and relaxation (diastole). Describe in simple terms what the PR interval and ST segment mean. Watch the video at https://study.sagepub.com/essentialchildnursing to enhance your understanding.

ACTIVITY ANSWER 31.1

VIDEO LINK 31.1: UNDERSTANDING

WATCH A VIDEO ONLINE!

Advanced monitoring supports more complex decision-making and includes continuous arterial blood pressure (ABP) and central venous pressure (CVP) monitoring. ABP requires arterial cannulation (arterial line). These are useful for regular blood sampling and provide the best source for arterial blood gas (ABG) analysis. This line requires specific care as patients can exsanguinate if it becomes disconnected. Arterial lines are visibly and clearly labelled as intra-arterial drug administration can have serious consequences and even be fatal (NPSA, 2008). Always compare ABP with non-invasive BP to determine its reliability.

CVP measures right heart preload (end-diastolic pressure). It is a surrogate marker for circulating volume. The CVP line requires cannulation of a central artery. The spare lumens on this line can be used for infusing toxic or vasoactive drugs – for example, adrenaline (epinephrine) or noradrenaline (norepinephrine). All these invasive lines must be checked, labelled and handled carefully.

In specific cases, specialised monitoring may be required. For instance, in traumatic brain injury, an intracranial bolt may be inserted surgically to measure raised intracranial pressure (RICP). Also a, patient's temperatures may be monitored using specialised invasive thermometry (e.g. rectal). This is part of an evidence-based 'neuro-protective' protocol which includes maintaining normothermia in these patients (Agrawal and Branco, 2016).

Cardiac patients may have left atrial (LA) lines (similar to CVP but on the left side) and NIRS (near infrared spectroscopy) – a non-invasive probe applied across the forehead. LA lines monitor left atrial pressure (LAP) and left heart pre-load (Horrock, 2002) whilst NIRS monitors cerebral perfusion pressure in cardiac patients. NIRS can also be used for monitoring blood flow in other organ systems – for example, abdomen (Scheeren et al., 2012).

Some of the more standard critical care monitoring tools are listed below.

- Three- or five-lead ECG
- RR, SpO_2 and PR
- Temperature
- $EtCO_2$
- Non-invasive or invasive arterial BP
- CVP

Patient alarms

High and low monitoring alarms are set to the child's age, weight and/or condition and predetermined goals, and alert staff to actual or impending problems. Although artefacts cause false alarms, all alarms must be attended to promptly. Unattended alarms compromise patient safety and contribute to sensory overload, alarm fatigue and child/family stress.

ACTIVITY 31.2: REFLECTIVE PRACTICE

Reflect on a time when you were either in a noisy, chaotic and confusing environment or even in your first placement when you were unsure of what to expect. How did you feel? This experience will be significantly worse for critically ill children and their families who have little control over their own environment on the PCCU.

ACTIVITY
ANSWER 31.2

Read Blaise Fenn's (2014) experience, as a 15-year-old ex-PICU patient, of PCCU alarms via https://study.sagepub.com/essentialchildnursing

WEBLINK: PCCU
ALARMS

ASSESSING AND CARING FOR PCC CHILDREN

A structured approach is used to assess and manage critically ill children. This chapter illustrates two models – ABCDE and a top-to-toe/front-to-back model.

Airway

If the child in the HDU has the ability to talk, babble or cry means the airway is patent. Drooling, gurgling or snoring and stridor are signs of airway problems. Noisy breathing that quietens or muffled and hoarse speech signals an airway emergency. Loss of airway reflexes, a weak cough or the inability to cough requires urgent airway protection.

Breathing (respiratory)

Respiratory assessment is the assessment of the patient's breathing pattern and work of breathing (WOB). This consists of observing the child's RR, SpO_2, HR, colour and use of accessory muscles – that is, work of breathing (WOB). Increased WOB is characterised by the use of accessory muscles (e.g. recession, nasal flaring, grunting) and can be the indicator for respiratory support. Not tolerating being handled, agitation and irritability are also signs of this need.

VIDEO LINK 31.2:
RESPIRATORY
SYSTEM

Cyanosis, a late sign, and the patient who is too breathless to speak, eat or drink is in significant respiratory distress. Gasping, cyanosis, bradypnoea/apnoea and fatigue or exhaustion all herald impending collapse. These symptoms must be effectively managed, using, for example, bronchodilators, oxygen therapy or other respiratory support. In the infant with bronchiolitis, for instance, high-flow nasal cannula oxygen or NIV has shown some benefit (Sinha et al., 2015). A new or rising trend in supplementary oxygen confirms the need for respiratory support.

Observing the breathing pattern and how the chest/abdomen moves and expands is an important part of the respiratory assessment. As different pathologies cause different patterns of breathing, it is important to observe and report these early. For instance, upper airway obstruction causes paradoxical (see-saw) breathing. A pneumothorax, pleural effusions or mucus plugs, may cause unequal chest wall expansion and could require chest drains and airway clearance manoeuvres. Metabolic acidosis causes comfortable tachypnea but requires correction of the metabolic acidosis. Patients with head injuries with irregular breathing patterns may be developing RICP – a life threatening condition. They require a CT scan urgently. Secretion management is a simple strategy for supporting airway and breathing difficulties but requires proper assessment of secretions/sputum. Management consists of regular physiotherapy, good humidification of gases, nebulisation and mucolytics. Severe cases may require specialist input – for example, bronchoscopy and/or broncho-alveolar lavage.

An essential part of bedside respiratory assessment is the auscultation of breath sounds (BS). Normal BS are clear from the apex to the bases. Practise this skill in your placement and if you hear adventitious sounds make a note of where you hear them and what they sound like. Note whether you hear them during inspiration, expiration or both. You may auscultate a variety of adventitious sounds in different conditions. For instance, coarse crackles are a feature of retained secretions and you may be able to palpate/feel this by placing your hand on the patient's chest. Fine crackles at lung bases suggest pulmonary oedema. A positive fluid balance and hepatomegaly in a young child may confirm this finding. Wheeze is an intrathoracic sound from narrowed airways.

For intubated patients, assessment and management of the endotracheal tube (ETT) or tracheostomy is essential. The artificial airway must remain patent, stable and secure.

DOPE(S) is a mnemonic to identify clinical emergencies causing hypoxia or desaturations in a patient with an artificial airway.

DOPES stand for:

- **D**isplaced or dislodged ETT or tracheostomy
- **O**bstruction: any causes of tube obstruction (e.g. secretions, kink in ETT)
- **P**neumothorax (ventilated patients, patients with fragile lungs or insertion of neck lines may cause this)
- **E**quipment failure or problem (e.g. malfunctioning ventilator, disconnection)
- **S**tomach (if too full of air or fluid will splint the diaphragm, hindering lung expansion and ventilation)

WEBLINK:
NTSP

Access the National Tracheostomy Safety Project via https://study.sagepub.com/essentialchild nursing and find out what equipment the emergency tracheostomy box should contain. Look up the emergency algorithm for blocked tracheostomies.

Loose ETT or tracheostomy tapes must be resecured without delay. This is a two-person procedure that requires access to an airway expert in case reintubation is required. For secure tubes, note the tube position (oral/nasal/tracheostomy), type and size of tube, whether it is cuffed or uncuffed and the volume of air in the cuff (if inflated). Cuff pressure should be checked with a cuff manometer every shift. High cuff pressure and mobile tubes cause tracheal damage and airway swelling. Blocked tubes are an airway emergency.

Mechanically ventilated patients can continue to breathe comfortably and synchronously on the ventilator. However, some patients become agitated and uncomfortable on this mode of support. This is known as asynchrony. Asynchrony is exhausting, distressing and uncomfortable for patients, and parents become upset when they observe this. Retained secretions, suboptimal sedation, pain and discomfort (e.g. from a full bladder) are some of the causes of asynchrony.

Asynchrony may be managed by sedating the patient but for problems like retained secretions, airway clearance manoeuvres are essential (Walsh et al., 2011). Airway clearance – which may include preoxygenation and manually ventilating the child, saline instillation, chest physiotherapy and suction – requires proper assessment. Unnecessary or routine procedures are counterproductive, even dangerous (Strickland et al., 2013). Evidence-based guidelines (Tume and Copnell, 2015) and the endotracheal suction assessment tool are valuable strategies for supporting this practice (Davis et al., 2017). You can learn more about airway clearance manoeuvres in placement by teaming up with physiotherapists who are experts in this field.

ACTIVITY 31.3: TEAM WORKING

An intubated baby has copious, tenacious and thick secretions and his oxygen saturations fall to 87 per cent. Following a systematic assessment, his nurse identifies ETT secretions to be the problem and prepares to perform an airway clearance maneouvre.

- Which members of the multidisciplinary team (MDT) should, or could, be involved in this baby and family's care during this episode of desaturation?

ACTIVITY
ANSWER 31.3

> " Spend some time alongside other members of the multidisciplinary team, for example dieticians, physiotherapists and pharmacists. Talk to parents and patients. Ask them about their experience and try to see what it would be like if you were in their shoes.
>
> **Staff nurse, paediatrics** "

The respiratory system can be supported invasively through mechanical ventilation (MV) or non-invasively (e.g. O_2 therapy/NIV). One simple, non-invasive strategy for optimising airway and breathing is effective positioning. This facilitates not only airway opening but also optimises lung expansion, ventilation-perfusion (VQ) matching and gas exchange (Johnson and Meyenburg, 2009). HDU patients with the ability to position themselves adequately will normally do this independently (e.g. tripod position). Dependent patients require assisted therapeutic positioning. For instance, in unilateral lung disease, dependent patients are positioned with the 'good' lung up (Davis et al., 1985). In bilateral lung disease, prone positioning may be beneficial (Wells et al., 2005). Prone positioning displaces the patient's abdominal and thoracic structures to make more space for the lungs to expand, recruits atelectatic lungs and promotes VQ matching and gas exchange (Messerole et al., 2002). Always perform a risk assessment taking into account contraindications and local moving and handling policies prior to these procedures.

It is important to advise families that prone positioning is a special ventilatory mode safe only on the PCCU where there is continuous monitoring. There is a recognised risk of sudden infant death syndrome in babies who are placed prone at home (Lullaby Trust, 2013).

Circulation

Circulatory/cardiovascular (CVS) assessment is vital for identifying deteriorating patients. Non-invasive measurements of circulation consist of assessing capillary refill time (CRT), skin warmth, colour (flushed, pale or cyanotic or mottled) and toe-to-core temperature gradients. These measures provide valuable information on cardiac output (CO) and circulating volume in deteriorating patients. It can help to differentiate compensating patients from decompensating children. A bounding pulse, flash CRT and flushed appearance in septic shock, for instance, shows a compensating patient with a high CO and increased stroke volume (SV) (i.e. vasodilated patients). A low volume, thready pulse, prolonged CRT and mottled and cool skin are features of low CO, vasoconstriction and hypoperfusion. These patients may appear pale or cyanosed and diaphoretic (i.e. decompensated). They are in circulatory failure and at risk of imminent collapse.

HR and rhythm assessment is an important parameter for deteriorating patients as it influences CO, SV and organ perfusion. Children under the age of 2 are particularly HR dependent for increasing

VIDEO LINK 31.3:
CARDIOVASCULAR
ASSEESMENT

VIDEO LINK 31.4:
PHYSIOLOGY OF
SHOCK

their CO as they cannot improve their SV to any great extent – hence early tachycardia in this group. However, very rapid HR (in excess of 200 beats/minute in young children) and serious arrhythmias (e.g. supraventricular tachycardia) will compromise CO in all age groups (Hazinski, 2013).

Mean BP (MAP) is a core haemodynamic parameter in PCC and requires skilled observation. It is a measure of perfusion pressure for organ function. Without adequate perfusion (i.e. MAP) organs will fail. If one organ fails, this is termed single-organ failure. If more than one organ fails, then the child is in multi-organ failure. Maintaining a good CO and perfusion pressure minimises the risk of organ failure, PCC complications and/or death.

Lack of perfusion is not only life-threatening but can also be life-changing. For instance, lack of perfusion to limbs and digits compromises the viability of that limb and may lead to amputations. This is a life-changing event for the child. If there is inadequate perfusion to the heart, myocardial dysfunction and life-threatening arrhythmias can occur. In traumatic brain injury, an adequate cerebral perfusion pressure is required to prevent secondary brain injury, swelling, herniation and brain-stem death. Common strategies for maintaining MAP in these patients who are no longer fluid responsive is to use vasopressor drugs. In severe cases, specialised mechanical support may be required such as Extra Corporeal Life Support (ECLS or ECMO). Units that provide these highly specialised interventions are defined as Advanced 5 PCCU (PICS, 2015) and is the highest level of care any PICU can provide.

Lactate is a very useful marker of poor CO and perfusion. Lactate can be monitored at the bedside when performing blood gases. As lactate is a by-product of anaerobic metabolism, poor CO will cause a rise in lactate. A rising lactate (normal < 2mmol/l) is associated with increased mortality (Wheeler, 2013). Some caution is required in interpreting this result in liver disease as lactate is cleared by the liver. Initial management of deranged lactate levels is fluid resuscitation and/or vasoactive drugs to optimise CO. Blood transfusions and oxygen therapy may be required to improve the oxygen content of the blood for aerobic metabolism (Wheeler, 2013).

One early marker of hypoperfusion is acute kidney injury (AKI). AKI results in poor urine output, deranged kidney function and acid-base imbalance. Early AKI can be detected at the bedside by closely monitoring urine output and fluid balances. Mild AKI may respond to volume resuscitation and vasopressors to improve CO and perfusion pressures and may be reversed if managed effectively. Severe AKI requires renal replacement therapy (RRT) in the form of peritoneal dialysis or haemofiltration.

Pulse pressure – the difference between systolic and diastolic BP – is another important early marker of deterioration in PCC. In dehydration, reduced pulse pressure is detected long before a drop in BP and hypotension. Unlike adults, hypotension is a late and pre-terminal finding in children and the pulse pressure provides valuable information prior to this pre-terminal event.

CVP (sometimes referred to as right atrial pressure) measures right heart (atrial) filling pressures and circulating volume. It provides information on how well patients are responding to fluid resuscitation and other interventions that aim to improve CO. Patients who respond to fluid resuscitation will sustain a higher CVP. High CVP (but not necessarily high LAP) is seen in overloaded patients and patients in right-heart failure. Hepatomegaly, basal lung crackles and a positive fluid balance chart will also support the diagnosis of fluid overload. Low CVP is associated with dehydration, hypovolaemia and low circulating volume (Darovic, 2002). A prolonged CRT, cool skin or poor skin turgor and a sunken fontanelle in the young child will also support this finding although in certain conditions (e.g. diabetic ketoacidosis) these classical signs may not be evident.

Disability

The assessment of disability focuses on neurological assessment and blood glucose monitoring. Neurological assessments comprise the assessment of mental state or behaviour, Glasgow Coma Scale, tone/flaccidity and pupils assessment. For patients with epidural analgesia, spinal drains and/or other neurological conditions or surgical interventions involving the brain and/or spine, sensation and motor function are also assessed. Young babies will very quickly present with poor tone and floppiness if unwell. In hypoxic, hypercapnia or other forms of encephalopathy, agitation, confusion, drowsiness, seizure activity or coma may be the presenting features.

Pupil assessment is a very important part of neurological assessment. For instance, fixed dilated and/or unequal pupils and a bulging or tensed fontanelle in infants is a sign of RICP, which may require emergency treatment and CT scan. Evidence-based 'neuro-protective' strategies (e.g. normothermia, normocapnia, adequate MAP and normoglycaemia) are life-saving strategies (Argrawal and Branco, 2016). In the sedated or opioid-managed child, sluggish or pin-point pupils can be a sign of over-sedation.

Pain and sedation are a part of neurological assessment and a PCC priority as sedated patients may still be able to experience pain. Various pain tools are used to assess pain in PCC (RCN, 2009) and the COMFORT scale is commonly used to assess comfort and sedation in MV patients (Ambuel et al., 1992; Harris et al., 2016). Suboptimal pain and sedation management are detrimental and compromise patient safety but too much sedation in MV patients will prevent patients from weaning their ventilation, induce withdrawal symptoms and prolong their stay in the PCCU (Grant et al. 2013).

Exposure

Patients must be exposed (preserving their dignity and warmth as much as possible) to assess them fully and comprehensively. Abdominal assessment, assessment of pressure areas, lines and wound sites, tubes or drains, and the assessment of patients' limbs for any abnormality require proper exposure.

Abdominal assessment consists of observing the abdomen for any abnormality (e.g. distension, discolouration or shape). In critical illness, hypoperfusion to abdominal organs can result in deranged function, ischaemia, necrosis, bleeding and/or perforation. The bowel, liver and other gastro-intestinal organs can become involved. Many of these complications may result in abdominal discomfort, abdominal discolouration and/or distention. As a distended abdomen reduces chest wall compliance and complicates MV weaning, you may be required to monitor distention by measuring abdominal girth. Auscultating for bowel sounds is part of the abdominal assessment and a core PCC nursing skill. Learn to auscultate bowel sounds in your placement.

Top-to-toe/front-to-back assessment

Hygiene and other personal and health needs are thoroughly assessed using the above approach. Meeting PCC patients' personal hygiene needs is a nursing priority not only for infection control purposes but it is also integral to patient dignity and welfare. It normalises the critical care process for children and provides opportunities for families to participate in the patient's care.

During this assessment, comprehensively assess all areas of the patient's skin and mucous membranes. Observe for any abnormality, pressure damage and/or tissue oedema. In babies and young children, the occipital area is very much at risk for pressure damage and in all critically ill children the ears, ETT and other pressure points are vulnerable. In sedated patients with poor blinking reflexes, the children's eyes should remain moist and closed to prevent complications such as corneal keratitis and other eye infections. One of the first signs of keratitis is pink-tinged eyes.

Tissue oedema is a common PCC complication. One of the causes of this complication is hypoalbuminaemia and increased vessel permeability which can be exacerbated by critical illness and positive pressure MV. Tissue oedema is not only a potential risk factor for pressure ulcer formation but it can also impede chest wall compliance and interfere with ventilation and weaning. It causes an 'ooziness' or leakiness at line, tube and punctures sites, prevents dressings from adhering to skin and is a potential contributor for infection and poor wound healing. It also causes parents much distress if their child's normal appearance changes. Reassure families that tissue oedema caused by PCC complications may be managed with fluid restriction and drugs (diuretics) and will usually resolve as the patient recovers.

Comprehensive assessment includes a thorough assessment of the child's limbs and other areas. Here, observe the child's limbs for any abnormality or deformity (e.g. swelling from IV lines) and perfusion. Assess colour, warmth, capillary refill, motor and sensory function. For patients who have had surgical grafts or flaps, you may be required to perform a hand-held Doppler assessment of peripheral pulses. Promptly report swelling, inflammation, tenderness or pain as femoral and other lines can cause complications (e.g. thrombus, infiltration or extravasation of drugs and fluids). Remove thromboembolic stockings (if applicable) and check calves. Signs of inflammation, swelling, warmth or erythema may be the early signs of deep vein thrombosis in older children. Demarcation, discolouration and coolness may be signs of hypoperfusion and rashes have various causes, some of it ominous (e.g. petechial rash in meningococcal infection or a complication known as disseminated intravascular coagulopathy (DIC) which some very severely critically ill patients develop).

DIC is caused by any factor that triggers a dysfunctional clotting system (e.g. sepsis, cancer or liver dysfunction). In septic shock, endothelial injury and microvascular damage activates the clotting system. This results in thrombus formation in small vessels, thrombocytopenia and depletion of clotting factors. The depletion of platelets and clotting factors and the activation of fibrinolysis place patients at risk of bleeding and haemorrhage, some of it severe, hence the acronym DIC: 'death is coming' (Moore et al. 2010). Thus, thorough and comprehensive assessment for signs of bleeding at line, tube and puncture sites and observing for signs of covert or internal bleeding are important features of PCC assessment.

SCENARIO 31.2: PEARL

PRACTICE
SCENARIO 31:
SAM

Fifteen-year-old Pearl, an oncology patient, is septic and has received 40mls/kg volume resuscitation and antibiotics on the ward according to sepsis guidelines (NICE, 2016). Pearl was unresponsive to this treatment so she was transferred to PICU for ongoing management. On PICU, Pearl received another 20ml/kg of fluid to support her blood pressure and normalise tachycardia (Dellinger et al., 2013).

Here are Pearl's assessment details.

Airway: Patent, weak cough

Breathing: RR: 47 breaths/minute, saturations: 98% on 15 litres oxygen via non-rebreathe bag. Comfortable but shallow, rapid breathing, BS: resonant, clear to lung bases. ABG: metabolic acidosis

Circulation: HR: 157 beats/minute. Radial pulse regular, high volume, bounding, ECG: sinus tachycardia, BP is hypotensive – 89/30 (mean: 50mmHg), Temperature: 39°C. Shivering (rigors), CRT: flash, hot to touch, dry skin, pink, flushed, appearance, Urine output: oliguria. Lactate 4mmol/l (high)

Disability: GCS: Responding to questions. $E_4V_5M_6$ (15/15), PERL size 4mm, moving all limbs, blood glucose: 4.0mmol/l, denies pain. Not agitated. Looks lethargic/exhausted

Exposure: No rashes. Hickman line site appears inflamed

Problem: Warm shock

Potential problem: Decompensated shock and organ failure

Goal: Pearl will respond to treatment and recover from this deterioration

- What actions can we take to help Pearl's parents cope with this crisis?

SCENARIO
ANSWER 31.2

PCC management

The journey for patients like Pearl can be painful, traumatic and unpredictable. These patients may have advanced and/or specialised monitoring and all septic patients will have the source of infection aggressively treated (e.g. antibiotics and removal of invasive lines, if line sepsis). Most ventilated patients will have an indwelling urethral catheter to monitor their urine output, kidney function and fluid balances. A central line may be inserted for high volume fluid resuscitation, infusing vaso-active drugs and CVP measurement. An arterial line is useful for regular blood sampling, ABG and continuous BP monitoring.

Unstable or severely deteriorating patients are always electively intubated and sedated to support their respiratory and cardiovascular status. Intubation and ventilation allows for additional sedation to be given to enable tolerance of invasive procedures and painful interventions. It also induces a neces-sary sense of amnesia for unpleasant events. Deep sedation is beneficial as it reduces the metabolic rate but it also compromises the patient's ability to protect their airway and depresses respiratory function – hence the need for airway support. Some patients (e.g. oncology patients) are very high-risk intubations as they can decompensate very quickly and the team must be prepared for this.

HOLISTIC AND CHILD/FAMILY-CENTRED CARE

All PCC interventions are underpinned by a holistic and child/FCC approach (Hakio et al., 2015). This approach facilitates child/parental involvement and empowerment. Reassurance, commu-nication, meeting parents' basic needs and their need for information is all part of FCC (Latour, 2011). Looking for opportunities to involve parents, such as teaching them how to provide eye and mouth care for their ventilated child, changing a nappy on the child with an indwell-ing catheter or other invasive lines, assisting with bed-bathing or repositioning the intubated child plus comforting the critically ill child, are supportive of the parental role and empowering (McGraw et al., 2012).

VIDEO LINK 31.5:
JORDAN'S
STORY

Negotiation is a key concept in child/FCC (Tume and Latour, 2015). On the PCCU, negotiate to retain as much of the patient's normal routines as possible. Find out about the child's likes and dislikes and remember that beneath all lines, tubes and technology is a child who is both an individual and someone's child. Despite being in a busy and technologically rich environment, aim to promote nor-mality, a child-friendly atmosphere and psychological security. Facilitating a normal circadian rhythm and providing protected rest periods during the day, increasing natural light and decreasing artificial light may all aid this process. Bear in mind that families also provide the emotional love and bond for the child, so create opportunities for open visiting and minimise family waiting times. Importantly, form therapeutic partnerships with families and critically ill children and within professional bound-aries do all you can to facilitate a sense of control for children and their families (NMC, 2015).

In some cases, however, parents may be too distressed to engage. This requires referral to a family counsellor, psychologist or faith chaplain with their consent. As stress and distress can be an ongoing issue, even following PCCU discharge, follow-up care in the community may be required.

Parents' views of helpful nurse behaviours (Harbaugh et al., 2004):

- Nurturing and protective
- Allowing access and proximity to their child
- Openly being affectionate and caring
- Reducing stress and uncertainty
- Including parents in care
- Appreciating the individuality of their child
- Conducting care in competent, coordinated manner
- Providing accurate information and reassurance

Parents' views of unhelpful nurse behaviours (Harbaugh et al., 2004; Brooten et al., 2012):

- Separation from child
- Exclusion from their child's care
- Poor communication of child's progress
- Nursing care without affection
- Nursing care without protection
- Conflict between staff and parents
- Inexperienced staff

ACTIVITY 31.4: REFLECTIVE PRACTICE

Give examples of your own behaviours that children and their families may have found helpful. List the actions and behaviours that may have been perceived as negative.

ACTIVITY
ANSWER 31.4

> Our nurses were amazing from the time we arrived, when we knew the least but needed them the most. I say our nurses as they were there for the whole family. We needed to trust that they cared as much as we did about the survival of our child. We physically could not be there 24 hours a day, and our nurses told us not to be, but the assurance and confidence of our nurses allowed us to rest, trusting that our child would be looked after. There were so many people involved in the care that came and went but the nurses were our constant. I would ensure I was there for every shift change so I would know who was looking after our child so I could then relax. I felt a bond with those nurses we had more than once.
>
> **Leah, Parent of 18-month-old girl with multi-organ failure**

VIDEO
LINK 31.6
LISTENING
TO PARENTS

Go to https://study.sagepub.com/essentialchildnursing and watch the video illustrating the importance of listening to parents of sick children.

SAFEGUARDING STOP-POINT

Always clarify safeguarding issues during handover and as the situation changes on the PCCU. You must be aware of how actively parents and other visitors are allowed to participate in care, with or without supervision, and who is visiting your patient and if there any restrictions to this.

WHAT'S THE EVIDENCE?

Some critically ill children and their families experience post-traumatic stress disorder (PTSD) following a PCCU admission and require follow-up care on discharge from the PCCU. Read Colville and Pierce's (2012) article 'Patterns of post-traumatic stress symptoms after paediatric intensive care'.

✓

- What are the potential causes of PTSD for critically ill children and their parents?

WHAT'S THE
EVIDENCE?
ANSWER 31.1

PCC OUTCOMES

Many children and their families look forward to leaving the PCCU. For a few, the prospect of leaving can be daunting (Keogh, 2001). Being able to visit the ward and meet ward staff beforehand is an ideal strategy for reassuring children and their families. Where this is not possible, effective communication, reassurance and sensitive 'deintensifying' or 'de-escalating' monitoring may be the only options. Some units will have an outreach team or discharge nurse to support discharge and a minority of patients will be prepared for home/community care (e.g. those with life-limiting, long-term or rehabilitation/complex needs). This process requires the involvement and coordination of many hospital and community teams.

SCENARIO 31.3: HASAN

Hasan, a two-month-old baby who was intubated and ventilated for bronchiolitis leading to respiratory failure, has been recently extubated (removal of ETT) and transitioned to high dependency unit (HDU) care. Hasan's assessment is highlighted below:

Observation: Lying comfortably on his back, breathing spontaneously and watching and interacting with his mum.

Airway/Breathing:

Inspection: Naris clear and patent, no excessive secretions, in room air saturating at 97%, RR: 42 breaths/min. No excessive WOB. No stridor or other signs of airway obstruction or swelling – a risk factor for recently extubated young children. Hasan's breathing is

(Continued)

(Continued)

synchronous and there is bilateral chest wall expansion (equal). He has a strong, intermittent and non-problematic cough. His colour is normal for his ethnicity

Palpation: No evidence of retained secretions on chest

Auscultation: Bilateral breath sounds clear to bases. No crackles or wheeze

Circulation: Stable. HR: 115 beats/min, sinus rhythm, afebrile, CRT < 2 seconds, normotensive, warm and well-perfused, urine output: 1.5 ml/kg/hr

Disability: All sedation discontinued; no signs of withdrawal. $E_4V_5M_5$ (14/15), appropriate for age, fixing and following, moving all limbs normally and has normal tone. PEARL 3mm. Blood glucose: 4mmol/L

Exposure: Hasan has an intravenous cannula on the right hand which is infusing maintenance fluids at a normal rate. A spigotted naso-gastric tube is in situ. He has a urethral catheter which can be removed

Problem/need: Hasan and his family need to feel prepared for ward discharge

Potential problem: Hasan is recently extubated and may deteriorate to the extent of needing reintubation or respiratory support. His family may feel anxious about his discharge

Goal: Hasan will continue his recovery. Hasan and his parents will feel fully prepared for his discharge

- How can we prepare Hasan and his parents for discharge?

SCENARIO
ANSWER 31.3

SEE ALSO
CHAPTER 24

Sadly, for some patients and their family, there is no positive outcome and end-of-life care is a reality. Discussion around palliation, futility of care, the need to limit or withdraw treatment (we never withdraw care) and organ donation is distressing, not least for the families involved (Griffiths and Danburry, 2015). Involving the palliative care team during this time is good practice (Truog et al., 2006), and the RCPCH (Larcher et al., 2015) provide guidelines for the medico-legal issues surrounding treatment withdrawal. Managing death in a hospice or at home may be more comforting for families and dignified for the child but requires intense preparation. These issues must be sensitively raised and handled with children and their families as appropriate.

HEALTH
PROMOTION 31:
CRITICALLY ILL
CHILDREN

> Do some reading before your placement so you are not so overwhelmed. Show you are interested and willing to learn. Ask the nurses if you can do things. They let you do a lot which helps you learn new skills.
>
> **Francesca, 3rd-year children's nursing student**

PLACEMENT
ADVICE 31:
CRITICALLY ILL
CHILDREN

Go to https://study.sagepub.com/essentialchildnursing for tips on preparing for placements and helth promotion when working with highly dependent and critically ill children.

CHAPTER SUMMARY

- The systems within which UK PCCUs operate and function
- How to skilfully assess deteriorating and critically ill children
- The nature of holistic and FCC in a technologically orientated environment
- How PCC interventions and management impact on patient outcomes and family experiences
- The role of the critical care children's nurse

BUILD YOUR BIBLIOGRAPHY

Books

- Crawford, D. and McNee, P. (2012) Chapter 16: 'Care of the family', in M. Dixon and D. Crawford (eds), *Paediatric Intensive Care Nursing*. Chichester: Wiley-Blackwell.

  This chapter provides you with a comprehensive and detailed view of the strategies nurses can use to facilitate FCC.

- Davies, J.H. and Hassell, L.L. (2007) Chapter 10: 'Handy hints for various conditions', in J.H. Davies and L.L. Hassell *Children in Intensive Care: A Survival Guide*, 2nd edn. London: Elsevier Churchill-Livingstone.

  This chapter provides a quick reference for the management of common conditions. Critical care is a complex area of nursing where not only do you come across many different conditions and injuries but its management can be difficult to understand.

- Dixon, M. and Teasdale, D. (2012) Chapter 3: 'Physiological monitoring of infants and children in the intensive care unit', in M. Dixon and D. Crawford (eds), *Paediatric Intensive Care Nursing*. Chichester: Wiley-Blackwell.

  This chapter describes PCCU monitoring. One of the core experiences you will come across in your placement is the range of monitoring systems available in the critical care setting.

Journal articles

Go to https://study.sagepub.com/essentialchildnursing for further free online journal articles related to this chapter.

- Colville, G., Kerry, S. and Pierce, C. (2008) 'Children's factual and delusional memories of intensive care'. *American Journal of Respiratory and Critical Care Medicine*, 77: 976-82.

  It is important to appreciate that critically ill children's true experiences may differ from the assumptions we make about what they may or may not remember about their critical care admission and management and continuing support following discharge. This paper explores how accurately children's perceptions reflect their critical care experiences and the support they may or may not require to recover.

- Carnevale, F.A., Benedetti, M., Bonaldi, A., Bravi, E., Trabucco, G. and Biban, P. (2011) 'Understanding the private worlds of physicians, nurses and parents: a study of life-sustaining treatment decisions in Italian paediatric critical care'. *Journal of Child Health Care*, 15 (4): 334-49.

  We may never know the true impact that critical illness has on all those who are closely involved in this process. This important study provides some insights into the emotional and psychological costs of caring for or being a parent of a critically ill child.

FURTHER
READING:
ONLINE
JOURNAL
ARTICLES

(Continued)

(Continued)

- LaFond, C.M., Van Hulle Vincent, C., Corte, C., Hersheberger, P.E., Johnson, A., Park, C.G. and Wilkie, D.J. (2015) 'PCCU nurses pain assessments and intervention choices for virtual human and written vignettes', *Journal Pediatric Nursing*, 30 (4): 580-90.

  It is morally, ethically and professionally important to ensure that pain is effectively and adequately managed in any setting, including on PCCUs where assumptions may be made about children's pain experiences. This article provides important insights into how pain may be viewed, assessed or managed in this medicalised setting.

Weblinks

FURTHER
READING:
WEBLINKS

Go to https://study.sagepub.com/essentialchildnursing for further weblinks related to this chapter.

- Children's Hospitals and Clinics of Minnesota, Pediatric Inten*sive Care Units*

  www.youtube.com/watch?v=X49hzjE9cLs

  PCCUs can be somewhat threatening in appearance to a novice. This video gives you an insight into how a PCCU may appear and help you to identify some of its structures before you commence your placement.

- The Guardian, Children's Lives in the Balance at NHS Paediatric Intensive Care Unit

  www.youtube.com/watch?v=picfVuZr93s

  Family-centred care (FCC) is an integral part of critical care nursing. This video will provide you with some strategies on how FCC may be facilitated in the critical care environment.

- St George's Healthcare NHS Trust, The Recovery Journey after a PICU Admission

  www.PCCUpsychology.net/docs/road%20to%20recoveryv2.pdf

  Many children and their families continue to be traumatised by the critical care experience even following their discharge from the PICU. This video on 'A recovery journey after a PICU admission' by Colville and Atkins, describes some of these families' anxieties and fears and provides you with an insight into their psychological and emotional wellbeing.

ACE YOUR ASSESSMENT

ONLINE
QUIZZES &
ACTIVITY
ANSWERS

Revise what you have learned by visiting https://study.sagepub.com/essentialchildnursing

- Test yourself with multiple-choice and short-answer questions
- Do the chapter activities in the book and check your answers online

REFERENCES

Ambuel, B., Hamlett, K.W., Marx, C.M. and Blumer, J.L. (1992) 'Assessing distress in paediatric intensive care environments, the COMFORT scale', *Journal of Pediatric Psychology*, 17 (1): 95–109.

Argrawal, S.T. and Branco, R.G. (2016) 'Neuroprotective measures in children with traumatic head injury', *World Journal of Critical Care Medicine*, 501: 36–46.

Brooten, D., Youngblut, JM., Seagrave, L., Caicedo, C., Hawthorne, D., Hidalgo, I. and Roche, R. (2012) 'Parent's perceptions of health care providers actions around child ICU death, what helped, what did not', *American Journal of Hospice and Palliative Medicine*, 30 (1): 40–9.

Colville, G. and Pierce, C. (2012) 'Patterns of post-traumatic stress symptoms after paediatric intensive care', *ICM* 38: 1523–31.

Darovic, G.O. (2002) *Haemodynamic Monitoring, Invasive and Non-invasive Clinical Applications*. London: WB Saunders.

Davis, H., Kitchman, R., Gordon, I. and Helms, P. (1985) 'Regional ventilation in infancy, reversal of adult pattern', *New England Journal Medicine*, 313: 1625–8.

Davis, K., Bulsara, M.K., Ramelet, A.S. and Monterosso, L. (2017) 'Audit of endotracheal tube suction in a pediatric intensive care unit', *Clinical Nursing Research*, 26 (1): 68–81.

Dellinger, R.P., Levy, M.M., Rhodes, A., Annane, D., Gerlack, H., Opal, S.M., et al. (2013) 'Surviving Sepsis Campaign: international guidelines for management of severe sepsis and septic shock, 2012', *Critical Care Medicine*, 41(2): 580–637.

Fenn, B. (2014) 'Coma alarm dreams on intensive care', *Intensive Care Medicine*, 40: 1568–9.

Grant, M.J.C., Balas, M.C., Curley, M.A.Q. and RESTORE investigation team (2013) 'Defining sedation-related adverse events in the PICU', *Heart and Lung*, 42 (3): 171–6.

Griffiths, S. and Danburry, C. (2015) 'Medico-legal issues for intensivists caring for children in a district general hospital', *Journal of the Intensive Care Society*, 16 (2): 137–41.

Hakio, H., Rantanen, A., Astedt-Kurki, P. and Suominen, T. (2015) 'Parents' experiences of family functioning, health and social support provided by nurses – a pilot study in paediatric intensive care', *Intensive and Critical Nursing*, 31: 29–37.

Harbaugh, B.L., Tomlinson, P.S. and Kirschbaum, M. (2004) 'Parents' perceptions of nurses' caregiving behaviours in the pediatric intensive care unit', *Issues in Comprehensive Pediatric Nursing*, 27 (3): 163–78.

Harris, J., Ramelet A-S., van Dijk, M., Pokorna, P., Wielenga, J., Tume, L., Tibboel, D. and Ista, E. (2016) 'Clinical recommendations for pain, sedation, withdrawal and delirium assessment in critically ill infants and children: an ESPNIC position statement for healthcare professionals', *Intensive Care Med*, 42: 972–86.

Hazinski, M.F. (2013) *Nursing Care of the Critically Ill Child*, 3rd edn. St Louis, MO: Mosby.

Horrock, F. (2002) *Manual of Neonatal and Paediatric Heart Disease*. London: Whurr Publishers.

Johnson, K.L. and Meyenburg, T. (2009) 'Physiological rationale and current evidence for therapeutic positioning of critically ill patients', *AACN Advanced Critical Care*, 20 (3): 228–40.

Keogh, S. (2001) 'Parents' experiences of the transfer of their child from the PICU to the ward: a phenomenological study', *Nursing in Critical Care*, 6 (1): 7–13.

Larcher, V., Craig, F., Bhogal, K., Wilkinson, K. and Brierley, J. (2015) 'Making decisions to limit treatment in life-limiting and life-threatening conditions in children: a framework for practice', *Archives Disease in Childhood*, 100 (Suppl.2): s1–26.

Latour, J.M. (2011) *Empowerment of Parents in the Intensive Care: a journey discovering parents' experiences and satisfaction of care*. Rotterdam: Erasmus Universiteit Rotterdam.

Lullaby Trust (2013) *Sudden Infant Death Syndrome: A Guide for Professionals*. London: The Lullaby Trust.

McGraw, S.A., Truog, R.D., Solomon, M.Z., Cohen-Bearak, M.P.H., Sellers, D.E. and Meyer, E.C. (2012) '"I was able to still be her mom": Parenting at end of life in the PICU', *Pediatric Critical Care Medicine*, 13 (6): e350–6.

Messerole, E., Peine, P., Wittkopp, S., Marini, J.J. and Albert, R.K. (2002) 'Clinical commentary: the pragmatics of prone positioning', *American Journal Respiratory Critical Care Medicine*, 165: 1359.

Moore,G., Knight, G. and Blann, A (2010) *Haematology, Fundamentals of Biomedical Science*. Oxford: Oxford University Press.

NICE (2016) *Sepsis, Recognition, Diagnosis and Early Recognition*. NICE NG51. London: DH.

NMC (2015) *The Code: Professional Standards of Practice and Behaviour for Nurses and Midwives*. London: Nursing and Midwifery Council.

National Patient Safety Agency (NPSA) (2008) *Problems with Infusions and Sampling from Arterial Lines*, Rapid Response Report, NPSA/2008RRRS006, From Reporting to Learning. National Patient Safety Agency.

Peate, I. and Gormley-Fleming, E. (ed.) (2015) *Fundamentals of Children's Anatomy and Physiology: A Textbook for Nursing and Healthcare Students*. Chichester: Wiley-Blackwell.

PICS (2015) *Standards for the Care of Critically Ill Children*, 5th edn, version 2. London: Paediatric Intensive Care Society.

RCN (2009) *The Recognition and Assessment of Acute Pain in Children*, Clinical Practice Guidelines, update of full guideline, London: Royal College of Nursing.

Royal College of Paediatrics and Child Health (RCPCH) (2014) *High Dependency Care for Children: Time to Move: A Focus on the Critically Ill Child Pathway beyond the Intensive Care Unit. A Set of Recommendations to Improve the Care of the Critically Ill Child*. London: RPCPH.

Scheeren, T.W.L., Schober, P. and Schwarte, L.A. (2012) 'Monitoring tissue oxygenation by near infrared spectroscopy (NIRS), background and applications', *Journal of Clinical Monitoring and Computing*, 26 (4): 279–87.

Sinha, I.P., McBride, A.K., Smith, R. and Fernandes, R.M. (2015) 'CPAP and high-flow nasal cannula oxygen in bronchiolitis', *Chest*, 148 (3): 810–23.

Strickland, S.L., Rubin, B.K., Dreschu, D.H., O'Malley, C.A., Volskot, A., Branson, R.D. and Hess, D.R (2013) 'AARG clinical practice guidelines: effectiveness of non-pharmacological airway clearance therapies in hospital patients', *Respiratory Care*, 58 (1): 2187–93.

Truog, R.D., Meyer, E.C. and Burns, J.P. (2006) 'Toward interventions to improve end-of-life care in the pediatric intensive care unit', *Critical Care Medicine*, 34 (11 Suppl): S373–9.

Tume, L.N. and Copnell, B.(2015) 'Endotracheal suctioning of the critically ill child', *Journal of Pediatric Intensive Care*, 4 (2): 56–63.

Tume, L.N. and Latour, J.M. (2015) 'Family involvement in PICU rounds: reality or rhetoric?' *Paediatric Critical Care Medicine*, 16 (9): 875–6.

Walsh, B.K., Hood, K. and Merritt, G. (2011) 'Pediatric airway maintenance and clearance in the acute care setting: how to stay out of trouble', *Respiratory Care*, 56 (9): 1424–44.

Wells, D., Gillies, D. and Fitzgerald, D. (2005) 'Positioning for acute respiratory distress in hospitalized infants and children', *Cochrane Database of Systematic Reviews*, 2.

Wheeler, D.S. (2013) Critical care of the pediatric patient, 60(3), June (epub).

CARE OF THE NEONATE

ELISABETH PODSIADLY AND MARY GOGGIN

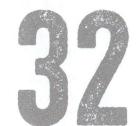

THIS CHAPTER COVERS

- Organisation and provision of neonatal care
- The term, pre-term and growth-restricted baby
- Environmental challenges to the infant
- Environmental stressors for the baby
- Environmental challenges to the family

> " The unexpected birth of my daughter at 28 weeks gestational age gave me a unique entry into the world of neonatal care. I had lived in this world as a nurse caring for babies and their families. Now I was to experience this as the recipient. During the next 12 weeks we occupied an environment that provided many noxious stimuli: light, noise, multiple care givers, occasional lack of understanding and insensitivity. The sense of loss of being unable to parent my daughter was overwhelming. The dependency on others, the unknown road ahead, the setbacks, the holding onto hope, the pain and discomfort – these were some of the experiences lived through on a daily basis. Setbacks knocked both hope and optimism. Parenting through this journey was conducted in a very public environment and always in the presence of others. The very environment that ensured her survival had also deprived me of privacy with my daughter. Developing friendship with other parents in the same situation was a source of support and joy. Throughout the journey staff unfailingly provided expertise, care, support, love to my daughter and to me. It is difficult to adequately articulate my gratitude and impossible to quantify it.
>
> **Kate, parent** "

Visit https://study.sagepub.com/essentialchildnursing to access a wealth of online resources for this chapter – watch out for the margin icons throughout the chapter.

INTRODUCTION

Neonatology – care given to a baby in its first four weeks of life – addresses the needs of infants born too soon (premature), too small (growth restricted) and ill. Care needs will vary depending upon the degree of prematurity and the condition of the infant and will identify what type of neonatal unit should provide infant and family care. Admission to a neonatal unit can be life-saving, but also exposes the vulnerable infant to an inappropriate environment for neurodevelopment during a critical time and can therefore have a lifelong impact on neurobehavioural outcomes.

This chapter explores the current provision of neonatal care to demonstrate its uniqueness in relation to other areas of child health and provide the setting for a comparison of the characteristics, problems/conditions and care of the term, preterm and growth-restricted baby. The chapter then considers the environmental challenges experienced by both the infant and family admitted to the neonatal unit with a focus on family-centred care to enable you to support a parent like Kate, the voice that introduced the chapter.

ORGANISATION AND PROVISION OF NEONATAL CARE

Providing care to infants and families in a neonatal unit requires you to have an understanding of how care is organised nationally and locally by network.

VIDEO
LINK 32.1:
INTRODUCTION
TO A NEONATAL
UNIT

Not all neonatal units are the same. The British Association of Perinatal Medicine (BAPM) represents neonatal healthcare professionals and is responsible for defining the levels/designation and categories of care that can be provided by neonatal units – the higher the level (1 to 3), the greater the complexity of care offered. Four categories of neonatal care have been identified (BAPM, 2011). These are, increasing in the order of care complexity: transitional care, special care, high dependency and intensive care. Since 2003, England has structured its neonatal care locally into managed clinical networks or organisational delivery unit networks. Scotland, Wales and Northern Ireland have followed suit. Such networks develop expertise in a small number of neonatal units which deliver all levels of care in order to improve infant morbidity and mortality. Not all units will provide all levels of care. Who provides what levels of care is negotiated and agreed within each network. A network will consist of special care units (SCUs), local neonatal units (LNUs) and usually one or two lead neonatal intensive care units (NICUs).

Ideally, infants requiring a higher level of care are delivered at the lead NICU. Transfer before delivery is known as an in-utero transfer. Some networks have arrangements whereby all mothers likely to deliver on or before, for example 26 weeks, do so in the maternity unit attached to the lead NICU. If an infant delivers before an in-utero transfer can be arranged, then the baby will be transported (ex-utero) to the network NICU for a higher level of care provided by a specialist team.

ACTIVITY 32.1: REFLECTIVE PRACTICE

Explore the provision of neonatal care in the hospitals affiliated with your university by using the 'Network Information' on the BAPM website (www.bapm.org/).

- What levels of care are available in your local network?
- How far would parents have to travel from an SCU or LNU to receive neonatal intensive care?
- What might be the emotional, social and financial impact on the family involved in a transfer for a higher level of care?

Your answers to the first two questions will vary enormously, depending on your location. Compare your answer to the last question with some of the potential responses given at https://study.sagepub.com/essentialchildnursing

ACTIVITY
ANSWER 32.1

WEBLINK:
BAPM WEBSITE

Neonatal infant and family care is mainly provided by neonatal nurses and paediatric doctors trained or undergoing training in the care of neonates. Nurses could be child or adult trained and, depending on where in the UK you are working, midwives. Neonatal nurses, who have undertaken further post-registration training and are identified as qualified in speciality (QIS), deliver and oversee all levels of care. Lower levels of care can be provided by nurses (not QIS), nursery nurses and/or healthcare assistants under supervision of a QIS nurse. Many neonatal units now have advanced neonatal nurse practitioners who often work as part of the medical team. Additional healthcare professionals contributing to neonatal care include pharmacists, physiotherapists, speech and language therapists, counsellors, family support nurses and paediatric surgeons, to name a few. Like many areas of nursing, neonatal units are experiencing staff shortages, particularly of staff that are QIS and are keen to recruit to 'grow their own' from both adult and child field-specific graduates.

WHAT'S THE EVIDENCE?

BLISS, the UK charity for babies that are born too soon, too small and too sick, published a report in October 2015 entitled *Bliss Baby Report 2015: Hanging in the Balance (England)*. This report explores the current state of nursing and medical staffing in neonatal units, why these units are under pressure and how they are coping. Read the report online via https://study.sagepub.com/essentialchildnursing

Compare the research findings with a neonatal unit affiliated with your university by organising a visit to speak with a neonatal nurse manager or a neonatal tutor/practice educator to discuss the following about medical and nursing staffing levels.

- Is the unit fully staffed?
- If not, which grades are they short of? What are the reasons for this?
- How is this affecting the unit's provision of care to infants and families?

WEBLINK:
BLISS BABY
REPORT

THE TERM, PRE-TERM AND GROWTH-RESTRICTED BABY

This overview presents a systems approach (rather than a nursing framework) to reflect the shared assessment approach used by the multidisciplinary (MDT) healthcare team in many neonatal units. The overview is followed by a diagrammatic representation of the interrelationships between neonatal systems to help you deliver holistic care (Figures 32.1–32.5).

The following tables (32.1–32.3) provide a concise introduction to the problem experienced by the pre-term, intrauterine growth-restricted and term infant requiring admission to the neonatal unit. The tables identify the system, problem, assessment and nursing action. Prior to assessment it is essential to understand the antenatal, intrapartum and resuscitation history to enable accurate assessment in context. Documentation of nursing observations and interventions must be completed in a timely manner.

Characteristics and problems associated with the small for gestational age infants (<10th centile on weight chart)

Small for gestational age (SGA) infants may be divided into two subgroups: small but appropriately and symmetrically grown (constitutionally small) and SGA due to growth restriction (IUGR). These infants present with asymmetrical growth.

Table 32.1 Overview: Characteristics and problems associated with the preterm infant (<37 weeks gestational age)

System	Characteristics and problems	Assessment skills	Nursing action
Neurological	Immature/fragile walls of cerebral blood vessels Less able to tolerate an asphyxia insult: risk of intraventricular haemorrhage (IVH) and periventricular leukomalacia Absent/immature suck swallow reflex Immature visual system: potential for the development of retinopathy of prematurity (ROP) Small muscle mass: inability to adopt flexed position conducive to development Poor muscle tone	Positioning Oxygen saturation appropriate to gestational age and oxygen requirement Method of feeding Susceptible to changing pressure	Appropriate position: head aligned with the body Nesting to maintain head aligned with body Physical boundaries Alternate positioning: supine, right lateral, left lateral Avoid prone position in the first week of life as head cannot be aligned with body
Respiratory	Immature lungs Lack of surfactant Apnoea of prematurity Transient tachypnoea of the newborn (TTN) Pneumonia Chronic lung disease (CLD) Signs of respiratory distress include the following: tachypnoea, nasal flaring, recession, grunting, asynchronous chest movement, cyanosis and apnoea	Stages of lung development Effect of lack of surfactant Pattern of breathing Assess need for degree of respiratory support Presence of apnoea and/or bradycardia	Assist with the administration of surfactant Monitor effects of surfactant Monitor O_2 saturation levels Adjust oxygen requirements in response to effects of surfactant Check blood gas in response to changes in ventilation: oxygen requirement, rising CO_2 Monitor respiratory function: colour, respiratory rate, work of breathing
Cardiovascular	Patent ductus arteriosus (PDA) with associated risk of IVH Low blood pressure (BP) Poorly oxygenated tissues: acidosis Bradycardia (<100)/tachycardia (>180)	Monitoring to include: – observe colour – SaO_2 level and variations – skin temperature – capillary refill time (CRT) – heart rate (HR) – note presence or absence of PDA – measure BP	Observe central and peripheral colour Continuous monitoring of oxygen saturation levels, respiratory and heart rate Note variations in oxygen saturation and bradycardia Take regular temperature measurements Use appropriate BP cuff and monitor blood pressure
Digestive	Immature gut motility limiting enteral intake Risk of necrotising enterocolitis (NEC) Limited enzyme activity Intermittent uncoordinated peristalsis	Pass oro/nasogastric tube (O/NGT) Check and monitor O/NGT; aspirate for volume, colour and pH Monitor tolerance Increase milk feeds slowly Observe abdomen for signs of distension/loopy bowels	Feed with colostrum initially then breast milk Trophic feeds Initiate small volume two hourly (once milk available) Increase as tolerated

System	Characteristics and problems	Assessment skills	Nursing action
Excretory	Feed intolerance due to immature gut motility Renal immaturity: inability to concentrate urine, inability to excrete acid load with low bicarbonate threshold resulting in metabolic acidosis	Observe abdomen for signs of distension, colour and presence of loopy bowels Monitor urinary output	Document status of abdomen Weigh nappies and measure urinary output (2-4mls/kg/hour) Test urine using clinistix reagent strips Document findings
Metabolic	Hypoglycaemia Lack of glycogen stores Immature gluconeogenic pathway Jaundice: high cell mass Immature liver: inadequate enzyme activity/immature enzymes	Assess glucose levels Issue that may increase energy consumption (e.g. infection, procedures, pain, respiratory distress, activity, handling, work of breathing) Assess serum bilirubin (SBR)	Monitor glucose levels Provide adequate glucose intake; i.e. breast milk, IV fluids, TPN Minimal handling to conserve infant energy Monitor SBR levels Plot levels on the appropriate treatment threshold graphs and initiate treatment when indicated (NICE Guidelines CG 98, 2016)
Skin	Immature skin Iatrogenic injury Transepidermal water loss	Daily assessment of skin Soft bedding to prevent pressure injury Check position of ears if infant wearing hat	Nurse in incubator set to 36°C Humidified environment (80-100%) Avoid use/minimise tape on infant's skin and where unavoidable use specialist tape (e.g. Siltape®) to secure dressings Use Apeel® to remove tape from immature skin Avoid the use of ECG electrodes on extremely immature skin (<26 weeks gestation) Nurse the very immature infant on 100% cotton or sateen sheets
Skeletal	Immature and soft bone Risk of metabolic bone disease Exacerbation of respiratory distress	Assess position	Promote bone mineralisation Administer vitamins and phosphate supplements as prescribed Use nests/rolls to support baby's position Ensure baby is in flexed position Position to help baby establish midline, hand to hand, and hand to mouth
Immunity	Relatively immature immune system (immunity transferred by mother in last trimester) Skin integrity breached by IV cannula/central lines	Documentation Prevent Assess for signs of infection and extravasation	Strict handwashing Universal precautions Weekly screening (as per local policy) Review stop date for antibiotics Hourly documentation of lines, sites and pump pressures Access 'plastics' team in the event of an extravasation injury Awareness of extravasation protocol Aseptic technique when accessing vascular devices

Infants who are SGA and are small but appropriately and symmetrically grown (constitutionally small) experience an insult in the first trimester, during embryogenesis. This results in a failure of growth which is sustained throughout pregnancy. The infant is undersized with fewer cells, but these cells grow normally. Causes include intrauterine infection, genetic abnormalities, smoking and alcohol. All can affect long-term prognosis.

Infants who are SGA due to growth restriction (IUGR) and who present with asymmetrical growth often experience an insult in the second to third trimester due to a lack of nutrition (starved). This results in slow/failure in weight gain, while head circumference is not affected. There is little subcutaneous fat, the skin may appear loose and thin, the muscle mass is greatly decreased, notably on the buttocks and thighs. The infant often has a wide-eyed anxious appearance. These infants can experience many potential problems (Table 32.2).

Term babies are admitted to the neonatal unit due to congenital abnormalities, antepartum/intrapartum events, maternal and environmental pregnancy related issues. A summary of conditions can be found in Table 32.3.

Table 32.2 Potential problems of the small for gestational age (SGA) infant due to growth restriction

Problems	Effect	Assessment	Nursing action
Perinatal asphyxia	Reduced oxygen is poorly tolerated and the impact may not be seen until later in life	Observation of vital signs, skin colour and capillary refill time (CRT) Appropriate positioning of saturation probe Observation of skin and frequent position change	Maintain oxygen saturation levels within the desired values for gestational age
Hypoglycaemia	Reduced energy to the brain and body tissues Apnoea and bradycardia	Assess glucose level Assess response to handling Assess physiological signs and behaviour that may increase energy expenditure	Ensure delivery of prescribed nutrition Monitor nutritional intake: 10% dextrose, TPN, enteral feeds Tolerance to enteral feeds Monitor glucose levels and document Initiate hypoglycaemia policy
Polycythaemia	Viscous circulation resulting in poor oxygenation to the tissues Low oxygen saturation levels Renal thrombi Blood in urine	Colour Temperature Peripheral temperature Blood gas SBR Hb/Haematocrit level	Monitor and document oxygen levels Test urine for the presence of blood Monitor SBR levels Plot levels on the appropriate treatment threshold graphs and initiate treatment when indicated (NICE Guidelines CG 98, 2016)
Thermal instability	Large surface area and small body mass increases risk of hypothermia, acidosis, hypoglycaemia and poor growth	Colour and temperature of peripherals Core temperature Assess temperature control Weight gain	Monitor closely to exclude other causes, i.e. infection Nurse infant in an incubator and maintain a neutral thermal environment to minimise energy and oxygen consumption Transfer to cot when infant is maintaining own temperature and achieving growth Ease the transition to cot by the initial use of heated mattress Monitor temperature and weight gain (aim for 15-25g/kg/day)

Table 32.3 Conditions of term babies requiring admission to the neonatal unit

Condition	Effect	Assessment	Nursing action
Congenital abnormalities			
Congenital diaphragmatic hernia (CDH)	Perforation of the diaphragm results in the abdominal organs (e.g. the stomach, liver, spleen, intestines) entering the chest cavity, causing compression of developing lungs May occur on left or right (most severe due to larger right lung) Difficult to achieve lung expansion due to pressure from organs in chest Air in the stomach may exacerbate the situation by reducing available space for lung expansion Resuscitation: infant is intubated; do not bag and mask Inflation breaths are given once infant intubated	Colour Chest movement Heart rate Dextrocardia	Stabilisation/pre-op care: – pass O/NGT (size 8Fr) and aspirate stomach contents, maintain on free drainage – no hand bagging Provide supportive care: – intubation and ventilation – paralysis and sedation – inotropic support – pain/discomfort management – IV fluids/TPN Blood gas monitoring Check glucose levels regularly Bilirubin measurement Monitor urinary output (2–4mls/ kg/hour)
Tracheoesophageal atresia/fistula	The upper part of the oesophagus ends in a blind pouch and does not connect to the lower oesophagus Swallowed saliva gathers in the upper pouch and if untreated may be aspirated If the baby feeds, milk fills the pouch overflowing increasing the risk of aspiration The oesophagus must grow to enable anastomosis of the upper and lower pouch; this may take many weeks Baby must remain hospitalised during this period of growth Nutrition is provided via a gastrostomy	Assess colour Presence of mucous at mouth Access success in passing O/NGT, if resistance felt stop procedure	Protecting the lungs by preventing aspiration of pouch contents is essential Pass an 8Fr. replogle tube into the pouch end, attach the end of tube to a continuous low suction (5KPa) Flush the replogle tube every 15 minutes with 0.5ml of NaCl 0.9% to prevent blockage of tube, documenting all flushes Monitor viscosity of mucous; if thick a larger flush may be required (1ml) Observe closely during flushing and ensure volume of flush is returned Prevent oral aversion by providing non-nutritive sucking
Antepartum/intrapartum events			
Perinatal asphyxia due to: – antepartum or intrapartum haemorrhage	Lack of oxygen delivered to the tissues results in: – brain deprived of oxygen – raised CO_2, raised lactic acid (>2mmol/L) – low glucose level (<2.5mmol/L)	Colour Tone Activity Chest movement Respiratory rate	Assist with resuscitation: – dry infant, consider passive cooling – maintain clear airway – provide inflation breaths

(Continued)

Table 32.3 (Continued)

Condition	Effect	Assessment	Nursing action
– foetal distress due to prolonged labour	– abnormal brain activity – possible seizures	Oxygenation status Glucose level Blood gas	– measure O_2 saturation levels – check blood gas and glucose level Once stabilised transfer infant to the NNU Initiate appropriate monitoring Provide respiratory support Provide nutritional support: IV fluids (10% dextrose initially) Commence cooling if infant meets the criteria Keep parents informed
Shoulder dystocia	Baby's head is delivered, but one shoulder becomes stuck behind the mother's pubic bone, delaying the birth of the baby's body Prolonged labour Brachial plexus injury (BPI) which may cause loss of movement to the arm Most common injury is Erb's Palsy, usually temporary and movement returns within hours or days Sometimes infants can suffer brain damage if they do not get enough oxygen due to delayed delivery	Colour Tone Activity Chest movement Respiratory rate Oxygenation status Tone, position and movement of affected limb	Support shoulder and arm Provide comfort measures Provide analgesia for pain Careful dressing of the infant to prevent discomfort Support and keep parents informed
Fractured clavicle	Sometimes shoulder dystocia can cause other injuries including fracture of the infant's arm or shoulder In the majority of cases these heal well	Use appropriate pain tool to assess level of pain/discomfort	Provide comfort measures Administer analgesia as required Reduce discomfort by carefully dressing and positioning Use figure of 8 support if indicated Support parents
Cardiac: acyanotic heart problems – patent ductus arteriosus (PDA) – atrial septal defect (ASD) – ventricular septal defect (VSD)	PDA results in increased pulmonary blood flow from the aorta across the ductus arteriosus into the pulmonary artery; this results in increased blood flow to the lungs (left to right shunt) Reduced systemic blood flow Increased oxygen requirement ASD less significant (atria are filling chambers) than VSD (ventricles are pumping chambers); mixing of arterial and venous blood more significant by lowering oxygen to the systemic circulation	Assessment is focused on cardiac output: – observe central and peripheral colour – assess CRT – oxygenation saturation levels – blood pressure	Maintain adequate gas exchange Monitor oxygen requirement Maintain saturation levels within the desired values (based on gestational age and oxygen dependency) Support parents

Condition	Effect	Assessment	Nursing action
Cardiac: Cyanotic heart problems e.g. Tetralogy of Fallot	Cyanosis Respiratory distress Acidosis	Colour Femoral pulses Four limb blood pressure	Respiratory support as required SaO_2 levels are prescribed Administer Prostaglandin E1 Monitor for apnoea Prepare infant and parents for transfer to the cardiac centre

Environmental and pregnancy related events

Condition	Effect	Assessment	Nursing action
Maternal diabetes which can be: – insulin dependent – gestational diabetes – type II diabetes	The foetus receives a higher than normal level of glucose from the maternal blood (via the umbilical vein) Foetal insulin axis is independent of the mother Infant produces a corresponding level of insulin to metabolise the glucose In the postpartum period the infant experiences a period of adaptation and is dependent on an exogenous supply of glucose while at the same time continues to produce high levels of insulin The effect is hypoglycaemia blood glucose level <2.5mmol/L, which if uncorrected may cause irreversible brain damage Increased risk of RDS, congenital abnormality, polycythaemia, hypocalcaemia and jaundice	Colour Tone Activity Heart rate Respiratory rate Glucose level	Check and monitor glucose levels at regular intervals to prevent hypoglycaemia Initiate hypoglycaemia policy Provide a suitable glucose supply Administer IV fluids (10% dextrose) Support mother to breastfeed or provide formula Cautious weaning of IV fluids to ensure maintenance of safe glucose levels Measure blood gas and bilirubin levels

Maternal substance abuse

Condition	Effect	Assessment	Nursing action
Neonatal abstinence syndrome most commonly due to: – alcohol – cocaine – heroin – cannabis	Withdrawal symptoms can affect all systems and signs and symptoms may include: – irritability – unsettled – high-pitched cry – difficult to console and settle – hyperactive – higher than normal demand for energy – high temperature – sneezing – seizures	Observe the baby at rest and post feed Note all activity at rest and when awake Frequency of feeds Vital signs	Appropriate environment: quiet part of the nursery with reduced lighting Loose clothing Comfort measures Nutritional support: baby may demand frequent feeds Complete withdrawal chart and monitor score Administer morphine as prescribed to manage symptoms Support parents and family Consider safeguarding issues MDT approach to discharge planning

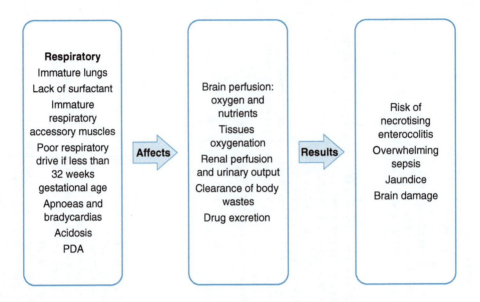

Figure 32.1   How a problem arising in the respiratory system can affect other systems

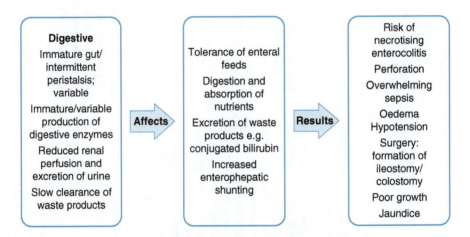

Figure 32.2   How a problem arising in the digestive system can affect other systems

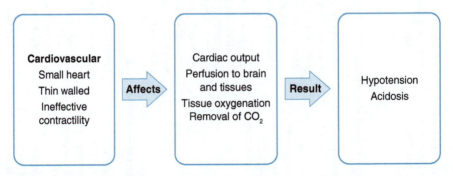

Figure 32.3   How a problem arising in the cardiovascular system affects oxygenation to the brain, tissues and removal of waste products

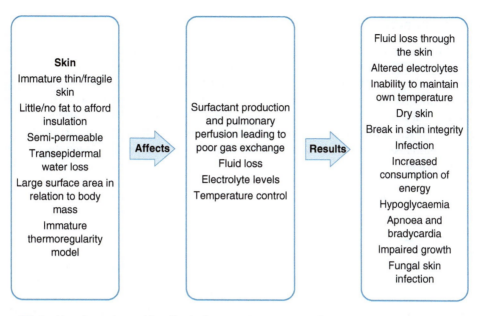

Figure 32.4 How immature skin affects temperature control, fluid loss, infection and energy consumption

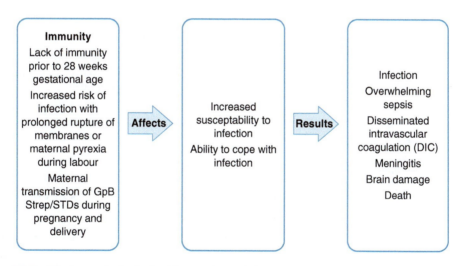

Figure 32.5 The impact of a lack of immunity on infant morbidity and mortality

ENVIRONMENTAL CHALLENGES TO THE INFANT

The neonatal environment compared to the intrauterine environment is hostile and provides the preterm and sick neonate with challenges. These challenges create risks and if not managed can impact on the infant and family journey through the neonatal unit by undermining treatment and increasing morbidity and mortality. These risks include infection and the influences of light and noise, and pain resulting from disease state and care interventions required to manage their condition.

Neonatal infection

Despite advances in neonatal care, neonatal infection remains a significant cause of neonatal morbidity and mortality, particularly for the IUGR and pre-term infant whose host defences are poor (Bedford Russell, 2015). The presentation of infection in the neonate is generalised or often expressed as non-specific (see Table 32.4). As a result we have difficulty diagnosing sepsis early. Treatment is based on a total reliance of killing the identified organism by using appropriate antibiotics (Bedford Russell, 2015). The consequences of neonatal infection can include meningitis, septicaemia, septic shock, disseminated intravascular coagulation (DIC), poor developmental and neurological outcome and death (see Figure 32.5).

Table 32.4 Signs of infection

System	Signs
Neurological	Irritability, listlessness/lethargy, sucks poorly, unresponsive, high-pitched cry, jitteriness, full or bulging fontanelle, hypo/hypertonic seizure activity, unstable temperature
Cardiovascular	Tachycardia, pale, mottled poor cutaneous circulation, capillary refill > 3 seconds
Respiratory	Tachypnoea, apnoea, nasal flaring, recession grunting, cyanosis
Gastrointestinal	Vomiting, diarrhoea, abdominal distension, poor weight gain, 'not interested in feeding'
Hepatic	Jaundice, altered coagulation, hypo/hyperglycaemia
Integumentary	Petechia, rash, heat and redness in an infected area
Immunological	Neutropenia, neutrophilia, thrombocytopenia, raised C-reactive protein (CRP)
Own learning	
Tacit or intuitive	'Just not right'; 'Handled better yesterday'

Table 32.5 Comparison of early and late onset infection

	Early onset infection	Late onset infection
Onset	<72 hours	>72 hours
Source	Mother's genital tract	Postnatal environment
		Mother's genital tract
Organism	Group B streptococcus	E. coli
	Listeriosis	Pseudomonas
		Klebsiella
		Group B streptococcus
Disease presentation	Fulminant	Insidious
	Multisystem	Focal
		Pneumonia frequent
		Meningitis frequent

A&P LINK

To remind yourself of the relevant anatomy and physiology, please view the A&P link: 'Intrinsic and extrinsic coagulation pathway' at https://study.sagepub.com/essentialchildnursing

A&P LINK 32.1:
COAGULATION
PATHWAY

SEE ALSO
CHAPTER 25

Three groups of infection have been identified: transplacental or congenital infections (e.g. toxoplasmosis, hepatitis, parvovirus, rubella, cytomegalovirus and herpes), intrapartum or early onset infections, and finally postpartum or late onset infections. See Table 32.5 for a comparison of early and late onset infection.

Nursing care is supportive. The key intervention in reducing nosocomial or late onset infection sepsis is to ensure all who interact with the infant adhere to the neonatal unit hand-washing policy in order to prevent cross-infection. Nurses need to lead by example and ensure that all who interact with infants follow unit guidelines. Parents taught how to correctly hand wash on their first visit generally go on to demonstrate good technique, ensuring all those who come into contact with their infant comply with unit policy.

ENVIRONMENTAL STRESSORS FOR THE BABY

The uterine environment is temperature consistent and dark, and as the foetus matures it provides a supportive positional environment with natural maternal noises and a muffled outside world. This environment ensures appropriate infant growth and development. When an infant is born prematurely or ill, the safe and nurturing environment is replaced by the neonatal unit which can be deemed hostile and not developmentally friendly. Increased survival and decreasing gestational age results in an infant less able to cope with the stresses of the neonatal environment, which include light, noise and pain.

Light

Circadian rhythms or how we respond to day and night are essential to wellbeing. They determine a range of biological activities including brainwave activity, hormone production, cell regeneration, sleep and feeding patterns (Robert, 2010). Fetal circadian rhythms are regulated by the mother, but lost if born early (Haumont, 2012). Pre-term eyes open more frequently and their thin lids are easily penetrated by the bright light of the neonatal environment (Robinson and Fielder, 1992). The bright and harsh lighting of this environment can lead to behavioural disorganisation, physiological instability, potentially ROP (Retinopathy of Prematurity) and disruption/deprivation of much-needed sleep (Haumont, 2012). Lighting in nurseries should be as natural as possible and adjustable, with directable procedural light available when needed. Many units now employ the use of cot covers and ensure periods when nursery lighting is dimmed if not off. These periods known as 'quiet time' or 'quiet hour' also address the other environmental stressor, noise.

Noise

Neonatal units provide 24-hour care and potentially 24 hours of varied but continuous noise. Unlike staff and parents, the infants cannot escape the sounds of the unit environment and are entirely dependent on us to regulate the levels of noise generated by equipment, care giving and talking. Intense and sustained noise may lead to physiological and behavioural instability, hearing deficits and delayed language acquisition (Brown, 2009). The nurse plays a key role in moderating noise levels in response to infant behavioural cues. Kuhl and Melzoff (1984) suggest that noise in the NICU may be a contributing factor in delayed parent–infant interaction as it masks meaningful sounds.

Neonatal pain

Neonates feel acute and chronic pain. The causes may be related to procedural activities, handling/care and of course illness itself. The infant's responses to pain are also influenced by gestational age, previous experience of pain and sleep state (Anand, 2015). Pain results in physiological and behavioural instability in the short term (Stevens, 1999) and potential long-term neurological damage, developmental delays and behavioural problems resulting in learning difficulties (Mitchell and Boss, 2002).

Pain assessment is central to good neonatal care (Anand, 2015). A large number of multidimensional pain assessment tools, for procedural and acute pain, are available to practice. These assess specific physiological and behavioural responses, but are also dependent on the caregivers' subjective assessment (Anand, 2015). Pain relief is dependent on using the correct tool and staff appropriately trained in its use.

Pharmacological and non-pharmacological interventions, together or alone, can be used to prevent, reduce or eliminate neonatal pain. Opiates, like morphine, continue to be the drug of choice for many ventilated or surgical neonates with moderate to severe pain. The use of opiates still creates anxiety about their short- and long-term side effects (Kariholu et al., 2014). Oral sucrose is frequently used to manage single-event procedural pain. In addition to modulating the neonatal environment by reducing light and noise, a range of non-pharmacological interventions can be used to alleviate pain during procedures, encourage behavioural organisation and general comfort. These measures give parents an active role and include non-nutritive sucking, breastfeeding, swaddling, facilitated tucking, kangaroo care and touch by means of containment holding.

SEE ALSO
CHAPTER 3

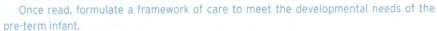

ACTIVITY 32.2: REFLECTIVE PRACTICE

WEBLINK:
CONFESSIONS
OF A PREEMIE

A neonatal nurse has assumed the voice of a pre-term baby in order to help parents understand the different needs of their pre-term infant. The advice offered is not only relevant to parents but will provide you with insight into the pre-term infant's developmental needs in light of the environmental stressors just discussed. 'Confessions of a preemie' can be found at https://study.sagepub.com/essentialchildnursing

Once read, formulate a framework of care to meet the developmental needs of the pre-term infant.

✓

ACTIVITY
ANSWER 32.2

ENVIRONMENTAL CHALLENGES TO THE FAMILY

The following section will explore, by means of a case study, the environmental challenges that are experienced by parents and the family. A series of questions relating to the case study will be asked to enable you to gain an understanding of the family experience and journey and identify appropriate supportive strategies.

CASE STUDY 32.1: THE HUNTER FAMILY

Louise, Ian and Ted (aged 18 months) were on holiday in Lanzarote. On their last day there, Louise, 24^{+5} weeks pregnant, went into premature labour. The family were transferred to Las Palmas, where Louise delivered Hugh. He weighed 660 grams, required ventilation, suffered an intraventricular haemorrhage and at 4 weeks required ligation of his patent ductus arteriosus. Hugh then developed necrotising enterocolitis (NEC), which was medically managed. His condition deteriorated and Hugh was baptised.

Hugh, 8 weeks old, was transferred to the UK for ongoing intensive care. Unfortunately, his local network NICU was closed to admissions, so Hugh transferred to a NICU outside the network for a few days, where Louise had her first cuddle with him.

Hugh's progress was slow. He made small steps forward and many large strides back. On arrival to his local NICU, complications from his original episode of NEC resulted in further bowel surgery. After three months Hugh was transferred to special care and appeared to be on the road to home. Due to further bowel complications and sepsis, Hugh moved back and forth between IC/HD and SC. On his third attempt he managed to stay in special care and make the required progress in feeding and growing to be considered for discharge. On day 246 Hugh was discharged home.

To celebrate Hugh's first birthday and as a thank you, Ian posted a video, which captures Hugh's and his family's journey. This can be seen at https://study.sagepub.com/essentialchildnursing Explore the feelings and needs of Louise, Ian and Ted on Hugh's various admissions and transfers to receive the appropriate level of care, by answering the following questions:

VIDEO LINK 32.2: HUGH'S JOURNEY

- What feelings might Louise and Ian be experiencing as a result of Hugh's unexpected arrival and subsequent admission to the neonatal unit in Las Palmas?
- What feelings and issues may arise for Louise and Ian when Hugh is re-patriated to the UK, and then as he moves between nurseries as his condition improves and deteriorates?

CASE STUDY ANSWER 32.1

An unanticipated early end to a normal pregnancy has resulted in Louise and Ian having to reappraise their expectations and adjust to a new reality. All babies born <26 weeks gestation should be cared for in a NICU. Once the baby is in the recovery stage a lower level of care is required. This can be delivered by transferring the baby within the unit to a special care nursery or transferring the baby to another hospital to deliver that lower level of care. Both transfers result in leaving a familiar environment and can result in a range of different emotions.

Supportive care offered to the family is informed by research which provides an understanding of the parent's reality. A key role of the neonatal nurse is to help minimise the impact of baby–family separation and role loss, and to promote parental adaptation.

ACTIVITY 32.3: REFLECTIVE PRACTICE

- Considering the case study of the Hunter family, what strategies can you employ to help the parent deal with their feelings?
- When and how would you promote parent-infant attachment?

ACTIVITY ANSWER 32.3

SEE ALSO
CHAPTER 1

> Family-centred care is at the heart of neonatal practice; every care is taken to involve the whole family in the care of their baby ... siblings are not ignored – they are encouraged to draw their new brother or sister pictures or bring in toys.
>
> **Sacha, 3rd-year children's nursing student**

PRACTICE
SCENARIO
32: SUNITA &
FAMILY

ACTIVITY 32.4: RELECTIVE PRACTICE

- What might be the impact of the neonatal environment on family-centred care?
- What strategies would you employ to involve the whole family in the care of their baby?

ACTIVITY
ANSWER 32.4

Health promotion commences on the admission of the baby and family to the unit and continues throughout to discharge. Handwashing, the first skill taught to the parents, is essential to infant well-being. Mothers require support to initiate and maintain breastfeeding. The feeding of expressed breast milk not only provides a milk best tolerated but the non-nutritional benefits play an important role in preventing conditions such as NEC. Health promotion materials should be widely available in a range of languages and should include guidance on newborn screening and the prevention of sudden infant death syndrome (SIDS).

VIDEO
LINK 32.3:
BUMP TO
BREAST FEEDING

ACTIVITY 32.5: REFLECTIVE PRACTICE

- How can you support Louise to initiate and maintain her lactation? You might find it helpful to watch the video *From Bump to Breastfeeding* via https://study.sagepub.com/essentialchildnursing
- What routine newborn screening takes place in the UK?
- What are the implications for screening an infant admitted to a neonatal unit? Access the screening website for health professionals via https://study.sagepub.com/essentialchildnursing
- What advice should be offered to Louise and Ian on how to prevent SIDS while Hugh is on the unit and in preparation for discharge? Access the Lullaby Trust website.

WEBLINK:
SCREENING
WEBSITE

WEBLINK:
LULLABY
TRUST

ACTIVITY
ANSWER 32.5

SAFEGUARDING STOP POINT

Safeguarding in a neonatal unit is less obvious than other areas where parents assume full responsibility and care for their children. All neonates are vulnerable and their needs must be considered and infant/family support provided throughout their journey to identify and mitigate problematic issues at the earliest opportunity. Clear-cut safeguarding situations include known maternal substance abuse and domestic violence.

- What early warning signs might alert you in parent behaviour/actions that there may be a safeguarding issue?

SAFEGUARDING
STOP POINT
ANSWER 32.1

Preparing parents for discharge commences on admission. Discharge planning is essential to ensure parents can make a seamless transition from hospital to community.

SEE ALSO
CHAPTER 29

ACTIVITY 32.6: REFLECTIVE PRACTICE

- What feelings might Louise and Ian have while preparing for and at the discharge of Hugh from the neonatal unit?
- What parentcraft and support are required to help make a smooth transition home?

ACTIVITY
ANSWER 32.6

Go to https://study.sagepub.com/essentialchildnursing for tips on preparing for placements and health promotion in neonatal care.

PLACEMENT
ADVICE 32:
CARE OF THE
NEONATE

CHAPTER SUMMARY

In this chapter we have looked at the care of a neonate. Key messages include:

HEALTH
PROMOTION 32:
NEONATAL
TERMS

- Neonatal care and service provision continues to evolve in order to optimise neonatal outcomes
- Neonatal nursing offers a challenging and rewarding career pathway. Quality care is ensured by ongoing professional development to achieve QIS status
- Delivery of appropriate and optimal care requires an understanding of the similarities and differences between infants born preterm, small for gestational age or with problems at term and knowledge of the interrelationships between the infant's body systems
- Neonatal care should be baby-centred, with parents the key caregivers working in partnership with and supported by the healthcare team

BUILD YOUR BIBLIOGRAPHY

Books

- Petty, J. (2015) *Bedside Guide for Neonatal Care: Learning Tools to Support Practice*. London: Palgrave.

  A useful bedside resource providing the student/novice neonatal nurse with the tools needed to support practice.

- Bliss (2011) *The Bliss Baby Charter Standards*, 2nd edn. London: Bliss Publications.

  A practical guide to help neonatal units provide the best possible family-centred care for premature and sick babies.

Journal articles

Go to https://study.sagepub.com/essentialchildnursing for further free online journal articles related to this chapter.

FURTHER
READING:
ONLINE
JOURNAL
ARTICLES

- Rossman, B., Kratovil, A.L., Greene, M.M., Engstrom, J.L. and Meier, P.P. (2013) '"I have faith in my milk": the meaning of milk for mothers of very low birth weight infants hospitalized in the neonatal intensive care unit'. *Journal of Human Lactation*, 29 (3): 359-65.

Mothers of pre-term infants are actively encouraged to express breast milk predominately for its therapeutic or non-nutritional benefits; this article explores the mother's perspective of the importance of her milk to her infant's well-being.

- Strandås, M. and Fredrikson, S-T.D. (2015) 'Ethical challenges in neonatal nursing'. *Nursing Ethics*, 22 (8): 901-12.

Advancements in neonatal technology and pharmacology combined with our understanding of neonatal pathophysiology have led to the survival of neonates at the edges of viability. Neonatal care provides many ethical dilemmas. This research article is useful as it provides insight into the ethical challenges that can face the neonatal nurse in her daily work, rather than the obvious life and death decisions associated with neonatal care.

- Stuart, M. and Melling, S. (2014) 'Understanding nurses' and parents' perceptions of family-centred care'. *Nursing Children and Young People*, 26 (7): 16-20.

Family-centred care is an essential component of neonatal care. Therefore, In order to work effectively together and facilitate optimal parental partnership, it is essential that you explore parental and nursing perceptions of the concept.

- Trajkovski, S., Schmied, V., Vickers, M. and Jackson, D. (2015) 'Using appreciative inquiry to bring neonatal nurses and parents together to enhance family-centred care: a collaborative workshop'. *Journal of Child Health*, 9: 239-53.

This article is useful as it considers strategies that can be used to enhance the delivery of family centred-care in the neonatal unit.

Weblinks

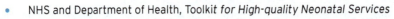

Go to https://study.sagepub.com/essentialchildnursing for further weblinks related to this chapter.

FURTHER READING: WEBLINKS

- NHS and Department of Health, Toolkit *for High-quality Neonatal Services*

http://webarchive.nationalarchives.gov.uk/20130107105354/www.dh.gov.uk/prod_consum_dh/groups/dh_digitalassets/@dh/@en/@ps/@sta/@perf/documents/digitalasset/dh_108435.pdf

The Toolkit, originally developed for England, now identifies the structure and principles need to deliver neonatal care across the four countries of the UK.

- Royal College of Nursing, *Career, Education and Competence Framework for Neonatal Nursing in the UK: RCN Guidance*

www.rcn.org.uk/professional-development/publications/pub-004641

A useful document to enable you to explore the possible career opportunities in neonatal nursing.

- Best Beginnings, *From Bump to Breastfeeding*

www.bestbeginnings.org.uk/from-bump-to-breastfeeding

A set of films following the journey of mothers wishing to breastfeed their babies, providing detailed information on how to breastfeed successfully.

- Best Beginnings, *Small Wonders*

www.bestbeginnings.org.uk/small-wonders

A set of 12 short films following 14 families through their neonatal unit journey.

ACE YOUR ASSESSMENT

Revise what you have learned by visiting https://study.sagepub.com/essentialchildnursing

- Test yourself with multiple-choice and short-answer questions
- Do the chapter activities in the book and check your answers online

ONLINE
QUIZZES &
ACTIVITY
ANSWERS

GREAT FOR
REVISION!

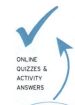

REFERENCES

Anand, K. (2015) 'Pain assessment in preterm neonates'. *Pediatrics*, 119 (3): 605–7.

Bedford Russell, A. (2015) 'Neonatal sepsis'. *Paediatrics and Child Health*, 25 (6): 271–5.

Bliss (2015) *Bliss Baby Report 2015: Hanging in the Balance (England)*. London: Bliss.

British Association of Perinatal Medicine (BAPM) (2011) *Categories of Care*, 3rd edn. London: BAPM.

Brown, G. (2009) 'NICU noise and the preterm infant'. *Neonatal Network*, 28 (3): 165–73.

Haumont, D. (2012) 'Environment and early development care', in G. Buonnocore, R. Bracci and M. Weindling (eds) *Neonatology: A Practical Approach to Neonatal Disease*. Milan: Spinger-Verlag.

Kariholu, U., Banerjee, J., Selkirk, L., Warren, I., Chow, P. and Godambe, S. (2014) 'Managing neonatal pain while rationalizing the use of morphine using a structured systematic approach'. *Infant*, 10 (1): 30–4.

Kuhl, P.K. and Meltzoff, A.N. (1984) 'The intermodal representation of speech in infants'. *Infant Behavior and Development*, 7 (3): 361–81.

Mitchell, A. and Boss, B. (2002) 'Adverse effects of pain on the nervous systems of newborns and young children: a review of the literature'. *Journal of Neuroscience Nursing*, 34 (5): 228–36.

NICE (2016) *Jaundice in Newborn Babies under 28 days*. Clinical guideline [CG98]. Available at: www.nice.org.uk/guidance/cg98?unlid=12491833120165225718 (last accessed 29 May 2017).

Robert, J. (2010) *Circadian Rhythm and Human Health*. Available at: www.photobiology.info/Roberts-CR.html (last accessed 29 May 2017).

Robinson, J. and Fielder, A.R. (1992) 'Light and the neonatal eye'. *Behavioural Brain Research*, 49 (1): 51–5.

Stevens, B. (1999) 'Pain in infants', in M. McCaffery and C. Pasero (eds) *Pain: Clinical Manual*, 2nd edn. St. Louis, MO: Mosby.

CARE OF CHILDREN AND YOUNG PEOPLE WITH A MALIGNANT CONDITION

33

JAYNE PRICE AND SUZANNE COULSON

THIS CHAPTER COVERS

- Childhood cancer
- Presentation
- Psychosocial impact of childhood cancer
- Treatment of childhood cancer
- Team working in childhood cancer care

> " We had to be strong at the time it was happening and just get on with it. The kindness of the hospital staff was really important to help us get through it. Until you've gone through something like this yourself it's really hard to understand how horrific your child being diagnosed with cancer really is.
>
> **Aimee, parent** "

Visit https://study.sagepub.com/essentialchildnursing to access a wealth of online resources for this chapter – watch out for the margin icons throughout the chapter.

INTRODUCTION

Cancer is a group of diseases in which cells grow uncontrollably and can spread from the originating site to another part of the body. Childhood cancer affects 1 in 500 children with approximately 1,600 children (under 15) in the United Kingdom (UK) diagnosed with cancer each year (CCLG, 2015).

The word 'cancer' is generally synonymous with death. Receiving such a diagnosis plunges children and families into a state of disarray and disruption. Great improvements in long-term survival have been noted in recent years, with estimates suggesting over 82 per cent of children are now cured, compared with fewer than 30 per cent between 1962 and 1971 (Macmillan, 2014). Improvements have been attributed to clinical trials and collaborative working regarding treatment protocols. Improvements in supportive care have also been noted, enhanced through some key publications. NICE (2005) produced guidance on the healthcare children with cancer should receive. Further, Children's Cancer Measures (2013) provide a benchmark for services throughout the UK aiming to improve care for patients and families. Cancer is classed as a 'life threatening' condition in that curative treatment can be feasible but can fail. While treatment is given from a Children's Cancer and Leukaemia Group (CCLG) treatment centre, supportive care is sometimes provided in shared care centres (hospitals more local to the child's home).

The parent voice cited at the beginning of the chapter indicates that despite increased survival rates the impact of childhood cancer is wide ranging, meaning children and families require intense care throughout treatment as well as ongoing support for years afterwards. This chapter is going to unravel the needs of children and families and highlight the nurse's role during diagnosis, treatment and beyond.

CHILDHOOD CANCER

Cancers in childhood often result from DNA changes in cells that take place very early in life, unlike adult cancers, which often have links to environmental or lifestyle factors. While causes of childhood cancer are generally unknown, certain genetic and familial traits are thought to influence the development of some cancers.

Childhood cancer generally falls into the following groupings:

- Haematological malignancies – arising in blood-forming tissue (leukaemia and lymphoma)
- Solid tumours – arising from tissue or organ (sarcoma, blastoma, germ cell)

The incidence of different types of childhood cancer is illustrated in Figure 33.1.

Haematological malignancies can spread out with the blood and lymph system into the cerebrospinal fluid (CSF) or occasionally cause skin lesions. Solid tumours may be confined to the primary site or may have local or distant metastatic spread. While metastatic disease can be cured, it is more challenging, and longer, more intense treatment is required.

Common childhood cancers

Leukaemia is the commonest form of childhood cancer, with approximately 400 new cases diagnosed each year within the UK. Leukaemia is the uncontrolled proliferation of immature blood cells (blasts) following an abnormality occurring during development in either the lymphoid or myeloid blood cell line. Acute lymphoblastic leukaemia (ALL) accounts for 80–85 per cent of diagnoses, and while it occurs in any age, it is most common in children under 4 years (Macmillan, 2014). Most of the remaining 15–20 per cent of children present with acute myeloid leukaemia (AML). Chronic leukaemia is very rare in childhood.

Brain tumours are the second most common childhood cancer and commonest solid tumour. They are usually named after the type of cells and area of the central nervous system (CNS) in which they develop. Most CNS tumours start in glial cells, the supporting cells of the brain. These tumours are known as gliomas and include astrocytomas, ependymomas and oligodendrogliomas. Another group arise from embryonal cells and include medulloblastomas and PNETs (primitive neuro-ectodermal tumours).

Main types of childhood cancer: children aged 0–14 years
United Kingdom 2001 to 2010
Based on data provided by National Registry of Childhood Tumours

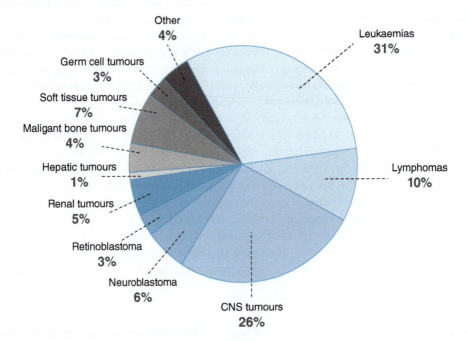

Figure 33.1 Incidence of types of cancer in children

Available at: www.childrenwithcancer.org.uk/childhood-cancer-types
Reproduced with permission of Children with Cancer UK

Other childhood cancers

A number of malignancies are seen almost exclusively in young children, others more often in the older child or young adult and some in both children and adults – though treatment and prognosis can be quite different (Table 33.1).

PRESENTATION

Children can present with a wide variety of symptoms depending on the condition and position of the tumour, its size and the impact on tissues and organs close by. In some cases reaching a diagnosis can be protracted. Symptoms can seem vague and taken in isolation may appear like regular childhood illnesses (see Figure 33.2).

Diagnostic tests aim to:

- Achieve an accurate diagnosis and establish the extent of disease
- Assess the child's general health status

Investigations performed are dependent on the type of cancer suspected. Some commonly used tests are listed below.

Table 33.1 Other types of childhood cancer

Type of cancer and age group	Common types	Organ or tissue of origin
Sarcomas – arising in bone and soft tissue All ages but especially older children and teenagers	Osteosarcoma	Bone, often the long bones
	Ewing's sarcoma and peripheral primitive neuroectodermal tumour (PPNET)	Bone or soft tissue
	Rhabdomyosarcoma	Primitive muscle cells, occurring in soft tissue almost anywhere in the body
Embryonal tumours (blastomas) – arising in immature embryonal tissue Mainly pre-school aged children	Neuroblastoma	Sympathetic nervous system pathway, often developing in the adrenal glands
	Retinoblastoma	Retina, small number of cases are bilateral
	Nephroblastoma (Wilm's tumour)	Kidney, small number of cases are bilateral
	Hepatoblastoma	Liver
Germ cell tumours	Germ cell tumours (GCT)	Immature tissue destined to become the ovaries or testes; include yolk-sac tumours, germinomas, embryonal carcinomas, teratomas and immature teratomas
Lymphoma	Non-Hodgkin's lymphoma	B or T lymphocytes – lymphoblastic, Burkitts and large cell
	Hodgkin's disease	Lymphatic system, distinguished by presence of Reed Steinberg cells
Rare tumours Occasionally in children – more common in adults	Carcinoma	Lining tissue (epithelial tissue) – possible sites include adrenal gland, nasopharynx, thyroid gland
	Melanoma	Arising in melanocytes, usually in the skin

The identification of risk factors is an increasingly important area enabling treatment protocols to be tailored more specifically for individuals who have, for example, genetic factors present that can influence overall prognosis (Bailey and Skinner, 2010).

Continued, unexplained weight loss

Headaches, often with early morning vomiting

Increased swelling or persistent pain in bones, joints, back, or legs

Lump or mass, especially in the abdomen, neck, chest, pelvis, or armpits

Development of excessive bruising, bleeding, or rash

Constant infections

A whitish colour behind the pupil

Nausea which persists or vomiting without nausea

Constant tiredness or noticeable paleness

Eye or vision changes which occur suddenly and persist

Recurrent or persistent fevers of unknown origin

Figure 33.2 Symptoms of childhood cancer

Source: Ped-Onc Resource Center (2015) *Signs of Childhood Cancer*. Available at: www.ped-onc.org/diseases/SOCC.html (last accessed 29 May 2017). Reproduced with permission.

Table 33.2 Diagnostic investigations (not exhaustive)

Investigation	Definition	Reason for investigation
Blood test (Full blood count (FBC)) and biochemistry	Peripheral blood sample	Presence of leukaemic (blast) cells Normal blood cell levels Biochemistry picture for renal and liver function
Bone marrow aspirate and trephine	Sample of bone marrow cells (aspirate) and segment of bone marrow (trephine) from hipbone. Performed under general anaesthetic	Presence, extent and type of leukaemia Presence of metastatic disease – solid tumours Also performed during treatment to monitor response
Lumbar puncture (LP)	Aspiration of cerebrospinal fluid (CSF) Performed under general anaesthetic	Establish if cancer cells have infiltrated the CSF in leukaemia or lymphoma Cytotoxic chemotherapy drugs can be given intrathecally during the LP
Ultrasound scan (U/S)	A non-invasive scan utilising high frequency sound waves to capture images inside the body, showing structure and movement of internal organs	Presence of a solid tumour or metastases Presence of testicular involvement in leukaemia
Chest X-ray	Ionising radiation used to take images of chest area	Presence of mediastinal mass, infiltrated lymph nodes (leukaemia or lymphoma) or tumour – primary or metastatic
CT (computerised tomography) scan	A CT scan using X-rays takes a series of images, providing a three-dimensional picture of organs inside the body. Provides more detail of internal organs, bones, soft tissues and blood vessels than ordinary X-rays	Presence, position and extent of primary tumour and existence of metastatic disease
MRI (magnetic resonance imaging) scan	Similar to CT but instead of X-rays MRI uses magnetism to build up a detailed picture of areas of the body. MRI is non-invasive but the machine noise can be frightening. A sedative or general anaesthetic may be used if the child will not lie still	Presence, position and extent of primary tumour, and existence of metastatic disease
Biopsy	Needle biopsy – a needle inserted through the skin into the tumour to remove a small part for examination. May be performed under local anaesthetic Open biopsy – under general anaesthetic an incision is made and a piece of tumour removed for examination	To identify the tumour type
Bone scan	A small amount of radioactive substance is injected into a vein and subsequently absorbed by the bones. Diseased bone is highlighted as it absorbs more than healthy bone	If a bone tumour is suspected or if a primary tumour may have spread to bones

When we first found out Jack had bone cancer I felt very guilty, thinking it was something I missed or did wrong.

Aimee, parent

SCENARIO 33.1: BELLE

Belle is 5 years old. Her mum had taken her to the GP repeatedly over the past six months. Initially Belle had a lingering ear infection, even after antibiotics. Mum then reported Belle being 'off form', with a poor appetite. She subsequently required further antibiotics for a sore throat. Mum felt the GP saw her as a paranoid mother. A few weeks later Belle experienced a nose bleed which settled spontaneously. Dad then noticed bruises on Belle's leg, but she explained she fell at school. Then Belle fell off her bike, complained of a painful wrist and her nose bled heavily again. Mum took Belle to the emergency department but felt under suspicion when the doctor, then the nurse, asked about the bruising. During a detailed history it was noted she was pale. Belle had her wrist X-rayed. An FBC was taken; her haemoglobin was low (anaemia), platelets were low (thrombocytopenia) and white cells raised. She was admitted to the children's ward and acute lymphoblastic leukaemia (ALL) was subsequently diagnosed. Mum and dad were in shock but felt angry that the diagnosis was delayed and that they were not listened to.

- Using knowledge of the physiology of blood, explain each of Belle's symptoms
- As well as FBC, what other investigations would be carried out?
- What might parental feelings be following the diagnosis? (The parent voice below may help you.)

CHECK YOUR
ANSWERS
ONLINE!

SCENARIO
ANSWER 33.1

ACTIVITY 33.1: REFLECTIVE PRACTICE

Remember, parents know their children. Professionals should hear and listen to their concerns. Think about how this could be applied to your practice.

SAFEGUARDING STOP POINT

Remember, children with low platelet counts in blood conditions such as leukaemia may present with bruising.

PSYCHOSOCIAL IMPACT OF CHILDHOOD CANCER

Communicating the news of the diagnosis is the point where the relationship with the team caring for the child commences and often continues over years.

The scenario about Belle and the parent voice above demonstrate how diagnosis of childhood cancer leads to profound emotional chaos for families. Practical disruption also occurs – for example, the immediate need to take time off work and reorganise routines around treatment. Such disruption instigates a change in family functioning, including reallocation or reorienting of roles.

SEE ALSO
CHAPTER 2

Family life was turned upside down. We were faced with the prospect of death of our precious child. There was nothing we could do. It was out of our control.

Aimee, parent

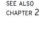

Reorganisation often involves the 'split family' (McCubbin et al., 2002) with, for example, one parent assuming responsibility for siblings while the other focuses on the sick child. This can be even more challenging for single parents or parents who may not have additional family to offer support.

> Having other children at home and having to leave them sometimes for 2–3 weeks at the start of Jack's treatment was really hard.
>
> **Aimee, parent**

Parenting the sick child becomes the parents' 'master status', influencing every aspect of life and somewhat overshadowing other roles. 'Master status' is described in sociological literature by Hughes (1945). The parent voice below demonstrates this effect.

> Everything we did and everywhere we went revolved around Greg's leukaemia and the restrictions and effects it had on him.
>
> **Aimee, parent**

ACTIVITY 33.2: CRITICAL THINKING

What social roles can become secondary when caring for their child with cancer becomes parents' master status?

ACTIVITY
ANSWER 33.2

Treatment and hospital become part of family life as families strive to create some sort of normality in an abnormal situation, alongside trying to 'battle' cancer (Price et al., 2012). Parents can feel isolated from their usual support networks (Jordan et al., 2015) and suffer exhaustion from juggling often competing demands of living through the uncertainty of their child's diagnosis and treatment (Rafii et al., 2014).

WHAT'S THE EVIDENCE?

Thoitis (1986) argued that social support helped families 'keep going' through cancer treatment and provided them with the practical resources, as well as the emotional sustenance, to keep strong amidst sustained uncertainty. Types of social support have been identified in the literature (for example Kaplan et al., 1977; Gottlieb, 1978; House, 1981). Commonalities indicate that three types are discernible:

- Informational - provision of advice, suggestions and information that a person can use to address problems
- Instrumental - involving the provision of tangible assistance and services that directly assist the person in need
- Emotional - involving the provision of empathy, love, trust and caring

WHAT'S THE
EVIDENCE?
ANSWER 33.1

ACTIVITY 33.3: CRITICAL THINKING

Chart the type of support needed to address each specific issue below.

- Mother becomes distressed during her child's first chemotherapy
- A sibling is asking questions about cancer; the parent is uncertain about what to say
- Parents do not feel ready to learn how to flush their child's central line
- A young person feels isolated during his treatment
- Parents express concerns about the financial implications of losing a salary and having to travel as a result of their child's cancer treatment

ACTIVITY
ANSWER 33.3

Remember that parents require support at different stages of their child's cancer journey, including on the completion of therapy and during the following months and years. Regular assessment is required.

> The end of treatment period can be fraught with emotions for parents: relief that treatment is over, gratitude to the team, anxiety that support is waning and fear that disease may return.
>
> **(Kirsty, ward manager)**

TREATMENT OF CHILDHOOD CANCER

Treatment takes the form of one or more of the following: chemotherapy, radiotherapy and surgery. For some children, high-dose chemotherapy followed by a haematopoietic stem cell transplant may be required. The role of immunotherapy is developing for certain conditions, for example neuroblastoma. Tests are required pre-treatment to ascertain organ function for toxicity monitoring. These will be repeated at regular intervals during and after treatment in order to establish any toxicity development, which may in turn require the adaptation of drugs or dosages or additional supportive care. The child will have a central line inserted (under general anaesthetic), enabling administration of drug therapy and supportive care. The disease and response to treatment is monitored at regular intervals.

Visit https://study.sagepub.com/essentialchildnursing to read about Riad and his treatment for rhabdomyosarcoma.

CASE STUDY
33. RIAD

Chemotherapy

Malignant conditions require cytotoxic chemotherapy, drugs which are toxic to cells and work by interfering with normal reproductive processes and cell division. Cytotoxic chemotherapy can be administered via oral and intravenous routes (bolus, short or continuous infusion) and occasionally intrathecally (given into the CSF). Children may require hospital admission for treatment or attend a day unit/outpatient department. Occasionally chemotherapy may be delivered at home; for example, children with ALL have ongoing oral medication for a number of months.

A&P LINK
33.1: CELL
CYCLE

The cell cycle is the formal process that all cells undergo in order to reproduce; including active stages where cells are dividing and a resting phase. To discover more about the cell cycle and cell division, please refer to the A&P link: 'Cell cycle' at https://study.sagepub.com/essentialchildnursing

Discover more about the cell cycle and cell division in the video on https://study.sagepub.com/essentialchildnursing

VIDEO LINK
33.1: CELL
DIVISION
CELL CYCLE

Cytotoxic drugs have different mechanisms and are active in different parts of the cell cycle. Consequently, several cytotoxic drugs are usually used in treatment protocols to complement each other's action. Standardised protocols have been developed, meaning that a child with a specific cancer would receive the same treatment regardless of their UK location.

As childhood cancer is rare, gaining insight into successful therapies is vital. Research conducted through clinical trials is incorporated into many treatment protocols.

ACTIVITY 33.4: TEAMWORKING

Read about the CCLG and the regional centres at www.cclg.org.uk. What is their role in treating children with cancer?

WHAT'S THE EVIDENCE?

Woodgate and Yanofsky (2010) uniquely examined parent perspectives (n=31) through qualitative interviews about decision-making and clinical trials when their child was diagnosed with cancer. Content analysis highlighted participation in decisions about clinical trials as a difficult and extraordinary experience that included six themes:

1. living a surreal event
2. wanting the best for my child
3. helping future families of children with cancer
4. coming to terms with my decision
5. making one decision among many
6. experiencing a sense of trust.

WHAT'S THE EVIDENCE? ANSWER 33.2

PREPARE FOR PRACTICE 33.1: CLINICAL TRIALS NURSE

In light of the findings in the Woodgate (2010) study, how might parents' needs be addressed?

You may find it useful to read about the role of the clinical trials nurse at https://study.sagepub.com/essentialchildnursing

Side effects of chemotherapy

The range of side effects experienced can vary, and as several drugs are usually used the number of potential complications is increased.

Cytotoxic drugs cannot differentiate between healthy and malignant cells, so normal fast reproducing cells within the body are also affected, resulting in some commonly seen and complex side effects (see Figure 33.3).

Side effects may be short term, lasting a number of days or weeks, or long term, continuing for a significant period of time, including after the completion of cancer treatment. While many are reversible, some may be lifelong (Table 33.3). It is important to remember that with all symptoms the child/parents need information and reassurance.

Dealing with some of the side effects of chemotherapy can be quite hard, but having the nurses and other people makes it a little easier to handle.

Aimee, parent

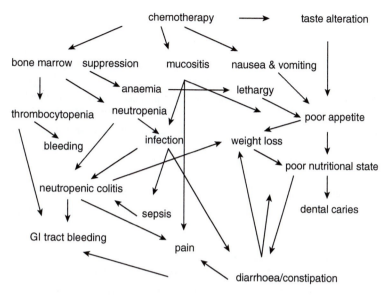

Figure 33.3 Complex effects of treatment

Table 33.3 Side effects of chemotherapy

Period	Potential symptoms	Supportive care
Immediate	Nausea/vomiting	Antiemetics pre-chemotherapy
	Allergic/sensitivity reactions	Pre-meds for agents known to increase risk of reaction; close monitoring
Short term	Alopecia	Provision of wig if desired
	Myelosuppression	Blood product support; treatment of suspected/identified infection
	Immunosuppression	Avoidance of infection risk factors and managing individual symptoms; use of prophylactic antibiotics and antivirals in certain protocols
	Nausea/vomiting	Antiemetics during and post-chemotherapy with adaptation if required; close monitoring
	Mucositis (painful inflammation and ulceration of the gastrointestinal tract)	Basic oral hygiene, analgesia, nutritional support
	Diarrhoea/constipation	Fluid and nutritional support, laxatives
	Organ toxicity	Close monitoring; adaptation of drug doses; additional intravenous fluids; oral/IV supplementation for altered blood chemistry (e.g. potassium)
	Haemorrhagic cystitis (blood in urine – certain cytotoxic agents)	Additional intravenous fluids and mesna to reduce irritation from cytotoxic drugs
	Fatigue	Change daily routine, enabling sleep and rest

(Continued)

Table 33.3 (Continued)

Period	Potential symptoms	Supportive care
Long term	Myelosuppression and immunosuppresssion	Avoidance of infection risk factors and manage individual symptoms
	Infertility	Involvement of reproductive specialists, sperm banking may be available pre-treatment for boys (post-puberty)
	Organ toxicity/failure	Close monitoring, involvement of specialist teams; organ transplant in rare cases
	Growth and development complications	Close monitoring via endocrine specialists
	Secondary cancers	Treat malignancy as appropriate
	Cardiomyopathy	Monitoring closely via cardiac specialists; transplant in rare cases

Children experiencing side effects may require significant levels of supportive care with further hospitalisation. Close monitoring is required in order to anticipate and identify problems and subsequently provide appropriate management. The production of healthy blood cells is also disrupted temporarily following many chemotherapy agents, leaving the child at risk of related side effects – anaemia, thrombocytopenia and neutropenia. While transfusions of red cells and platelets can be given to help manage the first two complications, neutropenia cannot be addressed as easily and the child will require antibiotics should infection be suspected or confirmed. As long-term immunity can also be affected they are at risk of opportunistic infections that can cause significant morbidity and occasional mortality.

Infection (confirmed or suspected) in the immunocompromised child should be treated as a medical emergency.

Long-term follow-up clinics for survivors continue for varying periods of time depending upon the presence or risk of complications.

Safety working with chemotherapy

Given such potentially hazardous side effects, precautions must be taken to protect handlers from cytotoxic chemotherapy. This includes staff and parents handling waste (i.e. urine, vomit). The NMC (2015) Code of Professional Conduct centres round four key areas, one being that we must 'preserve safety'.

Protecting the child, family and staff in the cytotoxic environment is crucial and requires a simple safe approach.

Spillage prevention.

Administration guidelines.

Follow protocol on correct disposal of waste including bodily fluids.

Extravasation recognition.

Ward sister, paediatrics

ACTIVITY 33.5: CRITICAL THINKING

Go to https://study.sagepub.com/essentialchildnursing and click on the link to the Health and Safety Executive website to read about the safe use of cytotoxic drugs.

• How would you, as a children's nurse, ensure safety was maintained in relation to handling of cytotoxic drugs and waste?

ACTIVITY
ANSWER 33.5

WEBLINK:
CYTOTOXIC DRUGS

Surgery

Surgery is often used in the treatment of solid tumours, the timing of which is dependent on the position and size of the tumour and its response to any earlier chemotherapy. If the tumour is too large or intricately involved with other organs or major blood vessels, chemotherapy is given first to shrink the tumour to make surgery less risky. In other situations, for example brain tumours, the tumour is removed first and chemotherapy given afterwards.

SEE ALSO
CHAPTER 16

Radiotherapy

Radiotherapy is the therapeutic application of radiation from high energy X-rays targeted at a tumour site in order to damage DNA causing cells to die or be unable to divide (Bailey and Skinner, 2010). This localised treatment is used with some solid tumours, especially brain tumours, and is administered daily over several weeks, usually as an outpatient. Tissue and organ damage can occur as radiation passes through to reach the target. Consequently, radiotherapy of the developing brain – under 3 years of age – is generally avoided.

Haematopoietic stem cell transplant

For some children the best hope of long-term survival is to receive very high-dose chemotherapy to eradicate any remaining disease. As this obliterates their bone marrow they then require haematopoietic stem cells – in the form of their own pre-harvested stem cells, a donor's bone marrow, or umbilical cord stem cells – to enable them to recover their own bone marrow function.

Side effects post stem-cell transplant are magnified due to the complete destruction of the child's bone marrow. During this time the child will be in protective isolation and require intense supportive care.

Go to https://study.sagepub.com/essentialchildnursing to read more about bone marrow transplantation.

WEBLINK:
BONE MARROW
TRANSPLANTATION

Immunotherapy

Immunotherapy involves using agents to enable the body's immune system and natural killer cells to recognise and attack cancer cells. Biological response modifiers are drugs, for example monoclonal antibodies, that work with the immune system to bring about malignant cell death in a number of ways: by attacking cancer cells, blocking signals that tell malignant cells to divide, blocking molecules that prevent the immune system from working correctly and by carrying cytotoxic drugs or radiation to cancer cells.

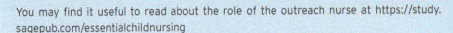

SCENARIO 33.2: BELLE

PREPARE FOR
PRACTICE
33.2:
OUTREACH
NURSE

CASE STUDY
33.1: NURSE
ROLES – A DAY
IN THE LIFE

Belle has undergone her first block of chemotherapy and is being discharged home. Her parents are both very anxious about her medications and central line and fearful about her risk of infection.

- What is the role of the nurse in discharge preparation?
- What are their likely needs for instrumental, informational and emotional support?
- Who might be the members of the team involved in Belle's care?

You may find it useful to read about the role of the outreach nurse at https://study. sagepub.com/essentialchildnursing

SCENARIO
ANSWER 33.2

Care of children with cancer is increasingly being carried out in the home. Parents usually take the lead in caring and often report feeling anxious and overwhelmed, and so require information, teaching and support, particularly following the first discharge (Flury et al., 2011). Some parents may be from medical backgrounds but they are parents first and foremost.

SEE ALSO
CHAPTER 30

> *The ward and clinic staff were very supportive knowing we were both 'medical' and understanding the added worries we had with extra medical knowledge but still treating us like the scared parents we ultimately were.*
>
> **Aimee, parent**

TEAM WORKING IN CHILDHOOD CANCER CARE

SEE ALSO
CHAPTER 5

Given the nature and duration of childhood cancer, care teams can be large, exist across care settings and members of the team can change over time. Such issues can cause problems to streamlined and quality care (NICE, 2005).

Many professionals and organisations provide care for children with cancer and their families, with each bringing their own individual expertise to ensure the physical needs of the child are met alongside the emotional, social and spiritual needs of the child and family. Charitable organisations also have an important role in supporting children with cancer and families, for example CLIC Sargent and Make A Wish.

The child is continuing to grow and develop throughout their treatment and associated care. Play and education therefore have a central role.

> *His school teachers were fantastic, ensuring he could still go to school by making sure he had a one-to-one support worker to help him cope when on steroids, which made him very emotional and unpredictable.*
>
> **Aimee, parent**

When everyone is using their abilities towards a common goal – the best care for each child and family – the results are greater than those achieved by a single person. These are the attributes of a team working within childhood cancer care:

Trust and respect for child and family and within team

Empathy and human approach

A high standard of individualised expert care

Meetings of team regularly

Well coordinated care that straddles hospital and home

Organisations from statutory and voluntary sector working together

Recognition that consistency and continuity are important

Key worker for each child to coordinate care

Information about team roles and contacts

Negotiation with parents as experts

Good communication (within and across teams)

The role of the children's nurse

The children's nurse is the professional who spends the most amount of time with the child and family, so they have a multifaceted role to play. Tedford and Price (2011) identified the children's nurse as supporter/facilitator, leader/manager, advocate for the child and family, teacher/educator and team player, in addition to their being the provider of physical care to the child.

> It's much better if the nurses are a little crazy and are willing to play with me.
>
> **Salisu, child**

Within the nurse's role as educator/teacher the nurse must educate the child and/or family about many aspects, ensuring an optimum level of health is promoted for the child and the family. Health education/promotion opportunities are wide ranging when a child has cancer. Remember these elementary ABCDEs of health promotion:

Avoid public areas

Beware of safe handling of body fluids whilst the child is undergoing chemotherapy

Care of central line and infection control management recognition

Discussion about vaccination status – no live vaccines when on treatment

Education regarding neutropenia and steps when child's temperature rises

Sun safety – some chemotherapy drugs make children particularly sensitive to the sun

Despite improved survival rates, childhood cancer can lead to the death of some children.

SEE ALSO
CHAPTER 35

Nursing students often express some anxiety about going to specialised cancer units or areas where children with cancer are cared for. They can express lack of certainty about the type of care they can be involved in and the learning opportunities available. Go to https://study.sagepub.com/essentialchildnursing for tips from a student on preparing for such placements.

PLACEMENT ADVICE 33: MALIGNANT CONDITIONS

PREP FOR PLACEMENT!

CHAPTER SUMMARY

This chapter has highlighted the main principles of caring for a child with cancer and their family:

- A collaborative approach to treatment through a centralised body – CCLG
- Care provision must be individualised and all-encompassing, addressing bio, psycho, social and spiritual elements
- Quality care for children with cancer and their families must be underpinned by the best available evidence
- Care must be individualised to the child and family centred
- There must be an interdisciplinary approach involving statutory and voluntary services across care settings
- Cure rates have increased over recent years but cure with least cost to the child is an essential consideration
- Long-term follow-up is an important part of childhood cancer care and continues for many years following completion of treatment

BUILD YOUR BIBLIOGRAPHY

Books

- Eiser, C. (2015) *Children with Cancer: The Quality of Life*. Oxfordshire: Routledge.

  Text examining how to ensure good quality of life for children with cancer and their families.

- Gibson, F. and Soanes, L. (eds) (2008) *Cancer in Children and Young People*. Chichester: John Wiley & Sons.

  A comprehensive book examining the principles of treatment and care of childhood cancer.

- Tomlinson, D. and Kline, N.E. (eds) (2010) *Pediatric Oncology Nursing*, 2nd edn. Berlin: Springer-Verlag.

  A book covering the conditions, treatment and supportive care for children with cancer.

Journal articles

FURTHER READING: ONLINE JOURNAL ARTICLES

Go to https://study.sagepub.com/essentialchildnursing for further free online journal articles related to this chapter.

- Fleming, C., Cohen, J., Murphy, A., Wakefield, C., Cohn, C. and Naumann, F. (2015) 'Parent feeding interactions and practices during childhood cancer treatment: a qualitative investigation'. *Appetite*, 89: 219-25.

  This paper presents a study examining the important issue of feeding difficulties and poor food intake, which are often experienced during childhood cancer treatment. The findings highlight a variety of child-parent interactions and practices relating to feeding.

- Ness, K.K., Armenian, S.H., Kadan-Lottick, N. and Gurney, J.G. (2011) 'Adverse effects of treatment in childhood acute lymphoblastic leukemia: general overview and implications for long-term cardiac health'. *Expert Review of Hematology*, 4 (2): 185–97.

  This paper examines the important issue of late effects of cancer treatment as experienced by children who were treated for ALL. The particular focus here is on the impact on the cardiac system.

- Wakefield, C., Butow, C., Fleming, S., Gunar, D. and Cohn, R. (2012) 'Family information needs at childhood cancer treatment completion'. *Pediatric Blood and Cancer*, 58 (4): 621–6.

  This study examines the important period after treatment for childhood cancer has been completed and examines the specific needs of the family in relation to information.

Weblinks

Go to https://study.sagepub.com/essentialchildnursing for further weblinks related to this chapter.

FURTHER
READING:
WEBLINKS

- Cancer Research UK, *Monoclonal Antibodies (MAB)*

  www.cancerresearchuk.org/about-cancer/cancer-in-general/treatment/biological-therapy/types/monoclonal-antibodies

  This website hosts four short videos about immunotherapy drugs and monoclonal antibodies.

- Macmillan Cancer Support, *Bone Marrow or Stem Cell Transplants for Children's Cancers*

  www.macmillan.org.uk/cancerinformation/cancertypes/childrenscancers/treatingchildrenscancers/bonemarrowstemcelltransplant.aspx

  Read more about bone marrow transplantation.

- Macmillan Cancer Support, *Radiotherapy for Children with Head and Neck Cancers*

  www.macmillan.org.uk/cancerinformation/cancertypes/childrenscancers/treatingchildrenscancers/radiotherapy/radiotherapyheadandneckcancers.aspx

  Read more about radiotherapy in children.

  Children with Cancer UK, *Patient Stories*

  www.childrenwithcancer.org.uk/stories/patient-story-lucy

  Meet Lucy and consider how she presented with a brain tumour, and the impact of treatment on her and her family.

- University Hospitals Birmingham NHS Foundation Trust, *Therapy Based Long Term Follow Up: Practice Statement*, 2nd edn

  www.uhb.nhs.uk/Downloads/pdf/CancerPbTherapyBasedLongTermFollowUp.pdf

  Read about long-term follow-up management for childhood cancer.

ACE YOUR ASSESSMENT

Revise what you have learned by visiting https://study.sagepub.com/essentialchildnursing

ONLINE
QUIZZES &
ACTIVITY
ANSWERS

- Test yourself with multiple-choice and short-answer questions
- Do the chapter activities in the book and check your answers online

REFERENCES

Bailey, S. and Skinner, R. (2010) *Paediatric Haematology and Oncology*. Oxford: Oxford University Press.

Children's Cancer and Leukaemia Group (CCLG) (2015) *Children's Cancer and Leukaemia Group*. Available at: www.cclg.org.uk (last accessed 29 May 2017).

Children's Cancer Measures (2013) *Manual for Cancer Services (version 3.0). National Cancer Peer Review*. London: National Cancer Action Team.

Flury, M., Caisch, U., Ullmann-Bremi, A. and Spichiger, E. (2011) 'Experiences of parents with caring for their child after a cancer diagnosis'. *Journal of Pediatric Oncology Nursing*, 28: 143–53.

Gottlieb, B.H. (1978) 'The development and application of a classification scheme of informal helping behaviours'. *Canadian Journal of Behavioural Science*, 10: 105–15.

House, J.S. (1981) *Work Stress and Social Support*. Reading: Addison-Wesley.

Hughes, E.C. (1945) 'Dilemmas and contradictions of status'. *American Journal of Sociology*, 50: 353–9.

Jordan, J., Price, J. and Prior, L. (2015) 'Disorder and disconnection: parent experiences of liminality when caring for their dying child'. *Sociology of Health and Illness*, 37 (6): 839–55.

Kaplan, B.H., Cassel, J.C. and Gore, S. (1977) 'Social support and health'. *Medical Care*, 15: 47–58.

Macmillan (2014) *Childhood Cancers*. Available at: www.macmillan.org.uk/Cancerinformation/ Cancertypes/Childrenscancers/Childrenscancers.aspx (last accessed 29 May 2017).

McCubbin, M., Balling, K., Possin, P., Frierdich, S. and Bryne, B. (2002) 'Family resiliency in childhood cancer'. *Family Relations*, 51: 103–11.

National Institute for Health and Clinical Excellence (NICE) (2005) *Improving Outcomes in Children and Young People with Cancer*. London: NICE.

NMC (2015) *The Code: Professional Standards of Practice and Behaviour for Nurses and Midwives*. London: Nursing and Midwifery Council.

Ped-Onc Resource Center (2015) *Signs of Childhood Cancer*. Available at: www.ped-onc.org/diseases/ SOCC.html (last accessed 29 May 2017).

Price, J., Jordan, J., Prior, L. and Parkes, J. (2012) 'Comparing needs of families of children dying from malignant and non-malignant disease: an in-depth qualitative study'. *British Medical Journal Supportive and Palliative Care*, 2(2):127–32.

Rafii, F., Oskouie, F. and Shoghi, M. (2014) 'Caring for a child with cancer: impact on mother's health'. *Asian Pacific Journal of Cancer Prevention*, 15 (4): 1731–8.

Tedford, J. and Price, J. (2011) 'Role of the nurse in family centred care'. *Cancer Nursing Practice*, 10 (2): 14–18.

Thoitis, P.A. (1986) 'Social support as coping assistance'. *Journal of Consulting and Clinical Psychology*, 54: 416–23.

Woodgate, R. and Yanofsky, R. (2010) 'Parents' experiences in decision making with childhood cancer clinical trials'. *Cancer Nursing*, 33 (1): 11–18.

CARE OF CHILDREN AND YOUNG PEOPLE WITH LIFE-LIMITING ILLNESS

34

ANTOINETTE MENEZES AND TRACIE LEWIN-TAYLOR

THIS CHAPTER COVERS

- What are life-limiting illnesses?
- The needs of children and families
- The role of children's hospices
- Care of children with a life-limiting illness
- Transition of young people supported by children's palliative care services to adult services

> " At that point we could not change what was going to happen to our family and most especially to Anouk. However, we were able to choose who was going to support us and to a certain extent how we were going to live during that time. We wanted to identify areas of our lives we did have some control over, to find partners who would empower us to make difficult choices, to enable us to be the best parents we could be to our daughters, to facilitate us to continue to live normal lives, and to permit us to continue to live our family life the way we wanted to.
>
> **Catherine, parent** "

Visit https://study.sagepub.com/essentialchildnursing to access a wealth of online resources for this chapter – watch out for the margin icons throughout the chapter.

INTRODUCTION

PREPARE FOR
PRACTICE 34:
CATHERINE

The quote above comes from a mother describing the moment they received the devastating news that their daughter would only live a few months or perhaps a year. You can read more about the nursing qualities and support services which this mother valued most in her own words at https://study. sagepub.com/essentialchildnursing

When a child is diagnosed with a life-limiting illness families like Anouk's need high-quality, flexible support designed to meet their individual needs. Community-based, interprofessional support is vital, and to achieve this professionals have to work collaboratively, ensuring the child and family are at the centre of everything they do.

This chapter unpicks the care of babies, children and young people with life-limiting conditions in partnership with their families. The needs of children and families are illustrated through two case studies, encouraging you to think from the child and family's perspectives.

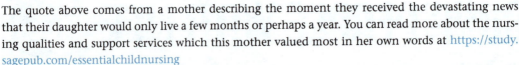

WEBLINK:
NCPC
GLOSSARY

You do not need prior knowledge to read the chapter although you may find the NCPPC *Glossary of Terms* (2014) will help to clarify terms you are not familiar with. You can access this via https://study. sagepub.com/essentialchildnursing The activities may be useful to reflect on later in your course – for example, when you have more relevant experience.

WHAT ARE LIFE-LIMITING ILLNESSES?

Life-limiting illnesses are those for which there is no reasonable hope of cure and from which children are likely to die before they reach adulthood. Experts have found it difficult to estimate the exact number of children in the UK with life-limiting illnesses (Ling et al., 2015). Many individual illnesses are extremely rare and in some cases they are inherited, so more than one child can be affected in the family. The exact number of children born per year with life-limiting illnesses is unclear because of the number of medical illnesses involved. The annual number of children aged 0–19, including neonates, likely to require access to palliative care services in the UK is estimated to be 23,500 (i.e. 16 per 10,000 population) (Department of Health, 2007). The number of neonates requiring access to palliative care services is estimated to be 1,473 (i.e. 1 per 10,000 population) (Department of Health, 2007).

A number of issues make caring for children with life-limiting conditions and their families complex. First, many rare life-limiting illnesses can affect children, some so unusual that only a handful of children are affected in this country or the world.

Second, the unpredictable nature of the conditions involved mean that many of the children have complex needs and require constant, complete care, punctuated by long tiring journeys to care and treatment centres. Such life-limiting illnesses can cause progressive deterioration, so the child becomes increasingly dependent on parents and carers.

PRACTICE
SCENARIO
34: JANET

PLACEMENT
ADVICE
34: LIFE-
LIMITING
ILLNESS

ACTIVITY 34.1: CRITICAL THINKING

Have you cared for a life-limited child? Reflect on how you felt during this experience or on any concerns you have if you have not cared for a child or family in this situation. Even if you have not yet cared for a child with a life-limiting condition, consider how you would feel and what anxieties you may experience.

Go to https://study.sagepub.com/essentialchildnursing for tips on preparing for placements with children with life-limiting illnesses, and a parent's prespective.

THE NEEDS OF CHILDREN AND FAMILIES

Babies, children and young people affected by life-limiting illnesses have a spectrum of physical/emotional needs.

Some have a clear understanding of their condition but suffer from declining physical abilities. Others have complex learning difficulties and very limited insight into their own situation. Rasmussen and Grégoire (2015) describe the range of neurological symptoms which can occur, discussing evaluation and management. Some of the children communicate non-verbally and sensory support can enable them to explore their world and express themselves.

SEE ALSO CHAPTER 2

Each child and family has individual needs, which must be accurately assessed and provided for. Sometimes different family members – for example, fathers (Nicholas et al., 2016), mothers, grandparents and siblings (Read et al., 2010; Malcolm et al., 2014) need particular care and support as described in the quote below.

> We prepared Matthias and his three brothers every step of the way by being open and honest … We felt strongly that the children were to know everything but felt it was important for the siblings to know and understand after Matthias had been told and had the chance to share his thoughts and emotions first with my husband and myself. In my experience parent lead/guided care was imperative, by a process of osmosis we were seeing and learning acceptance of our child's death.
> Honesty, openness, freedom to speak, planning and preparation were key to the children's understanding of cancer diagnosis, treatment, palliative care and death.
>
> **Rosie, parent**

ACTIVITY 34.2: CRITICAL THINKING

Think about the needs of life-limited children before you read on. Create a mind map of the needs of life-limited children that you can think of with branches for these headings:

- Physical needs
- Emotional needs
- Spirituality (Here we refer to spirituality as related to being human, how you nurture yourself as an individual – for example, some people do yoga, others go for a walk in the countryside (Llewellyn et al. (2015) and Crisp (2016) discuss these issues)
- Social needs and interaction with peers

CHECK YOUR ANSWERS ONLINE!

ACTIVITY ANSWER 34.2

THE ROLE OF CHILDREN'S HOSPICES

Life-limited children and their families need support from hospitals and different community-based health, social and education providers.

Children's hospices are one important component of care for this group of children and their families.

PREPARE FOR
PRACTICE 34:
CATHERINE

In some ways it was [to] the rest of the extended family that the children's hospice gave invaluable assistance, not provided by any other service. The wonderful play therapist visited Neave weekly, ensuring she felt valued and important at a time in our lives when despite our best intentions life did revolve around our youngest daughter.

Catherine, parent

SEE ALSO
CHAPTER 1

Children's hospices were first established in the UK in the early 1980s when Helen House opened in Oxford. Today there are over 40 services in the UK. Each provides a comparable but slightly different range of support. Children's hospice care is generally provided by interprofessional teams which include disciplines such as consultants and doctors, nurses, counsellors, play and music therapists, physiotherapists and occupational therapists as well as healthcare assistants. Some provide care in the child's home and some offer short breaks and symptom care as well as end-of-life care and post-bereavement support. Although some receive statutory funding they are primarily supported by charitable donations. Children's hospices share a child- and family-centred approach focusing on holistic care to meet the specific needs of each child and their family. The voices of children with life-limiting illnesses are critical to enhance our understanding of their needs and experiences (Menezes, 2010).

WHAT'S THE EVIDENCE?

Ling et al. (2016) found that families participating in their qualitative study most wanted support at home but also had concerns about the potential effects on family life and siblings of community care services and professionals visiting their home.

Read this article and write a reflection about why you think families might want support in their own home, highlighting the specific concerns outlined in this paper.

WHAT'S THE
EVIDENCE?
ANSWER 34.1

Palliative care for children differs from adult provision in a number of ways. Where referrals are made to the children's hospice close to diagnosis the child and family are offered support over long periods of time, perhaps years. The emphasis is on long- term support for families as well as symptom care, end-of-life care and bereavement support for families.

Together for Short Lives (2012) provide this definition:

VIDEO LINK
34.1: WE'RE
HAVING A
BABY

palliative care for children and young people with life-limiting conditions is an active and total approach to care, from the point of diagnosis or recognition, embracing physical, emotional, social and spiritual elements through to death and beyond. It focuses on enhancement of quality of life for the child/young person and support for the family and includes the management of distressing symptoms, provision of short breaks and care through death and bereavement.

Palliative care is therefore multifaceted and complex. The case studies below will help you unravel some of the components and complexities inherent in providing palliative care.

Watch the videos about children's hospices available at https://study.sagepub.com/essentialchildnursing

VIDEO LINK
34.2: CASE
STUDIES

CARE OF CHILDREN WITH A LIFE-LIMITING ILLNESS

Many children's hospices accept referrals pre-birth and the scenario below shows an example of an in utero referral to a hospice service.

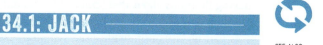

SCENARIO 34.1: JACK

Jack was diagnosed in utero with anencephaly when his mum was 36 weeks gestation. The local maternity and neonatal team referred Jack's mum to a hospice service because his diagnosis met the hospice referral criteria.

Jack's parents visited the hospice with the hospice at home team alongside the symptom care team. Jack was born at 41 weeks gestation and survived for 14 hours after delivery. His parents decided to remain at the hospital for care. The hospital team followed the individualised symptom care plan to manage Jack's end of life which was written by the symptom care team. Jack's parents decided to donate his heart valves, which had already been discussed and planned for as part of advance care planning (ACP), which is a process of discussion between an individual and their care provider and often those close to them. Jack was then transferred to the hospice for care after death. His parents were able to access bereavement support via the hospice. Jack had access to a 24/7 paediatric specialist care team who would act as a central point to coordinate and lead his end-of-life care (Department of Health, 2008a).

- Think of a time when you have worked with a family that may not have been offered these choices. What do you think are the benefits of having open discussions with families?
- How do you think the needs of parents for an in utero referral may differ from parents of a child?

SCENARIO
ANSWER 34.1

SEE ALSO
CHAPTER 32

A&P LINK

To remind yourself of the relevant anatomy and physiology, please read the A&P link: 'Anencephaly' at https://study.sagepub.com/essentialchildnursing

A&P LINK 34.1:
ANENCEPHALY

It is often hard to predict what the future holds for babies and children requiring palliative care. Parallel planning is paramount in paediatric palliative care, to plan for life and death. It is important for families to be given choices. These include place of care, place of death, place of care after death, and emotional and bereavement support. Putting the child and family at the centre of decision-making is a priority in producing a care plan that is right for them. The actual place of death may be less important than has been argued; the opportunity to place location of death may be a better proxy of high-quality end-of-life care than actual location.

SEE ALSO
CHAPTER 35

Communication is always paramount in providing the best care possible. Relationship building, demonstration of effort and competence, information exchange, availability, and appropriate level of child and parent involvement are valued by families (Hsiao et al., 2007).

Mitchell and Dale (2015) highlight how ACP for life-limited children can improve care for the child and their family. The *End of Life Care Strategy* (Department of Health, 2008b) clearly states that ACP and clarity about resuscitation decisions are essential to quality care. ACP may also lead to actions such as advance statements about wishes and preferences and withdrawal of treatment. For children and families this will include decisions relating to care in the case of acute deterioration and may also address preferences for organ and tissue donation (McNamara, 2013). Popejoy (2015) found that making decisions about their child's life was difficult and painful but as parents their input is vital and should be elicited by professionals during the early stages of decision-making.

As part of ACP an individualised symptom care plan is written. These plans are used to manage symptoms and support end-of-life care whether this is in hospital, hospice or at home. These plans are shared with the multiprofessional team to keep everyone who is involved informed.

WEBLINK:
NEONATAL
CARE
PATHWAY

WHAT'S THE EVIDENCE?

Download and read the Together for Short Lives' neonatal care pathway from https://study.sagepub.com/essentialchildnursing and review this case study with evidence-based practice.

Download and read Mancini et al. (2014) *Practical Guidance for the Management of Palliative Care on Neonatal Units* from https://study.sagepub.com/essentialchildnursing

WEBLINK:
PALLIATIVE
CARE
PRACTICAL
GUIDANCE

SAFEGUARDING STOP POINT

As a nursing student you will be in a unique position to observe signs of abuse, neglect or changes in behaviour which may indicate that a child is being abused or neglected. Safeguarding issues can arise for life-limited children and their families. Make sure you know who to ask for help if you have safeguarding concerns wherever you are working.

FIND OUT MORE!

TRANSITION OF YOUNG PEOPLE SUPPORTED BY CHILDREN'S PALLIATIVE CARE SERVICES TO ADULT SERVICES

The second case study will discuss a further scenario dealing with a young person who receives palliative care. Palliative care requires a total and active approach with agreed provision of appropriate and proportionate care (Thompson, 2015).

SCENARIO 34.2: MATTHEW

Matthew is 18, and has been known to a children's hospice service for many years. He has a diagnosis of epilepsy, scoliosis, cerebral palsy and a ventriculoperitoneal shunt (VP) in situ. He receives respite care from the hospice service both in house and from the hospice at home team. Matthew has had issues with recurrent chest infections which led to a deterioration and admission to an adult ward via Accident and Emergency. The hospital team informed his foster mother that Matthew was entering end of life; his medicines were discontinued and a 'do not attempt resuscitation' (DNAR) order was completed. Due to Matthew's age he needs to transition to adult services. The DNAR was replaced with an emergency care plan (ECP). The difference in these two documents is that there is discussion with families around things that they would like to be managed in an end-of-life event. The individualised symptom care plan can be helpful in managing anticipated symptoms. These plans are shared with all settings that Matthew uses or may use. He also has access to a 24/7 paediatric specialist care team (Department of Health, 2008a). The challenges for Matthew and his mother moving forward into adult services include whether services will be funded to support the family and the provision available to provide respite care to a young man like Matthew.

- Think about transition from childhood to adulthood and the need for young people to move from children's to adult services. What challenges do you think families face?

SCENARIO
ANSWER 34.2

A&P LINK

To remind yourself of the relevant anatomy and physiology, please read the A&P link: 'Scoliosis' at https://study.sagepub.com/essentialchildnursing

A&P LINK 34.2:
SCOLIOSIS

Most children and young people are cared for mainly in the community, with hospice care being a lifeline for respite care or more urgent supportive care beyond hospital or education settings. Sadly these families who are transitioning into adult settings face limited and under-resourced services due to limited funding and inexperience in working with young people with such complex needs. You may have experience yourself of an adult hospice and have seen the difference from children's hospices. Adult hospices are currently able to offer limited, if any, respite for families. This may see a change in the future.

Planning improves care; ACP enabled Matthew to have management of both reversible and non-reversible aspects of his condition that can be supported in any care setting. Care is integrally intertwined with other clinical, social, educational, therapeutic and voluntary services to ensure that families receive the care required throughout their journey. Matthew attends education and liaison between all services involved is important so that a clear plan can be put in place in partnership with families.

Children's services will plan and support the family as much as possible to achieve a seamless transition. Every young person should be appropriately supported in adult services, with a multiagency team fully engaged in facilitating care and support. There should be confidence from the young person, family and professional perspective in future planning and provision of care (McNamara, 2013). Activity 34.3 will help you reflect on learning from this case study.

ACTIVITY 34.3: CRITICAL THINKING

If you created a mind map about the needs of children with life limiting illnesses at Activity 34.2, use a new colour and add to each branch one or two things you think a young person might need.

WHAT'S THE EVIDENCE?

The *Moving to Adult Services: What to Expect* guide (Together for Short Lives, 2016) is free to download and shows evidence to support this case study and to help you complete Activities 34.2 and 34.3. You can find it at https://study.sagepub.com/essentialchildnursing

Read the evidence and consider how this compares with the points you added when you completed Activity 34.3.

Go to https://study.sagepub.com/essentialchildnursing for tips on preparing for placements with children with life-limiting illnesses, and a parent's perspective.

CHAPTER SUMMARY

- Life-limiting illnesses reduce the child's life expectancy to childhood or young adulthood and bring sustained uncertainty for the child and family. There are a wide range of life-limiting illnesses and many are extremely rare
- Children, young people and their families have diverse and often very complex needs
- Good communication with the family and between agencies is critical
- Symptom management and planning for emergencies are very important aspects of care
- Children's hospice and palliative care agencies provide child- and family-centred interprofessional support, often over years

BUILD YOUR BIBLIOGRAPHY

Books

- Dougherty, L. and Lister, S. (eds) (2015) *The Royal Marsden Manual of Clinical Nursing Procedures*, 9th edn. Chichester: Wiley-Blackwell.

  This provides detailed procedure guidelines for effective patient-focused nursing care. Information about the online edition at www.rmmonline.co.uk
- Royal College of Nursing (2012) *Palliative Care for Children and Young People*. London: RCN. Available at www2.rcn.org.uk/__data/assets/pdf_file/0012/488991/004_328.pdf (last accessed 30 May 2017).
- Downing, J., Ling, J., Benini, F., Payne, S. and Papadatou, D. (2013) *Core Competencies for Education in Paediatric Palliative Care*. Milan: European Association for Palliative Care. Available at: www.eapcnet.eu/LinkClick.aspx?fileticket=6elzOURzUAY%3D (last accessed 30 May 2017). The two publications above are about competencies in children's palliative care.

Journal articles

Go to https://study.sagepub.com/essentialchildnursing for further free online journal articles related to this chapter.

- Malcolm, C., Knighting, K., Forbat, L. and Kearney, N. (2009) 'Prioritization of future research topics for children's hospice care by its key stakeholders: a Delphi study'. *Palliative Medicine*, 23 (5): 398-405.

This is an interesting article which describes how families, hospice staff/volunteers and linked professionals identified and prioritised their future research priorities for children's hospice care.

- Malcolm, C., Forbat, L., Knighting, K. and Kearney, N. (2008) 'Exploring the experiences and perspectives of families using a children's hospice and professionals providing hospice care to identify future research priorities for children's hospice care'. *Palliative Medicine*, 22 (8): 921-8.

An article which explains how engaging families and care providers in the process of identifying research priorities resulted in the development of an extensive research agenda, which will contribute to quality hospice care for children and families.

- Hain, R.D.W. (2005) 'Palliative care in children in Wales: a study of provision and need'. *Palliative Medicine*, 19 (2): 137-42.

On how to establish incidence and prevalence of children needing palliative care in Wales.

Weblinks

Go to https://study.sagepub.com/essentialchildnursing for further weblinks related to this chapter.

FURTHER
READING:
WEBLINKS

- Together for Short Lives

  www.togetherforshortlives.org.uk

  UK charity representing life-limited children and their families. The website includes many professionals resources.

- Hospice UK

  www.hospiceuk.org

  National charity for hospice care offering information about courses, conferences and policy.

- Contact a Family

  www.cafamily.org.uk

  National charity for families with disabled children including an A-Z of medical conditions, some life limiting.

  Preparing for placement at a children's hospice: Before you go on placement look up the website for the hospice you will be attending.

──── ACE YOUR ASSESSMENT ────

ONLINE
QUIZZES &
ACTIVITY
ANSWERS

Revise what you have learned by visiting https://study.sagepub.com/essentialchildnursing

- Test yourself with multiple-choice and short-answer questions
- Do the chapter activities in the book and check your answers online

REFERENCES

Crisp, C.L. (2016) 'Faith, hope, and spirituality: supporting parents when their child has a life-limiting illness'. *J Christ Nurs*, 33 (1): 14–21.

Department of Health (2007) *Palliative Care Statistics for Children and Young Adults*. London: Department of Health.

Department of Health (2008a) *Better Care: Better Lives*. London: Department of Health.

Department of Health (2008b) *End of Life Care Strategy*. London: Department of Health.

Hsiao, J.L., Evan, E.E. and Zeltzer, L.K. (2007) 'Parent and child perspectives on physician communication in pediatric palliative care'. *Palliative & Supportive Care*, 5 (4), 355–65.

Ling, J., O'Reilly, M., Balfe, J., Quinn, C. and Devins, M. (2015) 'Children with life-limiting conditions: establishing accurate prevalence figures'. *Ir Med J*, 108 (3): 93.

Ling, J., Payne, S., Connaire, K. and McCarron, M. (2016) 'Parental decision-making on utilisation of out-of-home respite in children's palliative care: findings of qualitative case study research – a proposed new model'. *Child: Care, Health and Development*, 42: 51–9.

Llewellyn, H., Jones, L., Kelly, P., Barnes, J., O'Gorman, B., Craig, F. and Bluebond-Langner, M. (2015) 'Experiences of healthcare professionals in the community dealing with the spiritual needs of children and young people with life-threatening and life-limiting conditions and their families: report of a workshop'. *BMJ Support Palliat Care*, 5 (3): 232–9.

Malcolm, C., Gibson, F., Adams, S., Anderson, G. and Forbat, L. (2014) 'A relational understanding of sibling experiences of children with rare life-limiting conditions: findings from a qualitative study'. *J Child Health Care*, 18 (3): 230–40.

Mancini, A., Uthaya, S., Beardsley, C., Wood, D. and Modi, N. (2014) *Practical Guidance for the Management of Palliative Care on Neonatal Units*. London: Chelsea and Westminster Hospital NHS Foundation Trust.

McNamara, K. (2013) *Standards Framework for Children's Palliative Care*, 2nd edn. Bristol: Together for Short Lives.

Menezes, A. (2010) 'Moments of realization: life-limiting illness in childhood – perspectives of children, young people and families'. *Int J Palliat Nurs*, 16 (1): 41–7.

Mitchell, S. and Dale, J. (2015) 'Advance care planning in palliative care: a qualitative investigation into the perspective of paediatric intensive care unit staff'. *Palliat Med*, 29 (4): 371–9.

National Clinical Programme for Palliative Care (NCPPC) (2014) *Glossary of Terms*. Dublin: Health Service Executive. Available at: www.hse.ie/eng/about/Who/clinical/natclinprog/palliativecareprogramme/Resources/glossaryofterms.pdf (last accessed 30 May 2017).

Nicholas, D.B., Beaune, L., Barrera, M., Blumberg, J. and Belletrutti, M. (2016) 'Examining the experiences of fathers of children with a life-limiting illness'. *J Soc Work End Life Palliat Care*, 12 (1–2): 126–44.

Popejoy, E. (2015) 'Parents' experiences of care decisions about children with life-limiting illnesses'. *Nurs Child Young People*, 27 (8): 20–4.

Rasmussen, L.A. and Grégoire, M.C. (2015) 'Challenging neurological symptoms in paediatric palliative care: an approach to symptom evaluation and management in children with neurological impairment'. *Paediatr Child Health*, 20 (3): 159–65.

Read, J., Kinali, M., Muntoni, F. and Garralda, M.E. (2010) 'Psychosocial adjustment in siblings of young people with Duchenne muscular dystrophy'. *Eur J Paediatr Neurol*, 14 (4): 340–8.

Together for Short Lives (2012) *Definitions*. Available at: www.togetherforshortlives.org.uk/professionals/childrens_palliative_care_essentials/definitions (last accessed 28 June 2017).

Together for Short Lives (2016) *Moving to Adult Services: What to Expect*. London: Together for Short Lives.

CARE OF CHILDREN AND YOUNG PEOPLE AT THE END OF LIFE

35

JAYNE PRICE AND MELISSA HEYWOOD

THIS CHAPTER COVERS

- How do you know a child is nearing end of life?
- Assessment and planning in end-of-life care
- Symptom management
- Ethical issues when caring for a dying child
- The interdisciplinary approach inherent in caring for a child at the end of life and their family
- Self-care for professionals working with children at the end of life

> " Caring for a dying child is for me one of the most difficult parts of being a nurse but it is also the most rewarding. Having a family entrust the care of their child to you at this time is the greatest privilege and honour – there is a real pressure to get it right, there are no second chances.
>
> **Stephanie Minnis, staff nurse, neonatal intensive care** "

Visit https://study.sagepub.com/essentialchildnursing to access a wealth of online resources for this chapter – watch out for the margin icons throughout the chapter.

INTRODUCTION

Death of a child defies the expected order of life. No parent expects to outlive their child and such a life-altering event leads to profound and long-lasting grief (Price and Jones, 2015). Fortunately, childhood death is relatively rare. However, estimates indicate that approximately 6,000 children between the ages of 0–19 die within the UK annually (RCPCH, 2014). Whilst accidents are the most common cause of death, increasing numbers of children are dying as a result of life-limiting illness. Quality end-of-life care leading to a good death is essential, and is the right of every child (Davies, 2009).

End-of-life care is defined as:

> care [that] helps all those with advanced, progressive, incurable illness to live as well as possible until they die. It focuses on preparing for an anticipated death and managing the end stage of a terminal medical condition. This includes care during and around the time of death, and immediately afterwards ... It includes management of pain and other symptoms and provision of psychological, social, spiritual and practical support and bereavement support for the family. (Widdas et al., 2013, p. 39)

VEDIO
LINK 35.1:
AFTER A
CHILD DIES

The definition highlights the multifaceted nature of such care. The way a child dies can impact on the parents' bereavement (Gurkova et al., 2014) and is therefore another driving factor in ensuring a good death is achieved. You can watch the video on the impact of the loss of a child on the family via https://study.sagepub.com/essentialchildnursing

Caring for a child at the end of life can provoke feelings of anxiety for healthcare professionals (Cook et al., 2012), even those with experience. Such feelings can be attributed to the pressure professionals feel to 'get it right' for the child and family (Price et al., 2013). The quote at the beginning of the chapter highlights that caring for the dying child is difficult yet rewarding for the children's nurse. This chapter unravels some of the complexities associated with providing end-of-life care, drawing on best practice. If working through this chapter and the associated activities prove emotionally difficult or raise specific issues, you must seek help – for example, from your personal tutor or mentor.

ACTIVITY 35.1: REFLECTIVE PRACTICE

List your anxieties about providing end-of-life care for children.

ACTIVITY
ANSWER 35.1

> " One of the situations that most children's nursing students dread is encountering their first death. It is a difficult experience but ultimately teaches you new depths of compassion and caring which aid your professional growth. Every student copes with the death of a child differently.
>
> **Kate, 3rd-year children's nursing student** "

HOW DO YOU KNOW A CHILD IS NEARING END OF LIFE?

The dying process leads the body through many changes. Understanding physical and emotional changes may alleviate some of your fears and misconceptions about death. These are signs that may present when a child is approaching end of life:

- Profound weakness – the child may take to bed
- Respiratory changes – decreased and laboured breathing
- Decreased fluid intake – absence of a desire to drink or as a result of difficulty swallowing
- Skin colour – the child may become pale, bluish and/or mottled
- Organ failure – the body shutting down
- Agitation or decreased alertness

Concept of a 'good death'

The term 'good death' is one that has been used repeatedly, yet contested in the literature in relation to children (Welch, 2008). Given the individuality of a good death it has been suggested that it is difficult to define (Widdas et al., 2013). Hendrickson and McCorkle (2008) carried out a dimensional analysis, proposing a model of achieving a good death for children with cancer. The model proposes that aspects of care and quality of life come together to influence the dying process and are multidimensional in nature. Having someone present at the time of death was a component of the Hendrickson and McCorkle model (2008). In addition to 'being there', constituent properties of a good death included a peaceful death where the child was symptom free, the need to be cared for by familiar, caring professionals and dying in a place of the child's or parents' choosing.

ASSESSMENT AND PLANNING IN END-OF-LIFE CARE

Assessment is not a one-off activity and should be ongoing to address the changing needs/wishes of the child and family. Once it has been established that the child is at the end-of-life stage, planning care follows. A care pathway such as the one in Figure 35.1 (Together for Short Lives, 2013) can be used to guide care.

The pathway acts as a useful trigger to ensure the care addresses the physical, emotional, social and spiritual needs of the child and family. Planning must be centred round the needs and, where possible, wishes of the individual child and family:

- Collaborative approach with family and team
- A written plan agreed and shared amongst team
- Regular review of plan and alteration as necessary
- Explicit and honest communication with families
- Pain and symptom control as central
- Listen to child and family, supporting them in their choices
- Approach which ensures emotional and spiritual needs are met
- Necessity to promote quality of life and make memories
- Sibling and grandparents' involvement is important

Decision-making

Decision-making is a difficult task and should be seen as a collaborative process that involves the child (where possible), parents/family and healthcare team. All discussions should be considered a process and not an event (Heywood and Hynson, 2012). Families need time to process information, so decision-making occurs in stages: setting goals, gathering information, processing and making sense of the information, making choices and evaluation (Sharman et al., 2005).

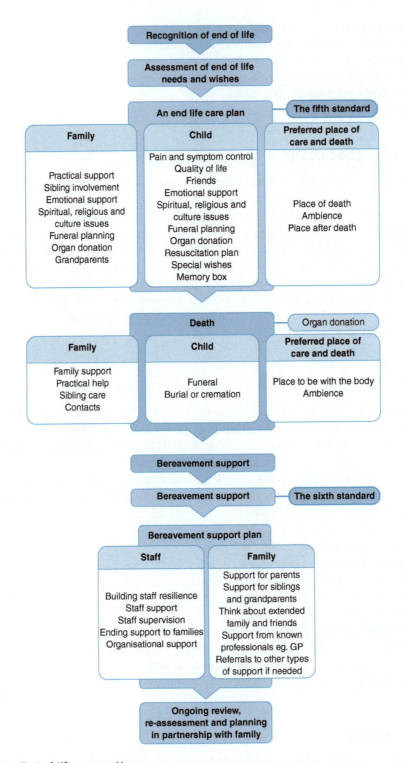

Figure 35.1 End-of-life care pathway

Widdas, D., McNamara, K. and Edwards, F. (2013) *A Core Care Pathway for Children with Life-limiting and Life-threatening Conditions* (3rd edn). Bristol: Together for Short Lives. Reproduced with permission.

The key to effective decision-making is establishing clear goals of care. Much of this planning should be undertaken prior to a crisis arising, with a clear focus on ensuring the child's comfort (Mack and Joffe, 2014). Difficult conversations are often part of such planning/decision-making, which may include resuscitation, organ donation, or location of end-of-life care (Widdas et al., 2013). It is important that families know that such decisions can and should be revisited (Popejoy, 2015). Involving parents in decisions and provision of their child's care is crucial (Gurkova et al., 2014) given their expert knowledge of their child, but also to enable them to feel they have some control of their child's life. One decision often faced is the place where their child's end-of-life care will be delivered.

SCENARIO 35.1: JESS

Colin and Jill's 1-year-old daughter Jess has an undiagnosed life-limiting condition and is being cared for in the hospice at the end of life. They have three other children aged 9, 7 and 2. Colin's parents live abroad. However, Jill's parents live close by and have been helping with Jess's care over the last year as well as the needs of the other children.

- What benefits would hospice care potentially have for this family?
- Colin seems less engaged in care and on the periphery – what would you do?
- How could you as the nurse address the potential needs of Jill's parents (Jess's grandparents)?
- Jill is anxious about the other children being around Jess, wanting to protect them. How would you guide her?
- Consider how you would promote memory-making in this case.

CHECK YOUR ANSWERS ONLINE!

SCENARIO ANSWER 35.1

WHAT'S THE EVIDENCE?

Melin-Johansson et al. (2014) carried out an integrative literature review exploring parents' experiences when facing their child's death. The review helpfully highlighted that parents in such a situation have five main desires and goals:

- Genuine communication
- Sincere relationships
- Respect as an expert
- Alleviation of the child's suffering
- Need for support

How could you incorporate the above evidence in your practice?

WHAT'S THE EVIDENCE? ANSWER 35.1

Parental coping

Parents living through the death of a child experience both emotional and practical chaos (Price et al., 2011). Parents can display a number of emotional responses, including disbelief, fear, anger, despair and hopelessness. Parents often experience guilt, particularly around their perception that they are neglecting their other children (Giovanola, 2005), as caring for their dying child takes precedence. Keeping busy and 'doing' for their child in terms of providing care appears to enable parents to cope with some of their emotional responses (Price et al., 2011).

WHAT'S THE EVIDENCE?

The seminal work by Lazarus and Folkman (1984) identifies two different approaches to coping (which can be applied to parents coping with their child's end-of-life care):

- Problem-focused coping (a direct approach where the problem is evaluated and action is taken to avoid/change the situation)
- Emotion-focused coping (this approach is much more indirect, with the focus on reducing the emotional consequences of stressful or potentially stressful events)

Considering Lazarus and Folkman's coping strategies, which do the following parental actions indicate? Jot these down.

WHAT'S THE EVIDENCE? ANSWER 35.2

Parental action	Lazarus and Folkman's approach
Organising grandparents to collect siblings from school	
Talking about feelings to staff nurse	
Surfing the net about symptom management	

Other family members

Within the ethos of family-centred care, the needs of siblings and grandparents as highlighted within the end-of-life pathway should be addressed (Widdas et al., 2013). Grandparents play important supportive roles and should not be forgotten during the end-of-life period. Grandparents suffer a double effect of loss in that they experience the pain of living through the loss of their grandchild, but in addition, they are watching their own child suffering (Gilrane-McGarry and O'Grady, 2011). Parents can feel unsure about how to deal with the needs of their other children and often attempt to protect them from the truth around their sibling's death. In reality, siblings themselves indicate their need to be involved, and need for information, communication and reassurance (Lövgren et al., 2016).

Addressing the needs of siblings is essential. Consider how the children's nurse could work in partnership with parents to meet sibling need. You can watch the video on the story of Marmaduke's family via https://study.sagepub.com/essentialchildnursing

VIDEO LINK 35.2: MARMADUKE'S FAMILY

SYMPTOM MANAGEMENT

Effective symptom management is vitally important and should include non- pharmacological strategies as well as pharmacological. The subcutaneous route of administration (via a syringe driver) is probably the most frequently used with children at the end of life.

ACTIVITY 35.2: LEADERSHIP AND MANAGEMENT

Consider the benefits of using the subcutaneous route for children at the end of life.

ACTIVITY ANSWER 35.2

Expertise and support regarding symptom management should be available 24 hours a day, regardless of the place of care.

> Effective symptom management is about anticipating possible symptoms likely to occur for that child and preparing for their management to ensure comfort. As a child's death is not the end of the journey for their family, it is therefore also about creating positive memories as they begin the grieving process. No one wants the last moments of a child's life to be of suffering and distress.
>
> **Anne O'Reilly, specialist transition nurse, children's hospice**

The more commonly encountered symptoms include pain, dyspnoea, nausea and vomiting, constipation, restlessness, anxiety and agitation, fatigue and seizures (Rajapakse and Comac, 2012). However, despite some challenges, the majority of symptoms can be adequately managed (Feudtner et al., 2011). Nurses should proactively assess symptoms by observing the child, asking the child and asking the parents. Other barriers that contribute to lack of recognition of symptoms include the child's inability to report and describe their symptoms, the child denying symptoms to protect parents or failure of the clinicians to utilise appropriate assessment tools (Rajapakse and Comac, 2012). Challenges in pharmacological symptom management in children at the end of life include:

- Drugs may be unlicensed for use in children
- Conditions in childhood, and consequently symptoms, can be rare
- Limited research regarding symptom management in some non-malignant conditions
- Myths and fears about the use of certain drugs (e.g. morphine)
- Preparations may not always be suitable for use in children

---

ACTIVITY 35.3: REFLECTIVE PRACTICE

You are caring for a child at the end of life and the issue of starting a syringe driver for his pain relief has been raised. Mum is anxious that this will hasten death, so she wants to wait a few days.

- Consider the management of this challenging issue.

ACTIVITY
ANSWER 35.3

Pain

Pain is the symptom most commonly associated with suffering at end of life. Children and parents often fear that pain will be unrelieved at this time (Collins et al., 2011).

Thorough assessment should:

- Recognise the child's age and developmental stage
- Always involve language appropriate to the child's developmental level
- Empower the child and family, by allowing some choice and control where possible
- Involve investing time in developing trust with the child and family. This might mean spending some time drawing, reading or chatting with them

SEE ALSO
CHAPTER 3

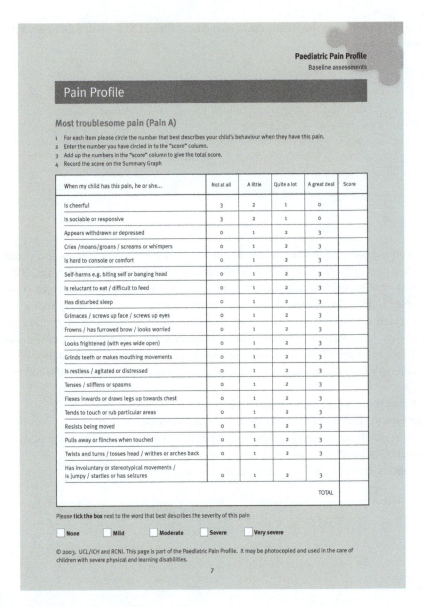

Figure 35.2   Paediatric Pain Profile

Hunt, A., Goldman, A., Seers, K., Crichton, N., Mastroyannopolou, K., Moffat, V. et al. (2003) 'Clinical validation of the paediatric pain profile', Dev Med Child Neurol, 46(1): 9-18. Reproduced with permission of UCLB. Available at https: //xip.uclb.com/i/health care_tools/ppp.html

Of particular note is that a large percentage of children requiring end-of-life care have conditions that affect them cognitively, so their ability to communicate may be impaired. For this group of children observation is key. Observe the child's vocal sounds, facial expression, mood, eating, sleeping, movement and posture (Hunt, 2012). The Paediatric Pain Profile (see Figure 35.2) is a tool that is designed for assessing this particular group of children.

ACTIVITY 35.4: CRITICAL THINKING

Which professionals may work collaboratively to assess and manage the pain of a child at the end of life?

ACTIVITY
ANSWER 35.4

Following an accurate assessment, a plan of care to manage the symptoms can be formulated and implemented. A number of key principles should prevail:

1. Assess the pain (involve the child's parents)
2. Discuss the management strategy/plan – always address potential parental anxieties
3. Use multimodal approaches – pharmacological and non-pharmacological approaches including massage, positioning, distraction
4. Utilise the least invasive route of medication administration – never intramuscular with children
5. Administer prescribed analgesics regularly
6. Minimise the number of doses
7. Plan ahead
8. Prescribe regular laxatives (only when using opioids)
9. Monitor the response, evaluate and reassess regularly

Other symptoms

In addition to pain, other symptoms may be experienced, requiring assessment and management (see Table 35.1).

Table 35.1 Other symptoms and associated multimodal treatment/care (not an exhaustive list)

Symptoms	Explanation	Treatment options	Specific nursing care tips
Dyspnoea (shortness of breath)	Relatively common symptom in paediatrics Causes considerable anxiety in the child and family if not controlled Very subjective sensation and reported symptoms may not match respiratory signs	Identify and treat any underlying cause Opioids are very effective - e.g. morphine The use of benzodiazepines can be appropriate Some children find oxygen therapy helps alleviate dyspnoea	Dyspnoea is a very frightening experience for a child Provide reassurance and involve family Utilise a fan - a cool draft of air can be very helpful in reducing the feeling of breathlessness Utilise breathing exercises Appropriate positioning (upright) and relaxation may be useful

(Continued)

Table 35.1 (Continued)

Symptoms	Explanation	Treatment options	Specific nursing care tips
Seizures	Experienced by children with: • primary or metastatic tumours of the brain • metabolic and genetic conditions	Anticonvulsant medications will be prescribed as maintenance treatment for seizures All families should have seizure management plan for emergency treatment of seizures including what medications should be administered and how long a seizure can be left before intervention	Maintaining child safety and dignity during seizure is essential
Restlessness, agitation and delirium	Not always an apparent cause but uncontrolled pain, hypoxia, anxiety and medications can be contributing factors	Use of medications to reduce symptoms where necessary – e.g. intranasal or buccal midazolam Midazolam is the sedation of choice and can be added into a syringe driver with other drugs	Nurse the child in a quiet and safe environment Reassure families that these symptoms can often be part of the dying process Acknowledge it is very difficult to witness but that it is often not distressing to the child
Nausea and vomiting	Identify the cause and then target anti-emetics according to their mode of action	Utilise anti-emetic medications as required – these can be added to drugs in the syringe driver (if the child has one) Identify causes that can be corrected and managed – e.g. pain, infection, drugs	Avoid strong smells and odours - eg perfume, foods Keep meals small and frequent if the child's appetite/condition allows Regular mouth care
Urinary retention	Some children with neurodegenerative disorders may experience difficulties with emptying their bladder Opiates can cause children to experience retention	Consider gentle bladder massage, warm baths or catheterisation	The family may value the opportunity to bath the child
Fatigue	Is a debilitating factor and can compromise quality of life Contributing factors – anaemia, depression, dehydration, malnutrition, insomnia and medications	Often a reflection of disease progression Eg Attend school for shorter periods and at times of favourite classes/subjects Planned activities can give the child a sense of wellbeing	Help child and family set realistic expectations and goals Encourage families to plan activities around the fatigue (when child has more energy)
Constipation	A number of factors can lead to constipation, including inactivity, weakness, poor food and fluid intake and reduced mobility; drugs such as opioids can cause constipation	Laxatives Rectal preparations should be avoided in children who are neutropenic/thrombocytopenia	Provide privacy when using the toilet or, if the child wears a nappy, ensure appropriate hygiene and skin care

(Information from Rainbow Children's Hospice (2011))

SCENARIO 35.2: DECLAN

Declan is a 4-year-old with metachromatic leukodystropy (MLD). He is non-verbal, has global developmental delay, epilepsy and frequent muscle spasms. Declan receives all his nutrition via gastrostomy and requires frequent oral suction. Mum carries out all Declan's care at home with some input from carers.

In recent months Declan has had multiple admissions to hospital. Most of the admissions are a result of Declan's increasing chronic lung disease and his susceptibility to chest infections.

Declan begins to experience an increase in his seizure activity. He has increased secretions, which have become thick and green and difficult for him to cough up. He is more agitated, restless and irritable.

- How would you assess Declan's pain?
- How would you manage the symptoms described?
- How would you address Declan's emotional needs?
- In what ways would you ensure Declan's care is child and family centred?
- What other care would you provide to ensure Declan is comfortable and that the complications of reduced mobility are minimised?
- What symptoms could you anticipate in the future?

Note: Declan's case is developed further at https://study.sagepub.com/essentialchild nursing to help you examine bereavement care.

CASE STUDY 35.1: DECLAN

HELPFUL FOR ASSIGNMENTS!

SCENARIO ANSWER 35.2

ETHICAL ISSUES WHEN CARING FOR A DYING CHILD

Given the complexity of care at the end of life and the fact that many decisions are central to planning care, it is not surprising that a range of ethical issues can arise (see Table 35.2 and Scenario 35.3: Richard).

Table 35.2 Potential ethical challenges

Ethical challenge	Example
Child as decision-maker	The child's ability to make informed choices – developmental level and life experience are major factors
Decision-making regarding treatment plan and goals	This includes: Life-sustaining inventions – ventilation, going to ICU Provision of hydration and nutrition Advance care planning
Treatment/procedure that appears to cause more burden to the child than benefit	Continuing chemotherapy in the last days of life
Parental refusal to utilise medication for symptom management	Morphine for pain relief and child is suffering
Parents refusing to tell child that they are dying	Anxious adolescent asking questions about if they are dying

There are number of factors that contribute to this:

SEE ALSO
CHAPTER 8

- The child's inability to make decisions
- Uncertainty often surrounds a young person's ability to make competent decisions
- The reliance on parents as surrogate decision-makers
- Tenseness of situation and emotions surrounding the child/family at this time

SCENARIO 35.3: RICHARD

Richard is 10 years old. He has Ewing's sarcoma and had a previous above-knee amputation. He has endured many years of treatments. Recently he has relapsed with no further treatment available. It is anticipated that he only has months to live. His parents do not want him to know he is dying, but are keen to get him home as soon as possible.

You are the registered nurse on night duty. It is 2am and you wander in to check on him. You find Richard awake and he says he is worried and can't sleep, and he then asks, 'Am I going to die?'

- Applying ethical principles, how would the nurse address this issue?
- Consider and jot down the potential benefits of care at home for Richard as the end of life draws near

SCENARIO
ANSWER 35.3

THE INTERDISCIPLINARY APPROACH INHERENT IN CARING FOR A CHILD AT THE END OF LIFE AND THEIR FAMILY

SEE ALSO
CHAPTER 5

To provide holistic care at the end of life, it is essential that a team approach be implemented to ensure planning, coordination and clear communication.

Team members consist of those with specific skills and expertise who are working towards a shared goal – that is, best care for the dying child and their family. Typically this team will consist of nursing, medical and allied health professionals. Voluntary as well as statutory services have an important role to play in caring for a child at the end of life and their family.

For many families there are a multitude of services and individuals to liaise with across a range of care settings (see Figure 35.3). The identification of a key worker to coordinate care and ensure all services are working together is important (Hynson et al., 2003; Heywood and Hynson, 2012).

SELF-CARE FOR PROFESSIONALS WORKING WITH CHILDREN AT THE END OF LIFE

When my child died my world changed forever. Seeing the nurses who cared for us for five weeks in intensive care shed a tear provided us with such comfort at the most difficult of times. It helped us see that our son was important and loved by others too.

Leyla, parent

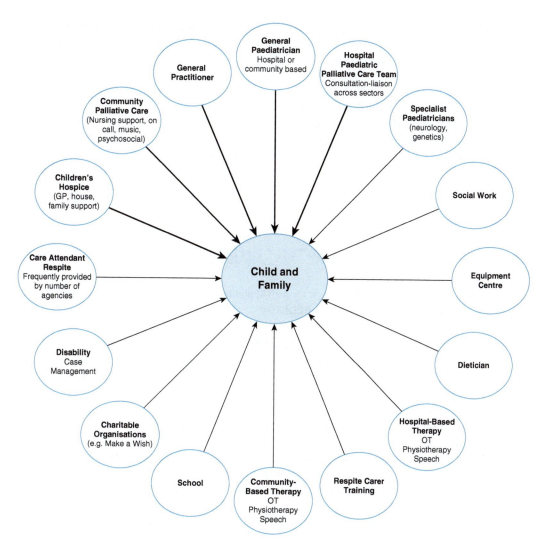

Figure 35.3 Interdisciplinary approach to caring for the child and family

As caring for dying children and their families can be both emotionally and physically exhausting, it is essential to recognise that looking after yourself and your colleagues is integral to best practice for children and families (Morgan, 2009). Only when we look after ourselves and our colleagues can we provide children and families with care and support at end of life on a regular basis. Self-awareness is crucial, and as professionals we need to have a clear knowledge of our own beliefs and needs (Furingsten et al., 2015).

Providing care to a dying child and their family will bring stress, anxiety and suffering. It is important to understand and acknowledge the impact that your work has on the personal and professional areas of your life. Looking after oneself and developing self-care practices is imperative in ensuring best care is delivered to children and families (McCloskey and Taggart, 2010).

A variety of strategies can be employed to ensure optimum health for all staff caring for dying children and their families. We need to 'rescue' ourselves and to look out for members of our team. Strategies for the self care of staff include:

- Resources available within the organisation
- Reflect and debrief after the death of a child
- Respect and support the other members of the team
- Relevant training days may be useful
- Realise your own ways of coping (including identifying your strengths)
- Remember to take care of yourself physically, mentally and spiritually

Go to https://study.sagepub.com/essentialchildnursing for advice from a student regarding experienceing the death of a child while on placement.

PLACEMENT
ADVICE 35:
CARE OF THE
DYING CHILD

CHAPTER SUMMARY

To ensure that the main principles of care for a child and family at the end of life highlighted in this chapter are addressed, remember your **ABCDEFG**s:

- **A**sk – ask the child and/or family what you can do for them (individualised care)
- **B**e – be there, be with and be available (and tell the parents/child that you are available)
- **C**are – remember to care for the whole child, including physical, emotional, social and spiritual care. Be human and be empathetic
- **D**iscuss – discuss and explore arising ethical issues with sensitivity
- **E**nsure a team approach – recognise your limitations and draw on the expertise of others within the team
- **F**amily-centred care – be human and empathetic to parents, and remember siblings and grandparents (wider family can find themselves on the periphery)
- **G**arner support strategies – ensure you develop your own means of addressing your emotions (self care)
- **S**top, look and listen – reassess care plans regularly, while being flexible and responsive (child and family needs may change and this should be recognised and addressed)

BUILD YOUR BIBLIOGRAPHY

Books

The chapters cited in each of these books gives insights and guidance in caring for children after death.

- McNeilly, P. and Price, J. (2008) Chapter 44: 'Care of the child after death', in J. Kelsey and G. McEwing (eds) *Clinical Skills in Child Health Practice*. Oxford: Churchill Livingstone.
- Shapcott, J. (2015) Chapter 35: 'Last offices' in C. Delves-Yates (ed.) *Essentials of Nursing Practice*. London: Sage.
- Bennett, H. (2012) Section 4: 'Care of a child after death', in *A Guide to End of Life Care*. Available at: www.togetherforshortlives.org.uk/assets/0000/1855/TfSL_A_Guide_to_End_of_Life_Care_5_FINAL_VERSION.pdf (last accessed 30 May 2017).

Journal articles

Go to https://study.sagepub.com/essentialchildnursing for further free online journal articles related to this chapter.

FURTHER READING: ONLINE JOURNAL ARTICLES

- Garstang, J., Griffiths, F. and Sidebotham, P. (2014) 'What do bereaved parents want from professionals after the sudden death of their child? A systematic review of the literature'. *BMC Pediatrics*, 15 (14): 269–86.

  Gives insights into parents' needs after the sudden death of their child.

- Neilson, D. (2012) 'Discussing death with pediatric patients: implications for nurses'. *Journal of Pediatric Nursing*, 27 (5): 59–64.

  Gives insights into children's awareness of death and discusses developmental theories.

- Snaman, J.M., Torres, C., Duffy, B., Levine, D., Gibson, D. and Baker, J. (2016) 'Parental perspectives of communication at the end of life at a pediatric oncology institution'. *Journal of Palliative Medicine*, 19 (3): 326–32.

  This paper gives useful insights into communication.

- van der Geest, I.M., van den Heuvel-Eibrink, M.M., van Vliet, L.M., Pluijm, S.M., Streng, I.C., Michiels, E.M., Pieters, R. and Darlington, A.S.E. (2015) 'Talking about death with children with incurable cancer: perspectives from parents'. *The Journal of Pediatrics*, 167 (6): 1320–6. Further examination of the complex issue of talking to children about death.

- Wender, E. and the Committee on Psychological Aspects of Child and Family Health (2012) 'Supporting the family after the death of a child'. *Pediatrics*, 130 (4): 1164–9.
  Bereavement care explored.

Weblinks

Go to https://study.sagepub.com/essentialchildnursing for further weblinks related to this chapter.

FURTHER READING: WEBLINKS

- Rainbows, Jassal, S.S. (2011) *Basic Symptom Control in Paediatric Palliative Care*, 8th edn. Bristol: Rainbows Children's Hospice.

  www.rainbows.co.uk/wp-content/uploads/2011/06/Rainbows-Hospice-Basic-Symptom-Control-In-Paediatric-Palliative-Care-8th-Ed-2011-protected.pdf

  This resource provides in-depth information on symptom management of children at the end of life. It is used by practitioners in practice who need to review management of a symptom.

- Royal College of Nursing (RCN), RCN (2011) *Spiritual Needs in Nursing Care: A Pocket Guide*. London: RCN.

  www2.rcn.org.uk/__data/assets/pdf_file/0008/372995/003887.pdf (last accessed 30 May 2017).

  This resource has been produced to aid nurses in ensuring the spiritual needs of patients are being met. This usefully highlights that spirituality is not purely related to religion and encourages the nurse to think more widely about it.

- Winston's Wish

  www.winstonswish.org.uk

  A UK charity providing resources and support for bereaved children.

ACE YOUR ASSESSMENT

Revise what you have learned by visiting https://study.sagepub.com/essentialchildnursing

- Test yourself with multiple-choice and short-answer questions
- Do the chapter activities in the book and check your answers online

REFERENCES

Collins, J.J., Berde, C.B. and Frost, J.A. (2011) 'Pain assessment and management', in J. Wolfe, P.S. Hinds and B.M. Sourkes (eds) *Textbook of Interdisciplinary Pediatric Palliative Care*. Philadelphia: Elsevier Saunders.

Cook, K.A., Mott, S., Lawrence, P., Jablonski, J., Grady, M.R., Norton, D., Reidy, S., Liner, K.P., Cioffi, J., Hickey, P. and Connor, J.A. (2012) 'Coping while caring for the dying child: nurses' experiences in an acute care setting'. *Journal of Pediatric Nursing*. 27 (4): 11–21.

Davies, R. (2009) 'Care of the dying child', in J. Price and P. McNeilly (eds), (2009) *Palliative Care for Children and Families: An Interdisciplinary Approach*. Basingstoke: Palgrave Macmillan.

Feudtner, C., Hexem, K. and Rourke, M.T. (2011) 'Epidemiology and the care of children with complex conditions', in J. Wolfe, P.S. Hinds and B.M. Sourkes (eds), *Textbook of Interdisciplinary Pediatric Palliative Care*. Philadelphia: Elsevier Saunders.

Furingsten, L., Reet, S. and Forsner, M. (2015) 'Ethical challenges when caring for dying children'. *Nursing Ethics*, 22 (2): 176–87.

Gilrane-McGarry, U. and O'Grady, T. (2011). 'Forgotten grievers: an exploration of the grief experiences of bereaved grandparents'. *International Journal of Palliative Nursing*, 17 (4): 170–6.

Giovanola, J. (2005) 'Sibling involvement at the end of life'. *Journal of Pediatric Oncology Nursing*, 22 (4), 222–6.

Gurkova, E., Andrasckova, I. and Cap, J. (2014) 'Parents' experiences with a dying child with cancer in palliative care'. *Central European Journal of Nursing and Midwifery*, 6 (1): 201–8.

Hendrickson, K. and McCorkle, R. (2008) 'Dimensional analysis of the concept: good death of a child with cancer'. *Journal of Pediatric Oncology*, 25 (3): 127–38.

Heywood, M. and Hynson, J.L. (2012) 'Paediatric palliative care: the challenging dimensions'. *Grief Matters*, 15 (2): 28–31.

Hunt, A. (2003) *Paediatric Pain Profile*. London: GOSH and RCN. Available at: https://xip.uclb.com/i/healthcare_tools/ppp.html (last accessed 30 May 2017).

Hunt, A. (2012) 'Pain assessment', in A. Goldman, R. Hain and S. Liben (eds) *Oxford Textbook of Palliative Care for Children*, 2nd edn. New York: Oxford University Press.

Hynson, J.L., Gillis, J., Collins, J.J., Irving, H. and Trethewie, S.J. (2003) 'The dying child: how is care different?' *Medical Journal of Australia*, 179: S20–2.

Jassal, S.S. (UK) (2011) *Symptom Management Guidelines*, 8th edn. Bristol: Rainbows Children's Hospice. Available at: www.rainbows.co.uk/wp-content/uploads/2011/06/Rainbows-Hospice-Basic-Symptom-Control-In-Paediatric-Palliative-Care-8th-Ed-2011-protected.pdf (last accessed 15 February 2017).

Lazarus, R.S. and Folkman, S. (1984) *Stress, Appraisal and Coping*. New York: Springer.

Lövgren, M., Jalmsell, L., Eilegård Wallin, A., Steineck, G. and Kreicbergs, U. (2016) 'Siblings' experiences of their brother's or sister's cancer death: a nationwide follow-up 2–9 years later'. *Psycho-Oncology*, 25 (4): 435–40.

Mack, J. and Joffe, S. (2014) 'Parents communicating about prognosis: ethical responsibilities of pediatricians and parents', *Pediatrics*, S24–29.

McCloskey, S. and Taggart, L. (2010) 'How much compassion have I left? An exploration of occupational stress among children's palliative care nurses'. *International Journal of Palliative Nursing*, 16 (5): 233–40.

Melin-Johansson, C., Axelsson, I., Jonsson Grundberg, M. and Hallqvist, F. (2014) 'When a child dies: parents' experiences of palliative care. An integrative literature review'. *Journal of Pediatric Nursing*, 29 (6): 660–9.

Morgan, D. (2009) 'Caring for dying children: assessing the needs of the pediatric palliative care nurse'. *Pediatric Nursing*, 35 (2): 86–90.

Popejoy, E. (2015) 'Parents' experiences of care decisions about children with life-limiting illnesses'. *Nursing Children and Young People*, 27 (8): 20–4.

Price, J, Jordan, J., Prior, L. and Parkes, J. (2011) 'Living through the death of a child: a qualitative study of bereaved parents' experiences'. *International Journal of Nursing Studies*, 48 (11): 1384–92.

Price, J., Jordan, J. and Prior, L. (2013) 'A consensus for change: parent and professional perspectives on care for children at the end-of-life'. *Issues in Comprehensive Pediatric Nursing*, 36 (1–2): 70–87.

Price, J.E. and Jones, A.M. (2015) 'Living through the life-altering loss of a child: a narrative review'. *Issues in Comprehensive Pediatric Nursing*, 38 (3), 222–40.

Rajapakse, D. and Comac, M. (2012) 'Symptom in life-threatening illness: overview and assessment', in A. Goldman, R. Hain and S. Liben (eds), *Oxford Textbook of Palliative Care for Children*, 2nd edn. New York: Oxford University Press.

Royal College of Paediatrics and Child Health (RCPCH) (2014) *Why Children Die: Death in Infants, Children and Young People in the UK. Part A*. London: RCPCH.

Sharman, M., Meert, K. and Sarnaik, A (2005) 'What influences parents' decisions to limit or withdraw life support?' *Pediatric Critical Care Medicine*, 6 (5): 513–18.

Welch, S.B. (2008) 'Can the death of a child be good?' *Journal of Pediatric Nursing*, 23: 120–5.

Widdas, D., McNamara, K. and Edwards, F. (2013) *A Core Care Pathway for Children with Life-limiting and Life-threatening Conditions*, 3rd edn. Bristol: Together for Short Lives. Available at: www.togetherforshortlives.org.uk/assets/0000/4121/TfSL_A_Core_Care_Pathway__ONLINE_.pdf (last accessed 30 May 2017).

CARE OF CHILDREN AND YOUNG PEOPLE WITH LEARNING DISABILITIES

36

TRISH GRIFFIN AND JANE LOPEZ

THIS CHAPTER COVERS

- Changing ideas and value base around children with learning disabilities
- The care and educational pathways that children with a learning disability follow
- The changing nature of learning disability
- Challenges to children's health and wellbeing

> "
> Working alongside children with learning disabilities and their families is such a privilege. As a children's nursing student, I have learnt so much from spending time with children and their families. Their often complex and multifaceted health issues require a significant depth of knowledge and understanding to be able to provide high-quality care that is family focused.
>
> **Sarah, 3rd-year children's nursing student**
> "

Visit https://study.sagepub.com/essentialchildnursing to access a wealth of online resources for this chapter – watch out for the margin icons throughout the chapter.

INTRODUCTION

You could be forgiven for thinking that every child with learning disabilities has Down's syndrome: this could be due to the image often portrayed by the media and charities. This chapter seeks to dispel this misunderstanding by providing you with insights into children with learning disabilities and their families by explaining some of the key issues that shape their lives. Importantly, it seeks to enable you to focus on maximising the health of the child and not their disability.

This chapter suggests strategies you can adopt to support children with a learning disability across a range of settings and needs, including effective communication and inclusiveness (Beacock et al., 2015).

The opening quotation for this chapter acknowledges the complex and multifaceted health issues that shape the lives of children with learning disability and their families. With this in mind, the authors provide examples of the diversity of issues. You will be inspired to extend your knowledge and understanding. This will empower you to deliver first-rate child-centred professional care based on your Code of professional conduct (Nursing and Midwifery Council, 2015).

CHANGING IDEAS AND VALUE BASE AROUND CHILDREN WITH LEARNING DISABILITIES

Since the introduction of the NHS in the late 1940s significant influences have continued to shape the delivery of care and education services for children with learning disabilities. These changes gained momentum during the 1970s and 1980s with a dramatic move away from a medical model and segregated patterns of care based on the child's condition. The late 20th century heralded a cautious emergence of enlightened social policies focusing on a child-centred approach, developing each child to their fullest potential. Most notable were the education, health and social care initiatives that began to implement a range of new health, education and social care policies and legislation including:

- Education Act 1981
- Education Act 1996
- National Health Service and Community Care Act 1990
- Human Rights Act 1998
- *Valuing People: A New Strategy for Learning Disability for the 21st Century* (Cm 5086, 2001)
- Special Educational Needs and Disability Act 2001
- *Every Child Matters* (Cm 5860, 2003)
- Children Act 1989
- Children Act 2004
- Disability Discrimination Act 1995
- Disability Discrimination (Northern Ireland) Order 2006
- The Equality Act 2010
- *Working Together to Safeguard Children* (HM Government, 2013, 2015)
- Children and Families Act 2014

The politicisation of ideas such as human rights, normalisation, social role valorisation and integration were perceived as moving service emphasis towards child rights. Innovative thinking concerning inclusion and the removal of disabling social and environmental barriers challenged existing service provision (Mansell, 1997). Labels previously used to categorise children such as 'mentally defective', 'subnormal' or 'handicapped' were contested and seen as stigmatising.

The USA, Republic of Ireland and Australia use the term 'intellectual disability'. The term 'global development delay' is recognised internationally. British social policy uses 'learning disabled' and 'learning disability' with confusion arising as to how that differs from 'learning difficulties'. MENCAP (2016) describes learning disability as 'a reduced intellectual ability and difficulty with everyday activities – e.g. household tasks, socialising or managing money – which affects someone for their whole life'. Most learning disabilities arise from a condition before, during or shortly after birth/childhood. Public Health England (2015) add that one in 50 people in England have a learning disability and 'significantly poorer health and increased age-adjusted mortality than their non-disabled peers' and therefore, greater health inequalities. There can also be associated problems/issues as outlined below:

- Cognitive ability – that is, thinking and/or reasoning skills
- Communication skills
- Functional – that is, practical, organisational skills
- Learning and educational development
- Memory
- Physical coordination
- Physical and mental wellbeing
- Social behaviour

Whereas a learning difficulty constitutes a condition which creates an obstacle to a specific form of learning this does not affect the overall intelligence of an individual child. For example, a child with Retts syndrome is classed as having a learning disability but a child with dyslexia is classed as having a learning difficulty. There is obfuscation over both terms because the child is designated as having a statement of 'special educational needs/EHC Plan'. This therefore signposts the formal provision of additional services. Children are further categorised by their ability within the range of learning disability – mild, moderate or severe. Additionally, a number of children can have more complex needs; these children are defined as having profound and multiple disabilities (PMLD) (Emerson et. al., 2010, Public Health England 2015). Children with PMLD may also have:

- Profound Learning disabilities
- Physical disabilities (these may include restricted mobility)
- Sensory impairment
- Health issues (e.g. epilepsy, nutritional problems or respiratory problems)
- Challenging behaviours
- Communication difficulties
- Continence problems (The Scottish Government, 2013)

It is important that you have an idea of the different terminology and 'labels' as these define the way both children and adults are not only perceived but also the care and services they receive; they are not meant to be negative constructs.

THE CARE AND EDUCATIONAL PATHWAYS THAT CHILDREN WITH A LEARNING DISABILITY FOLLOW

Accessing services: The early years

Parents anticipate their baby reaching the early milestones. When this does not happen, it's a time of great anxiety. Some babies born with more complex developmental and sensory problems may be identified at birth: parents are often the first to notice delays in their baby's progress and usually seek help via their friends, wider family and professionals they trust.

Valuing People Now (HM Government, 2009) stated that for children with a learning disability, access to a health service designed around their needs, delivered to a consistently high standard with additional support needed, early diagnosis and intervention are crucial. Currently, under section 23 of the Children and Families Act 2014, responsibility for early identification, assessment, diagnosis, intervention and review of the child's needs rests with the health service; the children's nurse plays a central role.

Primary healthcare services generally include general practitioner (GP), health visitor (HV), specialist nurses (e.g. community learning disability nurses), speech and language therapists, dieticians, psychologists and physiotherapists. Often the professional most involved in the early years is the HV who has responsibility for checking the developmental achievements of the child as part of the universal Healthy Child Programme (Department of Health, 2009). Research from King's College London (Donetto et al., 2013) evidenced how the HV's coordination of care for the child contributed to parents being able to come to terms with and manage difficult circumstances.

HVs are well placed to advise parents about support in a growing voluntary sector. Charities such as MENCAP and the National Autistic Society provide a wide range of resources and information. Others formed around specific conditions such as Down's syndrome, Rett's syndrome and mucopolysaccharide disorders, where families (and professionals) came together to enable research, share expert information and pool resources to improve their child's future outcomes. (For more examples of charities and family groups see the table on https://study.sagepub.com/essentialchildnursing)

WEBLINK: CHARITIES & FAMILY GROUPS

When you are on placement with a community-based nurse, you will have valuable learning opportunities to gain insight into the heath, social, educational, cultural and leisure aspects of both the child and family's life. Each insight will be unique and enable you to develop clinical, professional and communication skills. Beacock et. al. (2015) and *Strengthening the Commitment* (Scottish Government, 2012) directs you to develop core knowledge and skills to work 'safely and appropriately' with people with learning disabilities.

VIDEO LINK 36.1: WORLD WITHOUT DOWN'S SYNDROME

SCENARIO 36.1: JOANNA

As a nursing student you are on a placement with the health visitor (HV). You have met Joanna, her son Simon aged 5 and her daughter Isabel aged 2. The HV has arranged to undertake Isabel's health and development review. Isabel was diagnosed with Rett's syndrome two months ago and is now having epileptic seizures and is proving very difficult to feed. Joanna admits to being concerned about the impact Isabel is having on the family and that she also feels lonely. Joanna also revealed that she finds Isabel's seizures absolutely terrifying. As you leave, Joanna argues with the HV that they – the professionals – must have got it wrong: Isabel will get better.

- Consider the psychosocial impact that a child with complex needs can have on family life
- What professional skills do you think that the HV can use to establish a partnership with Joanna and her family?
- How can the HV help Joanna manage both Isabel's seizures and her own anxiety about the seizures?

SCENARIO ANSWER 36.1

WEBLINK: RETT'S SYNDROME

WEBLINK: MUCOPOLY SACCHARIDE DISORDERS

FIND OUT MORE!

Parents begin the difficult journey by establishing the nature of their child's problems. Research undertaken in 2013 by the Scottish Government highlighted that the initial experience of how both the diagnosis and prognosis were revealed can have 'a long lasting influence on the parents ability to cope' with a wide range of professionals and services involved. It is also generally through the health sector that children are brought to the local authority's attention if they believe that a child under compulsory school age is disabled, and has, or probably has, special educational needs (SEN) (see Table 36.1).

Children may be referred to as having learning disabilities and/or SEN. Since 1981 successive educational reforms have as their intent the ideal of all children attending mainstream schools, recognising that

Table 36.1 Special educational needs

WEBLINK: SEN

WEBLINK:
LEARNING
DISABILITIES
DEFINITION

Children will be considered to have a learning disability if any of the following conditions are met:

1. That they have been identified within education services as having a special educational need (SEN) associated with 'moderate learning difficulty', 'severe learning difficulty' or 'profound multiple learning difficulty' (Public Health England, 2016)

2. That they score lower than two standard deviations below the mean on a validated test of general cognitive functioning (equivalent to an IQ score of less than 70) or general development although Holland (2011) suggests this is outdated

3. That they have been identified as having learning disabilities on locally held disability registers (including registers held by GP practices (e.g. QOF), community health services or at the local authority) (MENCAP 2017a)

for some the need for an educational environment that provides an individualised learning environment where they can thrive is key. Such schools are known as special schools, which pupils can attend until they are 16 and, in England, until they are 18. Young people with a learning disability – living in England and who have an Education, Health and Care (EHC) plan – may remain in education or training, free of charge, until they are 25 if agreed that it would be beneficial for them to do so (MENCAP 2017b).

When it is anticipated that a young person with an EHC plan will soon be leaving education or training, the local authority should agree in advance the support the young person might need to access and the support they might need to help them access it. The Department for Education's 2010 figures show that students with SEN in England increased from around 1.53 million (19 per cent of students) in 2006 to approximately 1.69 million (21 per cent of students) in 2010. Children with the most severe needs represent about 3 per cent of students (Hartley, 2010). Between 2004 and 2009, the numbers of children with severe learning disabilities (SLD) increased by 5.1 per cent, and children with profound and multiple learning disabilities (PMLD) rose on average by 29.7 per cent (Carpenter et. al., 2013).

McClusky and McNamara (2005) reported that government figures indicated that of the 700,000+ disabled children in Great Britain, '100,000+ are severely disabled and numbers are rising as a result of (early) medical interventions'. Tommy's 2015 (www.tommys.org/ funding research, saving babies' lives) reported a rise in survival of extremely pre-term babies born 26 weeks plus. There are approximately 1.5 million people in Britain living with learning disabilities and this number is likely to grow by 14 per cent between 2001 and 2021, which aligns with The Scottish Government's (2004) estimate of a prevalence of 0.05 per cent per 1,000 people and anticipating that numbers will increase with better survival rates.

For parents, meeting their child's needs becomes a paramount concern; it's vitally important that their concerns are heard by health professionals centrally placed to respond. The government continues to oblige the three major service providers to work together to meet the requirements and expressed wishes of the child and family. The most recent attempt came with the Children and Families Act 2014 which introduced the Education, Health and Care (EHC) plan, a carefully coordinated process to meet the assessed health, social and educational needs of the child. A child's EHC plan remains in place until they leave education and it is reviewed annually. Broadly speaking, Northern Ireland and Wales have similar systems and Scotland has articulated a clear commitment to support the child and their parents in removing barriers to services.

VIDEO
LINK 36.2:
PERSON-
CENTRED
THINKING

The school years

When a child with learning disabilities enters their school life, a key link for health and wellbeing is the school nurse (Wright, 2012). For a nursing student, a placement in a special school provides an

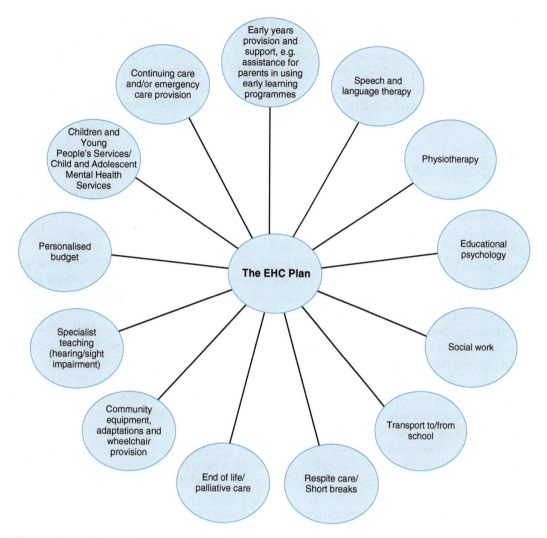

Figure 36.1 The EHC plan: services that may be included

opportunity to gain professional and clinical skills as well as working alongside nurses, therapists and teachers. School nurses work in partnership with the teaching team and support staff with children who require healthcare – e.g. medication. They play a major role in risk management (e.g. of epilepsy) and health promotion, and provide specific advice (e.g. on sexual health). This is an excellent opportunity for you to work closely with children who are not in a health setting and see at first hand how families, educational services and community- based services work together.

Crucially, school nurses can also identify emerging problems and make referrals to special services (e.g. Child and Adolescent Mental Health Services (CAMHS)). The prevalence rate of mental health problems amongst children with learning disabilities is thought to be much higher than amongst the mainstream school population, with 36 per cent having a diagnosable mental health condition (Mansell, 2010; NHS England, 2013).

Parents play the major role in supporting their child's health and development. McCann et al. (2015) indicated that there was clear evidence that mothers of children with learning disabilities, although feeling competent, disliked performing healthcare activities but enjoyed the other aspects of parenting.

There are clear role tensions for parents; parents need clear and easily understood health information. Health visitors, community learning disability nurses and school nurses are well placed to use their listening skills to hear parents' stories and children's voices and to respect differences in families e.g. cultural. This is an invaluable chance to observe skills that nurses use to establish clear two-way communication channels (e.g. school to home/home to school). The creation of opportunities for parents to share important aspects of their culture, concerns and expectations are vital for their child's wellbeing and to begin to prepare them for the transition into adult services.

VIDEO
LINK 36.3:
INTERVIEWS
WITH
PARENTS

THE CHANGING NATURE OF LEARNING DISABILITY

Not only have services and attitudes changed, the children you will meet are changing. Developments in healthcare alongside social change continue to impact on the nature of childhood learning disability. A hundred years ago, life expectancy for a child with Down's syndrome was 9 years (NHS Health Scotland, 2004). In contrast, people with Down's syndrome can now live into old age. Alongside care provision, legal changes in abortion laws and scientific developments in genetic screening have impacted on birth rates resulting in an acceptance of termination on detection of abnormalities. Inherited genetic conditions such as phenylketonuria and chromosomal abnormalities continue to result in children being born with a learning disability.

Improved public health measures have radically reduced the numbers of babies born to mothers who have had infections such as syphilis, toxoplasmosis or rubella during their pregnancy. Carpenter et. al. (2013) have researched extensively into children who are now requiring major adjustments in special educational provision to meet their complex needs. Crucially, those who have difficulties arising from very low birth weight have survived infancy due to advanced medical interventions. Other children are identified as born with learning disabilities arising from lifestyle factors such as parental substance and alcohol misuse.

The disorders that result in a child being born with or developing a learning disability are too numerous to catalogue in this brief chapter. It is nonetheless an opportunity to provide you with some examples of conditions that illustrate the dimensions of a child's life that can be affected:

- Complications before or during birth resulting in damage to the brain
- Premature birth
- Very low birth weight
- Mother's illness during pregnancy
- Congenital/genetic defects
- A debilitating illness or injury in early childhood affecting brain development – for example, meningitis, a road traffic accident or child abuse
- Contact with damaging substances (e.g. alcohol, drugs, lead or radiation)
- Neglect, and/or a lack of mental stimulation early in life (NHS Health Scotland, 2004)

In your practice, you are going to work with children, some of whom may have needs in addition to their learning disability. Here are some examples.

Children with cerebral palsy

Whilst not always resulting in a learning disability, cerebral palsy is a significant cause and the resultant degree of learning disability varies greatly. Approximately 1 in 400 children are diagnosed with cerebral palsy. One in fifty of these children have a degree of learning disability through reduced brain development during pregnancy and 1 in 10 as a result of damage during labour. Perinatal stroke is still a leading cause of cerebral palsy (Bemister et. al., 2015). Premature babies, especially those born before 26 weeks, are more likely to develop cerebral palsy.

Motor function problems are the distinguishing factor in cerebral palsy. Children may also have problems with sensory, communication and nutritional systems (particularly swallowing and aspiration). Hutton and Pharoah (2006) concluded that the more severe the impairments that the child has as a result of cerebral palsy the shorter the life expectancy. Their research also reported the major causes of mortality in children with cerebral palsy to be respiratory disease (1 in 5) and epilepsy (1 in 25). The National Institute of Clinical Excellence (NICE, 2017) have published guidance which will assist you when working with children with cerebral palsy, in particular regarding assessment and management.

To remind yourself of the relevant anatomy and physiology you can read chapters 12 and 16 in *Fundamentals of Children's Anatomy and Physiology: A Textbook for Nursing and Healthcare Students* (Peate and Gormley-Fleming (eds), 2015).

Children with foetal alcohol spectrum disorder (FASD)

FASD is caused by exposure to alcohol prior to birth, directly attributable to the mother's consumption of alcohol. Alcohol is a teragen and impacts on the growth and development of the embryo or foetus in the womb. Children may have a range of mild to severe intellectual and physical effects. The numbers of children born each year with FASD is difficult to determine. Mothers may not disclose their drinking and professionals may misdiagnose. In 2011, the World Health Organization suggested that 6,000–7,000 children are born with FASD in the UK each year. This is based on international research suggesting that 1 in 100 children are affected. It is important to note that whilst only a small proportion of these children will have learning disabilities, many will have neurocognitive defects that result in behavioural and learning difficulties (Cockburn, 2013).

ACTIVITY 36.1: CRITICAL THINKING

The UK has the highest teenage pregnancy and highest underage drinking rate in Western Europe.

Do you think that the government should take action to diminish the risks of foetal alcohol syndrome occurring and if so, how should public health agencies approach this? Discuss.

ACTIVITY
ANSWER 36.1

Children with Down's syndrome

Down's syndrome is most commonly caused by trisomy 21, an additional chromosome attached to chromosome 21 in every cell of the body. Children with Down's syndrome resemble their parents and siblings but with some physical characteristics that are recognisable – for example, eyes with an epicanthic fold, broad hands with stubby fingers and a simian crease. The number of children born with Down's syndrome, despite having declined since the introduction of screening, increased by 2009, attributed to more people opting to start families later. Interestingly, an increasing number of mothers who were given results that indicated the risk following screening chose to go ahead with their pregnancies. Current estimates are that 1 in every 1,000 babies (i.e. about 775) are born in England and Wales each year with Down's syndrome (Morris and Springett, 2014).

The Down's Syndrome Association (DSA) vision is to create conditions in which all people with Down's syndrome live full and rewarding lives. They are spearheading the 'Tell it Right® Start it Right' (Down's Syndrome Association, 2016) campaign to ensure health professionals (including nurses) continue to provide information about Down's syndrome in a non-biased manner – including non-invasive prenatal testing (NIPT). The DSA have reported that prospective parents can feel pressurised into a termination when being given a very pessimistic view of the life chances of someone with Down's syndrome, a view that is not always accurate.

SEE ALSO
CHAPTER 19

Children with Down's syndrome are more prone to respiratory problems; they are more likely to breathe through their mouths. Between 40 per cent and 60 per cent of babies with Down's syndrome have cardiac problems as a result of their congenital abnormality – for example, Fallots tetralogy (The Down's Syndrome Medical Interest Group, 2007).

Additionally, they are also at risk of hypothyroidism, atlanto axial instability, leukaemia, delayed milk teeth and subsequent dental problems, ear and eye infections and lower white cell count (NHS Health Scotland, 2004). This may sound negative, but with the correct approach and knowledge, you will assist the child and parents in navigating the healthcare system.

To remind yourself of the relevant anatomy and physiology please read the A&P link to *Fundamentals of Children's Anatomy and Physiology: A Textbook for Nursing and Healthcare Students* (Peate and Gormley-Fleming (eds), 2015), Chapters 5, 9 and 10.

Children with autism

Many children with learning disability are diagnosed/can be described as also being on the autistic spectrum, often experiencing difficulties making sense of their world and with their social imagination (National Autistic Society, 2016a). Because of these factors children diagnosed with autism can find their healthcare experience difficult. For children, interventions should focus on important aspects of their development. As a healthcare professional, you will play an important role in helping parents improve their ability to communicate and to 'focus on the individual child, not their diagnosis' (Jones, 2015). This statement is echoed by the mother of Danny, a young man of 15 years with autism and who lives a full, unique life based on an individualised care package. Go to https://study.sagepub.com/essentialchildnursing and watch the video on 'What is autism?'.

VIDEO LINK
36.4: WHAT IS
AUTISM?

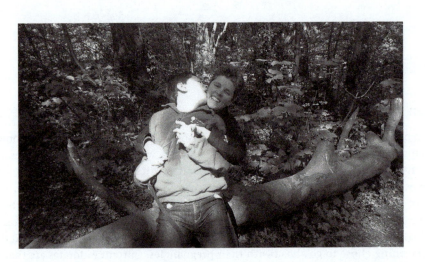

Figure 36.2 Danny

Autism spectrum disorder (ASD) is a lifelong developmental condition affecting the way the brain processes information. It occurs in varying levels of severity, is a lifelong condition with no single cause and about four times as many boys as girls are diagnosed (National Autistic Society, 2016a, 2016b). Gould and Ashton-Smith (2011) argued a case for missed diagnosis and misdiagnosis in females. ASD has a wide range of symptoms, often grouped into two main categories: problems with social interaction and communication, such as understanding other people's emotions and feelings, and restricted and repetitive patterns of thought, interests and physical behaviours (Jones, 2015). NICE suggest around half have an intellectual (learning) disability and approximately 70 per cent have at least one other mental or physical health problem, often unrecognised, including eating and sleeping problems, epilepsy, anxiety, depression, attention deficit hyperactivity disorder and dyspraxia (Jones, 2015).

SEE ALSO
CHAPTER 2

Signs of autism can be noticed in some children aged 2, becoming more noticeable as children grow. The role of the health visitor is crucial, as are nursery staff and teachers, to assist in assessment and early diagnosis, and appropriate intervention including social interaction, communication and cognitive skill development. A key point for you is that effective and appropriate communication is essential.

ACTIVITY 36.2: CRITICAL THINKING

What communication skills do you need to communicate effectively with a child who is on the autistic spectrum? Where can you seek assistance in refining these?

ACTIVITY
ANSWER 36.2

CHALLENGES TO CHILDREN'S HEALTH AND WELLBEING

Emerson et al. (2010, p. 2) claim that the 'risk of children being reported by their main carer (usually their mother) to have fair/poor general health is 2.5–4.5 times greater for children with learning disabilities when compared to their non-disabled peers'. This statement is crucial for health professionals – especially nurses who are often the first or main contact for a family – and highlights inequalities in health faced by many learning disabled people. Some health challenges that children with learning disabilities face are described below.

Respiratory problems

Children with PMLD are more at risk of developing a respiratory problem because the nature of their disability may make them more prone to aspiration. The risk of this happening needs to be fully assessed by the multidisciplinary team. Dysphagia is also a problem (Roberts, 2010). Where children have difficulties swallowing this may be compounded by difficulty in coughing, which may lead to fluid and food entering the lungs. The number of children with learning disabilities who have enteral feeding to manage their nutritional needs has increased. A side effect of non-oral feeding is increased saliva production, which in turn may lead to aspiration.

A&P LINK

To remind yourself of the relevant anatomy and physiology, please read the A&P link: 'Nutrition and enteral feeding' at https://study.sagepub.com/essentialchildnursing

A&P LINK 36.1:
NUTRITION
& ENTERAL
FEEDING

An increase in enteral feeding has resulted in fewer hospital admissions for children with respiratory disease. Importantly, parents have been found to have positive perceptions about their child's growth and development after enteral feeding has been introduced (Sullivan et. al., 2005). Other physical abnormalities can also contribute to poor respiratory function; children with specific syndromes or birth defects, spinal problems such as kyphoscoliosis and neuromuscular defects can prevent the child breathing normally. Children can have asthma and allergies that impact on their ability to breathe with ease.

Nutrition

You may be working with children who have difficulties with their nutritional status. A common cause of malnutrition is insufficient dietary intake because of feeding difficulties. Some may overeat as the result of an inherited condition (Emerson, 2004) of which Prader Willi Syndrome is a good example. A defect in chromosome 15 disrupts the functioning of the hypothalamus, which plays a part in the production of hormones but importantly in regulating appetite.

Children may have their ability to consume and enjoy food impaired by a number of factors: these may be physical, behavioural or both. Physically, some conditions (e.g. foetal alcohol syndrome and Down's syndrome) may result in the child having a deformity of their oral cavity or difficulties resulting in problems with sucking, chewing, swallowing, choking and aspiration. Detailed assessment by the multidisciplinary team of this may result in modifications, including how the child receives their nutrition.

Children with physical disabilities may be unable to move themselves into a position that makes eating a comfortable and enjoyable process. Functionally and behaviourally some children may struggle or never develop the skills to eat by themselves unaided. There are a range of utensils and devices available to enable children to learn to eat independently or more independently.

Behaviourally, some children have problems with attention or proximity, or disruptive conduct (i.e. spitting, screaming, refusing to sit and refusal of food) that maintaining their mealtimes can be challenging. It is essential that nurses caring for children with learning disabilities are alert to the problems of over- and under-nutrition and closely monitor the child's nutritional status (Caroline Walker Trust, 2007).

WHAT'S THE EVIDENCE?

Feeding children with cerebral palsy orally may encourage oral motor function, including language development skills. Enteral feeding may, however, be more effective in providing nutrition and hydration. Approaches to risk management for minimising the risk of aspiration is a key determinant in reaching a decision to provide an enteral intervention. (Arvedson, 2013). However, evidence suggests that this is not always beneficial to family life, and the debate continues about giving children the opportunity for oral taste and the social aspects of feeding experiences.

- How can children's nurses help empower the child and their family to make difficult choices that involve discussions about risk management in this situation?

WHAT'S THE EVIDENCE? ANSWER 36.1

Epilepsy

The Joint Epilepsy Council of the UK and Ireland (2011) stated that around one in five people with learning (or intellectual) disability have epilepsy. Not only does it manifest much earlier in childhood, the more severe the learning disability the greater the incidence. Some children may have epilepsy as part of their syndrome – for example, fragile X; some resulting from their condition – for example, cerebral palsy. Seizures are noted to be more difficult to manage with often a higher seizure frequency (Ockenden, 2007). The ketogenic diet (Epilepsy Society, 2016) may be tried when epilepsy does not respond to treatment. Read more about this at https://study.sagepub.com/essentialchildnursing Parents may be faced with taking decisions and administering emergency medication as well as managing regular medications. Enabling parents to make judgements and gain skills to manage their child's epilepsy requires you to be a skilled practitioner with advanced communication skills and clinical knowledge in what could be a life-threatening situation.

WEBLINK:
KETOGENIC
DIET

Children with learning disabilities and challenging behaviour

All children require individual approaches. Whilst not widely researched, the health and wellbeing of the family was found to be not only adversely affected by the demands of physical care but more so by the level of behavioural problems (Raina et al., 2005). Children who present with the most demanding behaviour problems can be referred to as having 'challenging behaviour'. This is broadly categorised in four ways: aggressive, destructive, or engaging in self-injurious behaviours or stereotypical behaviours. Examples of challenging behaviour that children with a learning disability can exhibit are listed below:

- Hurting self and/or others
- Head-banging, eye poking, hand biting
- Hair pulling, biting, scratching, hitting, head butting
- Destructive behaviours
- Throwing things, breaking things
- Tearing things up
- Eating inedible objects e.g. stones, pen tops, bedding, paper

Other behaviours:

- Spitting
- Smearing
- Repetitive rocking
- Running away
- Stripping (The Challenging Behaviour Foundation, 2016)

NICE estimates that around 41,500 children with learning disabilities display behaviour that challenges (NICE, 2015). McGill's blog (2012) suggests that difficult behaviours may manifest in all children during 'the terrible twos', but with the development of cognitive and communication skills these are usually resolved. Developmental delays impede the ability to communicate and understand, and the learning disabled child remains unable to progress to more acceptable behaviour. For children with learning disabilities it is essential to recognise that health and medical conditions can also be an underlying factor in challenging behavior – for example, particularly painful are irritating inflammatory conditions such as earache and toothache.

For parents the impact on the quality of life of the family may be very distressing. For professionals meeting the health, educational and social care needs of the child and family it demands a collaborative and effective approach. From the child's perspective it can put their personal safety at risk, disrupt home life and can lessen the child's ability to be included in ordinary social, educational and recreational activities. In turn this can further affect their development by causing problems with their learning and attainment; their behaviour may be not only disruptive but put other children at risk. The Royal College of Nursing (2010) raised in their draft consultation overreliance on the use of restrictive interventions in learning disability services and in some schools. Guidance for best practice has been commissioned by the Department of Health and emphasises strongly that some forms of restraint being used are not consistent with the UN Convention on the Rights of the Child (UN, 1989).

SCENARIO 36.2: RAVI

Ravi is currently on a children's ward whilst essential surgery is carried out to improve his bilateral cavorous feet. Ravi finds the hospital environment very difficult. Ravi has both severe learning disabilities and an autistic spectrum disorder. Ravi shouts repetitively, slaps his face and furniture, then laughs loudly at the noise he makes. Ravi is constantly active, climbing over the side of his bed. When staff attempt to return Ravi to his bed he screams, bites his arm and slaps his head. Ravi's mother suggests that the staff try tying him into the bed by his legs as this is what she does at home.

- What might be the impact of Ravi's behaviour on the other children and parents in the ward?
- Why may children display enhanced problem behaviours in the clinical environment?
- Suggest strategies that you could use to communicate with Ravi

SCENARIO
ANSWER 36.2

Communication and the child in the health setting

Seliner et. al. (2015) suggest that, overall, children with disabilities are hospitalised more often than healthy children. You are well placed to be supportive to both the child and the parents, by supporting and assisting them to face the daunting challenge of providing multifaceted care over a protracted length of time. Bemister et. al. (2015) revealed that the blame attached to the child's condition had a mediating effect on caregiver depression. It can be difficult to help any child make sense of what is happening to them in a health setting; those with a learning disability face a greater challenge. They require nurses and other staff to use their extensive interpersonal skills to create a relationship that comforts the child (and parents/family) and facilitates the care they require.

For many children with learning disabilities communicating can prove difficult. Parents and siblings often develop systems of understanding, picking up on cues of body language, using eye contact and facial expressions to interpret and convey meanings. Makaton and Picture Exchange Communication Systems (PECS) are widely used as augmentative communication systems to assist children in finding their voice. Technological advances in Voice Output Communication Aids (VOCA) provide wonderful opportunities for even the most severely disabled children to express their needs and interact. Books beyond Words have a range of health-related picture-only materials, including a selection for children with learning disabilities. Many apps are also available.

Communication and coordination of care on every level are crucially important. Where this does not happen, the consequences can be devastating. Following successive investigations into avoidable deaths amongst patients with learning disabilities (Heslop et al., 2013; Department of Health, 2014) in acute hospital settings, service providers have been developing strategies to improve the care and communication experiences. The initial work continues with an initial three-year Learning Disabilities Mortality Review (LeDeR) Programme commissioned by the Healthcare Quality Improvement Partnership (HQIP) on behalf of NHS England in June 2015 to review the deaths of people with learning disabilities.

WEBLINK: AUGMENTATIVE COMMUNICATION SYSTEMS

> A key part of the LeDeR Programme is to support local areas to review the deaths of people with learning disabilities aged 4 years and over, irrespective of whether the death was expected or not, the cause of death or the place of death. This will enable them to identify good practice and what has worked well, as well as where improvements to the provision of care could be made (University of Bristol, n.d.)

WEBLINK: HQIP

Wales spearheaded the 'Care Bundle' which sets out the steps to be taken to ensure the safety of patients of all ages who have a learning disability in hospital or in an Accident and Emergency department. This is used countrywide. Derriford Hospital uses a system of NHS mail alerts that notify GPs, community teams for learning disabilities and other key liaison staff when a child or young adult with a learning disability is admitted. Great Ormond Street Hospital has developed a 'purple dot' added to the child's notes to denote that they have a learning disability. In addition, the expertise of specialist groups such as the National Autistic Society has helped develop hospital passports that focus on individual needs – thus aiding communication with a child who, for example, does not like being touched – and gives their preferred name, how they eat, their health needs, etc.

ACTIVITY 36.3: REFLECTIVE PRACTICE

- Practise and learn eight Makaton signs that you consider essential to making a child feel reassured in an acute hospital setting
- Compile a list of questions that you consider essential to include in a health passport for a young child with PMLD or ASD
- How could you reassure a young child who is on the autistic spectrum and does not like having people in close proximity or being touched?
- Explore how 'Books Beyond Words' can assist you in communicating with children (or their parents) who have a learning disability

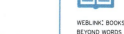

ACTIVITY ANSWER 36.3

WEBLINK: BOOKS BEYOND WORDS

VIDEO LINK 36.5: BOOKS BEYOND WORDS

Safeguarding

It is suggested that children with disabilities are three times more at risk of physical, sexual and emotional abuse and neglect than their non-disabled peers, boys being more at risk than girls. Although a contentious issue, research evidence suggests that disabled children also are more at risk of 'beliefs about evil spirits and witchcraft' in particular communities. For more information see Miller and Brown (2014). Children with learning disabilities are not a heterogeneous group; they manifest their problems and issues in many ways. Recognising that the children who are most at risk are children whose behaviours can be difficult to manage and challenge service provision helps to safeguard their welfare.

SEE ALSO CHAPTER 9

WEBLINK:
THE CODE

ACTIVITY 36.4: CRITICAL THINKING

In the previous scenario Ravi's behaviour is causing problems and Ravi's mother is using and suggesting a restrictive intervention that is unacceptable. She needs to be supported as a parent looking after a child with behaviours that challenge, and the ward manager needs to follow the organisation's safeguarding protocols. The Nursing and Midwifery Council provide guidance for students and registrants in *The Code*, which you can access via https://study.sagepub.com/essentialchildnursing The section on 'Preserving safety' is particularly relevant.

For nursing students the key requisites underpinning working with children who have learning disabilities is openness to learn about the the whole child, extending both the child's communication skills and their own. Each child is unique and every encounter is different. This chapter has as its intent to motivate nursing students to investigate the potential of the child with a learning disability despite their significant problems, and to design and deliver professional, competent nursing care and support.

PLACEMENT
ADVICE 36:
LEARNING
DISABILITIES

Go to https://study.sagepub.com/essentialchildnursing for tips on preparing for placements with children with learning disabilities.

CHAPTER SUMMARY

- Children with learning disabilities spend as much of their lives in an educational setting, where many of the child's needs are met, as in their home
- Effective communication is key to child-centred health, education and social care
- An extensive range of health, social and educational provision is available, delivered by experts with children's nurses at the centre – relationships become well established and knowledge is shared, problems are addressed and often creatively resolved

BUILD YOUR BIBLIOGRAPHY

Books

- Croghan, E. (2007) *Promoting Health in Schools: A Practical Guide for Teachers and School Nurses Working with Children Aged 3 to 11*. London: Sage.
  On how to promote health in schools.

Journal articles

FURTHER
READING:
ONLINE
JOURNAL
ARTICLES

Go to https://study.sagepub.com/essentialchildnursing for further free online journal articles related to this chapter.

- Bellamy, G., Croot, L., Bush, A., Berry, H. and Smith, A. (2010) 'A study to define profound and multiple learning disabilities (PMLD)'. *Journal of Intellectual Disabilities*, 14 (3): 221-35.
  To find out more on profound and multiple learning disabilities (PMLD).

- Emerson, E. and Hatton, C. (2009) 'The contribution of socio-economic position to the health inequalities faced by children and adolescents with intellectual disabilities in Britain'. *American Journal on Mental Retardation*, 112 (2): 140–50.

  On health inequalities in children and adolescents with intellectual disabilities in Britain.

- Emerson, E. and Hatton, C. (2007) 'The mental health of children and adolescents with intellectual disabilities in Britain'. *British Journal of Psychiatry*, 191: 493-9.
  British children and adolescents with intellectual disabilities and mental health.

Weblinks

Go to https://study.sagepub.com/essentialchildnursing for further weblinks related to this chapter.

FURTHER
READING:
WEBLINKS

- NSPCC, *'We Have the Right to Be Safe': Protecting Disabled Children from Abuse* (Miller and Brown, 2014)

  www.nspcc.org.uk/globalassets/documents/research-reports/right-safe-disabled-children-abuse-report.pdf

- NHS Choices, *Down's Syndrome*

  www.nhs.uk/Conditions/downs-syndrome/Pages/Introduction.aspx

ACE YOUR ASSESSMENT

Revise what you have learned by visiting https://study.sagepub.com/essentialchildnursing

ONLINE
QUIZZES &
ACTIVITY
ANSWERS

GREAT FOR
REVISION!

- Test yourself with multiple-choice and short-answer questions
- Do the chapter activities in the book and check your answers online

STATUTES

Children Act 1989
Children Act 2004
Children and Families Act 2014
Disability Discrimination Act 1995
Disability Discrimination (Northern Ireland) Order 2006
Education Act 1981
Education Act 1996
Human Rights Act 1988
National Health Service and Community Care Act 1990
Special Educational Needs and Disability Act 2001

REFERENCES

Arvedson, J. C., (2013) 'Feeding children with cerebral palsy & swallowing difficulties'. *European Journal Of Clinical Nutrition*, 67: S9-S12. Available at: www.nature.com/ejcn/journal/v67/n2s/full/ejcn2013224a.html (accessed 3 July 2017).

Beacock, S., Borthwick, R., Kelly, J., Craine, R. and Jelfs, E. (2015) *Learning Disabilities Meeting Educational Needs of Nursing Students*. The UK Learning and Intellectual Disability Nursing Academic Network (LIDNAN) and the UK Council of Deans of Health (CoDH). Available at: www.councilofdeans.org.uk/wp-content/uploads/2015/01/LD-Nursing-report-Jan-15-Final.pdf (last accessed 3 July 2017).

Bemister, T. B., Brooks, B. L., Dyke, R. H. and Kirton, A. (2015) 'Predictors of caregiver depression and family functioning after perinatal stroke'. *BMC Pediatr,* 15. Available at: www.ncbi.nlm.nih.gov/pmc/articles/PMC4502550/ (last accessed 3 July 2017).

The Caroline Walker Trust (2007) *Eating Well: Children and Adults with Learning Disabilities Nutritional and Practical Guidelines*. Available at: www.cwt.org.uk/wp-content/uploads/2015/02/EWLDGuidelines.pdf (last accessed 3 July 2017).

Carpenter, B., Cockbill, B., Wiggett, D. and Egerton, J. (2013) *Engaging Children with Complex Learning Difficulties and Disabilities in the Primary Classroom*. Available at: www.engagement4learning.com/wp-content/uploads/2016/11/Primary-Australian-article-Carpenter-et-al-2013.pdf (accessed 3 July 2010).

The Challenging Behaviour Foundation (2016) *Statement on restrictive physical interventions with children*. Available at: www.challengingbehaviour.org.uk/learning-disability-assets/statementonrestrictivephysicalinterventionswithchildren.pdf (accessed 3 July 2017).

Cm 5086 (2001) *Valuing People: A New Strategy for Learning Disability for the 21st Century*. London: Department of Health. Available at: www.gov.uk/government/uploads/system/uploads/attachment_data/file/250877/5086.pdf (last accessed 3 June 2017).

Cm 5860 (2003) *Every Child Matters*. London: TSO. Available at: www.education.gov.uk/consultations/downloadableDocs/EveryChildMatters.pdf (last accessed 3 June 2017).

Cockburn, F. (2013) 'Alcohol and health: A paediatrician's perspective (II)', in Foetal Alcohol Forum FASD The International Medical e-Network devoted to Foetal Alcohol Spectrum Disorders. Available at: www.nofas-uk.org/PDF/Forum%20Issue%209%20Final.pdf (accessed 3 July 2017).

Department for Education (2014) *Special Educational Needs in England: January 2014*. London: National Statistics. Available at: www.gov.uk/government/uploads/system/uploads/attachment_data/file/362704/SFR26-2014_SEN_06102014.pdf (last accessed 3 June 2017).

Department for Education (2014a) *Children and Families Act*. London: The Stationery Office. Available at: www.legislation.gov.uk/ukpga/2014/6/contents/enacted (last accessed 3 July 2017).

Department for Education and Department of Health (2015) *Special Educational Needs and Disability Code of Practice: 0 to 25 Years. Statutory Guidance for Organisations Which Work with and Support Children and Young People Who Have Special Educational Needs or Disabilities*. Available at www.gov.uk/government/uploads/system/uploads/attachment_data/file/398815/SEND_Code_of_Practice_January_2015.pdf (last accessed 3 June 2017).

Department for Education and Skills (2013) *Working Together to Safeguard Children*. London: The Stationery Office. Available at: www.gov.uk/government/uploads/system/uploads/attachment_data/file/417669/Archived-Working_together_to_safeguard_children.pdf (last accessed 10 January 2016).

Department of Health (2009) *Healthy Child Programme: The Two Year Review*. London: Department of Health. Available at: www.gov.uk/government/uploads/system/uploads/attachment_data/file/377800/dh_108329.pdf (last accessed 3 June 2017).

Department of Health (2014) *premature Deaths of People with Learning Disabilities: Progress Update*. London: The Stationery Office. Available at: www.gov.uk/government/uploads/system/uploads/attachment_data/file/356229/PUBLISH_42715_2902809_Progress_Report_Accessible_v04.pdf (accessed 10 January 2016).

Donetto, S., Malone, M., Hughes, J., Morrow, E., Cowley, S. and Maben, J. (2013) *Health Visiting: The Voice of Service Users – Learning from Service Users' Experiences to Inform the Development of UK Health Visiting Practice and Services*. London: National Nursing Research Unit, King's College London.

Available at: www.kcl.ac.uk/nursing/research/nnru/publications/Reports/Voice-of-service-user-report-July-2013-FINAL.pdf (last accessed 3 July 2017).

Down's Syndrome Association (2016) *Tell It Right Start It Right Campaign*. Available at: www.downs-syndrome.org.uk/about/campaigns/tell-it-right-start-it-right/ (last accessed 3 July 2017).

The Down's Syndrome Medical Interest Group UK and Ireland (2007) *Guidance for Essential Medical Surveillance: Cardiac Disease*. Available at: www.dsmig.org.uk/wp-content/uploads/2015/09/guideline-cardiac-5.pdf (last accessed 3 July 2017).

Emerson, E., Glover, G., Turner, S., Greig, R., Hatton, C., Baines, S., Copeland, A., Evison, F., Roberts, H., Robertson, J. and Welch, V. (2010) Improving health and lives: The Learning Disabilities Public Health Observatory. *Advances in Mental Health and Intellectual Disabilities*, 6(1): 26–32. Available at: https://doi.org/10.1108/20441281211198835 (last accessed 3 July 2017).

Epilepsy Society (2016) Ketogenic diet. Available at: www.epilepsysociety.org.uk/ketogenic-diet?gclid=CMfK0p_Lv9ICFdQ_GwodzycACA#.WLwiaW_yjIU (last accessed 03 July 2017).

Gould, J. and Ashton-Smith, J. (2011) 'Missed diagnosis or misdiagnosis: girls and women on the autistic spectrum'. *Good Autism Practice*, 12 (1): 34–41.

Hartley, R. (2010) *Teacher Expertise for Special Educational Needs: Filling in the gaps* (Research note: July). London: Policy Exchange.

Heslop, P., Blair, P., Fleming, P., Hoghton, M., Marriott, A. and Russ, L. (2013) *Confidential Inquiry into premature deaths of people with learning disabilities (CIPOLD)*. Norah Fry Research Centre University of Bristol. Available at: www.bristol.ac.uk/media-library/sites/cipold/migrated/documents/fullfinalreport.pdf (last accessed 3 July 2017).

HM Government (2009) *Valuing People Now: A New Three-year Strategy for People with Learning Disabilities*. London: The Stationery Office. Available at: http://webarchive.nationalarchives.gov.uk/20130107105354/http://www.dh.gov.uk/prod_consum_dh/groups/dh_digitalassets/documents/digitalasset/dh_093375.pdf (last accessed 03 July 2017).

HM Government (2015) *Working Together to Safeguard Children*. London: DfE. Available at: www.gov.uk/government/publications/working-together-to-safeguard-children--2 (last accessed 3 June 2017).

Holland, K. (2011) *Factsheet: Learning Disabilities*. British Institute for Learning Disabilities. Available at: www.bild.org.uk/EasysiteWeb/getresource.axd?AssetID=2522&type=full&servicetype=Attachment (last accessed 3 July 2017).

Hutton, J. L. and Pharoah, P. O. D. (2006) 'Life expectancy in severe cerebral palsy'. *Diseases in Childhood*, 91(3). Available at: www.ncbi.nlm.nih.gov/pmc/articles/PMC2065925/ (last accessed 3 July 2017).

The Joint Epilepsy Council of the UK and Ireland (2011) *Epilepsy Prevalence, Incidence and other Statistics*. Joint Epilepsy Council of the UK and Ireland. Available at: www.epilepsyscotland.org.uk/pdf/Joint_Epilepsy_Council_Prevalence_and_Incidence_September_11_(3).pdf (last accessed 3 July 2017).

Jones, S. (2015) 'Autistic Spectrum Disorder clinical update'. *Nursing Standard*, 29 (38):19.

Mansell, J. (1997) '"Better Services" 25 Years On' *Tizard Learning Disability Review*, 2 (1): 45–46. Available at: https://doi.org/10.1108/13595474199700009 (last accessed 3 July 2017).

Mansell, J. (2010) *Raising our Sights: Services for Adults with Profound Intellectual and Multiple Disabilities*. Tizard Centre, University of Kent. Available at: http://webarchive.nationalarchives.gov.uk/20130105195721/http://www.dh.gov.uk/prod_consum_dh/groups/dh_digitalassets/@dh/@en/@ps/documents/digitalasset/dh_117961.pdf (last accessed 3 July 2017).

McCann, D., Bull, R. and Winzenberg, T. (2015) 'Brief Report: Competence, Value and Enjoyment of Childcare Activities Undertaken by Parents of Children With Complex Needs'. *Journal of Pediatric Nursing*. Available at: www.pediatricnursing.org/article/S0882-5963(15)00339-5/abstract (last accessed 3 July 2017).

McCluskey, J. and McNamara, G. (2005) 'Children in need'. In C. Horton (ed.) *Working with Children 2006–2007: Facts, figures and information*. London: Sage.

McGill, P. (2012) *Understanding Challenging Behaviour*. Available at: www.challengingbehaviour.org.uk/learning-disability-files/01--Understanding-challenging-behaviour.pdf (last accessed 3 July 2017).

MENCAP (2016) *What is a Learning Disability? Our Definition*. Available at: www.mencap.org.uk/learning-disability-explained/what-learning-disability (last accessed 3 July 2017).

MENCAP (2017a) *Don't Miss Out*. Available at: www.mencap.org.uk/advice-and-support/health/dont-miss-out?gclid=EAIaIQobChMIpdiejKHt1AIVyantCh2yNwvhEAAYASAAEgJ6C_D_BwE (last accessed 3 July 2017).

MENCAP (2017b) *Transition into Adult Services*. Available at: www.mencap.org.uk/advice-and-support/children-and-young-people/education-support/transition-adult-services (last accessed 3 July 2017).

Miller, D. and Brown, D. (2014) *We Have the Right to be Safe: Protecting Disabled Children from Abuse*. Executive Summary NSPCC. Available at: www.nspcc.org.uk/globalassets/documents/research-reports/right-safe-disabled-children-abuse-report.pdf (last accessed 3 July 2017).

Morris, J. K. and Springett, A. (2014) *National Down's Syndrome Cytogenetic Register for England and Wales 2012 Annual Report*. Available at: www.binocar.org/content/annrep2012_final.pdf (last accessed 3 July 2017).

National Autistic Society (2016a) *Our Position on the Causes of Autism*. Available at: www.autism.org.uk/get-involved/media-centre/position-statements/causes.aspx (last accessed 3 July 2017).

National Autistic Society (2016b) *What is Autism?* Available at: www.autism.org.uk/about/what-is.aspx (last accessed 3 July 2017).

National Institute for Health and Care Excellence (2015) *Challenging Behaviour and Learning Disabilities: Prevention and interventions for people with learning disabilities whose behaviour challenges* NICE guideline 11. Available at: www.rcpch.ac.uk/system/files/protected/page/NICE%20CG%20Challenging%20behaviour%20and%20learning%20disabilities%20-%20full%20version%20PUBLISHED_0.pdf (last accessed 10 January 2016).

National Institute for Health and Care Excellence (2017) *Cerebral Palsy in under 25s: assessment and management* NICE guideline [NG62]. Available at: www.nice.org.uk/guidance/ng62 (last accessed 3 July 2017).

NHS England (2013) *Supporting and Meeting the Needs of People with Profound and Multiple Learning Disabilities – Top Tips*. Available at: www.devon.gov.uk/nhsenglandsouth_pmld_version2.pdf (last accessed 13 January 2016).

NHS Health Scotland (2004) *Health Needs Assessment Report – Summary People with a Learning Disabilities in Scotland*. Available at: www.healthscotland.com/uploads/documents/1676-LD_summary.pdf (last accessed 3 July 2017).

Nursing and Midwifery Council (2015) *The Code. Professional Standards of Practice and Behaviour for Nurses and Midwives*. London: Nursing and Midwifery Council. Available at: www.nmc.org.uk/globalassets/sitedocuments/nmc-publications/nmc-code.pdf (last accessed 3 July 2017).

Ockenden, J. (2007) 'Epilepsy and people with PMLD'. *PMLD Link*, 19, 3: 6-9. Available at: www.pmldlink.org.uk/wp-content/uploads/2015/09/PMLD-Link-Issue-58.pdf (last accessed 3 July 2017).

Peate, I. and Gormley-Fleming, E. (eds) (2015) *Fundamentals of Children's Anatomy and Physiology: A Textbook for Nursing and Healthcare Students*. Chichester: Wiley Blackwell.

Public Health England (2015) *The Determinants of Health Inequities Experienced by Children with Learning Disabilities*. Available at: www.gcad.info/media/294672/determinants_of_child_health_inequalities.pdf (last accessed 3 July 2017).

Public Health England (2016) *Learning Disabilities Observatory: People with learning disabilities in England 2015: Main report Version 1.0*. Available at: www.gov.uk/government/uploads/system/

uploads/attachment_data/file/613182/PWLDIE_2015_main_report_NB090517.pdf (last accessed 3 July 2017).

Raina, P., O'Donnell, M., Rosenbaum, R., Brehaut, R., Walter, S. D., Russell, D., Swinton, M., Zhu, B. and Wood, E. (2005) 'The health and well-being of caregivers of children with cerebral palsy. *Pediatrics*, 115(6): 26–36. Available at: http://pediatrics.aappublications.org/content/pediatrics/115/6/e626.full.pdf (last accessed 3 July 2017).

Roberts, J. (2010) 'Dysphagia: the challenge of managing eating and drinking difficulties in children and adults who have learning disabilities'. *Tizard Learning Disability Review*, 15(1): 14–16. Available at: www.emeraldinsight.com/doi/abs/10.5042/tldr.2010.0024 (last accessed 3 July 2017).

Royal College of Nursing (2010) *Royal College of Nursing Consultation Draft Guidance on the Minimisation of and Alternatives to Restrictive Practices in Health and Adult Social Care, and Special Schools*. Available at: www.rcpsych.ac.uk/pdf/Use_of_restrictive_practices_in_health_and_adult_social_care_and_special_schools_-_draft_guidance.pdf (last accessed 3 July 2017).

Scottish Government (2012) *Strengthening the Commitment: The Report of the UK Modernising Learning Disabilities Nursing Review*. Available at: www.gov.scot/resource/0039/00391946.pdf (last accessed 3 July 2017).

Scottish Government (2013) *The Keys to Life: Improving Quality of Life for People with Learning Disabilities*. Available at: www.gov.scot/Resource/0042/00424389.pdf (last accessed 3 July 2017).

Seliner, B. Wattinger, A. and Spirig, R. (2015) 'Experiences and needs of parents of hospitalised children with disabilities and the health professionals responsible for the child's health-care – A systematic review'. *Pflege*, 28(5): 263–76. Available at: www.ncbi.nlm.nih.gov/pubmed/26412679 (last accessed 3 July 2017).

Sullivan, P. B., Juszczak, E., Bachlet, A. M., Lambert, B., Vernon-Roberts, A., Grant, H.W., Eltumi, M., Mclean, L., Alder, N. and Thomas, A.G. (2005) 'Gastrostomy tube feeding in children with cerebral palsy: a prospective, longitudinal study'. *Developmental Medicine & Child Neurology*, 47(2): 77–85. Available at: http://onlinelibrary.wiley.com.ezproxy.kingston.ac.uk/doi/10.1111/j.1469-8749.2005.tb01095.x/pdf (last accessed 3 July 2017).

Tommy's (2015) *Premature Birth Statistics*. Available at: www.tommys.org/page.aspx?pid=387 (last accessed 3 July 2017).

The United Nations (1989) *The United Nations Convention on the Rights of the Child*. Available at: www.unicef.org.uk/Documents/Publication-pdfs/UNCRC_PRESS200910web.pdf (last accessed 3 July 2017).

University of Bristol (n.d) *Review of Deaths*. Available at: www.bristol.ac.uk/sps/leder/about/reviews-of-deaths (accessed 15 September 2017) .

Wright, J. (2012) *School Nurse Survival Guide*. London: Quay Books.

CARE OF CHILDREN AND YOUNG PEOPLE WITH MENTAL HEALTH ISSUES

37

ORLA McALINDEN AND JULIA PELLE

THIS CHAPTER COVERS

- Prevalence of some of the more common mental health and behavioural problems in children
- Recognition of some of the conditions, signs and symptoms
- Identifying areas of concern, risk and safeguarding guidance when caring for children with mental health problems

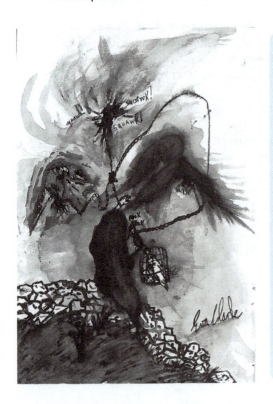

> " A girl had four birds. The first was named Depression, its wings vast, they could easily engulf her, trapping her in a suffocating embrace of feathers and keeping her there. The second was Anxiety, always flapping its wings and squawking, lodging its cries into the back of her head. The third was Stress, by being a parrot, it naturally repeats every worry the girl possesses. Nagging her until she cracks. The final being a woodpecker, named Hate. Hate taps venomous thoughts into her head, like jealously and doubt, until eventually she believes them. The girl loathed each bird! She wished they would stop encircling her, like vultures on the hunt. So, she took the advice of an old Peregrine, named Reason. 'Instead of be-ridding of your four birds, I will give you a fifth. A dove, named Forgiveness.' Said the Peregrine. The girl released the encaged dove. The dove broke the chains, to which the girl was ignorant of, and sat proudly upon her shoulder. Astonished, the girl allowed herself to forgive the birds and they flew away freely. As Forgiveness broke her chains, she gained strength. Most importantly she forgave herself, for chaining the birds to her. She grew wings, learning to fly on her own. The girl became a bird. A bird named Positivity.
>
> Eva Clarke, 13 years old, The Girl of Many Birds "

Visit https://study.sagepub.com/essentialchildnursing to access a wealth of online resources for this chapter – watch out for the margin icons throughout the chapter.

INTRODUCTION

The opening quotation illustrates the feelings of Eva, a young person, regarding mental illness and is reproduced in this chapter with her consent. Sadly, the number of children and young people like Eva who experience mental health issues is growing steadily, and these children continue to present at a much earlier age than previously.

Recent and ongoing media interventions and awareness from the younger British royal family members and high-profile individuals, plus people in general who are more willing to speak of their mental health issues, has cast a fresh spotlight on this dilemma including listening to children, reducing stigma and increasing access to support.

PREVALENCE OF SOME OF THE MORE COMMON MENTAL HEALTH AND BEHAVIOURAL PROBLEMS IN CHILDREN

Seventy per cent of children who experience mental health problems have not had appropriate interventions at a sufficiently early age. These are some of the most vulnerable people in our society (Green et al., 2005; Sempik et al., 2008; Children's Society, 2008; Bazalgette et al., 2015). Helping these children and recognising the impact their disability has on health and wellbeing and their educational and social progress is an ethical and professional imperative for all health and social care professionals in all settings. It could also be argued that in a civilised society it is a legal and ethical imperative to protect our young.

The preferred current approach to caring for a child with a mental health problem is to:

* Build resilience, capacity and inclusion
* Show respect
* Promote 'recovery capability' attitudes
* Minimise the stigma of mental illness
* Raise awareness of the importance and education of early detection, management and support for children who present with mental health issues

Common mental health and behavioural problems in childhood

The World Health Organization (WHO, 2015) estimate that, worldwide, 20 per cent of adolescents in any given year may experience a mental health problem, with the origin of the difficulty starting at a young age.

It is recognised that data for CAMHS in the UK are probably both outdated and difficult to capture accurately. Surveys carried out by the Office of National Statistics (ONS) (Bazalgette at al., 2015) found that 10 per cent of children (aged 5–16 years) already had clinically diagnosable mental health problems.

The same survey, which comprised 7,977 interviews with parents, children and teachers, found the prevalence of mental health problems in children (aged 5–16 years) to be: 78 – 4% for emotional problems (depression or anxiety) – 6% for conduct problems – 2% for hyperkinetic problems – 1% for less common problems (including autism, tic disorders, eating disorders and selective mutism).

Clearly these issues arise much earlier in the lifespan. However, there is a lack of robust information available about the prevalence of preschool mental health problems. This is significant when we consider the importance of early years development and progress.

SEE ALSO
CHAPTER 11

RECOGNITION OF SOME OF THE CONDITIONS, SIGNS AND SYMPTOMS

According to Bazalgette et al. (2015), the rates of mental health problems rise steeply in mid to late adolescence. Fink et al. (2015) carried out a study of 3,366 adolescents which found that, from 2009 to 2014, overall, adolescents experienced similar levels of mental health difficulties (i.e. emotional problems, peer problems, hyperactivity and conduct problems). There was, however, a significant increase in emotional problems in girls over time, and a decrease in mental health difficulties in boys. There are also clear associations between childhood psychological problems and the ability of affected children to live, work and earn as adults. This is not what we desire for our young people and not how they can become happy healthy adults. It is also in opposition to the aspirations of the United Nations Convention on the Rights of the Child (UN, 1989).

One in four adults and one in ten children are likely to have a mental health problem in any year, which can have a profound impact on the lives of tens of millions of people in the UK, and can affect their ability to sustain relationships, work, and life. It is estimated that only about a quarter of people with a mental health problem receive ongoing treatment, meaning the rest deal with their with mental health issues on their own (Mental Health Foundation, 2015).

SEE ALSO
CHAPTERS 11
AND 38

Both retrospective and prospective research has shown that most adulthood mental health problems begin in childhood and adolescence. This highlights further the importance of gaining understanding of the magnitude, risk factors and progression of mental disorders in youth (Ries Merikangas et al., 2009).

WEBLINK:
NATIONAL
SERVICE
FRAMEWORK

Go to https://study.sagepub.com/essentialchildnursing to access *A National Service Framework for Children, Young People and Maternity Services* (Department of Health, 2004**)**, a ten-year programme (which remains government policy) intended to stimulate long-term sustained improvement in children's health to ensure fair, high-quality integrated health and social care from pregnancy through to adulthood and *The Five Year Forward View for Mental Health* (Mental Health Taskforce to the NHS in England, 2016). The Children's National Service Framework is aimed at everyone who comes into contact with or delivers services to children.

WEBLINK:
FIVE YEAR
FORWARD

Contemporary issues in the field of child psychiatric epidemiology include: refinement of classification and assessment, inclusion of young children in epidemiologic surveys, integration of child and adult psychiatric epidemiology, and evaluation of both mental and physical disorders in children (Ries Merikangas et al., 2009).

Anxiety disorders

SEE ALSO
CHAPTERS 10,
11 & 13

Those experiencing disorders usually have recurring intrusive thoughts or concerns and may avoid certain situations out of worry. They may also have physical symptoms such as sweating, trembling, dizziness or a rapid heartbeat. Anxiety disorder is a common mental illness defined by feelings of uneasiness, worry and fear and whilst anxiety occurs for everyone sometimes, a person with an anxiety disorder feels an inappropriate amount of anxiety more often than is reasonable to expect.

VIDEO
LINK 37.1:
STRESS &
ANXIETY

Many people with an anxiety disorder do not realise they have a defined, treatable disorder and as a result anxiety disorders are thought to be underdiagnosed. The definition of an anxiety disorder also requires evidence of an impairment of day-to-day functioning. The child with an anxiety disorder often experiences a significantly reduced quality of life and anxiety disorders are also associated with other health-related issues (comorbidities). You can find out more about how the brain responds to stress and anxiety by watching the video accessible via https://study.sagepub.com/essentialchildnursing

Anxiety disorders are the most frequent conditions seen in children, followed by behaviour disorders, mood disorders (e.g. depression), and substance use disorders. About 290,000 children (3.3%) have an anxiety disorder.

Several types of anxiety disorders are identified in the *Diagnostic and Statistical Manual of Mental Disorders* (APA, 2013):

- Obsessive-compulsive disorder (OCD)
- Generalised anxiety disorder (GAD)
- Panic disorder
- Post-traumatic stress disorder (PTSD)
- Agoraphobia
- Social phobia, also referred to as social anxiety disorder

Specific phobia (also known as a simple phobia):

- Adjustment disorder with anxious features
- Acute stress disorder
- Substance-induced anxiety disorder
- Anxiety due to a general medical condition

Social phobia

This is the most common anxiety disorder and typically manifests before the age of 20. Specific, or simple phobias – such as a fear of snakes – are also very common with more than 1 in 10 people experiencing a specific phobia in their lifetime. Read about Aidan's experience below and consult https:// study.sagepub.com/essentialchildnursing for some suggested approaches to his situation.

SCENARIO 37.1: AIDAN

Aidan is 18 years old and due to complete his final year of A levels at sixth form college. Aidan lives with his mother Iris, a single mum and hotel manager, and a younger brother Jonathan aged 15.

Iris has observed a change in Aidan's behaviour since receiving results for his mock A level exams, in which he received good grades. Although his teachers report good progress, Aidan felt very disappointed with his results and has become very irritable. His brother Jonathan complains that Aidan doesn't come out with him to play football any more and gives the excuse that he is too tired and has to study for getting into university. Aidan's peers say that he has become very distressed, he has started to hyperventilate and asks to be excused from class more frequently. One of his teachers has suggests he goes to see the school nurse to get 'checked over'.

- What are the key signs and symptoms Aidan presents with?
- How does this affect his family life and school life?

PRACTICE SCENARIO 37: ADAM & CLAIRE

✓

SCENARIO ANSWERS 37.1

When I was at school nobody spoke about it at school. When I tried to go and get help from many different places they said I was young and they didn't understand how I could possibly be suffering from mental health conditions. There was a lot of stigma around it. They said, 'you are young, you don't have anything to worry about.' Even after I was diagnosed I had people saying to me, 'you don't want people talking about it, you don't want people knowing about it.' There was no education about it and no discussion about it. It made me feel worse, and prevented me from seeking help.

(Continued)

(Continued)

[I got help] initially from my GP. She referred me to mental health services. I had cognitive behavioural therapy and I was prescribed medication. Once I started to speak about it, I got support from family and close friends; the biggest thing that changed my outlook was cognitive behavioural therapy.

Lynne, (Malik, 2016)

What is the difference between fear and anxiety?

WEBLINK:
FEAR &
ANXIETY:
EXTREME
SPORT

Go to https://study.sagepub.com/essentialchildnursing to access the journal articles by Brymer and Schweitzer (2013) and Sylvers et al. (2011) on the subject.

Major depression

Major depression, also referred to as clinical depression, usually requires an occurrence of two or more episodes of significant depression. The number of young people aged 15–16 with depression nearly doubled between the 1980s and the 2000s (Beng Huat See and Gorard, 2013; Gorard and Beng Huat See, 2015).

In children, clinical depression needs to be distinguished from general 'growing pains', the emotions associated with child and adolescent development or normal everyday 'blues'. Depression can go unrecognised and untreated because it is passed off as the normal emotional and psychological experience of ongoing childhood growth and development.

Over 8,000 children younger than 10 years old suffer from severe depression (Green et al., 2005). About 8,700 children (0.2%) aged between 5 and 10 years old are seriously depressed. About 62,000 children (1.4%) between 11 and 16 years old are seriously depressed. Between 1 in 12 and 1 in 15 children deliberately self-harm (Mental Health Foundation, 2015) which is characterised by low mood and/or loss of interests or pleasure in life activities, continues for at least two weeks and includes five of the ten symptoms listed below:

- A low/depressed mood most of the day
- Diminished social interests or reduced pleasure in all or most activities
- Changes in appetite e.g. significant or unintentional weight loss or gain
- Changes in sleep patterns e.g. insomnia (lack of sleep) or sleeping too much
- Vocal angry outbursts or crying
- Agitation, irritability or psychomotor retardation noticed by others
- Physical complaints e.g. stomach aches, headaches that do not respond to medical treatment
- Fatigue or loss of energy and vitality
- Feelings of worthlessness or excessive guilt
- Diminished ability to think or concentrate, or indecisiveness

Signs and symptoms of depression can be masked by other symptoms such as angry behaviour. Although this can occur in younger children, most children experience depression in very much the same way as adults with feelings such as sadness, hopelessness and mood change.

Children may also begin using drugs and alcohol, particularly if they are over 12 years of age. If tearfulness or sadness become persistent or interfere with usual social activities, interests, schoolwork or family life then a depressive illness may be indicated.

Go to https://study.sagepub.com/essentialchildnursing to watch the video on depression and its treatment.

VIDEO LINK 37.2: DEPRESSION & TREATMENT

Suicide

Suicide is an increasingly serious and pervasive public health problem (see a selection of these websites: Samaritans, Papyrus, Mental Elf, YoungMinds, MindEd, Special Needs Jungle, NHS.uk/Livewell)

Early recognition and awareness of the likelihood of suicide is important (at all ages) as early awareness may help the individual to have a voice and feel listened to and cared for at this darkest of times. Increasingly, help is being made available by routes such as social media and apps which are more readily accessed by young people. Go to https://study.sagepub.com/essentialchildnursing to access two of these.

These are signs of suicidal thinking:

WEBLINK: SELF-HARM PREVENTION

- Many children will exhibit significant depressive symptoms
- Social isolation, particularly isolation from family and peers
- Talk of suicide, hopelessness, helplessness
- Increasing 'acting out' behaviours or engaging in particularly risky behaviours
- Frequent accidents, possibly associated with increased risky behaviours
- Experiencing and demonstrating high levels of stress or anxiety
- Substance misuse (alcohol, drugs, solvents, poisons)
- A focus on negative or morbid themes
- Talk about death and dying beyond the usual curiosity of children
- Increased crying or reduced/flat emotional affect
- Giving away possessions and/or making plans for death (BUPA, undated)

Self-harm

There has been a big increase in the number of young people being admitted to hospital or services because of self-harm. In recent years this figure has increased by 68% (YoungMinds) which indicates a crisis. This may be one of the first signs to be picked up by parents or carers and should be noted and sensitively explored in an appropriate and safe manner.

WEBLINK: SELF-HARM

IDENTIFYING AREAS OF CONCERN, RISK AND SAFEGUARDING GUIDANCE WHEN CARING FOR CHILDREN WITH MENTAL HEALTH PROBLEMS

——— SAFEGUARDING STOP POINT ———

Consider the role of the children's nurse in safeguarding children who may be considering suicide:

- How prepared would you be for having a discussion about a friend, family member or young person?
- Would you know how to contact assistance if you needed support/advice, at any hour of the day or night?

SAFEGUARDING STOP POINT ANSWER 37.1

Role of the children's nurse

First and foremost it is important to recognise that it is not possible to cover all mental and behavioural topics in such a short chapter, either in number or depth. The reader may therefore wish to explore some topics further. This includes issues around what to do if *you* have concerns about a child's mental health.

Please note that most mental and emotional disorders are likely to present either first or early on with the children's nurse. It is therefore essential to be aware of key indicators and how to liaise with and refer children for appropriate professional assessment. This may be community based or inpatient based depending on the type of disorder, its severity and availability of services locally.

Many children's nurses are in an excellent position to detect children's behaviours that are concerning, but may also feel that they lack the knowledge and skills to manage or assess the situation alone. It is timely to remind ourselves that working with others in the team and other agencies should be the first step in raising your concerns. The RCN (2014) document *Mental Health in Children and Young People: A Toolkit for Nurses Who Are Not Mental Health Specialists* is updated at intervals and is an excellent resource for those who are not 'experienced' in mental health.

Children's nurses usually have excellent interpersonal skills across the developmental stages and an ability to connect through a wide range of communication and play techniques. These skills should not be underestimated. Rather, they should reassure you that as a children's nurse you have an important part to play in early assessment and intervention. Working with and as part of the wider multidisciplinary team and across agencies and boundaries is part of what we do well.

SEE ALSO
CHAPTERS 8
AND 4

Remembering to act in the best interests of the child professionally, legally and proactively (NMC, 2015).

Responding in a non-critical way, listening actively and respecting the child's lived experience are important first steps in reducing the stigma which surrounds the topic of mental health and behavioural issues. Listening and risk assessment should precede formal intervention.

This first step done well will go a long way to improving the child's experience of seeking help, and will have a far-reaching effect on the process of recovery. *Note:* Children with a high assessed risk of suicide need to be seen as an emergency and *should not* be treated as low risk of self-harm or suicide.

CAMHS and mental health and behavioural expertise

For mental health practitioners to assess the signs and symptoms of clinical depression, they will need to take time to gather information about the individual before confirming a diagnosis. Tearfulness and sadness are not in themselves enough to indicate the presence of clinical depression. Equally important is the need to recognise how serious clinical depression can be, and to ensure that child and family members know that clinical depression is treatable.

A mental health evaluation should be carried out sensitively with parents or primary care giver alongside the child. Additional psychological assessment may be needed and may include an assessment by a CAMHS professional. Information will be gathered from teachers, friends and classmates to complete the mental health assessment. A diagnosis of severe depression could also increase the risk of suicide in children and young people. Girls are more likely to attempt suicide, but boys are more likely to kill themselves when they attempt suicide.

Children who come from families with a history of severe mental health problems and or substance misuse are more more likely to suffere with depression. This can also increase the risk of self-harm behaviours and suicide. Health practitioners need to ensure that parents and their children are aware of the side effects of antidepressant medication and what to do and who to call when unwanted side effects occur. Parents may deny the depression their child is experiencing and delay accessing mental health services due to the social stigma of mental illness – it is important to educate parents and other family members about the impact of depression on their child and encourage them to access the support available from mental health services. General awareness campaigns in media, schools, communities and in peer groups can help raise the profile of what is essentially an increasingly serious public health issue.

Whan assessing a child with depression it is important to provide age-appropriate information so that the child can understand the diagnosis and treatment options discussed. Ensuring that the child can collaborate with family and health professionals remains an essential professional approach, which respects the right of the child to be involved in decisions which affect their wellbeing and respects their autonomy and right to participate in their care (UNCRC, 1989).

> My advocate made me feel like I am someone, and that I have the right to be listened to. I will never forget this.
>
> **Zoe, child, Coram Voice, 2017**

SEE ALSO
CHAPTER 35

Autism

Autism is a lifelong, neurodevelopmental disorder, which is part of a group of disorders referred to as 'autistic spectrum disorders' (ASD). In the Diagnostic and Statistical Manual of Mental Disorders (DSM – 5, 2013), ASD is characterised by two main areas of impaired development, namely a) impaired social communication e.g. unable to maintain a flow of conversation and b) fixated interests and repetitive behaviours e.g. having quite fixed knowledge base and repeating that knowledge (Lauritsen, 2013).

The first documentation of the signs and symptoms of ASD occurred in the 1940s by both the psychiatrist Leo Kanner from the United States and a paediatrician, Hans Asperger from Austria. Kanner (1943) described the behaviour of eleven children who presented with delays in language and whom were socially distant. In the same period, Hans Asperger (1944) described very similar behaviour in four children, who were socially awkward, but sustained good vocabulary. Further epidemiological surveys of autism emerged in the 1960s. In 1989, Firth compared the work of Kanner and Asperger to form what is now considered a way of understanding the range of ASDs diagnosed in a population (Buxbaum and Hof, 2013).

Males appear to be more affected than females. Diagnosis of autism, along with another ASDS like 'Asperger's Syndrome' is more common today than in the past.

In children with ASD difficulty may arise in meeting social developmental milestones e.g. problems with following another person's shift in gaze during a conversation. They are often described by their teachers as 'loners' and when they do socialise, focussed on conversing with one person only – in a primary school setting, this could be a child who appears clingy to a teacher, and sees that teacher as the only focus of conversation, rather than the other children in the class or indeed other teachers.

In adolescence, ASD may present in the individual being unable to initiate and maintain meaningful conversation, demonstrating poor eye contact and limited gestures. This can negatively affect the development of social relationships with peers and others (Buxbaum and Hof, 2013).

VIDEO
LINK 37.3:
ADHD

One of the difficulties with the diagnosis of ASDs is that there is a high incidence of comorbidity with other mental health problems like anxiety, depression, obsessive compulsive disorder and ADHD to name a few. In addition, children and adolescence with autism may find it difficult to adapt to any change in environment e.g. having to move desks in a classroom setting.

Aetiology

The development of ASD is linked to genetics, some medical problems, complications of pregnancy and brain abnormalities (Buxbaum and Hof, 2013).

Management/Treatment

Treatment for ASDs usually involves a combination of medical and psychosocial interventions which fall into four main categories which include:

1. Social skills training where children and adolescents can be supported to develop speech and language skills e.g. turn-taking during a conversation.
2. Cognitive Behaviour Therapy can be used to help develop learning techniques for problem solving.
3. Drug therapy interventions tend to be used to manage some of more destructive signs and symptoms of anxiety, obsessive compulsive disorder (OCD) and Attention Deficit Hyperactivity Disorder (ADHD), which may present with ASD.
4. Family-based approaches which can help and support families/caregivers to cope with their child and adolescent who is diagnosed with autism.

WEBLINK:
AUTISM

The above approaches can be combined with specific educational interventions for use in a classroom environment and at home.

Conduct disorder

Conduct disorder (CD) is defined as a repetitive and persistent pattern of behaviour and forms part of a group of disorders, also referred to as antisocial behaviours. This is characterised by violation of the rights of others or major age-appropriate societal norms or rules for living. In DSM-5 (2013), there are specific criteria which indicate a diagnosis of conduct disorder. These criteria are categorised under four areas: (i) aggression towards people or animals; (ii) destruction of property; (iii) deceitfulness or theft and (iv) serious violation of rules. Further information to confer a diagnosis of conduct disorder include whether the presenting behaviour at onset of childhood or adolescence or is unspecified. An ongoing assessment of how the presenting behaviour impacts on the social, academic and occupational functioning of a child or adolescent forms an important part of the diagnosis of conduct disorder. Conduct disorder can be confused with another type of antisocial behaviour disorder known as Oppositional Defiant Disorder (ODD). Conduct disorders are more prevalent in males than females.

VIDEO
LINK 37.4:
ODD

Aetiology

There is more than one cause of conduct disorder which includes a specific genetic disposition to having the disorder; problems with learning socially acceptable behaviour, possessing an aggressive temperament and mood; hyperactivity psychology, problems with learning and reading and writing, sociocultural factors and the family environment (NHS England and HEE, 2017).

Management/Treatment

Treatment for CD involves a combination of medical and psychosocial interventions which fall into four main categories which include:

1. Cognitive behaviour therapy can be used to help develop learning techniques for problem solving.
2. Family-based approaches which can help and support families/caregivers to cope with their child and adolescent who is diagnosed with conduct disorder.

   - Parent management training
   - Functional family therapy
   - Multi-systematic therapy

3. Drug therapy interventions tend to be used to manage signs of hyperactivity and symptoms such as increased levels of frustration, anger and aggression.

The care of children and adolescents with conduct disorders, requires the combined work of health, social, educational and criminal justice agencies. Further information on the different management and treatment approaches can be accessed from the *National Institute for Health and Care Excellence Guidelines on Antisocial behaviour and conduct disorders in children and young people: recognition and management* (NICE, 2017).

SCENARIO 37.2: MIKE AND TOM

Mike, a senior nurse practitioner, schedules a home visit to a family whose youngest son Tom, 12 years, has oppositional defiant disorder (ODD) and has been exhibiting an escalation in verbally aggressive behaviour and throwing a vase at his father. Mike arranged for Tom and his parents to come to the CAMHS Unit for an initial assessment.

Go to https://study.sagepub.com/essentialchildnursing to see how Tom was supported.

SCENARIO
ANSWER 37.2

PLACEMENT
ADVICE 37:
MENTAL HEALTH
ISSUES

Go to https://study.sagepub.com/essentialchildnursing for tips on preparing for placements and health promotion with children with mental health issues.

HEALTH
PROMOTION 37:
MENTAL HEALTH
ISSUES

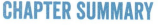

CHAPTER SUMMARY

- This chapter looks at the prevalence of common mental and behavioural disorders in children with a focus on anxiety, depression, conduct disorders and recognsing behaviour which may lead to self-harm and suicidal behaviour
- The resources available at https://study.sagepub.com/essentialchildnursing encourage the reader to explore these topics more deeply and widely and to look at other marginalised groups known to be at risk of poor mental health (e.g. LGBT, black and ethnic minority groups, children in care and leaving care, those in the juvenile criminal justice system and those who have a parent in prison)

──── BUILD YOUR BIBLIOGRAPHY ────

Books

- Buxbaum, J.D. and Hof, P.R. (2013) *The Neuroscience of Autism Spectrum Disorders*. Oxford: Academic Press and Elsevier.

- Matthys, W. and Lochman, L.E. (2017) *Oppositional Defiant Disorder and Conduct Disorder in Childhood*, 2nd edn. London: John Wiley and Sons.

  An extensive look at evidence-based assessments and intervention from ages 3–14.

- Bryant-Waugh, R. (2015) 'Feeding and eating disorders' in A. Thapar, D.S. Pine, J.F. Leckman, S. Scott, M.J. Snowling and E.A. Taylor (eds), *Child and Adolescent Psychiatry*. Chichester: John Wiley and Sons.

  A key interdisciplinary and international text on the topic of feeding problems and eating disorders.

Journal articles

FURTHER READING: ONLINE JOURNAL ARTICLES

FIND OUT MORE!

Go to https://study.sagepub.com/essentialchildnursing for further free online journal articles related to this chapter.

- Baranek, G.T., David, F.J., Poe, M.D., Stone, W.L., Linda, R. and Watson, L.R. (2006) 'Sensory Experiences Questionnaire: discriminating sensory features in young children with autism, developmental delays, and typical development'. *Journal of Child Psychology and Psychiatry*, 47 (6): 591–601.

  Provides a review of the sensory symptoms of autism and how these differ from sensory symptoms experienced in other health care problems – useful in assessment of autism spectrum disorders.

  On autism.

- Gondek, D., Edbrooke-Childs, J., Velikonja, T., Chapman, L., Saunders, F., Hayes, D. and Wolpert, M. (2016) 'Facilitators and barriers to person-centred care in child and young people mental health services: a systematic review'. *Clinical Psychology & Psychotherapy*, doi: 10.1002/cpp.2052.

  Explores some of the essential skills required by mental health practitioners in caring for children and young people with mental health problems.

- Simmons, M.B., Hetrick, S.E. and Jorm, A.F. (2011) 'Experiences of treatment decision making for young people diagnosed with depressive disorders: a qualitative study in primary care and specialist mental health settings'. *BMC Psychiatry*, 11: 194.

  Provides information on how 'partnership working' can be negotiated with both children and young people and their caregivers in the transition from primary care to specialist mental health settings.

Weblinks

FURTHER READING: WEBLINKS

Go to https://study.sagepub.com/essentialchildnursing for further weblinks related to this chapter.

- NICE, *Autism Spectrum Disorder in under 19s: Recognition, Referral and Diagnosis*. Clinical guideline [CG128].

  www.nice.org.uk/guidance/cg128

  This document is useful for assessment of autism spectrum disorders.

- NICE, *Autism Spectrum Disorder in under 19s: Support and Management*. Clinical guideline [CG170]
  www.nice.org.uk/guidance/cg170

- Place2Be and NAHT, *Children's Mental Health Matters: Provision of Primary School Counselling*
  www.place2be.org.uk/media/10046/Childrens_Mental_Health_Week_2016_report.pdf

- Department of Health, *Future in Mind: Promoting, Protecting and Improving Our Children and Young People's Mental Health and Wellbeing*.
  www.gov.uk/government/publications/improving-mental-health-services-for-young-people

  The report outlines a five-year vision for good mental health, recognising that everyone who works with children has a role in helping them to get the help they need.

ACE YOUR ASSESSMENT

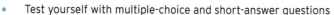

ONLINE
QUIZZES &
ACTIVITY
ANSWERS

Revise what you have learned by visiting https://study.sagepub.com/essentialchildnursing

- Test yourself with multiple-choice and short-answer questions
- Do the chapter activities in the book and check your answers online

REFERENCES

American Psychiatric Association (APA) (2013) *Diagnostic and Statistical Manual of Mental Disorders (DSM-5)*. Washington, DC: APA.

Bazalgette, L., Rahilly, T. and Trevely, G. (2015) *Achieving Emotional Wellbeing for Looked after Children: A Whole System Approach*. London: NSPCC.

Beng Huat See and Gorard, S. (2013) *What Do Rigorous Evaluations Tell Us about the Most Promising Parental Involvement Interventions? A Critical Review of What Works for Disadvantaged Children in Different Age Groups*. London: The Nuffield Foundation.

Brymer, J. and Schweitzer, R. (2013) 'Extreme sports are good for your health: a phenomenological understanding of fear and anxiety in extreme sport'. *Journal of Health Psychology*, 18 (4): 477–87.

BUPA (undated) *Depression in Children*. Available at: www.bupa.com.sa/english/healthandwellness/healthinformation/articles/pages/depression-in-children.aspx (last accessed 29 June 2017).

Buxbaum, J.D. and Hof, P.R. (2013) *The Neuroscience of Autistic Spectrum Disorders*, 1st edn. Oxford: Academic Press & Elsevier.

Children's Society (2008) *Mental Health of Looked After Children in the UK: Summary The 2008 Survey*. Available at: www.childrenssociety.org.uk/what-we-do/research/initiatives/well-being/background-programme/2008-survey (last accessed 25 April 2008).

Coram Voice (2017) *Mental Health Issues* [online]. Available at: www.coramvoice.org.uk/professional-zone/mental-health-issues (last accessed 15 November 2017).

Department of Health (DH) (2004) *A National Service Framework for Children, Young People and Maternity Services: Core Standards*. London: DH. Available at: www.gov.uk/government/uploads/system/uploads/attachment_data/file/199952/National_Service_Framework_for_Children_Young_People_and_Maternity_Services_-_Core_Standards.pdf (last accessed 4 June 2017).

Fink, E., Patalay, P., Sharpe, H., Holley, S., Deighton, J. and Wolpert, M. (2015) 'Mental health difficulties in early adolesecence: A comparison of two cross-sectional studies in England from 2009 to 2014'. *Journal of Adolescent Health*, 56, (5): 502–7.

Gorard, S. and Beng Huat See (2015) *Do Parental Involvement Interventions Increase Attainment? A Review of the Evidence*. London: The Nuffield Foundation.

Green, H., McGinnity, A., Meltzer, H., Ford, T. and Goodman, R. (2005) *Mental Health of Children and Young People in Great Britain, 2004*. Newport: National Statistics.

Malik, A. (2016) 'Suffering in silence: why the voices of young people on mental health must be heard', *Commonspace* [online]. Available at: www.commonspace.scot/articles/8829/suffering-silence-why-voices-young-people-mental-health-must-be-heard (last accessed 10 November 2017).

Lauritsen, M.B. (2013) 'Autism spectrum disorders', *European Journal of Child and Adolescent Psychiatry*, 22 (1): 37–42.

Mental Health Foundation (2015) *Fundamental Facts About Mental Health 2015*. London: Mental Health Foundation.

Mental Health Taskforce to the NHS in England (2016) *The Five Year Forward View for Mental Health*. Available at: www.england.nhs.uk/wp-content/uploads/2016/02/Mental-Health-Taskforce-FYFV-final.pdf (last accessed 4 June 2017).

National Institute for Health and Care Excellence (2017) *Guidelines on antisocial behaviour and conduct disorders in children and young people: recognition and management*. London: NICE.

NHS England and Health Education England (2017) *Children and Young People's Improving Access to Psychological Therapies Programme*. London: NHS England and Health Education England.

Ries Merikangas, K., Nakamura, E.F. and Kessler, R.C. (2009) 'Epidemiology of mental disorders in children and adolescents'. *Dialogues in Clinical Neuroscience*, 11 (1): 7–20.

Royal College of Nursing (RCN) (2014) *Mental Health in Children and Young People: A Toolkit for Nurses Who Are Not Mental Health Specialists*. Available at: www.rcn.org.uk/professional-development/publications/pub-003311 (last accessed 4 June 2017).

Sempik, J., Ward, H. and Darker, I. (2008) 'Emotional and behavioural difficulties of children and young people at entry to care', *Clinical Child Psychology and Psychiatry*, 13 (2): 221–233.

Sylvers, P., Lilienfeld, S.O. and LePrairie, J.L. (2011) 'Differences between trait fear and trait anxiety: a clinical review'. *Implications for Psychopathology*, 31 (1): 122–37.

United Nations (1989) *United Nations Convention on the Rights of the Child*. Available at: www.unicef.org.uk/what-we-do/un-convention-child-rights (last accessed 4 June 2017).

WebMD (undated) *Depression Guide*. Available at: www.webmd.com/depression/mental-health-depression-children?printing=true#1 (last accessed 29 June 2017).

World Health Organization (2015) *World Health Statistics: Factsheet on Adolescent Health*. Geneva: WHO.

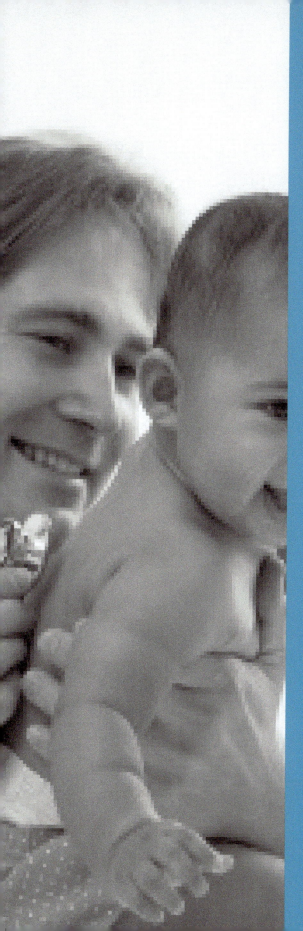

PART 5 ON BEING A PROFESSIONAL CHILDREN'S NURSE

38 Leadership and management in children
   and young people's nursing   591

39 Lifelong learning and continuing
   professional development for the
   children and young people's nurse   602

40 Decision-making and accountability
   in children and young people's nursing   616

41 Being politically aware and professionally
   proactive in children and young
   people's nursing   626

LEADERSHIP AND MANAGEMENT IN CHILDREN AND YOUNG PEOPLE'S NURSING

JACKIE PHIPPS

38

THIS CHAPTER COVERS

- Collective leadership for the promotion of sustainable quality healthcare for children and their families
- Ethical, authentic and transformational leadership styles for the promotion of quality healthcare for children and their families
- The NHS Healthcare Leadership Model for leadership development

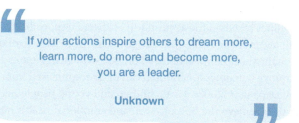

> If your actions inspire others to dream more, learn more, do more and become more, you are a leader.
>
> **Unknown**

Visit https://study.sagepub.com/essentialchildnursing to access a wealth of online resources for this chapter – watch out for the margin icons throughout the chapter.

INTRODUCTION

The concept of leadership within nursing is not a new one. As the opening quotation suggests, this is a complex concept. There is a clear connection between effective nursing leadership and quality patient care and positive patient outcomes (Wong et al., 2013). Within the context of developing and sustaining a culture of quality healthcare, collective, ethical, authentic and transformational leadership styles have been cited as appropriate leadership styles. However, there is a lack of clear direction for children's nurses as to how these styles of leadership can be applied in practice in order to promote and develop quality healthcare for children, young people and their families at the point of care. This chapter will first identify the nature of collective leadership for children's nurses. It will then explore the concepts of ethical, authentic and transformational leadership styles. Throughout, it will explore how the concepts of these leadership styles can be applied in practice by children's nurses to ensure the development of effective cultures for the planning, implementation and evaluation of quality healthcare that meet the unique needs of children and their families. Finally, it will examine the nature of the NHS Healthcare Leadership Model and how it can be applied by children's nurses for continuous leadership development in practice.

COLLECTIVE LEADERSHIP FOR THE PROMOTION OF SUSTAINABLE QUALITY HEALTHCARE FOR CHILDREN AND THEIR FAMILIES

Over the years, and often in the wake of investigations into high-profile cases of failures within the NHS, it has been highlighted that despite the many organisational and strategic changes that have been made in health and care services, there is much to be done to improve the health and care outcomes for children and young people (Kennedy, 2010; CYPHOF, 2013). It is against this background that there has been an emphasis on embracing a collective leadership approach, from government to children's nurses at the point of care, to ensure the development of effective cultures for the planning, implementation and evaluation of quality health and care that meet the unique needs of children and their families (Kennedy, 2010; CYPHOF, 2013). There is still much work to be done.

WATCH A VIDEO ONLINE!

VIDEO LINK 38.1: COLLECTIVE LEADERSHIP

Collective leadership is based on the assumption of shared responsibility and accountability for everyone working at all levels of the NHS, from the government to those working at the point of care, to assure a culture of quality health and care based on best evidence (West et al., 2014). Cultures of quality healthcare to improve outcomes for children can be conceptualised from three general principles of quality proposed by Darzi (DH, 2008). First, children and young people need effective evidence-based care to ensure that they achieve the best physical and emotional health outcomes both in childhood and into adulthood. Second, children and young people should be protected from harm from the perspective of the treatment that they receive and safeguarding them from maltreatment. Finally, they should experience health and care that is delivered in a way that takes into account the unique needs of a child according to their age and cognitive development (DH, 2004).

SAFEGUARDING STOP POINT

HM Government (2015) and the NMC (2015) set out the legislative requirements and the collective responsibility and accountability of children's nurses for raising a concern immediately if they believe a child is vulnerable or at risk of harm and in need of extra support and protection.

Whilst child health and social policy and philosophies, professional standards and guidelines set the terms of reference for a culture of quality healthcare for children and their families, they fall short of offering children's nurses guidance on the development of effective leadership frameworks and leadership styles at the point of care. There are a great number of leadership theories, concepts and styles that children's nurses can apply to their practice. However, they should be aware there is no one best leadership style that can be used on every occasion and that selection should be context sensitive (West et al., 2015).

ACTIVITY 38.1: CRITICAL THINKING

Leadership and Leadership Development in Health Care: The Evidence Base (West et al., 2015), which you can access via https://study.sagepub.com/essentialchildnursing, presents a review of leadership theory and research in general and as associated with healthcare. It describes a number of common leadership theories and examines the links between effective leadership and the development of positive cultures for the provision of quality healthcare.

WEBLINK:
LEADERSHIP
DEVELOPMENT

ETHICAL, AUTHENTIC AND TRANSFORMATIONAL LEADERSHIP STYLES FOR THE PROMOTION OF QUALITY HEALTHCARE FOR CHILDREN AND THEIR FAMILIES

Table 38.1 Leadership styles

Leadership style	Ethical leadership	Authentic leadership	Transformational leadership
Description	Knowing and doing what is right. Knowing what is right is associated with the moral characteristic of the leader based on the leader's internal values, attitudes and beliefs (Alvolio et al., 2004; Stouten et al., 2012). Doing what is right is associated with being a moral manager and behaving in a way that upholds the leader's values, attitudes and beliefs based on sound standards (Brown and Trevino, 2006).	Shares some similarities with ethical leadership style. It focuses on how leaders use behaviours grounded in staying true to their values, attitudes and beliefs based on sound ethical standards (Gardner et al., 2005; Wong and Cummings, 2009; Wong et al., 2010; Wong and Giallonardo., 2013).	Associated with how leaders use their characteristics and behaviours to influence others, based on their own internal values attitudes and beliefs (Parry and Proctor-Thomson, 2002; Doody and Doody, 2012; Lievens and Vlerick, 2014).

ACTIVITY 38.2: CRITICAL THINKING

The NMC Code (2015) contains the professional standards that registered children's nurses must uphold to demonstrate effective leadership. It can act as a focus to reflect on and become more self-aware of your own leadership values and behaviours associated with the principles of collective, ethical, authentic and transformational leadership.

- How do you think the principles of collective, ethical, authentic and transformational leadership are demonstrated within the Code?

PRACTICE
SCENARIO 38:
RUBY

✓

ACTIVITY
ANSWER 38.2

Gardner et al.'s (2005) model of leadership, based on the four components (then discussed in turn below) of internalised moral perspective, relational transparency, balanced processing and self-awareness can help children's nurses to apply the key principles of collective, ethical, authentic and transformational leadership to their practice at the point of care.

Internalised moral perspective

Knowing what is right based within this component involves children's nurses understanding the professional, political, legal and ethical principles of health and care for children.

Children's nurses can demonstrate effective leadership by role-modelling behaviours that demonstrate their responsibility and accountability for and commitment to promoting a culture of care which upholds these even when they are under considerable pressure (NHS Leadership Academy, 2013; NMC, 2015).

Children's nurses who role-model behaviours associated with the characteristics of honesty, integrity and fairness of decision-making while emphasising justice, equality and human dignity are more likely to be admired for their behaviours and are therefore more likely to influence similar values and behaviours in others (Wong et al., 2010; Storch et al., 2013; Makaroff et al., 2014). By fostering cooperation and modelling actions consistent with health and social policy and professional and legal standards, children's nurses are more likely to motivate others to new quality initiatives for the care of children (Parry and Proctor-Thomson, 2002; Doody and Doody, 2012; Lievens and Vlerick, 2014).

> I feel inspired by one nurse in particular with whom I have worked on many occasions. She has the ability to listen and make people feel comfortable. No individual is treated or deemed to be better or less important than others by her. I look to her as a role model, admiring her passion and commitment towards caring for children, young people and their families.
>
> **Rebecca, 3rd-year children's nursing student**

This reflection by Rebecca shows how demonstrating internalised moral perspective can inspire others to 'dream more, learn more, do more and become more'.

Relational transparency

Knowing what is right within this component involves children's nurses understanding how systems of health and care fit together and how children and families care use health and care systems. Children's nurses can demonstrate effective leadership behaviour by being responsible and accountable for assuring effective two-way formal and informal information channels with children and their families, colleagues and other health and care professionals who may be involved in their care (NHS Leadership Academy, 2013; CYPHOF, 2013). By being open and honest with colleagues, children and families – even when mistakes are made – children's nurses are more likely to win their trust and promote a culture of learning (Parry and Proctor-Thomson, 2002; Wong et al., 2010; Doody and Doody, 2012; Lievens and Vlerick, 2014; Makaroff et al., 2014; Storch et al., 2014).

SCENARIO 38.1: JAMES

James is a 14-year-old boy who has a rapidly deteriorating health condition. James's children's community nurse Pamela arranged for an end-of-life care meeting to take place between key health and care professionals and James's family. The purpose of the meeting was to agree an advanced care plan based on the essential care of James before, at the time of and after his death. Pamela took the lead role in managing and leading the meeting.

* What resources could Pamela have drawn upon to demonstrate effective leadership and management and relational transparency?

SCENARIO
ANSWER 38.1

> **"** The nurse created a really safe environment to discuss such issues as where we wanted end-of-life care for my son to take place, and even my fears over what would happen to his body after death. Her calm, authoritative and caring approach led the tone, ensured my own wellbeing and participation throughout.
>
> **Avril, parent** **"**

This reflection by Avril demonstrates how the environment of trust created by the children's nurse, through relational transparency, inspired her to 'learn more' about the resources and support for end-of-life care and to 'do more' to ensure that the end-of-life care plan met the individual needs of her son and the family.

Balanced processing

Knowing what is right, within this component, involves children's nurses understanding their responsibility and accountability for maintaining their knowledge and skills for effective evidence-based practice through the collection and analysis of a range of data from relevant sources (NHS Leadership Academy, 2013; NMC, 2015).

Leadership behaviours for children's nurses should include engaging in appropriate continuing professional development activities to maintain their knowledge and skills required to deliver, promote and advocate for quality health and care for children and their families. It should also involve engaging children and their families in meaningful engagement in decision-making at the point of care or for the development of future services (NHS Leadership Academy, 2013; NMC, 2015). Go to https://study.sagepub.com/essentialchildnursing and watch Julie Bailey's speech at the NHS Leadership Summit on ensuring that healthcare leaders listen to the voices of patients and their carers.

VIDEO LINK 38.2:
LEADERSHIP
SUMMIT

By applying the moral characteristics of being open to new ideas and opinions before making decisions about the care of children, children's nurses are more likely to be equipped to influence individuals and teams able to work collaboratively and make suggestions for transformational change for the children and families that they care for, based on best evidence (Parry and Proctor-Thomson, 2002; Wong et al., 2010; Doody and Doody, 2012; Lievens and Vlerick, 2014; West et al., 2014).

VIDEO LINK 38.3:
A CARER'S
PERSPECTIVE

Self-awareness

Knowing what is right, within this component, involves children's nurses understanding the importance of using effective feedback mechanisms and reflection for effective leadership development. Behaviours which demonstrate authentic leadership for children's nurses within this component include engaging with a wide range of appropriate approaches for seeking feedback from colleagues and children and their families. It also includes using evidence-based approaches of self-reflection and reflection on feedback from others (Gardner et al., 2005; Branson, 2007; Horton-Deutsch and Sherwood, 2008; Mackie, 2015).

From this component, children's nurses can demonstrate effective leadership through embracing the moral characteristic of commitment to open discussion about their leadership behaviours and performance in order to gain genuine and meaningful insight into their leadership strengths, limitations and future developmental needs (Densten and Gray, 2001; Horton-Deutsch and Sherwood, 2008; Mackie, 2015).

By gaining a strong sense of self and emotional intelligence, a genuine understanding of their own assumptions and considering the viewpoints of others about their leadership values, attitudes and behaviours and the impact on the wellbeing of colleagues, children and families, children's nurses are more likely to gain their trust (Gardner et al., 2005; Horton-Deutsch and Sherwood, 2008). By gaining the trust of colleagues, children and their families, children's nurses are more likely to successfully influence commitment to a collective vision of transformational change for the improvement of care to children and their families (Parry and Proctor-Thomson, 2002; Doody and Doody, 2012; Hutchinson and Jackson, 2013; Lievens and Vlerick, 2014).

WHAT'S THE EVIDENCE?

WEBLINK: LCAV

Following a survey of 9,000 people, NHS England (2016) presented ten commitments that should underpin nursing, midwifery and care staff leadership today for the transformational change for the improvement of health and care services.

Leading Change, Adding Value (NHS England, 2016) encompasses the assumptions of collective leadership for the transformation change based on the three quality objectives set out under the five-year forward view (NHS England, 2014)

- Better outcomes
- Better experiences
- Better use of resources

This framework can help children's nurses focus on leading transformational change based on the principles of collective, ethical, authentic and transformational leadership.

THE NHS HEALTHCARE LEADERSHIP MODEL FOR LEADERSHIP DEVELOPMENT

There are a number of interventions that can help children's nurses develop their leadership effectiveness.

The Healthcare Leadership Model (NHS Leadership Academy, 2013) was developed to help everyone who works in health and care to become a better leader – whether they have a formal leadership responsibility or not. The model is made up of nine leadership dimensions. For each of the dimensions there is a brief description of what the dimension is about and why it is important. Leadership behaviours, associated with each of the dimensions, are shown on a four-part scale which ranges from 'essential' through

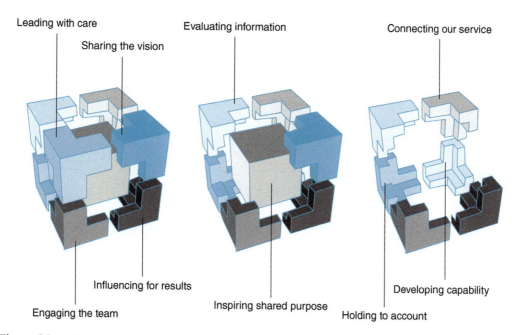

Leading with care

Sharing the vision

Evaluating information

Connecting our service

Influencing for results

Engaging the team

Inspiring shared purpose

Developing capability

Holding to account

Figure 38.1 The nine dimensions of the NHS Healthcare Leadership Model

Full colour version available at: www.leadershipacademy.nhs.uk/resources/healthcare-leadership-model

The Healthcare Leadership Model and associated graphics are ©NHS Leadership Academy, reproduced with permission.

'proficient' and 'strong' to 'exemplary'. Within these scales, the leadership behaviours themselves are presented as a series of questions. These are the questions that can be used to guide the thoughts of children's nurses and result in effective leadership behaviours commonly associated with the key principles associated with collective, ethical, authentic and transformational leadership theories. The Healthcare Leadership Model (NHS Leadership Academy, 2013) is a broadly progressive model. It can, therefore, be applied to all jobs that children's nurses work in, whether they have a formal leadership role or not.

WHAT'S THE EVIDENCE?

Ellis and Abbot (2014a, 2014b, 2014c, 2014d) present a series of articles which are a good place for children's nurses to begin to explore the content and nature of all nine separate yet inextricably linked dimensions of the Healthcare Leadership Model.

ACTIVITY 38.3: LEADERSHIP AND MANAGEMENT

Access the Healthcare Leadership Model at the Leadership Academy via https://study.sagepub.com/essentialchildnursing

Explore each of the dimensions to help you understand the leadership behaviours associated with collective, ethical, authentic and transformational leadership within the nine dimensions.

WEBLINK:
LEADERSHIP
MODEL

The NHS Leadership Academy have also developed a self-assessment tool to support the Healthcare Leadership Model. Children's nurses can utilise the process of self-assessment and subsequent reflection to help them understand their leadership behaviours and highlight areas of strengths and areas for development throughout their career in healthcare.

By reflecting on behaviours associated with collective, ethical, authentic and transformational leadership, within the nine dimensions of the model, children's nurses should be able to demonstrate how they can use effective leadership to influence and promote the development of a culture of high-quality health and care for children and their families.

WEBLINK:
ASSESSMENT

ACTIVITY 38.4: REFLECTIVE PRACTICE

Undertake the Healthcare Leadership Model self-assessment via https://study.sagepub.com/essential childnursing The interactive self-assessment tool is free to access. You will need to register for a free NHS Leadership Academy ID at https://nhsx.uk/register in order to access this resource. Once you have completed the self-assessment, through the process of reflection:

- Identify your leadership values and behaviours that demonstrate the principles of collective, ethical, authentic and transformational leadership
- Complete an action plan for your continuing leadership development

CHAPTER SUMMARY

- There has been a growing emphasis on the need for effective leadership to improve the quality of health and care services in the UK
- Children's nurses have a professional responsibility to manage, lead and promote quality healthcare for children and their families
- By applying the policies and philosophies, professional and legal standards and guidelines which set the terms of reference for children's nurses within the principles of collective, ethical, authentic and transformational leadership styles in practice, children's nurses can help to ensure the development of an effective culture for the planning, implementation and evaluation of quality health and care that meet the unique needs of children and their families
- Children's nurses can utilise the Healthcare Leadership Model for their continuing leadership development throughout their healthcare career

BUILD YOUR BIBLIOGRAPHY

Books

- Ellis, P. and Bach, S. (2015) *Leadership, Management and Team Working in Nursing*, 2nd edn. London: Learning Matters.

  Specifically tailored to the pre-registration nursing student, this text will help them understand how leadership fits with daily practice.
- Marquis, B.L. and Hudson, C.J. (2017) *Leadership Roles and Management Functions in Nursing: Theory and Application*, 9th edn. Philadelphia: Wolters Kluwer Health.

Focuses on leadership and evidence-based decision-making, covering a wide range of topics including patient safety and quality.

- Barr, J. and Dowding, L. (2015) *Leadership in Health Care*, 3rd edn. London: Sage.

Covers a wide spectrum of topics on leadership and management relevant to nurses at all levels.

Journal articles

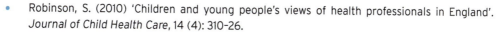

Go to https://study.sagepub.com/essentialchildnursing for further free online journal articles related to this chapter.

FURTHER READING: ONLINE JOURNAL ARTICLES

- Robinson, S. (2010) 'Children and young people's views of health professionals in England'. *Journal of Child Health Care*, 14 (4): 310-26.

This study provided an analysis of 31 studies which reported on CYP views about health professionals working in England. The study concluded that CYP wanted healthcare professionals to be familiar, accessible and available, to be informed and competent, to provide accessible information, to be a good communicator, to ensure privacy and confidentiality and to demonstrate acceptance and empathy.

- Coleman, A., Sharp, C. and Handscomb, G. (2015) 'Leading highly performing children's centres: supporting the development of the "accidental leaders"'. *Educational Management Administration & Leadership*, 44 (5): 1-19.

The article summarises research into the leadership of Sure Start children's centres. It includes discussion of how best to support the preparation and development of all leaders within health and care children's services.

- Fallatah, F. and Laschinger, H.K.S. (2016) 'The influence of authentic leadership and supportive professional practice environments on new graduate nurses' job satisfaction'. *Journal of Research in Nursing*, 21 (2): 1-12.

The aim of this study was to uncover new leadership approaches to attracting and retaining newly qualified nurses. The findings suggest that managers who demonstrate authentic leadership are more likely to enhance new graduate nurses' job satisfaction.

Weblinks

Go to https://study.sagepub.com/essentialchildnursing for further weblinks related to this chapter.

FURTHER READING: WEBLINKS

- The Kings Fund

www.kingsfund.org.uk

An independent charity working to improve health and care in England. Offers a wide range of resources and publications related to leadership and quality improvement.

- The Health Foundation

www.health.org.uk

An independent charity committed to bringing about better health and healthcare for people in the UK. Offers a wide range of resources and publications related to leadership and quality improvement.

- NHS Leadership Academy

www.leadershipacademy.nhs.uk

Offers a range of tools, models, programmes and expertise to support individuals, organisations and local academies to develop leaders.

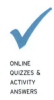

ACE YOUR ASSESSMENT

Revise what you have learned by visiting https://study.sagepub.com/essentialchildnursing

- Test yourself with multiple-choice and short-answer questions
- Do the chapter activities in the book and check your answers online

REFERENCES

Avolio, B.J., Gardner W.L., Walumbwa F.O., Luthans, F. and May, D.R. (2004) 'Unlocking the mask: a look at the process by which authentic leaders impact follower attitudes and behaviors'. *The Leadership Quarterly*, 15 (6): 801–23.

Branson, C. (2007) 'Effects of structured self-reflection on the development of authentic leadership practice among Queensland primary school principles'. *Educational Management Administration and Leadership*, 23(2): 225–46.

Brown, M.E. and Trevino L.K. (2006) 'Ethical leadership: a review and future directions'. *The Leadership Quarterly*, 17 (6): 595–616.

Children and Young People's Health Outcomes Forum (CYPHOF) (2013) *Children and Young People's Health Outcomes Forum Report for the Secretary of State for Health: Response to the Francis Inquiry Report*. Available at: www.gov.uk/government/uploads/system/uploads/attachment_data/file/307307/CYPHOF_Francis_report_-_final_23_Oct_13.pdf (last accessed 1 June 2017).

Densten, I.L. and Gray, J.H. (2001)'Leadership development and reflection: what is the connection?' *International Journal of Educational Management*, 15 (3): 119–24.

Department of Health (DH) (2004) *National Service Framework: Children, Young People and Maternity Services*. Available at: www.gov.uk/government/publications/national-service-framework-children-young-people-and-maternity-services (last accessed 13 October 2017).

Department of Health (DH) (2008) *High Quality Care for All: NHS Next Stage Review Final Report*. London: DH.

Doody, O. and Doody, C.M. (2012) 'Transformational leadership in nursing practice'. *British Journal of Nursing*, 21 (20): 1212–18.

Ellis, P. and Abbott, J. (2014a) 'An overview of the new NHS Healthcare Leadership Model'. *Journal of Renal Nursing*, 6 (1): 42–4.

Ellis, P. and Abbott, J. (2014b) 'Understanding the new NHS Healthcare Leadership Model'. *Journal of Renal Nursing*, 6 (2): 90–2.

Ellis, P. and Abbott, J. (2014c) 'Identifying goals with the NHS Healthcare Leadership Model'. *Journal of Renal Nursing*, 6 (3): 144–7.

Ellis, P. and Abbott, J. (2014d) 'The NHS Healthcare Leadership Model: the role of the renal manager'. *Journal of Renal Nursing*, 6 (4): 196–8.

Gardner, W.L., Avolio, B.J., Luthans, F.R., May, D.R. and Walumbwa, F. (2005) '"Can you see the real me?" A self-based model of authentic leader and follower development'. *The Leadership Quarterly*, 16 (20): 343–72.

Horton-Deutsch, S. and Sherwood, G. (2008) 'Reflection: an educational strategy to develop emotionally competent nurse leaders'. *Journal of Nursing Management*, 16: 946–54.

HM Government (2015) *Working Together to Safeguard Children: A Guide to Inter-agency Working to Safeguard and Promote the Welfare of Children*. London: DfE.

Hutchinson, M. and Jackson, D. (2013) 'Transformational leadership in nursing: towards a more critical interpretation'. *Nursing Inquiry*, 20 (1): 11–22.

Kennedy, I. (2010) *Getting it Right for Children and Young People: Overcoming Cultural Barriers in the NHS so as to Meet Their Needs*. London: Department of Health. Available at: www.gov.uk/government/uploads/system/uploads/attachment_data/file/216282/dh_119446.pdf (last accessed 1 June 2017).

Lievens, I. and Vlerick, P. (2014) 'Transformational leadership and safety performance among nurses: the mediating role of knowledge-related job characteristics'. *Journal of Advanced Nursing*, 70 (3): 651–61.

Mackie, D. (2015) 'Who sees changes after leadership coaching? An analysis of rater level and self-other alignment on multi-score feedback'. *International Coaching Psychology* Review, 10 (2): 118–30.

Makaroff, K.S., Storch, J., Pauly, B. and Newton, L. (2014) 'Searching for ethical leadership in nursing'. *Nursing Ethics*, 21 (6): 642–58.

NHS England (2014) *Five Year Forward View*. Available at: www.england.nhs.uk/wp-content/uploads/2014/10/5yfv-web.pdf (last accessed 1 June 2017).

NHS England (2016) *Leading Change, Adding Value: A Framework for Nursing, Midwifery and Care Staff*. Available at: www.england.nhs.uk/wp-content/uploads/2016/05/nursing-framework.pdf (last accessed 1 June 2017).

NHS Leadership Academy (2013) *Healthcare Leadership Model*. Available at: www.leadershipacademy.nhs.uk/wp-content/uploads/2014/10/NHSLeadership-LeadershipModel-colour.pdf (last accessed 1 June 2017).

Nursing and Midwifery Council (NMC) (2015) *The Code: Professional Standards of Practice and Behaviour for Nurses and Midwives*. London: NMC. Available at: www.nmc.org.uk/globalassets/sitedocuments/nmc-publications/nmc-code.pdf (last accessed 1 June 2017).

Parry, K.W. and Proctor-Thomson, S.B. (2002) 'Perceived integrity of transformational leaders in organisational settings'. *Journal of Business Ethics*, 35 (2): 75–96.

Storch, J., Makaroff, K.S., Pauly, B. and Newton, L. (2013) 'Take me to my leader: the importance of ethical leadership among formal nurse leaders'. *Nursing Ethics*, 20 (2): 150–7.

Stouten, J., van Dijke, M. and De Cremer, D. (2012) 'Ethical leadership: an overview and future perspectives'. *Journal of Personnel Psychology*, 11: 1–6.

West, M., Armit, L.L., Eckert, R., West, T. and Lee, A. (2015) *Leadership and Leadership Development in Health Care: The Evidence Base*. London: FMLM.

West, M., Eckert, R., Steward, K. and Pasmore, B. (2014) *Developing Collective Leadership for Health Care*. London: The King's Fund.

Wong, C. and Cummings, G.G (2009) 'Authentic leadership: a new theory for nursing or back to basics?' *Journal of Health Organization and Management*, 23 (5): 522–38.

Wong, C.A. and Giallonardo, L.M. (2013) 'Authentic leadership and nurse-assessed adverse patient outcomes'. *Journal of Nursing Management*, 21: 740–752.

Wong, C., Cummings, G.G. and Ducharme, L. (2013) 'The relationship between nursing leadership and patient outcomes: a systematic review update'. *Journal of Nursing Management*, 21: 709–24.

Wong, C.A., Spence Laschinger, H.K. and Cummings, G.G. (2010) 'Authentic leadership and nurses' voice behaviour and perceptions of care quality'. *Journal of Nursing Management*, 18: 889–900.

LIFELONG LEARNING AND CONTINUING PROFESSIONAL DEVELOPMENT FOR THE CHILDREN AND YOUNG PEOPLE'S NURSE

39

CLAIRE ANDERSON

THIS CHAPTER COVERS

- Examination of CPD for the children's nurse and why it is important
- Socio-political drivers for CPD
- The experience of nurses who have undertaken CPD
- Theories of learning and how they apply to CPD for the children's nurse

> "
> I have always been nervous about academic writing, lacking significantly in confidence… However I did have a passion for learning and teaching and fully appreciated that lifelong learning is an essential part of not only my personal and professional development, but also that of others.
>
> **Judy, children's nurse**
> "

Visit https://study.sagepub.com/essentialchildnursing to access a wealth of online resources for this chapter – watch out for the margin icons throughout the chapter.

INTRODUCTION

Once registered, nurses shift by shift gain more and more confidence in their ability to nurse. In contrast, many nurses lose confidence in their academic ability. The quotation above describes how one registered nurse feels about continuing her education. She is nervous and lacks confidence in her academic ability but at the same time recognises why continuing to learn as a nurse is so important. Continuing your development after you register as a nurse is referred to as 'continuing professional development'.

The Nursing and Midwifery Council (NMC) defines continuing professional development (CPD) as 'taking parting in appropriate and regular learning and professional development activities that aim to maintain and develop your competence and performance' (NMC, 2017c).

Nurses do need to know how to practise, and throughout their pre-registration education equal emphasis is placed on academic and practice achievement. After registering as a children and young people's nurse this balance between learning in practice and learning formally through academic study remains important. CPD is more than just academic development. While understanding the evidence that supports nursing practice is key, nurses also need to develop their nursing skills. This includes specific skills or updates that may be an employment or professional requirement.

In this chapter three nurses describe their CPD experience and it is clear that, while they have all achieved academic success, for some nurses the experience of CPD is not always easy.

EXAMINATION OF CPD FOR THE CHILDREN'S NURSE AND WHY IT IS IMPORTANT

Historically there was an expectation that all nurses would maintain a portfolio that outlined all the different types of activities that they had undertaken as CPD. This process has been made more formal and in order to revalidate their registration with the NMC all nurses are required to provide evidence of their continuing practice and their continuing development (NMC, 2017a):

- 450 practice hours over three years (or 900 hours if you have dual registration as a midwife and a nurse)
- 35 hours CPD, including 20 hours participatory learning
- A minimum of five pieces of practice-related feedback
- A minimum of five written reflective accounts on your CPD, and/or practice-related feedback, and/or an event or experience in your own professional practice and how this relates to The Code
- A reflective discussion with another NMC registrant covering your five written reflective accounts
- Health and character declaration
- Declaration that you have a professional indemnity arrangement
- Third-party confirmation that you have complied with the revalidation requirements

Many nurses begin their CPD by studying the role of a mentor and some nurses find both the academic and practice process of mentoring a challenge. As registered nurses you have a role in developing the future nursing workforce. This means you are expected to mentor students and support junior nursing colleagues in developing confidence and skills in their nursing practice. While some nurses find this highly rewarding, the process of mentoring has been described as challenging and even an intimidating experience. Undertaking the CPD required for nurses to mentor student and junior nursing colleagues is sometimes seen as a 'badge of honour'. However, for some, it is an additional burden to add to their workload (Willis, 2015). It is helpful to remember your own experience as a nursing student when developing your mentoring skills. Rather than being challenged by mentoring it is useful to consider what role the mentor had in helping you develop your nursing skills or perhaps you can remember a mentor who you can model your own mentorship style on.

However, the role of the mentor is changing and, while all nurses continue to have a role in supporting the development of nursing students, the current approaches to mentorship do not reflect the changes happening to the healthcare workforce. New approaches to mentoring could include a lead mentor or facilitator with other nurses acting as 'coaches' to support the practical application of learning for students. It is anticipated that these changes could begin shortly after the new standards for pre-registration nursing are announced in early 2018.

SOCIO-POLITICAL DRIVERS FOR CPD

There are also many political drivers for developing the future workforce, which have some influence on CPD. These include the mandate from the government to Health Education England (DH, 2016) which identifies the need to educate the workforce with the right skills, 'developing a workforce fit for purpose' (Addicott et al., 2015). The case studies outline the personal opportunities and challenges the nurses had when undertaking CPD, but with changes to funding for pre-registration nurses (Your guide to NHS Student Bursaries, 2016) there is a potential impact on how much funding there will be for CPD. With a reduction in resources for CPD it is important that the focus now, more than ever, is about developing the nursing workforce. Developing a workforce with the right skills often means developing specialist skills. As such, CPD needs to be more than mandatory training. It should be about developing children's nurses to deliver high-quality healthcare to children. The nurse undertaking CPD must value the experience and relate it to how it impacts on their practice. Employing organisations need to value the nurse and recognise how their CPD achievements will enhance the care they deliver.

CPD is about taking the newly registered nurse on the journey from their graduation and forward throughout their career. It is also about recognising that there is an existing workforce of nurses who need to maintain their skills. There is an international shortage of nurses and the nurses who are in practice and specialised are an aging population (Griffith, 2012). CPD is about motivating this workforce to remain in nursing, valuing their existing knowledge and building on this knowledge to reflect and respond to the dynamic nature of nursing in the 21st century.

ACTIVITY 39.1: CRITICAL THINKING

WEBLINK:
FIVE YEAR
FORWARD

Access *NHS Five Year Forward View* (Mental Health Taskforce to the NHS in England, 2016) via https://study.sagepub.com/essentialchildnursing and consider how it outlines developing a workforce fit for purpose.

In the section on workforce development the *Five Year Forward View* suggested new roles should be developed to create a 'flexible workforce that can provide high quality care wherever and whenever the patient needs it' (p.30).

- Can you think of any new roles that have been developed that may have an impact on how nurses practice?

ACTIVITY
ANSWER 39.1

Just as the nature of nursing is a dynamic ever-changing process so is how we learn. One constant is that nurse education has always been about practice alongside knowledge and so the learning environment is not always in the classroom. It is important that nurses develop academically so that they are equipped with an understanding of the complexities of healthcare and that their contribution to this healthcare as a profession is valued and respected. However, alongside the formal learning there is a range of learning opportunities that are employed. Simulation of clinical practice has been used in nursing studies for some time and it is particularly relevant to CPD. The registered nurse often has to learn new skills and practise them competently. With simulated learning the student practises and is assessed in an environment that represents the clinical workplace, but not with real patients. There is some evidence that the student being assessed in a safe environment practising their clinical skills in scenarios using high-fidelity simulation is more likely to become confident and competent (McCaughey and Traynor, 2010; Bradley, 2012).

Another relatively recent approach to learning is through social media sites. We live in a technological society and these sites offer a different mode of communication. The debate arises from when they are used without caution. Our priority must be the need to be professional when communicating via social media. When 'instagramming', tweeting, snapchatting or posting on Facebook we need to recognise the risk that these are public spaces and we must protect the confidentiality of children and their families, organisations and fellow professionals. Despite the cautionary advice (Nursing and Midwifery Council (2017b), social media sites used in the right way are effective contemporary approaches to learning and offer the support of peer networks. Try the @WeCYPnurses Twitter feed and joining @WeCommunities.

WEBLINK:
TWITTER

SAFEGUARDING STOP POINT

We need to protect the confidentiality of children and families when using social media sites, as per the NMC social networking guidance available via https://study.sagepub.com/essentialchildnursing
The principles of safeguarding should underpin our CPD:

WEBLINK:
SOCIAL
NETWORKING
GUIDANCE

Health Education England must ensure that the principles of safeguarding are integral to education and training curricula for health professionals. (NHS England, 2015, p. 21)

This chapter aims to identify why CPD is important for chilren's nurses and has begun by outlining socio-political drivers for this but will now explore the real-life experiences of nurses who have undertaken CPD. The case studies below refer to the three nurses mentioned earlier. They all undertook CPD to gain their degree as they had registered before all pre-registration courses were graduate level. Each of them describes the challenges of CPD but also how it has made them feel and how they will carry on in their CPD journey.

THE EXPERIENCE OF NURSES WHO HAVE UNDERTAKEN CPD

Below are three examples of registered nurses who are continuing their studies; two of them are completing their degree as they registered having completed a Diploma or Advanced Diploma in Nursing. This will not be the case for nurses completing their registering qualification today. All the examples relate to CPD and include what the nurses find challenging, how they feel and what they think they are achieving.

CASE STUDY 39.1: JUDY

Judy works as a practice educator and was completing a degree after qualifying as a children's nurse with a Diploma. She begins by describing her motivation to become a children's nurse:

> I knew from a very young age that I wanted to work with children and was very interested in the art of nursing. I grew up with a sibling who spent a lot of time as a child being cared for in hospital by children's nurses. I remember being fascinated with them, how hard they worked and how caring they were ... a true inspiration. I wanted to be just like them, making sick children's lives better in every way possible.

As she reflects on her experience of CPD it is clear that she sees how it has impacted on her practice and how she will use the experience to influence other nurses.

> I want to specialise in practice education because by following this path, I am not only able to develop and influence my own practice for the better but am able to positively influence the care of many children and young people through the continued support, education, skills and knowledge of many nurses, parents and children and young people themselves, thus ensuring evidence-based practice and patient safety for all.

- What motivated you to become a children and young people's nurse?

CASE STUDY 39.2: JON

PRACTICE
SCENARIO 39:
ANDI

Jon works in a clinical research facility and 'topped up' his non-honours degree. Like all nurses he had to meet the professional requirements of maintaining his NMC status but was also under some pressure to complete his degree and work towards a Masters qualification.

> After working as a healthcare assistant with children with learning disabilities the move to study nursing seemed like the next logical career step after this so I began my studies in 2005 at the age of 25 and I graduated with a non-honours degree. I have found that I am passionate about children's nursing and I have moved through the ranks and I have just moved from practice educator to a research facility.

- In a healthcare climate where there are shortages of nurses and employers are finding it difficult to retain the nurses that they have, what would motivate you to remain in an organisation?
- What would motivate you to undertake CPD as a nurse?

CASE STUDY 39.3: HARPREET

Harpreet works in a bone marrow transplant specialist ward. She also talks about her motivation to become a children's nurse but is aware of the specialist nature of the type of nursing she does and the importance of developing practice with evidence.

I was raised in a medical family and would often see the passion my parents had for their careers. I wanted to care for people and offer reassurance, kindness and support whilst they are experiencing some of the worst times of their lives. Unwell children along with their families need advocates and need to gain trust in care professionals. I wanted to be that for them and aim to make a horrible situation easier. I wanted to specialise in bone marrow transplants because the ongoing research and medication is the future to curing some of the worst conditions in the world.

She refers to research that will change how the children in her specialty are being treated.

- Can you think of an example of evidence-based practice that has changed since you started nursing? This does not need to be specialist research; it could be something quite straightforward such as the research behind the importance of hand washing but still makes a big difference to how we practise.

THEORIES OF LEARNING AND HOW THEY APPLY TO CPD FOR THE CHILDREN'S NURSE

There are several theoretical approaches to learning that can be used in nursing.

Malcolm Knowles' andragogy model

The principles of andragogy, introduced by Malcolm Knowles in 1980 and developed further in 1984, emphasise the learning strategy of facilitating autonomous learning. Rather than a passive approach to learning, the learner has to seek out the new knowledge for themselves. They may be aided in doing so by lecturers signposting their way but the responsibility is their own. In this approach the nurse makes sense of what they learn by applying this knowledge to their practice. Many nurses find it easier to learn if they can make sense of their learning. An example might be that a nurse learns the theory related to caring for a child who is pyrexial and the debate about the use of antipyretic medication when a child is pyrexial. It makes more sense and they are able to recall details only after they have been involved in the care of a child who is pyrexial (Shann et al., 2003; Wragg et al., 2014). Their experience adds to the resources they have to draw from. The andragogical learner has to see the relevance and value in their learning experience.

WHAT'S THE EVIDENCE?

Malcolm Knowles (1984) describes five assumptions about the adult learner:

1. *Self-concept*: The adult learner differs from the child learner as they become more self-directed
2. *Adult learner experience*: The adult learner has more resources available to them through their own experiences
3. *Readiness to learn*: As a mature adult this relates their learning to the development of their social roles
4. *Orientation to learning*: The learner moves from focus on the subject to focus on a problem-solving approach

(Continued)

(Continued)

5. *Motivation to learn*: An adult learner motivates themselves to learn using an andragogical approach to learning, that is, using your own experience to inform but also as an autonomous learner seeking out the evidence you need

Answer the questions below:

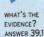

WHAT'S THE EVIDENCE? ANSWER 39.1

- What does the evidence say about using antipyretics when a child is pyrexial?
- What is your experience of managing pyrexia in children?

Judy discusses how she initially lacked confidence but developed this during her studies, and not only gained in her own confidence but how she could use this to enable others to study.

I have always been nervous about academic writing, lacking significantly in confidence. I also was not overly confident with teaching and assessing others and had not quite discovered my own teaching style or developed an appreciation for the different learning styles there are…

Judy, children's nurse

Harpreet also can see how by learning she is more confident in teaching:

Since completing this module, I have continued to grow comfortable and confident in the art of teaching and assisting others, both patients, their families as well as my colleagues to learn new skills, assessing their understanding and competence as a progressive experience.

Harpreet, children's nurse

The constructionist or experiential approach

A different learning theory, the constructionist or experiential approach to learning, also recognises the value of experience. The learner uses their own experience and knowledge to develop and acquire more. Kolb's experiential learning style theory is typically represented by a four-stage learning cycle, as you can see in Figure 39.1.

An approach often used in constructionist learning is case-based learning or problem-based learning where students work as a group or a team to explore a case or problem and which reflects the reality of the healthcare workforce. It is not without its challenges, as we can see from Harpreet's description of an experience when she was studying with a group of colleagues more senior to her:

I found this module extremely challenging – especially the anatomy and physiology of the acutely ill. The classroom sessions were interactive but I was studying alongside some very senior staff members which made me self-conscious and unconfident in answering questions.

Harpreet, children's nurse

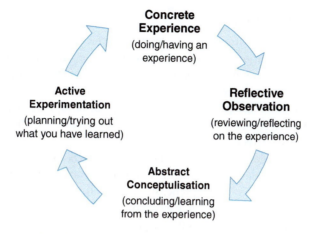

Figure 39.1 Adaptation of Kolb's learning cycle

Source: www.simplypsychology.org/learning-kolb.html

Case-based learning

Case-based learning is an established process of learning in healthcare. Bob Price, using Knowles' philosophy of andragogy (Knowles, 1984) introduced the concept of problem- or enquiry-based learning (Price, 2003). This approach included group communication etiquette as part of the process. Harpreet said she lacked confidence in asking questions; a problem-based learning approach would encourage active participation from all students, recognising that each student has a wealth of different experiential resources to offer. The list below outlines the process of problem-based learning:

1. Appraisal of the problem (also, what do you understand and know?)
2. What do you not understand, what do you not know?
3. Gathering of information about the problem – each group member may be allocated a distinct aspect of the problem to explore
4. Analysing the information – this is done individually and then as a group
5. Repeat stages 3 and 4 as often as necessary
6. Reach an understanding about a response to the problem

ACTIVITY 39.2: CRITICAL THINKING

Drawing on an experience from your practice, use Kolb's (1984) experiential learning cycle as an individual to explore and understand it better.

As a group you can do the same with a case or problem from practice (do you recognise that this is what we do every day in practice as part of the multi-professional group?)

ACTIVITY
ANSWER 39.2

Go to https://study.sagepub.com/essentialchildnursing and watch the video addressing the issues of concept-based curriculums.

VIDEO
LINK 39.1:
CONCEPT-
BASED
CURRICULUMS

Preferences in learning styles

Felder and Solomon (n.d.) identified differing learning styles that students may prefer. This does not mean that a student cannot have more than one style or that they are not able to adapt a preferred learning style to suit the learning experience. They described styles that were often opposite from each other, so an active learner needs to apply their learning while a reflective learner needs to make sense of what is being learnt by thinking it through. A sensing learner needs accuracy and factual information while an intuitive learner learns through identifying possibilities or relationships between concepts.

Visual learners prefer images to learn from and verbal learners prefer written words. Sequential learners prefer to learn in steps, each step adding to previous learning while global learners prefer a more random approach. This is not a comprehensive list of learning styles but it is meant to demonstrate the individual nature of learning. Being aware of the theory that supports learning and of our own preferred learning style helps to demystify the process and leads us to succeed in our CPD.

ACTIVITY 39.3: REFLECTIVE PRACTICE

Spend half an hour reflecting on something you studied in the last year and how this has changed how you practise as a nurse today - you might find this easier if you use a model such as John Driscoll's (2007).

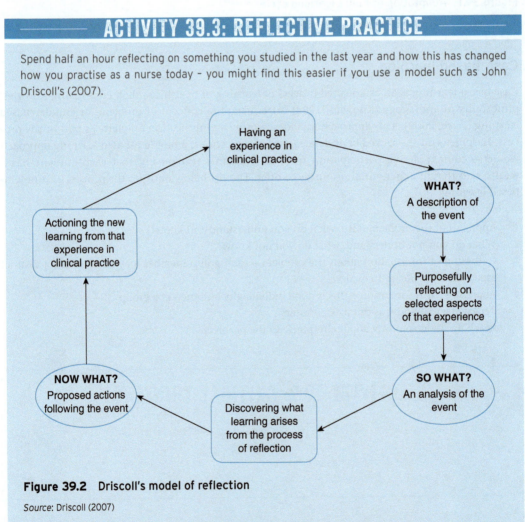

Figure 39.2 Driscoll's model of reflection

Source: Driscoll (2007)

- *What?* What did you study or, perhaps more accurately, what did you learn? What was the easiest thing about this learning experience or what did you enjoy the most during the time you were learning? Conversely, what was hardest or most challenging about the learning experience?

- *So what?* How are you using what you learnt in your practice today?
- *What next?* Have you shared the knowledge you learnt with anyone else – taught other students or perhaps the child or their family? How will you continue to develop and build on what you learnt?

Theory and practice

Here the case studies develop and demonstrate how the theories we have looked at apply to Harpreet, Judy and Jon's experiences.

Harpreet works in a very specialist area and described how it was intimidating when studying alongside her senior colleagues:

> The classroom sessions were interactive but I was studying alongside some very senior staff members which made me self-conscious and unconfident in answering questions.
>
> **Harpreet, children's nurse**

This was case-based learning where students work as a group or a team to explore a case or problem which reflects the reality of the healthcare workforce (constructionist/experiential).

Harpreet also describes her experience of undertaking a module related to research and how she now applies this knowledge to her practice:

> Before this module I was unfamiliar with how to find and critically appraise research. I now feel confident in searching and learning, being able to teach students and provide the highest, safest care to my patients. My clinical practice has benefited from the module as I will read routinely, search articles and discuss with colleagues.
>
> **Harpreet, children's nurse**

The learner has to seek out the new knowledge for themselves. They may be aided in doing so by lecturers signposting their way but the responsibility is their own. In this approach the nurse makes sense of what they learn by applying this knowledge to their practice (andragogy).

Judy, in the first excerpt, was reflecting on her learning whilst undertaking a module related to mentoring students:

> I have always been nervous about academic writing, lacking significantly in confidence. I also was not overly confident with teaching and assessing others and had not quite discovered my own teaching style or developed an appreciation for the different learning styles there are. However, I did have a passion for learning and teaching and fully appreciated that lifelong learning is an essential part of not only my personal and professional development but also that of others.
>
> **Judy, children's nurse**

The learner has to seek out the new knowledge for themselves. They may be aided in doing so by lecturers signposting their way but the responsibility is their own. In this approach the nurse makes sense of what they learn by applying this knowledge to their practice (andragogy).

Later, Judy describes their experience of undertaking a module exploring research methods and processes:

> Before completing this module, I really did not have a great knowledge base to enable me to confidently locate and interpret strong research to support my clinical practice. I knew the very basics of research interpretation, however this module enabled me to advance and build on those basic skills and knowledge. It really has, and will continue to have, a significant impact on every aspect of my nursing care, future study and role in practice development, strengthening my clinical judgement and confidence in passing this evidence-based knowledge and skill onto nursing students, parents/families and colleagues alike and most importantly keeping my clinical expertise as relevant as possible.
>
> **Judy, children's nurse**

The learner uses their own experience and knowledge to develop and acquire more (constructionist/experiential).

Finally, Judy comments:

> The course gave me the confidence to start thinking about my own professional future and which direction to go.
>
> **Judy, children's nurse**

The learner uses their own experience and knowledge to develop and acquire more (again constructionist/experiential).

Jon was under pressure to gain an honours degree and also appears conscious of the professional requirements to study:

> They prove that I have continuously worked to further my knowledge and skills since qualification as well as complying with the minimum amount of study time needed every year to remain registered.
>
> **Jon, children's nurse**

The learner has to seek out the new knowledge for themselves (andragogy).

There are many factors that motivate but it is reassuring that Jon recognised that the learning experience was far more than simply meeting professional requirements:

> Together these three modules have given me a much wider and more comprehensive understanding in relation to surgical nursing as well as giving me the skills and knowledge to teach and assess students and junior nurses in the clinical setting.
>
> **Jon, children's nurse**

The learner uses their own experience and knowledge to develop and acquire more (constructionist/experiential).

ACTIVITY 39.4: CRITICAL THINKING

What is your preferred learning style? Think about the last time you learnt something – this could be formally, such as a module at university, or it could be more applied, such as how to do a wound dressing. What learning styles did you use, and if you use these suggestions as examples of your own learning, did you use the same style each time?

CHAPTER SUMMARY

After reading this chapter you should:

- Be aware that CPD can enable you to inform and improve your practice, remembering that it is not only formal academic learning that counts as CPD
- Recognise that we work in a changing and complex healthcare system and this reflects the society that we live in
- Be aware that the way the children's nurse learns is informed and supported by learning theories such as andragogy and experiential learning theories. These are not abstract concepts – they help us make sense of how we learn

---

BUILD YOUR BIBLIOGRAPHY

Books

- Knowles, M., Holton, E. and Swanson R. (2005) *The Adult Learner*, 6th edn. Burlington MA: Elsevier.

  Many nurses use Kolb's learning cycle but this text explains how it was developed and the principles of learning that underpin the learning cycle.

- Price, B. (2003) *Studying Nursing Using Problem-based and Enquiry-based Learning*. New York: Palgrave Macmillan.

  This is a seminal text on the process of problem-based learning. Not only does it explain the approach but also how to facilitate learning.

Journal articles

Go to https://study.sagepub.com/essentialchildnursing for further free online journal articles related to this chapter.

- Driscoll, J. and Teh, B. (2001) 'The potential of reflective practice to develop individual orthopaedic nurse practitioners and their practice'. *Journal of Orthopaedic Nursing*, 5: 95-103.

  This article outlines how reflective models have developed and how they can help you with your CPD.

- Burbach, B., Barnason, S. and Hertzog, M. (2015) 'Preferred thinking style, symptom recognition, and response by nursing students during simulation'. *Western Journal of Nursing Research*, 37 (12): 1563-80.

  This study explored the link between thinking styles rather than learning styles of students in a high-fidelity simulation scenario. They found that students' thinking was more rational rather

FURTHER
READING:
ONLINE
JOURNAL
ARTICLES

(Continued)

(Continued)

than intuitive; that is, they would choose the most pragmatic solution rather than considering an instinctive response.

- Condon, B. (2015) 'Politically charged issues in nursing's teaching-learning environments'. *Nursing Science Quarterly*, 28 (2): 115-20.

This paper explores the relationship between politics and education in the USA but has real relevance to the debate in the UK also.

- Feil, M. (1999) 'Preceptorship: the progression from student to staff nurse'. *Journal of Child Health Care*, 3 (3): 13-18.

This is now quite old and it is important to look at more recent work also, but it is interesting to see that the issues have not changed very much. The nurse that is newly qualified and is not supported through this transitionary period will often leave nursing.

Weblinks

FURTHER
READING:
WEBLINKS

Go to https://study.sagepub.com/essentialchildnursing for further weblinks related to this chapter.

- The King's Fund, Addicott R., Maguire D., Honeyman M., Jabbal J., (2015) *Workforce Planning in the NHS*.

www.kingsfund.org.uk/publications/workforce-planning-nhs

This is a very readable outline of NHS policy and plans.

- We Communities

www.wecommunities.org

This is an exciting online resource which allows you to contribute to the community of children's nurses. It has blogs and discussions which you are encouraged to participate in or you can ask questions and be offered support from your peers in this speciality of nursing.

- Nursing Times

www.nursingtimes.net

This is a valuable resource for the nursing profession and reports on breaking news developments for nurses. They are keen for nurses to write for them and there is guidance if you want to contribute to the journal.

ACE YOUR ASSESSMENT

ONLINE
QUIZZES &
ACTIVITY
ANSWERS

GREAT FOR
REVISION!

Revise what you have learned by visiting https://study.sagepub.com/essentialchildnursing

- Test yourself with multiple-choice and short-answer questions
- Do the chapter activities in the book and check your answers online

REFERENCES

Addicott, R., Maguire, D., Honeyman, M. and Jabbal, J. (2015) *Workforce Planning in the NHS*. Available at: www.kingsfund.org.uk/publications/workforce-planning-nhs (last accessed 2 June 2017).

Bradley, C. (2012) 'The role of high-fidelity clinical simulation in teaching and learning in the health professions'. Available at: www.kcl.ac.uk/study/learningteaching/kli/research/hern/hern-j4/claire-bradley-hernjvol4.pdf (last accessed 2 June 2017).

Department of Health (2014) *Delivering High Quality, Effective, Compassionate Care: Developing the Right Skills and the Right Values*. Available at: https://hee.nhs.uk/sites/default/files/documents/WES_DH_HEE_Mandate.pdf (last accessed 29 June 2017).

Department of Health (2016) *A Mandate from the Government to NHS England: April 2015 to March 2016*. Available at: www.gov.uk/government/publications/nhs-mandate-2015-to-2016 (last accessed 29 June 2017).

Driscoll, J. (2007) *Practising Clinical Supervision: A Reflective Approach for Healthcare Professionals*, 2nd edn. Edinburgh: Bailliere Tindall Elsevier.

Felder, R.M. and Soloman, B.A. (n.d.) Learning styles and strategies. Available at: www4.ncsu.edu/unity/lockers/users/f/felder/public/ILSdir/styles.htm (last accessed 25 June 2016).

Griffith, M.B. (2012) 'Effective succession planning in nursing: A review of the literature'. *Journal of Nursing Management*, 20 (7): 900–11.

HM Government (2015) *Working Together to Safeguard Children*. London: DfE. Available at: www.gov.uk/government/publications/working-together-to-safeguard-children--2 (last accessed 2 June 2017).

Knowles, M. (1984) *Andragogy in Action*. San Francisco: Jossey-Bass.

Kolb, D.A. (1984) *Experiential Learning*, Englewood Cliffs, NJ: Prentice Hall.

McCaughey, C.S. and Traynor, M.K. 'The role of simulation in nurse education'. *Nurse Education Today*, 30: 827–32.

Mental Health Taskforce to the NHS in England (2016) *The Five Year Forward View for Mental Health*. Available at: www.england.nhs.uk/wp-content/uploads/2016/02/Mental-Health-Taskforce-FYFV-final.pdf (last accessed 2 June 2017).

NHS Business Services Authority (2016) *Your Guide to NHS Student Bursaries 2016/17*. Available at: www.nhsbsa.nhs.uk/sites/default/files/2017-06/guide-to-nhs-student-bursaries-2016-17.pdf (last accessed 1 June 2017).

NHS England (2015) *Safeguarding Policy*. Available at: www.england.nhs.uk/wp-content/uploads/2015/07/safeguard-policy.pdf (last accessed 19 September 2017).

Nursing and Midwifery Council (NMC) (2017a) *Revalidation: What You Need to Do*. Available at: http://revalidation.nmc.org.uk/what-you-need-to-do (last accessed: 2 June 2017).

Nursing and Midwifery Council (2017b) *Social media guidance*. Available at: www.nmc.org.uk/standards/guidance/social-networking-guidance/ (last accessed 7 February 2017).

Nursing and Midwifery Council (NMC) (2017c) *Standards for Competence for Registered Nurses*. Available at: www.nmc.org.uk/standards/additional-standards/standards-for-competence-for-registered-nurses (last accessed 2 June 2017).

Price, B. (2003) *Studying Nursing Using Problem-based and Enquiry-based Learning*. New York: Palgrave Macmillan.

Shann, F., Curtis, N. and Mulholland, K. (2003) 'Evidence on the use of paracetamol in febrile children'. *Bulletin of the World Health Organization*, 81 (5): 367–72.

Willis, Lord (2015) *Raising the Bar. Shape of Caring: A Review of the Future Education and Training of Registered Nurses and Care Assistants*. Available at https://hee.nhs.uk/sites/default/files/documents/2348-Shape-of-caring-review-FINAL.pdf (last accessed 1 June 2017).

Wragg, E., Francis, J. and Amblum, J. (2014) 'Managing paediatric patients with pyrexia'. *Emergency Nurse*, 22 (8): 20–3.

DECISION-MAKING AND ACCOUNTABILITY IN CHILDREN AND YOUNG PEOPLE'S NURSING

LORRAINE HIGHE

--- **THIS CHAPTER COVERS** ---

- Decision-making in clinical practice
- Who are the decision-makers in children and young people's health care?
- How can children's nurses improve their decision-making?

> " During my third year of training I worked on a burns unit. On one shift, a child came in for an outpatient dressing change and I assisted the nurse. Due to a miscommunication between myself and the nurse I brought her the wrong solution to irrigate the burn. I left the room and went to ask the nurse in charge why we used that solution instead of others. It was here that I realised my mistake and told the nurse in charge what had happened. Thankfully she was able to re-irrigate the wound and prevent any harm from occurring. This incident taught me the importance of being honest when I make mistakes and always double check when I am unsure. Moreover, I became more aware of my accountability to both my patients and colleagues. I learnt the importance of acting within my own limitations and that it is better to say when I cannot complete a task than for it to be administered in a potentially unsafe manner.
>
> **Sophie, 3rd-year children's nursing student** "

Visit https://study.sagepub.com/essentialchildnursing to access a wealth of online resources for this chapter – watch out for the margin icons throughout the chapter.

INTRODUCTION

Decision-making is arguably one of the most difficult and important processes a health professional has to undertake. The process requires skills in problem solving, critical thinking, reflective practice and sound judgement, alongside knowledge of scientific evidence-based practice, ethical values and professional accountability. This chapter will discuss what we mean by clinical decision-making and how our clinical decisions display our professional accountability.

Pre-registration nursing courses are designed to foster critical thinking and analytical reflection (NMC, 2010); however, the nature of the decisions made by a children's nursing student will depend upon the stage of the course they have reached, the clinical placement and the preferences of the child or young person in their care. Throughout this chapter you will have the opportunity to identify who the decision-makers are in children's nursing and appraise theoretical models of decision-making in order to enable you to make decisions which promote safe and effective care.

DECISION-MAKING IN CLINICAL PRACTICE

Making decisions is something we do every day. Sometimes we make decisions that are not in our own best interests, but we choose to take a risk based on our judgement of a particular course of action. For example, I should have an apple for lunch, but I choose the chocolate biscuit despite knowing this is not the healthiest option. Professional decision-making involves the same process of balancing the pros and cons of a given situation (although the apple is healthier, the biscuit I conclude has a superior taste), but crucially as we are now making decisions that impact on children we can be held accountable.

One of the most important factors in clinical decision-making is that of accountability. Accountability means being answerable to a higher authority for your actions. You may consider your actions are justifiable and in the best interests of your patient, but as a nurse, higher authorities can ask us to justify our actions.

Dimond (2015) claims that there are four spheres of accountability for children's nurses:

- The profession through statute law
- Children and young people through tort law
- Society through public law
- The employer through the contract of employment

Go to https://study.sagepub.com/essentialchildnursing and watch the four-minute video on decision-making in nursing.

WATCH A VIDEO ONLINE!

VIDEO LINK 40.1: DECISION-MAKING

Profession

Our professional accountability is clearly outlined in The Code as set out by the NMC (2015) whose standards state we should: 'always practise in line with the best available evidence' (p.9); 'recognise and work within the limits of your competence' (p.11) and 'take measures to reduce as far as possible the likelihood of mistakes' (p.14). The Code stresses that these standards also incorporate the expectations of our patients and the general public.

Watch the video made by the Royal College of Nursing to help nurses and healthcare assistants understand their roles and responsibilities in relation to accountability available at https://study.sagepub.com/essentialchildnursing

VIDEO LINK 40.2: ACCOUNTABILITY

Children and young people

Nurses are also accountable to the individual patients and families under their care. The tort or civil law system allows a patient to seek compensation if they believe harm has been caused through negligence or a failure to uphold our duty of care. As a children's nurse it is important to be aware that a child who has suffered a personal injury has no time barrier to bringing an action against you, until they reach the age of 18 years. For example, you may need to rely on your nursing notes that are 21 years old because a newborn who suffers an injury has three years from their 18th birthday to present a civil action claim.

Society

Society holds you to account through public law. Examples for nurses would be the Medicine Act 1968 and the Mental Health Act 2007. It is possible to breach a public general act as a consequence of a decision you have made in your clinical practice. In these circumstances you would be asked to account for your actions in a criminal court of law.

Employer

Finally, a nurse who is employed by the NHS or another organisation is accountable to their employer through their contract of employment. The contract sets out the terms and conditions of employment and the standard of work expected of the employee. Nurses who breach NHS guidelines or local policies can expect to be held to account, through reasonable disciplinary procedures.

Professional judgement and decision-making is therefore open to scrutiny by a range of people, including children and young people, parents, colleagues, other professional staff and the public. My colleagues may comment on my poor choice of lunch, but this everyday decision will not be scrutinised by external criteria as outlined above through legal, clinical or procedural guidelines and standards.

WHO ARE THE DECISION-MAKERS IN CHILDREN AND YOUNG PEOPLE'S HEALTHCARE?

When decisions have to be made concerning a child's health, in the initial stages three parties are involved: the child, the parents and healthcare professionals. This section will discuss the role of each party and identify some of the challenges each party faces when contributing to healthcare decisions.

PRACTICE
SCENARIO 40:
ABU

SCENARIO 40.1: REENA

Reena is a 13-year-old girl with febrile neutropenia who refused to be transferred to the high-dependency unit (HDU) because the nurses in that ward are 'mean and uncaring'. Reena's parents are keen for her to be transferred where additional care and support can be obtained immediately. Following a long consultation with Reena and her parents the medical and nursing team respected Reena's wishes and agreed a treatment plan if Reena's condition was to deteriorate.

Two hours later Reena called over the nurse-in-charge to state that she had changed her mind, and agreed to be transferred to the HDU to 'satisfy her parent's wishes'.

- Who is the primary decision-maker in this case?
- What is your role as a nursing student?

SCENARIO
ANSWER 40.1

Involving children and young people in decision-making

There are many reasons for involving children in decisions about their own healthcare and treatment. The ethical principle of autonomy or self-determination (Beauchamp and Childress, 2013) applies to children as well as adults. When children are given the opportunity to be part of the decision-making process this can give them a sense of control, which can in turn enhance their positive adjustment to the treatment plan. Watch the video at https://study.sagepub.com/essentialchildnursing on ethical issues to explore this further. As illustrated in the scenario, Reena is unlikely to engage with the staff and care in the HDU as she does not agree with the transfer taking place.

VIDEO LINK 40.3: ETHICAL ISSUES

The greatest challenge to involving children and young people in decision-making is their competence or ability to make a decision. Adults are assumed to be competent decision-makers, children are presumed to be incompetent and are therefore required to prove their competence. Reena's capacity to make a decision is not only a function of her age (as indicated by law) but also a reflection of her cognitive ability and personal experience. For example, Reena who has previous experience of hospitalisation and treatment is usually more competent to decide about a new treatment plan than less experienced children of a similar age and maturity.

Having frequent operations throughout my life is frustrating and I hope things improve one day. Whilst my mum is very thorough questioning the doctors, she now encourages me to ask about my surgeries too and tries to explain afterwards things I'm not sure about. Some doctors can talk over me like I'm not there and forget I'm not a young child anymore!

Jordan, patient

SAFEGUARDING STOP POINT

Imagine a slightly different scenario, in which Reena refuses to remain in hospital for treatment due to her dislike of the hospital. As a competent child what actions can be taken in such a situation?

The Children Act 1989 (s 25) allows the use of secure accommodation to restrict the liberty of a child for 72 hours in any 28-day period. Secure accommodation is not specifically defined by the Children Act, but in practical terms the Act would advocate for locking the entrance to the ward (see Re B (A Minor) (Treatment and Secure Accommodation [1997]). Before restricting the liberty of a child or young person the team must be satisfied that the child or young person has a history of absconding, is likely to suffer significant harm or that they are likely to injure themselves or other persons if they were to have their treatment in an alternative location.

Parents

Parents are used as proxies when their child is judged as not competent or do not have the legal right to make a decision. This parental responsibility is defined within the Children Act 1989, s 3(1) in which parents have a duty to act in the child's best interests. According to Beauchamp and Childress (2013), a surrogate decision-maker – in this scenario Reena's parents – must determine the highest net benefit among available options, assigning different weights to the interest Reena has in each option. Parents themselves must therefore have the ability to make reasoned judgements for which they require adequate knowledge and information, emotional stability and the ability to balance the best interests of their child or young person.

Parents are usually the most suited to judge what is in the best interests of their child. The assumption is based upon the premise that parents know more than anyone else about their children due to their constant, close proximity. However, as in this scenario, a parent's own distress regarding their child's condition or belief that they have to protect their child from upsetting information and decisions may prevent them from giving due attention to the child's needs and wishes. This does not mean that they are bad parents, just that they need support to make decisions at distressing times.

> As parents of a child with complex medical needs we are often faced with having to make difficult decisions on Matthew's behalf. Being kept fully informed is key, however upsetting the medical information is to receive, to help us prepare ourselves and Matthew to overcome the challenges ahead. We always seek professional advice where our knowledge is limited to ensure we can make informed decisions together with the medical professionals and Matthew now he is a teenager.
>
> **Ava, parent**

WHAT'S THE EVIDENCE?

Read the article 'Children's participation in decision-making: balancing protection with shared decision-making using a situational perspective' by Coyne and Harder (2011), accessible via https://study.sagepub.com/essentialchildnursing

This article provides a synopsis of the research, which identifies reasons why adults wish to protect children and provides a summary of children's competence to participate in decision-making. Whilst reading the article, consider the following:

- What are the possible barriers to shared situational decision-making?
- What are the possible consequences for children or young people's healthcare if they do not participate in shared decision-making?

WHAT'S THE EVIDENCE? ANSWER 40.1

WEBLINK:
CHILDREN'S
PARTICIPATION

FIND OUT MORE!

Health professionals

Health professionals continue to self-regulate their standards of practice but as outlined earlier in this chapter, practitioners are increasingly held to account through public and employer scrutiny. As a result, the healthcare professional's role is to provide clinical judgements, decisions and interventions that are clearly explained, justified and defended when challenged either by children or young people and their parents. Children's nurses in particular are responsible for passing on healthcare information in a manner which can be understood and retained by children or young people and their family.

Judicial review

When a collaborative healthcare decision cannot be made, a fourth party involving our judicial system can be invited to make the final decision for a child or young person. The courts through their inherent jurisdiction exercise a supervisory role over healthcare decision-making. For example, in cases where those with parental responsibility strongly oppose the giving or withholding of treatment by a health professional the matter will be referred to the court for a decision. In a similar approach to parental responsibility, Lord Donaldson in the case of Re J (A minor) [1992] made it clear that the best interests of the child should always be sought when assessing any course of action to be taken.

WHAT'S THE EVIDENCE?

The test for determining the best interests of a child has developed over time as new cases have been brought to court. Thirty-five years ago, in the case of a child born with Down's syndrome who needed urgent surgery for an intestinal blockage, the court limited its consideration of the best interest test to the life expectancy of the child [Re B (a minor) 1981]. Thirty-two years later Baroness Hale of Richmond in Aintree University Hospitals NHS Foundation Trust v James [2013] asserted that in considering the best interests, decision-makers must look at the child's welfare in the widest sense, not just medical but social and psychological; they must consider the nature of the medical treatment in question and try to put themselves in the place of the individual patient.

• What factors would you consider when determining the best interests of a child?

WHAT'S THE
EVIDENCE?
ANSWER 40.2

HOW CAN CHILDREN'S NURSES IMPROVE THEIR DECISION-MAKING?

To be accountable when making decisions you require knowledge and understanding, an ability to rationalise, the skills to carry out required actions and the ability to make decisions. This final part of the chapter will explore decision-making models, which can be utilised to facilitate effective decision-making in practice.

SCENARIO 40.2: JOSHUA

Joshua is a 5-month-old infant who has been admitted to your ward for observation following a diagnosis of bronchiolitis. Currently his clinical observations are within normal parameters for his age, but his work of breathing has increased and the medical team are concerned he may deteriorate in the next few hours. The mentor you are working with appears concerned about Joshua, advising you to monitor his observations every 30 minutes. You ask your mentor about her decision-making process.

• Why do you think your mentor is concerned about Joshua?
• How do you determine the frequency of clinical observation monitoring for each child in your care?

SCENARIO
ANSWER 40.2

Banning (2008) identified three models of clinical decision-making. All three models can be used when working in the clinical environment. The scenario of Joshua will be used to demonstrate these models in action.

The information-processing model

This model uses a scientific (hypothetical–deductive) approach to assist cognitive reasoning. The approach involves multiple stages:

- Cue recognition
- Hypothesis generation
- Cue interpretation
- Hypothesis evaluation (Tanner et al., 1987)

As a student nurse you may consciously use scientific information such as a protocol or guideline for bronchiolitis (cue interpretation) to enable you to recognise and interpret Joshua's vital signs and symptoms (cue recognition) to formulate a plan of care (hypothesis generation). By contrast, an experienced qualified children's nurse may work from the hypothesis (hypothesis generation) and then collect the information (cue recognition) to either confirm or refute the efficacy of the care decision (hypothesis evaluation). The way in which the decision-making stages are applied can therefore depend upon the nurse's knowledge and experience of caring for children with bronchiolitis.

The strength of the information-processing model is the certainty and reliability it can provide when clinical decisions are made. Decision-tree algorithms based upon this model have been found to significantly improve the decision-making ability of nurses (Aspiuynall, 1979). There are, however, significant drawbacks to this model as it assumes existing knowledge is available and accurate. In clinical practice the decisions we make often possess an element of uncertainty as nursing knowledge is not static but continuously advances with every decision and discovery we make.

ACTIVITY 40.1: REFLECTIVE PRACTICE

Can you identify a situation in which you have made a nursing decision using the information-processing model?

The intuitive–humanistic model

Benner (1984) describes a model where inexperienced nurses tend to use procedures and guidelines to make decisions, while the experienced nurse may use intuitive decision-making processes. The intuitive decision-making occurs when experienced nurses appear to make sense of a situation without relying on processing analytical principles. Through unconscious thought processing and pattern recognition a decision is often expressed as a 'gut feeling' or 'sixth sense'. For example, an experienced nurse as in the scenario above may decide to increase the monitoring of an infant like Joshua, due to a 'gut feeling' that they may tire and clinically deteriorate despite his clinical observations being within the normal range for his age.

ACTIVITY 40.2: CRITICAL THINKING

Now that you have read about two decision-making models, what factors can influence children or young people care-related decisions?

ACTIVITY
ANSWER 40.2

The clinical decision-making model

The use of intuitive knowledge for the purpose of decision-making has been challenged, as without analysis and evaluation it is more difficult to explain, justify and defend clinical judgements. This hybrid model (O'Neill et al., 2004) is based around a computerised decision-support system which uses hypothetical deduction (information-processing model) and pattern recognition (intuitive–humanistic model) as a basis of decision-making. Patient-specific data (e.g. case notes and clinical observations) are used as a tool to help the nurse anticipate health risks to their patients. The degree of risk of each potential problem is ranked and then the nursing action is implemented to reduce the most threatening of risks.

In the absence of a computerised decision-making system, the nurse caring for the infant with bronchiolitis can adopt the principles of this hybrid model by using both subjective and objective data to decide what actions are needed to prevent respiratory deterioration for Joshua. The knowledge, experience and the ability of the nurse to care for a child or young person whose condition can change rapidly are all elements that are considered in O'Neil et al.'s (2004) multidimensional model. As your nursing knowledge and clinical experience increase, your ability to make clinical decisions will become more refined and intricate.

PLACEMENT ADVICE 40: DECISION-MAKING & ACCOUNTABILITY

Go to https://study.sagepub.com/essentialchildnursing for advice on decision-making and accountabilty during placements.

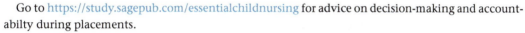

CHAPTER SUMMARY

- We all make decisions every day, but professional decision-making has an additional element in that the decisions we make as nurses are open to scrutiny by a range of people, including children and young people, parents, professional colleagues and the general public
- Delivering understandable information and active engagement with a child or young person and their family in the decision-making process is essential
- There are several decision-making theories which attempt to capture the complexity of making decisions in clinical practice
- Theoretical knowledge and clinical experience impact on the decision-making strategies of children's nurses

BUILD YOUR BIBLIOGRAPHY

Books

- Aston, L., Wakefield, J. and McGow, R. (2010) *The Student Nurse Guide to Decision Making in Practice*. Maidenhead: Open University Press.

  Chapter 4: 'Getting the most out of your mentor' provides you with tips and advice about how to gain the most of the time you spend with your mentor to develop your decision-making skills.

- Benner, P. (1984) *From Novice to Expert: Excellence and Power in Clinical Nursing Practice*. Menio Park: Addison Wesley.

(Continued)

(Continued)

This book is useful in assisting you to understand and appreciate your journey from a novice nurse to an expert practitioner. You will find examples of how nurses develop their decision-making skills through skill acquisition.

Journal articles

FURTHER READING: ONLINE JOURNAL ARTICLES

Go to https://study.sagepub.com/essentialchildnursing for further free online journal articles related to this chapter.

- O'Brien, I. Duffy, A. and O'Shea, E. (2010) 'Medical futility in children's nursing: making end-of-life decisions'. *British Journal of Nursing*, 19 (6): 352-6.

  In this article the authors discuss the concepts of parental autonomy and the child's best interests when making end-of-life decisions for infants.

- Twycross, A. and Powls, L. (2006) 'How do children's nurses make clinical decisions? Two preliminary studies'. *Journal of Clinical Nursing*, 15 (10): 1324-35.

  This preliminary research reveals how the analysis of verbal protocols obtained using the think aloud technique suggested that all the children's nurses in the sample used a hypothetical-deductive (analytical) model of decision-making.

Weblinks

FURTHER READING: WEBLINKS

Go to https://study.sagepub.com/essentialchildnursing for further weblinks related to this chapter.

- The King's Fund, Make Shared Decision Making a Reality: No Decision About Me, Without Me (Coulter and Collins, 2011)

  www.kingsfund.org.uk/sites/files/kf/Making-shared-decision-making-a-reality-paper-Angela-Coulter-Alf-Collins-July-2011_0.pdf

  The Government wants shared decision-making to become the norm in the NHS. This report by the King's Fund clarifies the concept and outlines the actions needed.

─── ACE YOUR ASSESSMENT ───

ONLINE QUIZZES & ACTIVITY ANSWERS

Revise what you have learned by visiting https://study.sagepub.com/essentialchildnursing

- Test yourself with multiple-choice and short-answer questions
- Do the chapter activities in the book and check your answers online

CASES

Aintree University Hospitals NHS Foundation Trust v James [2013]

Re B (A Minor) (Wardship: Medical Treatment) [1981] 1 WLR 1421

Re B (Minors) (Residence Order) [1992] Fam 162

Re B (A Minor) (Treatment and Secure Accommodation) [1997] 1 FLR 618

Re J (A Minor) [1992] All ER 614

STATUTES

Children Act 1989
Medicine Act 1968
Mental Health Act 2007

REFERENCES

Aspiuynall, M. (1979) 'Use of a decision tree to improve accuracy of nursing diagnosis'. *Nursing Research*, 28: 182–5.

Banning, M. (2008) 'A review of clinical decision making: models and current research'. *Journal of Clinical Nursing*, 17 (2): 187–95.

Benner, P. (1984) *From Novice to Expert: Excellence and Power in Clinical Nursing Practice*. Menlo Park, CA: Addison Wesley.

Beauchamp, T. and Childress, J. (2013) *Principles of Biomedical Ethics*, 7th edn. Oxford: Oxford University Press.

Coyne, I. and Harder, M. (2011) 'Children's participation in decision-making'. *Journal of Child Health Care*, 15 (4): 312–19.

Dimond, B. (2015) *Legal Aspects of Nursing*, 7th edn. Harlow: Pearson Education.

Nursing and Midwifery Council (NMC) (2010) *Standards for Pre-registration Nursing Education*. London: NMC.

Nursing and Midwifery Council (NMC) (2015). *The Code: Professional Standards of Practice and Behaviour for Nurses and Midwives*. London: NMC.

O'Neill, E., Dluhy, N., Fortier, P. and Howard, E. (2004) 'Knowledge acquisition, synthesis and validation: a model for decision support systems'. *Journal of Advanced Nursing*, 47 (2): 134–42.

Tanner, C., Padrick, K., Westfall, U. and Putzier, D. (1987) 'Diagnostic reasoning strategies for nurses and nursing students'. *Nursing Research*, 36 (6): 358–63.

BEING POLITICALLY AWARE AND PROFESSIONALLY PROACTIVE IN CHILDREN AND YOUNG PEOPLE'S NURSING

JIM RICHARDSON

THIS CHAPTER COVERS

- The nature of a political issue and its impact on children today
- Policy and law
- Principles of political activity and lobbying
- Means of influencing and persuading

> "
> One really clever tip which young people are being told is that if they are at risk of being taken from the country against their will they should hide a teaspoon in their clothing. This will cause the detection equipment at the airport to alarm. The security personnel will want to carry out a further check and this is the last opportunity to tell someone that they are being forced to travel.
>
> **Anonymous**
> "

Visit https://study.sagepub.com/essentialchildnursing to access a wealth of online resources for this chapter – watch out for the margin icons throughout the chapter.

INTRODUCTION

This chapter will address the factors involved in nurses becoming involved with political questions and the advantages to be gained from this (Porter-O'Grady and Malloch, 2013). The nature of health-related politics will be explored and how it might be exploited to produce positive change. The potential for good in political activity will be demonstrated and, therefore, its relevance to children's nurses. A topical subject will be used as a vehicle to illustrate these concepts. The subject to be used is forced child marriage. Nurses form a large professional group and are respected in society as professionals. This makes them potentially highly effective as a lobbying group in influencing and persuading individuals and organisations (Hart, 2004) in a position to bring about change which will have a positive impact on the health and wellbeing of children. Nurses are also in a strong position to identify factors affecting child health and they are powerful enough to bring about change for the better (McKenna, 2010). What follows in this chapter will indicate ways in which nurses might be able to achieve change and the insights they need to enable them to do so.

THE NATURE OF A POLITICAL ISSUE AND ITS IMPACT ON CHILDREN TODAY

ACTIVITY 41.1: CRITICAL THINKING

Research the history of the introduction of cycling helmets for children to reduce the risk of serious head injuries and the introduction of the perinatal sickle cell anaemia screening which allows early identification and treatment of this disorder. In both of these cases it was children's nurses who were highly influential in securing the change.

ACTIVITY
ANSWER 41.1

CHECK YOUR
ANSWERS
ONLINE!

In the conversation below, Robin is a final year children's nursing student who is visiting the Students' Union to renew her travel insurance when she sees Mason, the union's equalities officer, putting up a poster about child forced marriage. She is immediately intrigued as she has no idea what child forced marriage is.

SCENARIO 41.1: ROBIN AND MASON

Robin (R): That looks interesting, Mason. What's it about?

Mason (M): We're running a campaign this semester to raise awareness of forced marriage and make sure that anyone who is at risk of this knows where they can get help and support.

R: I've never heard of forced marriage. What is it?

(Continued)

(Continued)

M: Well, that tells you why we need a campaign to raise awareness. Forced marriage happens all over the world and involves a marriage to which one or both individuals did not give free consent. It is illegal in Britain and can be very harmful indeed to the people affected. Sometimes one of the people involved is under 18 and that would be seen as child abuse.

R: Oh my, I had no idea. I think everything must be done to prevent this. How common is it?

M: The people we got this poster from are the Forced Marriage Unit at the Home Office and they estimated that in 2015 they dealt with 1,220 cases, 80 per cent of them involving girls but the figure worldwide runs into millions. It can be enormously damaging to those affected both physically and psychologically. It's really a human rights issue that we should be working to eliminate.

R: Millions? That's dreadful, we must do something about this; it just can't continue.

M: That, Robin, is the point of the awareness campaign. Would you like to join the team!?

R: Count me in but I need to find out more about this.

- This encounter illustrates how raising awareness of political issues is the first step in securing support. Can you think of other issues which children's nurses could campaign on in the political sphere (e.g. faith-based child mistreatment, children being used as beggars, older female children being kept from school to care for younger siblings, etc.)?

WHAT'S THE EVIDENCE?

Forced marriage (Forced Marriage Unit, undated) can be defined as a marriage that has taken place without the express consent of one or both parties involved (Phillips and Dustin, 2004). This may be because they have been coerced by the threat of or actual violence by their family and/or community. Equally, if they are not competent to give consent because of a factor such as an intellectual disability then that would be regarded in the eyes of the law as being a forced marriage. Forced marriage is often explained by communities who practise it as being intended to protect those involved and strengthen the family as a whole (e.g. by bringing in money or property). Some believe that they are following a cultural or religious belief (Gangoli et al., 2008). However, all of the major religions are adamant that freely given consent must be given before marriage and, therefore, they all condemn forced marriage (The Scottish Government, 2011; HM Government, 2014a, 2014b).

Eighty per cent of forced marriages concern girls and women but it should also be borne in mind that 20 per cent involve the male partner. An estimate has been made that 5,000–8,000 people a year are at risk of being forced unwillingly into marriage (UK All-Party Parliamentary Group on Population, Development and Reproductive Health, 2012). The Forced Marriage Unit at the UK Home Office reports contact with 1,220 potential victims in 2015, with around 350 calls a month being received (Home Office, 2017). This report adds that 27 per cent of the victims are under the age of 18 and as such are, by definition, children.

Many forced marriages are held abroad, often under pretence of a family holiday. These situations can involve extreme coercion and violence and can ultimately lead to killing. This gives a sense of how severe a crime this is. It is worth noting that in 14 per cent (175 cases) of the victims coming to the notice of the Forced Marriage Unit the activity took place entirely in Britain.

The forced marriage of children, sometimes as young as 8, has a range of very damaging consequences for all children but particularly girl children. These include early motherhood with short gaps between pregnancies before the girl is physically ready, leading to health-damaging complications. This leads this group of girls to have higher than expected mortality and morbidity rates. Also, these girls may be at greater risk of other culturally determined harmful practices such as female genital mutilation (FGM) and so-called 'honour-based' violence. Early forced marriage also almost always leads to their being withdrawn early from education. This severely limits these girls' life opportunities, including their ability to escape this situation.

It is important to draw a distinction between forced marriage and arranged marriage. Arranged marriage is also a culturally driven practice but the participants have given full and free consent and may refuse at any point.

POLICY AND LAW

In the UK, there is a legal framework for the prevention of forced marriage, which makes it a crime (Anitha and Gill, 2009). It has taken some time for forced marriage to be fully recognised for the harmful practice it is and the legal framework prohibiting it has evolved over time. The Children Acts of 1989 and 2004 set out the principles of the primacy of the best interests of children, and recognising and responding to the needs and the prevention of harm of children. The Forced Marriage (Civil Protection) Act 2007 extended the Family Law Act (1996) to protect from forced marriage those unable to consent. It also made provision for the Forced Marriage Protection Order which is a form of legal injunction. In 2005 the Mental Capacity Act 2005 laid down protection for those unable to give full and free consent because they lack competence or the ability to do so, and the procedures to be followed to protect people in that situation. This is vital protection for people with, for example, an intellectual disability. The Anti-Social Behaviour, Crime and Policing Act 2014 updates and unites these principles in one piece of legislation covering England and Wales, making forced marriage a criminal offence. The Forced Marriage etc. (Protection and Jurisdiction) (Scotland) Act 2011 fulfils the same purpose in Scotland.

The Forced Marriage Unit was set up in 2005 as a joint agency of the Foreign and Commonwealth Office and the Home Office. The Unit provides specialist advice and support for people at risk of forced marriage and those who are helping them. The unit publishes annual statistics of its activities, which helps to give a picture of the scale of the problem (Home Office, 2017). An important part of the Forced Marriage Unit's work is raising awareness of forced marriage and the legal framework forbidding it as well as the penalties available for those forcing the marriage.

The voluntary and charitable sector play a very important role in protecting people from forced marriage and other harmful traditions at a grassroots level. These organisations are particularly effective when they arise from within communities with these traditions and have full insight into the issues involved and the pressures which serve to perpetuate them. They are also able to offer services which are culturally appropriate and in a range of community languages.

—————————— **SAFEGUARDING STOP POINT** ——————————

If a child is in danger of being forced to marry, how might safeguarding processes be used to protect this young person from harm? You might think of using the flow charts in your local child protection procedures to help you address this question in a structured way. This will also help you to understand the part that you might play in this process.

The rights context of children

The United Nations Convention on the Rights of the Child provides a very useful framework for ensuring that the child's protection from any harm is in the forefront of everyone's mind. The Convention was published in 1989 and was ratified by the UK government in 1991, meaning that the government is bound to uphold all of the rights laid down in the convention (United Nations, 1989). Only two countries in the world have not to date ratified the Convention: Somalia and the United States of America.

Article 19 states, 'Governments should ensure that children are properly cared for, and protect them from violence, abuse or neglect by their parents or anyone else who looks after them.' This very clearly includes the harmful practice of forced marriage.

The very particular needs of the child with a disability are covered by article 23 of the Convention, 'If you have a disability, you should receive special care and support so that you can live a full and independent life.'

The very nature of forced marriage breaches article 12 of the Convention which states: 'You should have the right to say what you think should happen when adults are making decisions that affect you, and to have your opinions taken into account.'

Article 30 provides an interesting example of how any article in the Convention can be superseded by the need to protect the child from harm, which is the overriding principle, 'You have the right to learn and use the language and customs of your family whether or not these are shared by the majority of the people in the country where you live.' Forced marriage, which is a harmful practice, would, therefore, not be covered by the right expressed in this article.

Article 36 presents an overarching right which can be applied to the practice of forced marriage, 'You should be protected from any activities that could harm your development' (CEWC Cymru, 2012).

ACTIVITY 41.2: CRITICAL THINKING

Take a look at the UN Convention on the Rights of the Child (www.unicef.org.uk/what-we-do/un-convention-child-rights) and consider which other articles would be breached by taking a young person out of the country in order to carry out a forced marriage.

PRINCIPLES OF POLITICAL ACTIVITY AND LOBBYING

Engaging in activity in order to change the opinion of prominent people such as politicians might be seen as a process of influencing and persuading in order to achieve a goal. In our case that would be to take all steps necessary to eliminate as far as possible the practice of forced marriage.

The City of Portland, Oregon (2011) has prepared an interesting document outlining what they call the Ten Principles of Lobbying which gives a framework for effective political action.

Do your homework

This is important as you must get the facts right. If you make an error with the basic facts you not only look foolish but you have done nothing to advance your cause and you have potentially misled the people whose support you have enlisted. All in all, it is vital that you are factually accurate.

Be patient and flexible

Decision-makers have full agendas; plans change and availability alters so you need to be fairly fleet of foot to make the best of opportunities to persuade and influence as they occur.

Tell the truth

There is a risk of losing all credibility if you are untruthful. You will not look trustworthy if you make things up as you go along. If you don't have the precise facts at your fingertips and you are asked a direct question it is absolutely fine to answer that you don't know. However, it will certainly advance your cause if you can follow that up after the event by finding out what the answer is to that question and passing it on to the questioner. Also, you are more likely to influence if you undertake to find information that you follow that through by actually doing so.

Keep it simple

You are unlikely to persuade or influence anyone if you cannot state clearly and concisely what your objective is and the rationale for it. Long, convoluted and muddled explanations have no impact and are likely to make the listener feel bored and disinterested.

Take your friends where you find them

You are more likely to impress if you have recruited visible allies. The other side of this coin is avoiding making enemies – as you never know when you might need that person's support in the future.

Know your opponents

It is important to know who is likely to oppose your campaign and to try to understand their position. It is not helpful simply to dismiss opposition as this would rule out any potential future compromise.

Think big but be realistic

It is useful to be ambitious in your ambitions! That way you will still have a good chance of achieving something even if you have to compromise a little along the way towards your objective.

Build coalitions

Allies are always important in any campaign. You can easily supplement your efforts by identifying groups who share your interests and values and with whom you could effectively work in common cause. This could include professional organisations and trade unions.

Work at the local level

Working at the local level makes contact with the principal decision-makers easier so they are more susceptible to influencing and persuading. It also ensures that what is being attempted remains relevant to the local community.

And, always thank the people who help you!

This is common courtesy and might well strengthen opportunities to form alliances.

PRACTICE
SCENARIO 41:
LEE

ACTIVITY 41.3: CRITICAL THINKING

Consider how these steps could be used to support a campaign in the community to raise awareness of and eradicate the practice of forced marriage. Work through each principle in turn and take notes as you go to build up a complete picture of what might make the campaign effective.

MEANS OF INFLUENCING AND PERSUADING

There are a number of approaches to influencing and persuading decision-makers (Kunaviktikul, 2014). One way is to secure the support of others in producing, for example, a petition. This persuades key people that the issue being promoted has the support of a significant numbers of people – who also happen to be voters! Currently, there is a mechanism whereby if 10,000 people sign a petition the government must provide a response while if 100,000 people sign a petition then that will automatically trigger a debate in the House of Commons. This could result in a rapid processing of the matter with a quick response which could include new legislation.

ACTIVITY 41.4: CRITICAL THINKING

Research the events of spring 2016 when attempts were made by lobbyists to have the Meningitis B vaccine extended to all children, not just 3-5-month-old infants. What methods were used in this campaign? Consider how these methods might influence political decision-makers.

The political demonstration has a long history and can be very effective in persuading. However, if the matter which has brought the protest about is emotive it can lead to feelings running very high with the risk of it getting out of hand and spilling over into behaviour which does nothing to advance the cause.

Producing information materials such as the poster Robin saw from the Forced Marriage Unit can be helpful in raising awareness of the issue and potentially recruiting supporters to the cause as well as influencing influential people.

How to improve future health and wellbeing

Engaging with organisations with significant lobbying experience and power such as the Royal College of Nursing or any other union or professional body can be highly effective in making a campaign successful. The important point here is that the activist should work to get the issue onto the agenda of that organisation. Another key alliance which can be very helpful is to work with voluntary sector and charitable groups to increase the impact of the campaign. In the case of forced marriage, groups such as Girls not Brides (www.girlsnotbrides.org) and Plan International UK (www.plan-uk/act-for-girls/because-i-am-a-girl) are very active in this area.

ACTIVITY 41.5: CRITICAL THINKING

Spend some time looking at the websites of Girls not Brides and Plan International UK and access the resources they provide to gain a sense of the strategies these groups are using to further their objectives.

WEBLINK:
GIRLS NOT
BRIDES

WEBLINK:
PLAN-UK

Go to https://study.sagepub.com/essentialchildnursing for advice on being politically aware and professionally proactive during placements.

PLACEMENT
ADVICE 41:
BEING
POLITICALLY
AWARE

CHAPTER SUMMARY

- This chapter has examined some of the perspectives relating to how a children's nurse can work to influence and persuade key decision-makers to improve an issue which has an impact on children's health and wellbeing
- The example of forced child marriage was used as an example of a current and significant topic which is suitable for political influencing and identified some of the main actors in this arena
- All of these taken together will give you indications of how you can take this important issue forward

BUILD YOUR BIBLIOGRAPHY

Books

- Altschuler, J. (2016) *Migration, Illness and Health Care*. London: Palgrave.

  This book examines the impact of acculturation on the health and wellbeing of people recently relocated from their homeland.

- MacBain, S., Dunn, J. and Luke, I. (2017) *Contemporary Childhood*. London: Sage.

  A versatile text examining a range of modern factors in society which have potential impacts on children.

- Nicholson, B. (2016) *Global Health*. London: Sage.

  This book introduces the range of factors affecting health in an age of geographically mobile populations.

Journal articles

Go to https://study.sagepub.com/essentialchildnursing for further free online journal articles related to this chapter.

- Baines, E. (2014) 'Forced marriage as a political project: sexual rules and relations in the Lord's

FURTHER
READING:
ONLINE
JOURNAL
ARTICLES

(Continued)

(Continued)

> Liberation Army'. *Journal of Peace Research*, 51 (3): 405–17.
>
> An investigation in Africa showing clearly how power and dominance can affect women and girls.

- Chantler, K. (2012) 'Recognition of and intervention in forced marriage as a form of violence and abuse'. *Trauma, Violence and Abuse*, 13 (3): 176–83.

  An analysis of UK-based research studies on forced marriage.

- Bergan, D.E. (2009) 'Does grassroots lobbying work? A field experiment measuring the effects of an e-mail lobbying campaign on legislative behaviour'. *American Politics Research*, 37 (2): 327–52.

  A study and analysis of the impact of an email campaign on the voting intentions of law makers.

FURTHER
READING:
WEBLINKS

Weblinks

Go to https://study.sagepub.com/essentialchildnursing for further weblinks related to this chapter.

- Girls Not Brides, *No to Child Marriage, Yes to Education for Girls in India*

  www.girlsnotbrides.org/video-no-to-child-marriage-yes-to-education-for-girls-in-India

  A video illustrating the importance for girls to be given improved life chances through education by eliminating forced child marriage.

- Girls Not Brides, '*Waylowaylo! Changing Attitudes on Girls' Education to Delay Marriage in Senegal*

  www.girlsnotbrides.org/waylowaylo-girls-education-marriage-senegal

  This video explores the range of harmful effects of forced child marriage and the benefits of eliminating this custom.

- ForwardUK, *See, Hear, Speak*

  www.youtube.com/watch?v=J8T3edt1R8A

  A flash mob on female genital mutilation (FGM) and forced marriage. This footage shows a contemporary means to highlight a societal problem, raise awareness and engage supporters in the campaign to end these practices.

ONLINE
QUIZZES &
ACTIVITY
ANSWERS

—— ACE YOUR ASSESSMENT ——

Revise what you have learned by visiting https://study.sagepub.com/essentialchildnursing

- Test yourself with multiple-choice and short-answer questions
- Do the chapter activities in the book and check your answers online

REFERENCES

Anitha, S. and Gill, A. (2009) 'Coercion, consent and the forced marriage debate in the UK'. *Feminist Legal Studies*, 17: 165–84.

CEWC Cymru (2012) *What Rights? Summary of the United Nations Convention on the Rights of the Child.* Cardiff: CEWC Cymru.

City of Portland (2011) *Ten Principles of Lobbying*. Available at: www.portlandoregon.gov/oni/article/338655 (last accessed 3 June 2016).

Gangoli, G., McCarry, M. and Razak, A. (2008) 'Child marriage or forced marriage? South Asian communities in North East England'. *Children & Society*, 23: 418–29.

Hart, C. (2004) *Nurses and Politics: The Impact of Power and Practice*. Basingstoke: Palgrave Macmillan.

HM Government (2014a) *The Right to Choose: Multi-agency Statutory Guidance for Dealing with Forced Marriage*. London: Cabinet Office.

HM Government (2014b) *Multi-agency Practice Guidelines: Handling Cases of Forced Marriage*. London: Cabinet Office.

Home Office (2017) *Forced Marriage Unit Statistics 2016*. London: Home Office. Available at: www.gov.uk/government/statistics/forced-marriage-unit-statistics-2016 (last accessed 29 June 2017).

Kunaviktikul, W. (2014) 'Moving towards the greater involvement of nurses in policy development'. *International Nursing Review*, 64 (1): 1–2.

McKenna, H. (2010) 'Nurses and politics: laurels for the hardy'. *International Journal of Nursing*, 47 (4): 397–8.

NMC (2015) *The Code: Professional Standards of Practice and Behaviour for Nurses and Midwives*. London: Nursing and Midwifery Council.

Phillips, A. and Dustin, M. (2004) 'UK initiatives of forced marriage: regulation, dialogue and exit'. *Political Studies*, 52: 531–51.

Porter-O'Grady, T. and Malloch, K. (2013) *Leadership in Nursing Practice: Changing the Landscape of Healthcare*. Burlington, MA: Jones & Bartlett.

The Scottish Government (2011) *Forced Marriage: Statutory Guidance*. Edinburgh: The Scottish Government.

UK All-Party Parliamentary Group on Population, Development and Reproductive Health, (2012) *A Childhood Lost: A Report on Child Marriage in the UK and the Developing World*. London: UK All-Party Parliamentary Group on Population, Development and Reproductive Health.

United Nations (1989) *United Nations Convention on the Rights of the Child*. Geneva: United Nations.

INDEX

1001 Critical Days, The 170

ABCDE approach
  emergency department 234–5
  fever 228–9
  health promotion 525
  respiratory assessment 272
  seizures 234
abdominal assessment 483
abdominal pain 439–41
abdominal ultrasound scans 447
abdominal X-rays 446
ABO blood group 391, *392*
abuse 141
  domestic 141
  emotional 135
  fractures 135
  physical 135
  sexual 135
abusive head trauma (AHT) 310
accidents *see* unintentional injury
accountability 125
  children and young people 618
  employers 618
  professional 617
  society 618
  spheres of 617
acidosis 263, 334
acne 57, 404–5
acquired brain injury (ABI) 310
  long-term outcome 311–12
  non-traumatic brain injury 311
  traumatic brain injury (TBI) 310–11
acquired immunity 352
activities of daily living (ADLs)
  activities
    breathing 83, 419
    communication 83, 419
    controlling temperature 83, 420
    death and dying 83, 421
    eating and drinking 83, 419
    elimination 83, 420
    expressing sexuality 83, 421
    maintaining a safe environment
      83, 419
    mobilisation 420
    sleeping 83, 421
    washing and dressing 83, 420
    working and playing 83, 421
acute epiglottis 279
acute kidney injury (AKI) 482
acute lymphoblastic leukaemia (ALL) 513
acute myeloid leukaemia (AML) 513
acute needs
  ABCDE approach
    emergency department 234–5
    fever 228–9
    seizures 234
  assessment of 226
  dehydration 230–2
  diarrhoea 231
    intravenous fluids 232, 233
    oral rehydration salt (ORS) 233
    stool specimens 232
  fever
    antipyretic interventions 229
    assessment of 227–8
    measurement of 228
    pharmacological interventions 230
    physical interventions 229
    serious illness, risk of 229
  gastrointestinal disturbance 230
  seizures 233–5
  sepsis 235–6
    Paediatric Sepsis 6 procedures 237
    Red Flag Sepsis 236–7
    urgent intervention 237–8
  unintentional injury 238
    falls 240
    first aid 241
    fractures 240–1
    head injuries 242
    prevention 239–40
    risk 238–40
  vomiting 231
    intravenous fluids 232, 233
    oral rehydration salt (ORS) 233
    stool specimens 232
acute pain 37
acute renal failure 325

acyanotic heart problems 500–1
adapted rules of nines 411
Adelaide Scale 307
adhesions 443
adolescence 57, 185
  diabetes and 338
adrenal insufficiency 332
adult hospices 535
adult learning 607–8
adulthood 7
advanced care planning (ACP) 533, 534
  individualised symptom care plans 534, 535
adverse childhood events (ACEs) 166
aerosol spray injuries 410
agency, concept of 7
Ages and Stages Questionnaire (ASQ) 215
agitation 548
AIDS (acquired immune deficiency syndrome) 356
air trapping 273
alarms, patient 478–9
albumin 394
allergic reactions 521
allergy tests *280*
allodynia 375
alopecia 521
ambiguous genitalia 320
ambulatory assessment units (AAU) 92
Ammentorp et al. 25
amoxicillin 59
amplified musculoskeletal pain syndrome (AMPS)
      366, 375
anaemia 388, 522
anaesthesia 258, 263, 264
analgesia 42–3
anaphylaxis 353
andragogy model 607–8
angiotensin-converting enzyme
      (ACE) inhibitors 297
anorectal anomaly 443
anti-epilepsy drugs (AEDs) 312
Anti-Social Behaviour, Crime and Policing Act
      (2014) 629
antibiotics 277, 297
  azithromycin 278
antibodies 351, 353
  see also immunoglobulins
anticoagulants 297
antigens 353
antipyretic interventions 229
antisocial behaviours 584
anxiety disorders 578–9
aplastic anaemia 388
apnoea 273, 479
appendicitis 440
appetite 566
arranged marriage 629
arrhythmias 291–3, 434
arterial blood pressure (ABP) monitoring 478
arterial lines 478

ASD (autistic spectrum disorder) 24, 565, 583–4
Asperger, Hans 583
Asperger's Syndrome 583
assessment 84–5
  of abdominal problems 483
  of acute needs 226
  on admission 85
  baseline observation and recording of data 85
  circulatory/cardiovascular (CVS) 481–2
  community nursing 103, 104–5
  discharge planning 457–61
  end-of-life care 541–4
  of fever 227–8
  of growth 339–41
  of head injuries 242
  identifying deteriorating health 85
  importance of 84
  of mental health problems 582–3
  of neurological problems 482–3
  of patients 86–7
  of pupils (eyes) 483
  of respiratory problems 271–4
  of risk 87
  on shift handover 85
  tools 86–7
    behavioural pain assessment 38
    PEWS 87, 262, 265, 274, 324
    SBAR 87, 236, 262, 265, 324
    for thermal injuries 411–12, 414
  top-to-toe/front-to-back 483–4
  Type 1 diabetes 338–9
  see also Common Assessment Framework
      (CAF); Early Help Assessments (EHAs) pain
      assessment and management
Assessment Framework 197, 200, 202
associative play 28
asthma 44, 275–6
asynchrony 480
atopic eczema 399, 406
  diagnosing 399–400
  treating 400–2
attachment theory 175, 187, 201
attention 22
attention deficit hyperactivity disorder
      (ADHD) 584
Audit Commission 238, 240
auscultation 273, 480
authentic leadership 593
autism 564–5
  aetiology 584
  autism spectrum disorder (ASD) 24, 565, 583–4
  management/treatment 584
  mental health problems 583–4
autoimmune conditions 444
autonomous learning 607–8
autonomy 111, 161
autosomal dominant patterns 158, 159
autosomal recessive patterns 159, *159*
azithromycin 278

baby bonds 172–3
Baby-Friendly Hospital Initiative (BFHI) 198
bacteria 351, 405
bacterial endocarditis 290
bacterial meningitis 227
bad news, breaking 29–31
balanced processing 595
barium enema 447
Barnardo's 205
baseline bloods 262, 265
baseline observations 262, 265
Beauchamp, T.L. and Childress, J.F. 160
behavioural pain assessment tools 38
behaviour(s)
    antisocial 584
    challenging behavior 567–8
    indicators of pain 38–9
    of nurses 486
    types of 22
beneficence 160
bereavement 540
beta blockers 297
bilateral lung disease 481
biological response modifiers 523
biopsies 447, 516
blackheads 405
bladder extrophy 320
blastomas 515
BLISS 495
blood
    beliefs about 387
    bleeding disorders 387, 388–9, 390–1
    composition of 387
    transfusions
        compatibility 392
        consent 393
        haemolytic reactions 393
        hypersensitivity reactions 394
        observations 393
        platelets 393
        potential changes in blood groups 392
        red blood cells 393
blood clots 263
blood cultures 280
blood disorders 387, 388–9, 390–1
blood gas tests 446
blood glucose 334, 335, 336
    hypoglycaemia 335, 337
blood groups
    ABO 391, 392
    potential changes in 392
    Rh 392
blood pressure 39, 263, 324
    raised 304
    vital sign observation 294
blood tests 342
body image 57, 319, 322, 324
Bolam test 125, 126
bone marrow tests 516

bone marrow transplantations 355
bone scans 516
bowel obstruction 277, 441
Bowlby, J. 5
bradycardia 304
    see also sinus bradycardia
bradypnoea 273, 479
brain injuries 310–12
brain tumours 314, 513
breaking bad news 29–31
breast milk 198, 352, 449, 496,
    497, 508
breastfeeding 169, 176, 198, 215, 229, 231, 431,
    444, 445, 501, 508
breathing see respiratory system/problems
breathing rates 39
British National Formulary for Children (BNFC)
    61, 403
Broca's area 307
bronchiolitis 274–5, 622
    red flags 274–5
bronchitis 479
bronchoscopy 280
bruising 389, 390
Burkholderia cepacia 277
Burn Care Review 410
burn injuries 410
    see also thermal injuries

C-reactive protein (CRP) tests 446
calcinuerin inhibitors 403
Caldicott Review (1997) 96
CAMHS Professionals 582
cancer see childhood cancer
cancer treatment, endocrine effects of 333
capillary refill 294
car safety 112
carcinoma 515
cardiac arrhythmias 434
cardiac catheterisation 287, 288
cardiac output (CO) 481–2
cardiomyopathy 290–1, 522
cardiopulmonary bypass 287
cardiovascular problems 286
    acquired heart disease
        cardiomyopathy 290–1, 522
        infective endocarditis 290
        Kawasaki disease 228, 291
        rheumatic heart disease 291
    affecting oxygenation 502
    arrhythmias 291–2, 434
        heart block 293
        long QT syndrome 293
        sinus bradycardia 292
        sinus rhythm 292
        sinus tachycardia 292
        supraventricular tachycardia (SVT) 292
    congenital heart disease (CHD) 286–9
        coarctation of the aorta 287

complexity of defects 286–7
  tetralogy of fallots (TOF) 288
  transposition of the great arteries
    (TGA) 288
  ventricular septal defect (VSD) 287
heart, significance of 286
nursing considerations 293
  child safety 294–5
  common diagnostic tests 296
  discharge planning 295
  general 294
  interprofessional team 297
  medication 297
  mobilisation 295, 296
  nutrition and fluid 295
  positioning 295
  post-surgery care 296
  vital sign observation 294
preterm infants 496
care
  care decisions
    children and young people's involvement in 4,
      6, 7–9, 14
    children's nurses 4
    family involvement in 4, 6, 9–13, 14
    future directions 15
    key skills required 13–14
    levels of involvement 11
    social and political contexts 4–6
  hierarchy of care 11
  holistic approaches to 195
  in non-hospital settings 102–15
Care Act (2014) 74, 75
Care Bundle initiative 569
care by parents units 11–12
care cordinators in IPW 72
care in the community
  cardiovascular problems 295
  gastrointestinal problems 452–3
  respiratory problems 282
  seizures 234
care integration 72–4
  in England 73
  in Northern Ireland 73
  in Scotland 73
  in Wales 73
care needs
  child protection plans 90
  Common Assessment Framework (CAF) 89
  Early Help Assessments (EHAs) 89–90, 93
  identifying and planning 87–90
  integrated care pathways (ICPs) 89
  problems and goals 87, 88–9
  risk assessment 87
care plans
  community nursing 103–4
  in community settings 90–1
  delegation of 90
  delivery of 90

  implementing and evaluating 90–4
  reassessment 91
  recording and documenting 91
  referrals 91–4
Care Quality Commission (CQC) 74
  From the Pond to the Sea report 70
carers 6, 62, 105, 251, 415, 452, 457
  decision-making 189
  IPW and 74
  legal rights in decision-making 71, 72
  listening to concerns of 226
case-based learning 608–9
catheters 326
CD4 cell counts 356
CD4 glycoproteins 356
cell cycles 519
central venous access devices (CVADs) 451
central venous pressure (CVP) monitoring 478, 482
cerebral palsy 314, 562–3
cerebral spinal fluid (CSF) 302, 309
  shunt devices 309
cerebral vascular abnormalities 314
challenging behaviour 567–8
Charter for Children in Hospital (ASC, 1991) 5
chemical thermal injuries 410
chemotherapy 519–20
  safety working with 522
  side effects of 520–2
chest X-rays 280, 516
Child Accident Prevention Trust 240
Child and Family-centred Healthcare
  (Smith and Coleman) 84
child-centred care 84, 485–7
child development 21, 170–1
  community resources, access to 205
  family functioning 202–3
  health 197–200
  housing 203–4
  income and employment 204–5
    poverty 204–5
  key stages of 183–5
  Piaget's theory of 196
  promoting effective parenting
    programmes 200–1
  resilience 200, 202
  social integration 205
  wider family 203
  see also health
Child Exploitation and Online
  Protection Centre (CEOP) 139
child forced marriage 627–8
  girls 629
child-parent psychotherapy 173
Child Poverty Action Group 204
child protection 111, 128, 134
  definition 134
  see also safeguarding
child protection plans 90
Child Psychotherapy Trust 170

child sexual exploitation (CSE) 32, 92, 94, 139–40
Child Transitional Communication Model 26–7
childhood 7, 184–5
childhood cancer 513
  brain tumours 513
  diagnostic investigations 516
  haematological malignancies 513
  haematopoietic stem cell transplant 523
  home care 524
  immunotherapy 523
  incidents of types of 514
  leukaemia 513, 514, 516
  long-term survival 513
  presentation 514–17
    diagnostic tests 514–15
  psychosocial impact of 517–19
    social support 518–19
  radiotherapy 523
  sarcomas 515
  solid tumours 513
  surgery 523
  symptoms 515
  team working 524–6
    role of children's nurses 525–6
  treatment 519
    chemotherapy 519–22
  tumours 513, 514, 516
childhood disease 5–6, 188
childhood immunisations 353
Children Act (1989) 106, 134, 189, 211, 619, 629
Children Act (2004) 629
Children and Families Act (2014) 559, 560
Children and Young People (Scotland) Act (2014) 72, 73
Children and Young People's Mental Health Taskforce (DH) 174
Children's Cancer and Leukaemia Group (CCLG) treatment centres 513, 520
Children's Cancer Measures 513
children's cardiac nurse specialists 297
children's centres 171
children's community care
  context of 102–3
  health promotion and education 112–13
  information sharing 110–11
  multiagency activity and partnerships 106–8
  pathways 103
  school nursing 113–15
  supervision 111
  visiting and personal safety 111–12
  see also Common Assessment Framework (CAF); community children's nurses (CCNs); community nursing
children's hospices 531–3
Children's National Service Framework 578
children's nurses
  as advocates for children and young people 9, 57, 61
  agency, concept of 7

breaking bad news 29–31
care and care decisions 4
changing role of 4–5, 6
childhood cancer care 525–6
children at play, observing 27–9
children's mental health problems 582
communication with children and young people 21, 24, 26
communication with children with ASD 24
dilemmas 8
family-centred care 13
interpreting clinical information 86–7
mastering complex skills 121
negligence in medication administration 61
numerical ability 61
as preventative health champions 94
record keeping 96
relationships with parents 25
responses to infants' crying 23
skills 86–7
  communication 86
  observational 86
  understanding of human physiology 86
supervision and support for 190
surgical nursing care 261–3
  anaesthesia 263
  children's play 261
  consent 263
  fasting 263
  negotiating with children/families 262
  preparation for theatre 262
  promoting recovery in postoperative period 265–7
toddlers and 23
working with parents 11
wound healing, understanding 266
see also community children's nurses (CCNs); CPD (continuing professional development); decision-making; leadership
children's rights 402, 557
  forced marriage 630
  see also United Nations Convention on the Rights of the Child (UNCRC)
Children's Society 187
CHIVA statement 357
Choosing Health (DH, 2004) 112
chromosomes 154
chronic pain 37
chronic renal failure (CRF) 326
circadian rhythms 505
circle of security 172
circulation 481–2
circulatory/cardiovascular (CVS) assessment 481–2
City of Portland, Oregon 631
clavicle, fractured 500
Climbié, Victoria 70, 406
clinical decision-making model supervision 623
clinical dehydration 431

clinical depression 580–1, 582–3
Clinical Negligence Schemes for Trusts (CNST) 82
clinical shock 431
clitoridectomy 142
close head injuries 310
closed-loop communication 457–8
clotting factor deficiencies 390
club foot 366, 372–4
coagulation 391
codeine 46
coeliac antibodies 447
coeliac disease 444
cognitive behaviour therapy 584, 585
colostomy 451
Common Assessment Framework (CAF) 72, 90,
       108–11
  consent 109
  core features of 109–10
  information sharing 110–11
  multiagency meetings 110
  purpose of 109, 110
  team around the child 109, 110
communicating hydrocephalus 309
communication
  breaking bad news 29–31
  with children and young people 184
  children with learning disabilities 568–9
  closed-loop 457–8
  development of skills 15
  developmental aspects of 21–4
    developmentally appropriate communication
       23–4
    in infancy 21–2
    intentional communication 22
    linguistic communication 22–3
    symbolic communication 22
  discharge planning 457–8, 459
  effective 14, 20–33
  family-centred care and 24–7
  formal and informal 21
  hospital transfers 465–6
  lack of 4
  life-limiting illnesses 534
  play and 23, 27–9
  skills of nurses 86
  technology and social media 31–2
  verbal and non-verbal language 21, 31
  visible-ness in 26–7
  written 461
community care 102
  evolution of 102
  see also children's community care
community children's nurses (CCNs) 107
  empowering children and families 105
  future of 103
  information sharing 110
  lone worker policy 112
  record keeping 128
  relationship with families 110
  responsibilities of 102
  role of 103, 111
  teams 102
  visiting and personal safety 111–12
community mental health nurses (CMHNs) 108
community nursing
  assessment 103, 104–5
  evaluation 104, 106
  intervention 104, 105
  planning 103–4, 105
  working together 106–8
community paediatricians 108
comodenes 405
compensation 273
competence 619
complement system 352
compliance in medication 56
concordance with medication 56–7
conduct disorder (CD) 584
  aetiology 584–5
    management/treatment 585
confidentiality 129
  health information 190
  MASH activity 138
  using social media 605
conflict 202
congenital adrenal hyperplasia 332
congenital diaphragmatic hernia (CDH) 499
congenital heart disease (CHD) 286–9
congenital hyperinsulinism 331
congenital hypothyroidism 332, 344–5
congenital talipes equinovarus (CTEV)
       366, 372–3
  treatment 373–4
consciousness 306
consent 109, 110, 125
  blood transfusions 393
  marriage and 628
  surgical procedures 263
  theatre preparation 262
constipation 104–6, 439–40, 548
constructionist approach to learning 608–9
containment 48
continuing professional development (CPD) see
       CPD (continuing professional development)
controlled drugs (CDs) 59–60
  administration to children and
       young people 60
  stock levels 60
  storage of 60
convulsions 233
cooperative play 28
coping styles 187–8
Cork et al. 399
corticosteroids 403
cow's milk protein allergy (CMPA) 445
CPD (continuing professional development) 111
  case studies 606–7
  definition 603

evidence of 603
funding for 604
mentoring 603–4
purpose of 604
simulated learning 605
social media sites 605
socio-political drivers for 604–5
theories of learning
  case-based learning 608–9
  constructionist/experiential
    approach 608–9
  Knowles' andragogy model 607–8
  preferences in learning styles 610–11
  theory and practice 611–13
crackles/crepitations 273
cradle cap 404
cranial nerves 308
cranial ultrasound 305
creon (enzyme capsules) 277
Crime and Disorder Act (1998) 141
Crohn's disease 444
croup 279
crushing injuries 311
crying 22, 23
CT scans 304–5, 516
cue interpretation 622
cue recognition 622
Cushing's syndrome 332
Cushing's triad 303, 304
cyanosis 273, 479
cyberbullying 31, 32
cyclooxygenase (COX) 43
cystic fibrosis (CF) 188, 276–9
  treatment for 277
cytokines 351
cytotoxic chemotherapy 519, 520, 522

DDH (developmental dysplasia of the hip)
    see developmental dysplasia of the hip (DDH)
debridement 417
decision-making
  accountability
    to children and young people 618
    to employers 618
    professional 617
    to society 618
    spheres of 617
  carers 189
  in clinical practice 617–18
  decision-makers 618
    children and young people 619
    health professionals 620
    judicial review 620–1
    parents 619–20
  end-of-life care 541–3, 549
  legal rights of parents/carers 71, 72
  models
    clinical decision-making model 623
    information-processing model 622

intuitive-humanistic model 622
  needs of children 188–9
  shared 15
Declaration of Montréal (IASP, 2015) 37
decompensation 273
dehydration 230–2, 334, 426, 429–30,
    432, 435, 482
  clinical 431
delirium 548
dentritic cells 352
Denver Developmental Screening Test 215
depression 580–1
dermal burn depth 414
dermatological problems 398
  acne 404–5
  affects of immature skin 503
  atopic eczema 399, 406
    diagnosing 399–400
    treating 400–2
  dermatitis 399
  discoid eczema 403–4
  eczema herpeticum 404
  history taking and skin assessment 405–6
    food allergies 406
  physiology of the skin 398–9
  preterm infants 497
  seborrhoeic eczema 404
dermatophytes 405
dermis 398
Derriford Hospital 569
developmental dysplasia of the hip (DDH) 365
  diagnosis 370
  hip spica care 370
  risk factors 367
  surgery 370
  treatment 367–9
    Pavlik harness 367, 368, 369–70
diabetes insipidus 333
diabetes mellitus 154–5, 325
  CF-related 277
  Type 1 diabetes 331, 334–7, 338–9
    symptoms 334–5
  Type 2 334
diabetic ketoacidosis (DKA) 334,
    335, 429
Diagnostic and Statistical Manual of
    Mental Disorders (APA, 2013) 579
diagnostic tests 280, 296
dialysis 326–7
diaphragmatic hernia 259
diarrhoea 231
  dehydration 429, 432
  gastroenteritis 429, 430
  haemolytic uraemic syndrome (HUS) 322
  hypokalaemia 434
  intravenous fluids 232, 233
  milk and 233
  non-specific toddler 233
  oral rehydration salt (ORS) 233

prolonged 233
side effect of chemotherapy 521
stool specimens 232
dieticians 297
digestive problems
impact on other systems 502
preterm infants 496
dimercaptosuccinic acid (DMSAs) scans 321
directing attention 22
directive therapeutic play 28
disability 482–3
discharge planning 457
assessment 457
communication and knowledge sharing 457–8, 461
family-centred care and partnership working 459–60
processes to aid communication and knowledge sharing 459
cardiovascular problems 295
care-pathway-led discharge 467
complex discharge 462–7
processes and systems 466–7
criteria-led discharge 467
gastrointestinal problems 452–3
neonates 509
nurse-led discharge 467
record keeping 459
respiratory problems 282
simple discharge 460–1
written communication 461
transfers 464
from children's services to adult services 464–5
from hospitals in other countries 465–6
transition 464–5
discoid eczema 403–4
topical corticosteroids 403
disseminated intravascular coagulation (DIC) 391, 484, 503, 504
distraction therapy 28, 47
diuretics 297
DNA (deoxyribonucleic acid) 154
epigenetic alterations 154–5
gene therapy 158
DNAR (do not attempt resuscitation) orders 534–5
documentation 262, 265
domestic abuse 141
domestic violence 202
DOPES 480
Down's syndrome 339, 344, 444, 557, 559, 562, 563–4
Down's Syndrome Association (DSA) 564
drain care 296
dressings, wound 417
Driscoll's model of reflection *610–11*
drugs administration *see* medication administration
dry heat thermal injuries 410

duodenal atresia 259
duty of candour 123
duty of care 123, 129
dyads, communication 15, 24, 26
dying process 540, 541
dysphagia 565
dyspnoea 273, 547

e-health 95, 189
early childhood 167–8
Early Help *see* Common Assessment Framework (CAF)
Early Help Assessments (EHAs) 89–90, 93
early warning tools 87
early years interventions 138, 166, 167, 169, 170–1, 171–4
East Cheshire NHS Trust 61
ECG (electrocardiography) monitoring 477, 478
ecological systems theory 175
eczema 397, 398
see also atopic eczema; discoid eczema
eczema herpeticum 404
education *see* CPD (continuing professional development)
Education, Health and Care (EHCs) plans 560, *561*
effective communication *see* communication
electrical thermal injuries 410
electrolyte imbalance *see* fluid and electrolyte imbalance
electrolytes 428
embryonal tumours 515
emergency care plans (ECPs) 535
emergency surgery 258
emollients 400–1, 403
emotion-focused coping 544
emotional abuse 135
emotional warmth 199–200
emotional wellbeing 166–8, 267
employment 205
empowerment 105
end-of-life care 488, 533
assessment and planning 541
decision-making 541–3
other family members 544
parental coping 543–4
definition 540
end-of-life signs 540–1
ethical issues 549–50
good death, concept of 541
interdisciplinary approach 550, *551*
self-care for professionals 550–2
symptom management 544–5
challenges 545
other symptoms 547–8
Paediatric Pain Profile 546
pain 545–7
plan of care 547
End of Life Care Strategy (DH) 534
end-tidal CO2 (EtCO2) monitoring 477

endocrine problems
  conditions 331–3
  congenital hypothyroidism 344–5
    newborn screening 344–5
  major endocrine organs 333
  short stature 339
    causes of 341–3
    growth assessment 339–41
    growth hormone 342, 343
    growth hormone deficiency 342
  Type 1 diabetes 334–7
    hypoglycaemia 335, 337
    interference with normal adolescence 338
    knowledge and psychosocial aspects 339
    long-term management 337–9
    regular assessments 338–9
endocrinology 331
endoscopies 447
endotracheal tubes (ETTs) 480
enteral feeding 449, 565–6
  types of 449
enuresis 324–5
epidermal burn depth 414
epidermis 398, 399, 400, 414
epidural pain relief 267
epigenetics 152, 167
  alterations in DNA 154–5
  concept of 154
epilepsy 312–13
  children with learning disabilities 567
  seizures 233, 234–5, 312, 313
  terminology 312–13
epilepsy syndrome 312
epispadias 320
ethical leadership 593
Eurochild 171
Every Child Matters 106
evidence summaries (ESUOMs) 56
Ewing's sarcoma 515, 550
excision 142
excretory problems, preterm infants 497
exomphalos (omphalocele) 442
experiential approach to learning 608–9
expertise, sharing 70–1
expiration 272
exploitation 143
exposure 483–4
  abdominal assessment 483
  disseminated intravascular
      coagulation (DIC) 484
  hygiene assessment 483
  limbs assessment 484
  tissue oedema 483–4
Extra Corporeal Life Support (ECLS) 482
eye opening tests 307

faces pain scales 40, 41
facilitated tucking 48
falls 240

families
  involvement in care and care decisions
      4, 6, 9–13
  promoting child development 202–3
  wider family 203
family-centred care (FCC) 10, 11, 12–13, 507
  communication and 24–7
  discharge planning 459–60
  as nursing model 84
  PCC children 485–7
  perioperative care 261–2
Family Centred Care (Smith and Coleman) 84
Family Health Needs Assessment (FHNA) 212,
    214–15
Family Law Act (1996) 629
Family Nurse Partnership (FNP) 172, 174–8
  evidence for 175
  results 175
Family Nurse Partnership National Unit 174–5
family nurses (FNs) 175, 176
family pedigree 155–7
  drawing with symbols 155–6
fasting 263
fat-soluble vitamin supplementation 277
fathers 170
fatigue 521, 548
febrile convulsion 312
female genital mutilation (FGM) 141–2, 629
fever 227–30
filaggrin 399
first aid 241
fit for practice 130
Five Year Forward View for Mental Health (Mental
    Health Taskforce to the NHS in England, 2016)
    73, 578, 604
FLACC (Face, Legs, Activity, Cry, Consolability)
    scale 40, 41
fluid 440
fluid and electrolyte imbalance 427
  dehydration 426, 429–30, 435
  gastroenteritis 430
    fluid prescription charts 431
    intravenous therapy 431–2
    treatment and management 430–1
  homoeostasis 427
    electrolytes 428
    fluid balance 427
    normal electrolyte values 428–9
    normal fluid requirements 427–8
  potassium imbalance 433–5
  sodium imbalance 433, 434
fluid prescription charts 431
fluid therapy/balance 262, 265, 295
Flying Start programmes 213
foetal alcohol spectrum disorder (fasd) 563
following attention 22
food allergies 406
forced marriage 628–9
  policy and law 629

political activity and lobbying 630–2
rights context of children 630
voluntary and charitable sector 629
see also child forced marriage
Forced Marriage (Civil Protection) Act (2007) 629
Forced Marriage Protection Order 629
Forced Marriage Unit 628, 629
foundation years, importance of 120
fractures 240–1, 380–2
    first aid 241
    treatment of 241
fragmentation 371
Francis Report (2013) 70, 123
Freedom of Information Act (2000) 96
Freud, Sigmund 165
friction rub 273
frostbite 410
fuel poverty 205
full blood count (FBC) 280, 324, 446, 516
full thickness burn depth 414
functional/idiopathic constipation 440

gastric irritation 44
gastric sphincters 443–4
gastritis 441
gastro-oesophageal reflux disease (Gord) 444
gastroenteritis 233, 430–2, 440
gastrointestinal disturbance 230
gastrointestinal problems 439
    autoimmune disorders
        coeliac disease 444
        Crohn's disease 444
        ulcerative colitis 444
    care in the community 452–3
    common conditions
        abdominal pain 439–41, 441–2
        appendicitis 440
        constipation 439–40
        gastritis/peptic ulcer 441
        gastroenteritis 440
        intussusception 441
        peritonitis 440
    congenital abnormalities
        adhesions 443
        anorectal anomaly 443
        exomphalos (omphalocele) 442
        gastroschisis 442
        Hirschsprung's disease 443
        malrotation 443
        oesophageal atresia (OA) 442–3
        tracheo-oesophageal fistula 442–3
        volvulus 443
    cow's milk protein allergy (CMPA) 445
    discharge planning 452–3
    gastric sphincters
        gastro-oesophageal reflux disease
            (Gord) 444
        pyloric stenosis 443
    lactose intolerance 445

liver problems 445–6
necrotising enterocolitis (NEC) 444–5, 508
nursing management of 446–7
    diagnostic tests 446–7
nutrition 447–51
    enteral feeding 449, 565–6
    malnutrition 447
    parenteral nutrition (PN) 449, 451
parasite/worm infection 445
stoma management 451–2
gastroschisis 259, 442
gastrostomy-jejunostomy tube 449
gene therapy 158, 355
general practitioners (GPs) 108
genetic counselling 152, 160
genetics 152–3
    concept of 154
    family pedigree 155–7
    growth and 339
    nurses' use of genetic information 152
    risk 158–60
    testing 160, 161
genomics 152
    concept of 154
    ethical and legal implications 160–1
    Human Genome Project (HGP) 153–4
genotypes 154
genu valgum (knock knees) 363, 366
genu varum (bow legs) 363, 366
germ cell tumours (GCT) 515
germ cells 158
Getting It Right for Children, Young People and
    Families (DH, 2012) 114
Getting it Right for Every Child (GIRFEC) approach
    72, 73, 75
Giardia lamblia 445
Gillick competent 125
Giretzlehner et al. 413
Girls not Brides 633
Glasgow Coma Scale (GCS) 306
    modified forms 307
gliomas 513
Global Clubfoot Initiative 374
glomerulonephritis 322
glucose 334, 335
glucose-6-phosphate dehydrogenase (G6PD) 389
glucose monitoring 277
gluten 444
good death, concept of 541
good parenting 200
Graves' disease 332
Great Ormond Street Hospital 569
grief 540
growing long bone *381*
growth
    in childhood 340
    in infancy 340
    in puberty 340
growth hormone 342, 343

deficiency 332, 342
   insufficiency 332
grunting 273
guided imagery 47
Guillain-Barré syndrome 394
Guthrie test *344*

haemaglobinopathies 388
haematological problems *see* blood;
   blood disorders
haematopoietic stem cell transplant 523
haematopoietic stem cells 387
haemodialysis 326–7
haemolytic anaemia 389
haemolytic uraemic syndrome (HUS) 322–3
haemophilia 390, 391
haemorrhagic cystitis 521
Hall Report 212
harm 134
head bobbing 273
head injuries 242
   assessment and treatment of 242
health
   changes, coping with 188
   children's concept of 195–6
   and children's wellbeing 5
   concept of 187
   definition 195
   parenting capacity 197–201
      basic care and nutrition 198–9
      social interaction and emotional warmth
         199–200
   and social care
      health predictors 92
      integration of services 72–4, 92
   see also child development; illness
Health and Social Care Act (2012) 92, 94
Health Education England 605
*Health Inequalities and the Social Determinants of
   Health* (RCN, 2012) 195
health information and education 189–90
   e-health 189
   lifestyle choices 189
   privacy and confidentiality 190
   written information 189
health professionals 6, 620
   children's views of 7
   collaboration with parents 12, 13–14, 15
   ethical issues of genetics 160–1
   guidelines for 37
   listening to children and young people 9
health promotion 253
   ABCDE approach 525
   behaviours 196
   and education 112–13, 185
   immunisation 353–4
   neonatal care 508
Health Protection (Notification)
   Regulations (2010) 431

health services
   children as users of 5
   historic access to 92
health visitors (HVs) 108, 211–12, 559
   12-month review 215–16
      aims of 215–16
      competencies of practitioners 216
   flexibility of 217
   health visiting model
      4-level service model 214, 215
      high-impact areas 214, 215
      mandated visits 214, 215
   needs assessments 214
   response to 'Hall 4' 212–13
Healthcare Commission (2007) 37
Healthcare Leadership Model (NHS Leadership
   Academy, 2013) 596–8
   self-assessment tool 598
Healthcare Quality Improvement Partnership
   (HQIP) 569
Healthy Child, Healthy Future Programme 213
Healthy Child Programme 170–1, 175, 212,
   213, 559
   Family Health Needs Assessment (FHNA) 212,
      214–15
Healthy Child Wales Programme 213
Healthy Lives, Brighter Futures (DH and
   DCSF, 2009) 103
Healthy Lives, Healthy People (DH) 114
heart block 293
heart disease *see* cardiovascular problems
heart rates 39
heat transference sources 410
height velocity 340
Henoch Schönlein purpura (HSP) 323
hepatoblastoma 515
herd immunity 353
hereditary spherocytosis 388
herpes simplex encephalitis 227
herpes simplex virus HV1 404
Heslop et al. 68
high calorie diet 277
highly active antiretroviral treatment
   (HAART) 356
hip dysplasia *see* developmental dysplasia
   of the hip (DDH)
hip spica casts 370
Hirschsprung's disease 260, 443
histones 154
HIV (human immunodeficiency virus) 356–8
   stigma 357
   young people's voices 357
Hodgkin's disease 515
holistic care 71, 195
   PCC children 485–7
home visits 111–12
homoeostasis 427–9
hormones 331
   growth hormone (GH) 339

hospices
  adult 535
  children's 531–3
hospitals
  children attending 5, 10
  children's experiences in 9, 10, 249–51
    dislocation 251
    fright 251
    isolation 250–1
    separation anxiety 250
  early 5
  information about surgical conditions 258
  play in 28, 252
  preparation for 258
    pre-admission programmes 258
  safety and comfort 252
    context and timing 252
    information sharing 252, 253
    whole-family education 253
housing 203–4
HR and rhythm assessment 481–2
Human Genome Project (HGP) 153–4
human trafficking 142–4
hydrocephalus 260, 305, 308–9
hydronephrosis 320
hyperalgesia 375
hyperglycaemia 334, 498
hyperkalaemia 433–4
hypernatraemia 433, 434
hypernatraemic dehydration 231
hypernoea 273
hyperosmolality 334
hypnosis 47
hypo-pigmentation 404
hypoglycaemic episodes 335, 337
hypokalaemia 433, 434
hyponatraemia 433, 434
hypoperfusion 481, 482, 483
hypospadias 320
hypotension/hypovolemia 263, 482
hypothermia 263
hypothesis generation 622
hypothyroidism 344–5
hypoventilation 273
hypoxaemia 273
hypoxia 263, 273

ibuprofen 43
ice/salt challenge 410–11
identification and documentation (theatre
    preparation) 262
identity 188
ileostomy 451
illness 196, 226
  children's understanding of 196
    sources of information 196
  concept of 187
immune (idiopathic) thrombocytopenia (ITP) 389
immune system

anatomy and physiology 351–4
  acquired immunity 352
  health promotion 353–4
  herd immunity 353
  innate immunity 352
childhood immunisations 353
components of 351–2
HIV (human immunodeficiency virus) 356–8
ineffective 351
preterm infants 497
primary immune deficiencies (PID) 354–5
  categories of 354
  treatment 354–5
problems impacting on infant morbidity and
    mortality 503
types of immunity 352
immunogens 353
immunoglobulin therapy 354
  care plans 355
immunoglobulins 323, 351, 387, 394
  see also antibodies
immunosuppression 521, 522
immunosuppressive therapy 388
immunotherapy 523
imperforate anus 443
Improving Children and Young People's Health
    Outcomes: A System Wide Response
    (DH, 2013) 92
income 204
incontinence 324–5
Incredible Years model 173
infant mental health (IMH)
  children's centres 171
  concept of 165
  definition 165
  early intervention 166, 167, 169, 170–1
    baby bonds 172–3
    evidence for 171–4
    Family Nurse Partnership (FNP) 172, 174–8
    secure attachment 171
  emotional wellbeing 166–8
  influences on 165–6
    placenta 165, 166
  investment in 169
  skilled professionals 171
  strategies for improving 168–70
  timeframes for 165
An Infant Mental Health Service (2012) 170
infants/infancy 184
  communication development 21–2
    intentional communication 22
    crying 22, 23
    social interaction 22
infections 351
infective endocarditis 290
infertility 522
infibulation 142
infirmaries 5
inflammatory bowel disease (IBD) 444

information
  communication of 4
  mutual exchange of 15
  online resources 15
  sharing of 70, 96
    Common Assessment Framework (CAF) 110–11
    in hospitals 252, 253
    MASH teams 138
    safeguarding 140–1
  see also health information and education
information-processing model of
    decision-making 622
inhaled foreign body 279
inhalers 275
  technique 276, 282
inheritance, genetic
  patterns of 159
  variation in 155–7
innate immunity 352
inotropes 297
Inside the Ethics Committee (BBC) 161
inspiration 272
Institute for Patient- and Family-Centered Care 12
insulin-like growth factor(IGF-1) 339
insulins 334, 335
  injections 336
integrated care 72–4
Integrated Care Partnerships (ICPs) 73
integrated care pathways (ICPs) 72–3, 89
Integrated Joined Boards 73
intentional communication 22
inter-hospital transfers (IHTs) 464
intermediate-acting insulin 336
internal arcuate fasciculus 307
International Burn Injury Database 411
International Union of Immunological
    Societies Expert Committee for Primary
    Immunodeficiency 354
Internet 31–2
interprofessional working (IPW) see IPW
    (interprofessional working)
interventionism 7
interventions
  antipyretic 229
  community nursing 104, 105
  drug therapy 584, 585
  early 138, 166, 167, 169, 170–1
    evidence for 171–4
  effective parenting programmes 200–1
  infant mental health (IMH) 166, 167, 168–9
  pharmacological 230
  physical 229
  urgent 237–8
intracranial pressure (ICP) 302
  compensatory mechanisms 302
  raised 302
    causes of 303
    early signs and symptoms of 303–4
    late signs of 303–6

intravenous drugs 62
intravenous fluids 232, 233, 306
  access 262, 265
intravenous (IV) osmotic agents 305
intravenous therapy 431–2, 433
intubation 480, 483
intuitive-humanistic model 622
intussusception 260, 441
IPW (interprofessional working) 67
  benefits of 70–1
  challenges of 69–70
  core elements of 67–9
  current practice 71–2
  health and social care integration 72–4
  key policies around 72
  key roles in 72
  multiagency teams 107–8
  at an organisational level 69
  team working in transition 74–5
iron deficiency 388

James Coma Scale 307
jaundice 389, 445–6
Jenner, Edward 353
joined-up working 68, 69, 73, 74, 75
  children's needs 106–7
  sharing information 96
joint attention 22
Joint Epilepsy Council of the UK and Ireland 567
Joint Strategic Needs Assessment 204
Joseph Rowntree Foundation 204
judicial reviews 620–1
justice 160

Kanner, Leo 583
Kawasaki disease 228, 291
Kennedy Report (2010) 70
keratitis 483
ketogenic diet 567
key workers in IPW 72
kidneys see renal conditions
King's Fund 69, 71, 73–4
Kirk et al. 152
knowledge sharing 457–8, 459
Knowles, Malcolm 607–8
Kolb's experiential learning style theory 608, 609

lactate 482
lactose intolerance 445
Lambert at al. 26–7
Laming Report (2009) 111
language
  development of 21–3
  skills 22
laser doppler imaging 414
law
  Bolam test 125, 126
  care delivery and 122–3
  children home alone 127

consent 125–6
definition 121
duty of candour 123
duty of care 123
minimum expected standards 122
nursing and healthcare 120
rights of children 189
Lazarus, R.S. and Folkman, S. 544
lead professionals in IPW 72
leadership
balanced processing 595
collective leadership approach 592–3
concept of 592
internalised moral perspective 594
NHS Healthcare Leadership Model 596–8
relational transparency 594–5
self-awareness 596
styles
authentic 593
ethical 593
transformational 593
*Leadership and Leadership Development
in Health Care: The Evidence Base*
(West et al.) 593
Leading Change, Adding Value
(NHS England, 2016) 596
learning disabilities 557, 562
arising from lifestyle factors 562
associated problems/issues 558
autism 564–5
autism spectrum disorder (ASD) 565
cerebral palsy 562–3
changing ideas and value base 557–8
Down's syndrome 339, 344, 444,
557, 559, 562, 563–4
early years 558–60
diagnosis and prognosis 559
health visitors (HVs) 559
primary healthcare services 559
requirements of families 560
special schools 560
Education, Health and Care (EHCs) plans 560, *561*
foetal alcohol spectrum disorder (fasd) 563
growing numbers of children with 560
health and wellbeing
challenging behaviour 567–8
communication in a health setting 568–9
epilepsy 567
nutrition 566
respiratory problems 565–6
safeguarding 569–70
PMLD (profound and multiple disabilities) 558,
560, 565
policies and legislation 557
Rett's syndrome 559
school years 560–2
mental health problems 561
role of parents 561–2
school nurses 560–1

SEN (special educational needs) 559, 560
SLD (severe learning disabilities) 560
social change 562
terminology and labels 557–8
Learning Disabilities Mortality Review (LeDeR)
Programme 569
learning disability nurses 108
learning styles 610–11
Leeds Acne Grading system 405
left arterial (LA) lines 478
Legg–Calvé–Perthes disease (LCPD) 366, 370–1
stages of 371
treatment 372
shelf acetabuloplasty 372
varus derotation femoral osteotomy 372
leukaemia 513, 514, 516
libertarianism 7
life-limiting illnesses 530
advanced care planning (ACP) 533, 534
care of children 533–4
children's hospices 531–3
communication 534
definition 530
needs of children and families 531
palliative care 530, 532–3
parallel planning 533
transitioning to adult services 534–5
lifelong learning *see* CPD (continuing professional
development)
lifestyle choices, healthy 189
light 505
limb lengthening 375–80
Precice nail 376, 377, 379, 380
limb responses, assessment of 308
linguistic communication 22–3
listening skills 86
liver problems 445–6
lobbying 630–2
means of influencing and persuading 632–3
local neonatal units (LNUs) 494
local outcome improvement plans (LOIPs) 73
local safeguarding children boards (LSCBs) 136
Locke, John 119
long-acting analogues 336
long QT syndrome 293
Loughton, Tim 167
low platelets (thrombocytopenia) 388, 389, 517
LSCB (London Safeguarding Children Board) 141
lumbar punctures (LPs) 305, 516
Lund and Browder chart 412
lymphocytes 351
lymphoid progenitor cells 387
lymphomas 514, 515

macrophages 351
major depression 580–1, 582–3
major histocompatibility complex (MHC) 351
Makaton 568
Making a Difference (DH, 1999) 112

Making Every Contact Count (MECC) 113
malignant conditions *see* childhood cancer
malnutrition 566
malrotation 259, 443
Manchester and Salford Ladies Sanitary Reform
    Association 211
MARAC (multiagency risk assessment
    conferencing) 138
Mary Sheridan assessment tool 215
MASE (multiagency sexual exploitation meeting)
    139–40
MASH (multiagency safeguarding hub) 137–8, 140
maternal diabetes 501
mature long bone *381*
maturity onset diabetes in the young (MODY) 155
MDT (multidisciplinary teams) 68, 311, 327, 375,
    380, 495, 565, 566
    burn care 416, 422
    educational program for Type 1 diabetes 335
    meetings 463
    reducing surgical risks 264
    team around the child 110
    see also multiagency teams
Mean BP (MAP) 482
mechanical ventilation (MV) 481
meconium ileus (bowel obstruction) 277, 441
medical ethics 160
medication administration
    cardiovascular problems 297
    drug calculation 63
    drug therapy interventions 584, 585
    errors and adverse reactions 60–2
    issues
        compliance versus concordance 56–7
        covert administration of medication 58
        unlicensed and off label medication 56
    legislation 58
        controlled drugs (CDs) 59–60
        general storage of medication 58–9
    nurses' training 56
    oral or IV 267
    parental role in 62–3
    postoperative care 266
    procedure in hospitals 58
    six rights of 61, 62
    theatre preparation 262
Medicines Act (1968) 58, 618
Medicines and Health Regulatory Agency (MHRA)
    58, 61
Medicines Commission 58
medium- and long-action insulins 337
medulla oblongata 304
melanoma 515
MENCAP 558, 559
meningococcal disease 227
Mental Capacity Act (2005) 629
mental disorder 205
Mental Health Act (2007) 618

*Mental Health in Children and Young People:
    A Toolkit for Nurses Who Are Not Mental
    Health Specialists* (RCN) 582
mental health problems
    approaches to caring 577
    autism 583–4
        aetiology 584
        management/treatment 584
    common problems 577
    conditions, signs and symptoms 578
        in adolescents 578
        anxiety disorders 578–9
        major/clinical depression 580–1, 582–3
        self-harm 581
        social phobia 579–80
        suicide 581
    conduct disorder (CD) 584
        aetiology 584–5
        management/treatment 585
    evaluation and assessment 582–3
    prevalence of 577
    role of children's nurses 582
mentoring 603–4
mercaptoacetyltriglycine scans (MCUGs) 321
Mersey burns application 412
metabolic acidosis 479
metabolic problems, preterm infants 497
metachromatic leukodystropy (MLD) 548
methylation 154
milk 233, 406, 496, 499
    cow's milk protein allergy (CMPA) 445
    see also breast milk
Minding the Baby study 173, 201
Mistry, Ravi 7
Misuse of Drugs Act (1971) 59
mixed analogue 337
mixed insulin 337
monitoring equipment 95
Monro-Kellie Doctrine 302, 303
morbidity 324
morphine 46, 60
motor imitation 22
motor response tests 307
movement disorder 313
MRI scans 516
Ms. MN, case of 70
mucopolysaccharide disorders 559
mucositis 521
multiagency safeguarding hub (MASH) 137–8, 140
multiagency teams 106–8
    CAF/Early Help 110
    composition of 107–8
    safeguarding 136–7
        models 137–41
    service delivery 106–7
    see also MDTs (multidisciplinary teams)
multidisciplinary teams *see* MDTs
    (multidisciplinary teams)

multimodal analgesia 42–3
musculoskeletal (MSK) problems 362
  amplified musculoskeletal pain syndrome
    (AMPS) 366, 375
  assessment 362–3
  bone deformity 366
  bone health 363–5, 364
    rickets 364–5
  common orthopaedic conditions 365–7
  congenital talipes equinovarus (CTEV) 366,
    372–3
    treatment 373–4
  developmental dysplasia of the hip (DDH) 365
    diagnosis 370
    hip spica care 370
    risk factors 367
    surgery 370
    treatment 367–9
  fractures 380–2
    Salter Harris (SH) classification 381, 382
  genu valgum (knock knees) 363, 366
  genu varum (bow legs) 366
  Legg–Calvé–Perthes disease (LCPD) 366, 370–1
    stages of 371
    treatment 372
  limb lengthening 375–80
    Precice nail 376, 377, 379, 380
  slipped capital femoral epiphysis 366
  trauma 367
myeloid progenitor cells 387
myelosuppression 521, 522

nasal cannula *281*
nasal flaring 273
nasogastric tubes 448, 449
nasojejunal tubes 449
nasopharyngeal aspirate (NPA) 280
National Association for the Welfare of
    Children in Hospital (later
    Action for Sick Children (ASC)) 5
National Autistic Society 559, 569
National Child and Maternal Health
    Network 171
National Genetics and Genomics
    Education Centre (NGGEC) 155
*National Guidance for Child Protection
    in Scotland*, (Scottish Government, 2014) 136
National Institute for Health and Care Excellence
    (NICE) *see* NICE (National Institute for Health
    and Care Excellence)
National Paediatric Neuroscience
    Benchmarking Group 308
*National Service Framework for Children,
    Young People and Maternity Services*
    (DfES and DH, 2004) 5, 6, 9, 578
National Society for the Prevention of Cruelty to
    Children (NSPCC) 127
National Tracheostomy Safety Project 480

natural killer cells 351
nausea 46, 548
NCPPC *Glossary of Terms* (2014) 530
necrosis 371
necrotising enterocolitis (NEC) 444–5, 508
needs of children 183
  decision-making 188–9
  health information and education 189–90
  key developmental stages of childhood and
    adolescence 183–5
  therapeutic child-centred relationships 186–8
neglect 135, 201, 218
negotiation 485
neonatal abstinence syndrome 501
neonatal care
  environmental challenges 503
    to the family 506–9
    neonatal infection 504–5
  environmental stressors
    light 505
    noise 505–6
  neonatal pain 506
  organisation and provision of 494–5
    neonatal nurses 495, 507
  preterm infants
    cardiovascular problems 496
    dermatological problems 497
    digestive problems 496
    excretory problems 497
    immune system 497
    metabolic problems 497
    neurological problems 496
    respiratory problems 496
    skeletal problems 497
  small for gestational age (SGA) infants 332,
    495, 498
    growth restriction (IUGR) 498, 504
    hypoglycaemia 498
    perinatal asphyxia 498
    polycythaemia 498
    thermal instability 498
  term babies 498
    acyanotic heart problems 500–1
    congenital diaphragmatic hernia
      (CDH) 499
    fractured clavicle 500
    maternal diabetes 501
    neonatal abstinence syndrome 501
    perinatal asphyxia 499–500
    shoulder dystocia 500
    tracheoesophageal atresia/fistula 499
neonatal diabetes 155
neonatal intensive care units (NICU)s 494, 507
neonatal jaundice 445–6
neonatal nurses 495
neonatal thyrotoxicosis 332
neonates 46, 48
  life-limiting illnesses 530

neonatology 494
nephroblastoma (Wilms' tumour) 323–4, 515
nephrotic syndrome 322
neural tube defect 260
neurobiology 167
neuroblastoma 514, 515
neurodegenerative disorders 314
neurological assessments 482–3
  pupil assessments 483
neurological problems
  acute and long-term conditions
    acquired brain injury (ABI) 310–12
    brain tumours 314
    cerebral palsy 314
    cerebral vascular abnormalities 314
    epilepsy 312–13, 313
    hydrocephalus 308–9
    neurodegenerative disorders 314
    spinal cord abnormalities 313
  intracranial physiology
    compensatory mechanisms 302
    intracranial pressure (ICP) 302
    raised intracranial pressure (RICP)
      302, 303–6
  neurological observations
    best motor response 307
    best verbal response 307
    consciousness 306
    eye opening 307
    frequency of 308
    Glasgow Coma Scale (GCS) 306–7
    limb responses, assessment of 308
    physical stimulus 307–8
    pupils, assessment of 308
  preterm infants 496
neutropenia 44, 522
neutrophils 352, 388
New Birth Visit 214
Newborn Screening Programme 277
NHS at Home: Children's Community
  Nursing Service (DH, 2011) 103
NHS Choices 240
NHS Digital Technology 95
NHS England 174, 596
NHS Five Year Forward View for Mental Health
  (Mental Health Taskforce to the NHS in
  England, 2016) 73, 578, 604
NHS Leadership Academy 598
  Healthcare Leadership Model 596–8
NHS trusts 96
NICE (National Institute for Health and Care
  Excellence) advice/guidelines 56, 240
  azithromycin 278
  cerebral palsy 563
  challenging behaviour 567
  constipation 104, 440
  dehydration 231–2
  diseases 227
  eczema 399–400

evidence-based guidance 432
fluid prescription charts 431
gastro-oesophageal reflux disease
  (Gord) 444
gastroenteritis 431
head injuries 242–3
healthy lifestyle choices 189
intravenous therapy 433
kidney damage 320
pregnancy guidelines 441
PSHE education 114
risk stratification for sepsis 236
standards for referrals 92
thermal injuries 414
unintentional injury 238
vitamin D supplements 364
Nightingale, Florence 82, 83, 247
nil by mouth (NBM) 262, 263
NIRS (near infrared spectroscopy) 478
NMC (Nursing and Midwifery Council)
  care guidelines 90
  Code 96, 111
    best possible standards 122
    law 120
    principles-based approach 122
    professional standards 593
    record keeping 459
    safety 522
    section 10 96
  consideration of genetic and
    environmental factors 152
  CPD (continuing professional development) 603
  Professional Standards of Practice and
    Behaviour for Nurses and
    Midwives 56, 120
noise 505–6
non-accidental injury (NAI) 310
non-communicating hydrocephalus 309
non-directive therapeutic play 28
Non-Hodgkin's lymphoma 515
non-invasive prenatal testing (NIPT) 564
non-maleficence 160
non-nutritive sucking (NNS) 48
non-rebreathe facemasks 281
non-selective NSAIDs
  action of 43
  common side effects of 44
non-specific toddler diarrhoea 233
non-steroidal anti-inflammatory drugs (NSAIDs)
  see NSAIDs (non-steroidal anti-inflammatory
  drugs)
non-traumatic brain injury 311
non-verbal communication 31
Noonan syndrome 331
NSAIDs (non-steroidal anti-inflammatory drugs)
  43, 241
  non-selective 43–4
Numerical Rating Scale (NRS) 40, 41
nummular eczema 403–4

Nurse Family Partnership (NFP) model 174–8
nurse specialists 108
nurses
    see also children's nurses
    community children's nurses (CCNs)
        see community children's nurses (CCNs)
    family nurses (FNs) 175, 176
    practice nurses 108
    school nurses 560–1
    specialist community public health nurses
        (SCPHNs) 211
Nursing and Midwifery Order (2001) 121
nursing assessment 84–5
nursing process
    application to families, groups and communities
        103–6
    assessment 84–7
    care plan for immunoglobulin therapy 355
    components of 103, 104
    cyclical approach 82, 88, 355, 355
    identifying and planning care needs 87–90
    nursing models 82–4
        child-centred care 84
        family-centred care 84
        key concepts 83
        medical model of care 83
        Partnership model 84
        patient-focused model 83
        system-based approach 83
    see also community nursing
nutrition 198–9, 265, 295
    children with learning disabilities 566
    gastrointestinal problems 447–51
    growth and 339
    malnutrition 447
    parenteral nutrition (PN) 449, 451

obesity 333
observations
    baseline 262, 265
    neurological 306–8
    observational skills 86
    vital signs 294
obsessive compulsive disorder (OCD) 579, 584
occupational therapists 108
oedema 319, 322, 323, 324
oesophageal atresia (OA) 442–3
off label medication 56
Office of National Statistics (ONS) 577
ondansetron 440–1
onlooker play 28
open-ended questions 86
open or penetrating injury 311
operating department practitioners (ODPs) 264
opiates 506
opioids 45, 45, 267
    morphine 46
    tramadol 45–6
oppositional defiant order (ODD) 584, 585

oral antibiotics 59
oral rehydration salt (ORS) 233, 430, 431
oral sucrose 506
organ toxicity 521, 522
orthopaedic conditions 365–7
osmotic diuresis 334
osteosarcoma 515
ostomy 451–2
Ounce of Prevention 170
out-of-hospital care see community care
Oxford Parent Infant Project (OXPIP) 173
oxygen saturation 39, 40, 272, 274
    vital sign observation 294
oxygen therapy 274, 277, 279, 281

pacing wires 296
paediatric critical care (PCC) children see PCC
    (paediatric critical care) children
paediatric critical care units (PCCUs) see PCCUs
    (paediatric critical care units)
paediatric early warning systems (PEWS) charts see
    PEWS (paediatric early warning score) charts
paediatric endocrinology 331
    conditions 331–3
Paediatric Intensive Care Society (PICS) 476
paediatric intensive care units (PICUs)
    305, 476
    See also PCCUs
Paediatric Pain Profile 546
Paediatric Sepsis 6 procedures 237
pain assessment and management
    amplified musculoskeletal pain syndrome
        (AMPS) 375
    behavioural indicators of pain 38–9
    behavioural pain assessment tools 38
    end-of-life care 545–7
    guidelines 37
    importance of 37
    neonatal pain 506
    non-pharmacological management of pain
        47–8
        behavioural strategies 48
        cognitive strategies 47
    PCC children 483
    pharmacological management of pain 42–6
        multimodal analgesia 42–3
        NSAIDS 43
        opioids 45–6
        paracetamol 43–4
        tramadol 45–6
    postoperative care 266, 267
    postoperative period
        individualised strategies 267
        tools for 267
    psychological indicators of pain 39
    self-report tools 38
    stages of 38, 38
    strategies for 37–9
    theatre preparation 262

thermal injuries 417–18
validated pain assessment tools 39–41
    faces pain scales 40, 41, *41*
    FLACC (Face, Legs, Activity, Cry,
        Consolability) scale 40, 41, *41*
    Numerical Rating Scale (NRS) 40, 41, *41–2*
    Premature Infant Pain Profile (PIPP) 40
palliative care 488, 530, 532, 533
    transitioning to adult services 534–5
PAMIS (Promoting a More Inclusive Society) 68
panhypopituitarism 333
paracetamol 43–4, 230
    absorption of 44
    specific clinical conditions 44
parallel play 28
parasite/worm infection 445
parental responsibility 189
parenteral nutrition (PN) 449, 451
parenting capacity 197–201
    good parenting 200
parenting programmes 200–1
parents
    administering medication 62–3
    of children with learning disabilities 561–2
    as decision-makers in children and young
        people's healthcare 619–20
    helpful nurse behaviours, views of 486
    involvement in care and care decisions 4, 6,
        9–13
    legal rights in decision-making 71
    master status 518
    participation in care 11, 12
    as primary carers 462
    priorities of 25
    relationships with nurses 25
    role in children's earliest years 170
    secure attachments with children 171
    unhelpful nurse behaviours, views of 486
Parents Early Education Partnership (PEEP) 173
partnership in care 11–12
    model of paediatric nursing 12
partnerships
    across agencies 69, 70, 106–8
    discharge planning 459–60
    nurses and parents 11
        negotiation 12
passive bystanders 25, 26
paternalism 7
patient alarms 478–9
patient-centred care 15
patient confidentiality 129
Pavlik harness 367, 368, 369–70
PCC (paediatric critical care) children 476
    assessing and caring for
        airway 479, 480, 481
        breathing 479–81 *see also* respiratory system
        circulation 481–2
        disability 482–3
        exposure 483–4

PCC management 485
    tissue oedema 483–4
holistic and child/family-centred care
    485–7
monitoring 477–8
pain assessment 483
PCC outcomes 487–9
PCCUs (paediatric critical care units)
    definition 476
    learning opportunities 475
    monitoring
        arterial blood pressure (ABP) 478
        central venous pressure (CVP) 478
        end-tidal CO_2 ($EtCO_2$) 477
        left arterial (LA) lines 478
        NIRS (near infrared spectroscopy) 478
        specialised 478
    negotiation 486
    nursing practice 476–7
        essential bedside equipment 476
        patient alarms 478–9
    PCC monitoring 477–8
peak expiratory flow meters *280*
peptic ulcer 441
per-nasal swab 280
percutaneous endoscopic gastrostomy (PEG)
    449, 450
percutaneous endoscopic jejunostomy (PEJ) 449
perfusion pressure 482
peri-and postoperative period
    children's play 261
    collaborative approach 264–7
        transfer to theatre 264–5
    emotional wellbeing 267
    role of children's nurse perioperatively
        261–3
        anaesthesia 263
        consent 263
        fasting 263
        preparation for theatre 262
    role of children's nurse postoperatively
        265–7
    specific care 258–61
        emergency surgery 258
        pre-admission preparation programmes 258
        surgical conditions 258, 259–60
perinatal asphyxia 498, 499–500
peripheral neurovascular deficit 382
peripheral primitive neuroectodermal tumour
    (PPNET) 515
peritoneal dialysis 326
peritonitis 440
personal safety 111–12
Perthes *see* Legg–Calvé–Perthes disease (LCPD)
pertussis 279
petitions 632
PEWS (pediatric early warning score) charts 87,
    262, 265, 274, 324
pH study 447

pharmacology 42–6
phenotypes 154
physical abuse 135
physical growth 185
physical stimulus testing 307–8
physiological genu varum (bow legs) 363, 366
physiotherapists 108, 297
physiotherapy 277, 390
Piaget, Jean 196
Picture Exchange Communication Systems
    (PECS) 568
Pinderfield Scale 307
Plan International UK 633
plasma 387
platelet function 44
platelets 393
    low platelets (thrombocytopenia) 388, 389, 517
Platt Report (*The Welfare of Children in Hospital*,
    1959) 5, 11, 457
play
    associative 28
    in children's nursing 27–9
    communication and 23, 27–9
    developmental aspects of 27
    in hospitals 252, 261
    pretend 27
    symbolic 22
    types of 28
play specialists 28, 297
pneumonia 227, 279
policy, definition 121
political activity 630–2
    means of influencing and persuading 632–3
        improving future health and
            |wellbeing 632–3
political demonstrations 632
political issues, raising awareness of 627–8
    see also child forced marriage
polycythaemia 498
polydipsia 334
polyuria 334
Ponseti method 373–4
positioning 281, 295
positive psychology (PP) 166–7
post-traumatic stress disorder (PTSD) 487
posterior urethral valves 260
postnatal depression (PND) 200
postoperative care 265–6
potassium imbalance 433–5
poverty 204–5
    impacts on children 205
    in Wales 213
practice nurses 108
Precice nail 376, 377, 379, 380
pregnancy 441–2
Premature Infant Pain Profile (PIPP) 40
prescriptions 58
    prescription only medicines (POMs) 58
pretend play 27

preventative inhalers 275
Primary Care Dermatology Society 405
primary immune deficiencies (PID) 354–5
Principles of Good Transitions 3 (ARC Scotland,
    2017) 74
privacy 190
problem-based learning approach 609
problem-focused coping 544
procedure, definition 121
profound and multiple learning disabilities (PMLD)
    558, 560, 565
Promotion of Breastfeeding Intervention Trial
    (PROBIT) 198
prone positioning 481
prophylactic antibiotics 354
Propionibacterium acnes 405
prostaglandins 44
proteins 154
pruritus 46
pseudohyperkalaemia 433
Pseudomonas aeruginosa 277, 278
PSHE (personal, social, health and economic
    education) 114
psychological indicators of pain 39
puberty 340
    delayed 332
    early 332
Public Bodies (Joint Working) (Scotland)
    Act (2014) 73
Public Health (Control of Disease) Act (1984) 431
Public Health England (PHE) 199, 240, 558
public, protection of the 122
pulmonary oedema 480
pulmonary stenosis 288
pulse pressure 482
pulse, vital sign observation 294
pupils (eyes), assessment of 308, 483
pyloric stenosis 260, 443
pyrexia 324
pyruvate kinase deficiency 389

qualified in speciality (QIS) 495
quality healthcare 592–3
quality of life (QOL) 288–9

radiation 305
radiation thermal injuries 410
radiotherapy 523
raised blood pressure 304
raised intracranial pressure (RICP) 302
    causes of 303
    early signs and symptoms 303
    late signs of 303–4
        abnormal breathing pattern 304
        investigations for 304–5
        medical management 305
        nursing management 305–6
        raised blood pressure 304
    pronounced bradycardia 304

rapid-acting analogues 336
rashes 399
RCN (Royal College of Nursing) 96, 568
recession 273
record keeping 96
  by CCNs 128
  by children's nurses 96
  discharge planning 459
records
  paper-based 96
  paperless 96
  patients' legal right of access to 96
red blood cells 388, 393
referral management schemes (RMS) 92
referrals 91–4, 115
  ambulatory assessment units (AAU) 92
  NICE standards 92
  pathways 92
  process 93
  referral to treatment (RTT) 94
  SMART 92
Registered Child Nurses 183
rehabilitation 311
relational transparency 594–5
relative poverty 204
reliever inhalers 275
remodelling (Perthes disease) 371
renal blood flow 44
renal conditions 319
  acquired renal conditions
    ambiguous genitalia 320
    bladder extrophy 320
    general care 324
    glomerulonephritis 322, 323
    haemolytic uraemic syndrome (HUS) 322–3
    henoch Schönlein purpura (HSP) 323
    hydronephrosis 320
    hypospadias and epispadias 320
    nephrotic syndrome 322, 323
    reimplantation of ureters 321
    urinary tract infections (UTIs) 320–1
    Wilms tumour 323–4
  anatomy of renal system 319
    embryological errors 319
  escalating concerns to appropriate staff
    acute kidney injury (AKI) 325
    chronic renal failure (CRF) 326
    enuresis 324–5
    haemodialysis 326–7
    peritoneal dialysis 326
reossification 371
resilience 200, 202
respiratory depression 46
respiratory rates 85, 86
respiratory syncytial virus (RSV) 274
respiratory system/problems 271, 565–6
  abnormal breathing pattern 304
  airway clearance 480

assessment
  auscultation 273
  common terminology and descriptors 272–3
  depth and expansion 272
  deteriorating children 274
  effort (work of breathing) 272
  normal rates of breathing 271
  oxygen saturation 272
  physical appearance 272
  rate of breathing 272
  regularity 272
  sounds 272
  structured approach 272
asynchrony 480
breath sounds (BS) 480
chest wall expansion 479
children with learning disabilities 565–6
common conditions
  acute epiglottis 279
  asthma 275–6
  bronchiolitis 274–5
  croup 279
  cystic fibrosis (CF) 276–9
  diagnostic tests 280
  inhaled foreign body 279
  pertussis (whooping cough) 279
  pneumonia 279
  viral induced wheeze 279
conditions 271
cyansis 479
discharge planning 282
distress 272
DOPES 480
endotracheal tubes (ETTs) 480
invasive support 481
non-invasive support 481
nursing care and management 281
paradoxical breathing 479
preterm infants 496
problems impacting on other systems 502
tracheostomies 480
vital sign observation 294
restlessness 548
reticular formation 306
retinoblastoma 514, 515
Rett's syndrome 559
Rh blood group 392
rhabdomyosarcoma 515
rheumatic heart disease 291
rhonchi 273
rickets 333, 364–5
right atrial pressure 478, 482
rights, children's 8, 70–1, 120, 170
  see also United Nations Convention on the Rights of the Child (UNCRC)
risk
  analysing and assessing 138
  assessment of care needs 87

genetics 158–60
serious illness 229
unintentional injury 238–40
risk-taking behaviour 57
RNA (ribonucleic acid) 154
changes 154
Robertson, James 5, 249–50
Roper et al. 83, 415
roundworm 445
Royal College of Nursing (RCN) 96, 568
Royal College of Paediatrics and Child Health
(RCPCH) 238, 476
Royal Society for the Prevention of Accidents
(RoSPA) 411
rule of palms (1% rule) 412

safeguarding
abuse 241
administering medication 58
bruising 389
child protection plans 90, 466
children with learning disabilities 569–70
confidentiality using social media 605
cyberbullying 32
definition 134
domestic violence 202
emotional abuse 135
female genital mutilation (FGM) 141–2
fractures 382
head injuries 242
information sharing 140–1
life-limited children 534
malnutrition 447
multiagency safeguarding models
multiagency risk assessment conferencing
(MARAC) 138
multiagency safeguarding hub (MASH) 137–8, 140
multiagency sexual exploitation meeting
(MASE) 139–40
multiagency working 136–7
neglect 135, 201, 218
neonates 508
pain management 37
parenting capacity 201
physical abuse 135
policies and procedures 128
responsibilities for 134
screening activities 218
sexual abuse 135
Shaken Baby Syndrome 310
supervision 111
thermal injuries 411
trafficking 142–4
see also child protection
safety
in the home 239
in hospitals 252–4
cardiovascular problems 294–5
during theatre 264

salt supplementation 277
Salter Harris (SH) classification *381*, 382
sarcomas 515
SBAR (situation/background/assessment/
recommendation) tool 87, 236, 262, 265, 324
scalds 411
scarring 414
Schedule of Growing Skills (SOGS) 215
school nurses 114–15, 560–1
school nursing 113–15
role of school nurses 114–15
school readiness 217
scoliosis 260
Scottish Child Health Programme 213
screening 115, 212
see also universal screening
sebaceous glands 404
seborrhoeic eczema 404
sebum 404, 405
secondary cancers 522
secretion management 479–80
secure accommodation 619
secure attachment 171, 200
sedation 483, 485
seizure disorder 313
seizures 233–5, 548
in the community setting 234
in the emergency department 234–5
epileptic 233, 234–5, 312, 313
self-awareness 596
self-efficacy 201
self-empathy 201
self-esteem 4, 199, 205, 324, 338
self-harm 581
self-image 338
self-injuring activities 410
self-regulation 185
self-reporting of pain 38
SEN (special educational needs) 559, 560
separation anxiety 250
sepsis 235–6
Paediatric Sepsis 6 procedures 237
parenteral nutrition (PN) 451
Red Flag Sepsis 236–7
urgent intervention 237–8
septic arthritis 227
septic shock 484
septicaemia 440
serial halving 412
service hubs 110
severe learning disabilities (SLD) 560
sex development, disorders of 332
sexual abuse 135
sexual exploitation, child 32, 92, 94, 139–40
Shaken Baby Syndrome 310
sharing attention 22
shelf acetabuloplasty 372
Shelter 203
short-acting insulins 336, 337

short Q-T syndrome 156
short stature 339–43
shoulder dystocia 500
sickle cell disease 388, 389
silent chest 273
single points of care (SPOC) systems 92
single points of entry (SPE) systems 92
sinus bradycardia 292
sinus rhythm 292
sinus tachycardia 292
SIRS (systemic inflammatory response syndrome) 235
six rights of medication administration 61, 62
skeletal problems, preterm infants 497
skin care 324
skin grafts 417
skin problems *see* dermatological problems
slipped capital femoral epiphysis 366
small for gestational age (SGA) infants 332, 495, 498, 504
smallpox vaccine 353
SMART goals 89
SMART referrals 92, 94
Social Care (Self-directed-Support) (Scotland) Act (2013) 73
Social Determinants of Health (RCN) 195
social integration 205
social interaction 199–200
social media 31–2, 605
social media watch 176
social phobia 579–80
social skills 22
social support 518–19
sodium imbalance 433, 434
solitary play 28
Sousa et al. 10
spacer devices *276*
special care units (SCUs) 494
special schools 560
specialist community public health nurses (SCPHNs) 211
speech and language therapists (SaLTs) 108, 297
spinal cord abnormalities 313
sputum 280
stature
   short 331
   tall 332
status asthmaticus 275
status epilepticus 313
statutory services 70
stem cells 154, 388
stepping stones approach 462
steroid therapy 277
steroids 403
stoma 451–2
   care 266
stool culture tests 446
stool specimens 232
strangers 252

stratified squamous epithelium (skin) *see* dermatological problems
Strengthening the Commitment (Scottish Government, 2012) 559
stridor 273
subcutaneous insulin 335
subcutaneous tissue 398
sucrose therapy 48
suctioning 281
suicide 581
supervision 111
support groups 295
supraventricular tachycardia (SVT) 292
surgical conditions/principles 258, 259–60
Surgical Safety Checklist (WHO) 264
swaddling 48
sweat tests *280*
symbolic communication 22
symbolic play 22
systemic inflammatory response syndrome (SIRS) 235

T helper lymphocytes 353, 356
tachypnoea 272
tapeworms 445
technology
   communication through 31–2
   organisation of care and 95–6
temperature, vital sign observation 294
text messaging 31
theatre
   preparation for 262
   safe transfer to 264–5
therapeutic child-centred relationships 186–8
therapeutic play 28
therapeutic positioning 481
thermal injuries 410, 415–6, 419–21
   definition 410–11
   depth of 414–15
      assessment tools 414
      laser doppler imaging 414
      surgical intervention 414
   detailed history and clinical examinations 411
   extensive 418–22
      activities of daily living (ADL) care plan 418–22
   pain management strategies 417–18
      pharmacological and non-pharmacological approaches 418
   size of 411–13
      assessment tools 411–12
      credit card tool 413
   treatment options and considerations
      activities of daily living (ADL) 415–16
      burn care team 416
      debridement 417
      healing 415
      recovery phases 416
      skin grafting 417

thermal instability 498
thermoregulation 262, 264, 265
Think Family approach 90
third endoscopic ventriculostomy 309
third-party stories 23
third sector services
   core role in integrated care 73
   essential support 70
threadworms 445
thrombocytopenia 388, 389, 522
thrombosis 391
thyroid hormones 339
thyroid stimulating hormone (TSH) 344, 345
thyrotropin releasing hormone (TRH) 344
tinea 405
tissue oedema 483–4
toddlers 23
Together for Short Lives 532–3, 541
topical corticosteroids 402, 403
Townsend, P. 204–5
tracheoesophageal atresia 499
tracheoesophageal fistula (TOF) 259, 442–3, 499
tracheostomies 480
trachycardia 292
traffic-light system (NICE) 229
trafficking 142–4
tramadol 45–6
transfers 464
   from children's services to adult services
      464–5
   from hospitals in other countries 465–6
   in-utero 494
transformational leadership 593
Transforming Your Care (2011) 73
transfusions, blood 392–4
transition 74–5, 464–5
trauma 367
traumatic brain injury (TBI) 310–11
   closed head injury 310
   crushing injuries 311
   open or penetrating injury 311
triad of communication 24–7
   limited contribution of young people 26
triage system 87
tumours 513, 514, 516
   radiotherapy 523
   surgery 523
Turner syndrome 331
Type 1 diabetes 331, 334–7, 338–9

UK Children's Commissioners (2015) 72
UK Cross Party Manifesto 170
UK PID Registry 354
UK Sepsis Trust *238*
ulcerative colitis 444
ultra long-acting analogues 337
ultrasound scans 516
Understanding Needs of Children in Northern
   Ireland (UNOCINI) 72

UNICEF 142, 143
   breastfeeding initiative 198
unilateral lung disease 481
unintentional injury 238
   falls 240
   first aid 241
   fractures 240–1
      treatment of 241
   head injuries 242
      assessment and treatment of 242
   prevention 239–40
   risk 238–40
United Nations Convention on the Rights of the
   Child (UNCRC) 8, 70–1, 120, 170, 218, 251,
   568, 578, 630
   participation 248
   promotion 248
   protection 248
   see also children's rights
Universal (health visiting service) 214, 215
Universal Partnership Plus (health visiting service)
   214, 215
Universal Plus (health visiting service) 214, 215
universal screening
   12-month review 215–16
   delays 217
   evidence underpinning practice of 212–13
   New Birth Visit 214
   programmes in the UK 213–15
      in England 213
      Family Health Needs Assessment (FHNA)
         214–15
      in Northern Ireland 213
      in Scotland 213
      in Wales 213
   three-year review 217–18
   value of 212
   see also health visitors
University of California, San Francisco
   (UCSF) 68
unlicensed medication 56
unoccupied play 28
upper GI contrast study 447
urea and electrolytes (U&E) tests 446
ureters, reimplantation of 321
urinalysis 446
urinary retention 548
urinary tract infections (UTIs) 227, 320–1, 325
urine 319
ursodeoxycholic acid 277
in-utero transfers 494

vaccinations 353–4
Valuing People Now (HM Government, 2009)
   558–9
variation in inheritance 155–7
varus derotation femoral osteotomy 372
vasodilator antihypertensive 297
ventilation 483

ventilation requirements 262, 265
ventricular septal defect (VSD) 287, 288
ventriculo peritoneal (VP) shunt device *305*, 309
verbal language 21
verbal response tests 307
viral load 356
virtual reality (VR) 47
viruses 351
visible-ness 26–7
vital signs
    changes to 303
    observation of 294
vitamin D
    deficiency 363–4
    supplements 364–5
Voice Output Communication Aids (VOCA) 568
volvulus 443
vomiting 46, 231
    dehydration 432
    electrolyte imbalance 428
    end-of-life symptoms 548
    gastroenteritis 429, 430, 440–1
    hypokalaemia 434
    intravenous fluids 232, 233
    oral rehydration salt (ORS) 233
    side effect of chemotherapy 521
    stool specimens 232
von Willebrand disease (vW) 391

Welfare of Children and Young People in Hospital
    report (DH, 1991) 5
wellbeing 165
    children's 5
    emotional 166–8, 267
    improving 632–3
    learning disabilities and 565–70
    see also child development; health

Wernicke's area 307
wet heat thermal injuries 410
wheeze 273
    viral induced 279
white blood cells 388
whiteheads 405
whole-family education 253
whooping cough 279
wider family 203
Wilms' tumour 323–4, 515
Wolff-Parkinson-White syndrome 292
work of breathing (WOB) 479
in-work poverty 205
Working Together to Safeguard Children (HM
    Government, 2015) 134, 136, 197
World Health Organization (WHO) 43,
    195, 240
    Baby-Friendly Hospital Initiative
        (BFHI) 198
    childhood immunisations 353
    HIV (human immunodeficiency virus) 356
    mental health problems 577
    quality of life (QOL) 288–9
wound care 265, 266
    cleansing and dressings 417
    postoperative 296
    wound healing process 266

X chromosomes 154
x-linked recessive inheritance 390
X-rays 280, 446, 516

Your Community (health visiting
    service) 214, 215
Yura, H. and Walsh, M.B. 82, 87

Zero to Three 165